PHYSICAL DIAGNOSIS

BEDSIDE EVALUATION OF DIAGNOSIS AND FUNCTION

PHYSICAL DIAGNOSIS

BEDSIDE EVALUATION OF DIAGNOSIS AND FUNCTION

JANICE L. WILLMS, M.D., PH.D.
INSTITUTE OF MEDICINE AND HUMANITIES
ST. PATRICK HOSPITAL AND THE UNIVERSITY OF MONTANA
MISSOULA, MONTANA

HENRY SCHNEIDERMAN, M.D., F.A.C.P., F.C.C.P.
ASSOCIATE PROFESSOR OF MEDICINE (GERIATRICS) AND PATHOLOGY
UNIVERSITY OF CONNECTICUT HEALTH CENTER
FARMINGTON, CONNECTICUT

PAULA S. ALGRANATI, M.D., F.A.A.P.
ASSISTANT PROFESSOR
DEPARTMENT OF PEDIATRICS
UNIVERSITY OF CONNECTICUT HEALTH CENTER
FARMINGTON, CONNECTICUT

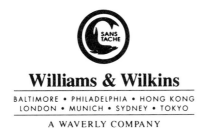

Williams & Wilkins

BALTIMORE • PHILADELPHIA • HONG KONG
LONDON • MUNICH • SYDNEY • TOKYO

A WAVERLY COMPANY

Editor: Patricia A. Coryell
Copy Editor: Bill Cady
Designer: Dan Pfisterer
Illustration Planner: Ray Lowman
Production Coordinator: Anne Stewart Seitz

Copyright © 1994
Williams & Wilkins
428 East Preston Street
Baltimore, Maryland 21202, USA

Accurate indications, adverse reactions, and dosage schedules for drugs are provided in this book, but it is possible that they may change. The reader is urged to review the package information data of the manufacturers of the medications mentioned.

Printed in the United States of America

Library of Congress Cataloging-in-Publication Data

Willms, Janice L.
    Physical diagnosis : bedside evaluation of diagnosis and function
 / Janice L. Willms, Henry Schneiderman, Paula S. Algranati.
        p.   cm.
    Includes bibliographical references and index.
    ISBN 0-683-09110-7
    1. Physical Diagnosis. I. Schneiderman, Henry, 1951–   . II. Algranati, Paula S.
III. Title.
    [DNLM: 1. Physical Examination. 2. Medical History Taking. WB 200 W737p
1994]
RC76.W55 1994
616.07´54—dc20
DNLM/DLC
for Library of Congress   92-48556
                                                                              CIP

94 95 96 97 98
1 2 3 4 5 6 7 8 9 10

This effort was stimulated by, and carried forth for, the women and men who must continuously incorporate expanded knowledge and skill into already "overloaded circuits." May this text contribute a bit of order and pleasure to their lifelong process of becoming healers.

JAN WILLMS, M.D., PH.D.

For giving me what it took to make my contribution to this book, among many other reasons, I am infinitely grateful to my parents Betty and Moe Schneiderman, who did not live to see their son catch fire in Medicine as he had in Classics; to the many who have taught me physical diagnosis, including my patients and the generous patients of other physicians; to the American College of Physicians, whose Teaching and Research Scholarship launched me toward mavenhood in physical diagnosis; and above everything and everybody, to my wife Ro and our son Joseph quibus omnia.

HENRY SCHNEIDERMAN, M.D., F.A.C.P., F.C.C.P.

To Charlie, Emily, and Bar, for their unconditional love and support in this and all ventures. In the end, they are the reason.

PAULA ALGRANATI, M.D., F.A.A.P.

Preface

The nihilists claim that the fine art of physical assessment will soon be rendered obsolete by technology. Highly specialized electronic techniques allegedly surpass the sensitivity of auscultation, palpation, and percussion in the location of hidden pathology. The course of disease may be monitored at a substantial distance from the bedside. In all these statements there is, of course, a grain of truth. But can healing be accomplished without a human intermediary—without hearing, seeing, and feeling the minds and the bodies of the sick and wounded? The answer is a resounding "No!" And thus we offer tools to empower every visit to the bedside, for purposes of evaluating the patient who requests help from the medical practitioner.

It would be foolhardy to disregard any technology that contributes to the care of our patients. But each such advance supplements rather than replaces the basic skills of hearing and interpreting the patient's illness narrative in the context of his life and of diligently reading with our well-trained senses the information his body provides. The human interaction of diagnostician and subject, of healer and patient, must not be undermined by inadequate preparation of the early learner or incomplete maintenance of skills by the experienced clinician.

The approach and organization of this book were conceived as a result of the our experience teaching interviewing, medical history acquisition, and physical examination skills to preclinical medical students, clinical clerks, interns, residents , and faculty in a variety of settings, including medical schools, university hospitals, and community teaching hospitals. In attempting to help our students acquire the primary database (medical history and physical examination) in the most effective, efficient, and accurate manner possible, we have found a number of problems that needed to be addressed.

Our major frustration was the lack of a textbook of clinical assessment that paralleled the progressive building blocks of basic science and clinical information as they are sequentially acquired in the medical training process. For example, a first- or second-year medical student who has neither completed basic science training nor had significant clinical exposure requires a different set of learning objectives and a different approach than does the experienced clinician who, facing difficult settings and situations, might want to review or study specialized examination techniques. It is the goal of this text, therefore, to sequence learning in modules appropriate to the knowledge base of the learner.

Acknowledgments

The authors wish to thank the many colleagues and friends who have been instrumental in the preparation of this book. To the support staffs of the Departments of Medicine and of Pediatrics goes our gratitude for their patience and assistance rendered in the hard work of collecting and processing information used in the text. Dixie McLaughlin at the Institute of Medicine and Humanities in Missoula, Montana, coordinated the long distance efforts among authors.

From the patient instructors ranks of the Clinical Skills Assessment Program at the University of Connecticut came the models for Greg Kriss's superb photographs. Joyce Lavery turned our crude sketches into finished line drawings.

Finally, to our families and associates who stood by us through the whole process, we express our special love and gratitude.

An Invitation

We extend an invitation to the reader as contributor: This work of improving physical diagnosis is not finished, not for you and us as adult learners, not for us as authors, and not for our profession. If you find novel, undescribed, or obscure signs or exceptions or counterexamples to the precepts and rules herein, please write to one of us. Dr. Schneiderman's address is University of Connecticut Health Center, Farmington, CT 06030-3940; Dr. Willms' address is Institute of Medicine and Humanities, St. Patrick Hospital, Missoula, MT 59806; and Dr. Algranati's address is Department of Pediatrics, University of Connecticut Health Center, Farmington, CT 06030 -3940.

For this purpose, we want to see a good paragraph or three of clinical data about the patient, a clear description of the surprising finding, and information about any steps taken to investigate its source and to confirm a revised diagnosis—even something as simple as a radiograph or a smear. We also welcome your thoughts about why or how the process formed an outlier. Clearly, this sometimes requires doing some homework, since we are not interested in learning, for example, that a hypertrophic cardiomyopathy murmur decreased with the Valsalva maneuver (that "atypical behavior" has been well documented in a substantial series published in 1986 in the *Annals of Internal Medicine*). Rather, we avidly seek anything that contradicts any of our flat assertions or that lends new insight about any physical sign.

It is the job of the entire medical community to increase the group wisdom about both the power and the limitations of physical examination. And we are happy to serve as a filter and a resource when a sign makes no sense or deviates wildly from conventional teaching.

Contents

Atlas

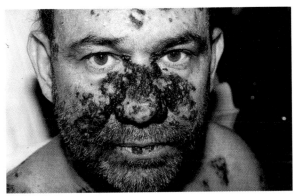

A. Striking destruction of facial skin and lips in pemphigus vulgaris. Patient recovered completely. See Chapter 3.

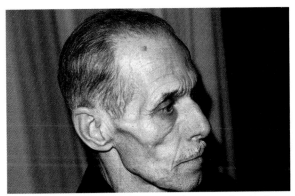

B. Temporal and masseter atrophy in cachexia from carcinomas of pancreas. See Chapter 2.

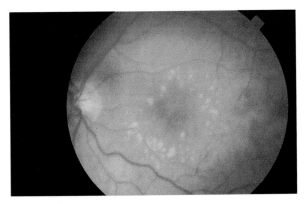

C. Peripheral retinal "exudates" in macular degeneration. See Chapter 4. (Courtesy of Robert Fagan.)

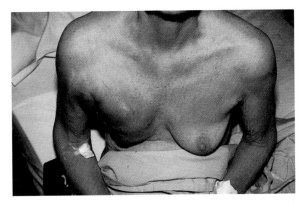

D. Erythema marks inflammation where an advanced untreated breast cancer has ulcerated. See Chapter 3.

Atlas

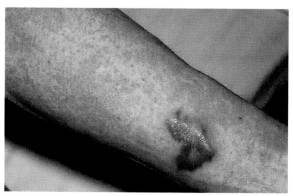

A. Raised "ecchymosis of Kaposi sarcoma in AIDS. Background skin shows coincidental maculopapular drug rash. See Chapter 3.

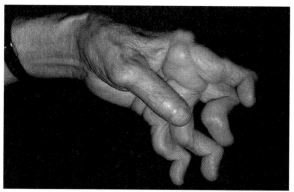

B. Extreme boutonniére, Z- and swan-neck digital deformities in advanced rheumatoid arthritis. See Chapter 10.

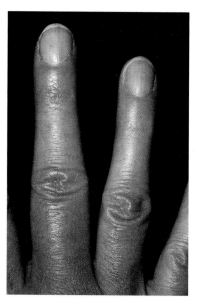

C. Tight shiny skin of distal fingers constitutes sclerodactyly in systemic sclerosis. See Chapter 10.

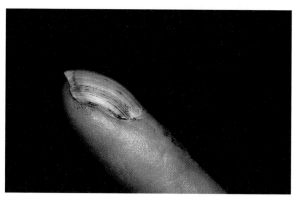

D. Digital clubbing in pulmonary fibrosis. The most proximal part of the nail is all that counts for this. See Chapter 3.

Atlas

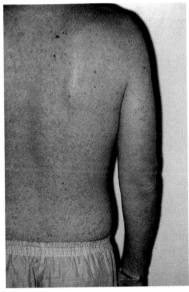

A. Maculopapular drug rash produces partially confluent pink-red discoloration that is minimally raised. See
Chapter 3.

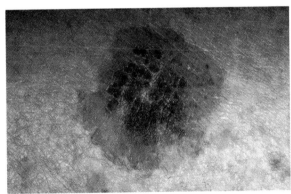

B. Large lesion with irregular dark pigmentation mandates biopsy to exclude malignant melanoma. See
Chapter 3.

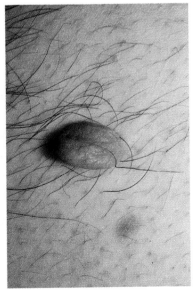

C. Papule. This one is an innocuous skin tag; an unrelated tiny brown macule is nearby. See Chapter 3.

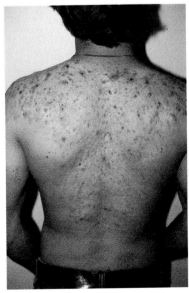

D. Upper-body cysts, erosions, papulopustules, and
excoriations of severe acne vulgaris. See Chapter 3.

Atlas

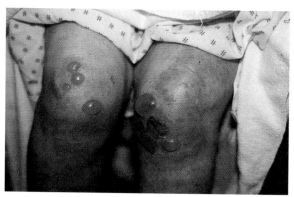

A. Bullae full of straw-colored fluid near the knees in bullous pemphigoid; and irregular background erythema. See Chapter 3.

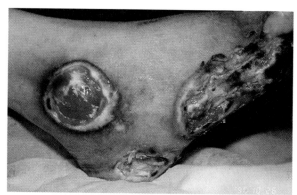

B. Deep pressure ulcers (bedsores) delineate pressure sites on an immobile patient's foot. See Chapter 3.

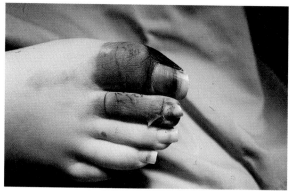

C. Dry gangrene on two toes, most fully developed at tip of hallux, in a young diabetic (at autopsy). See Chapter 3.

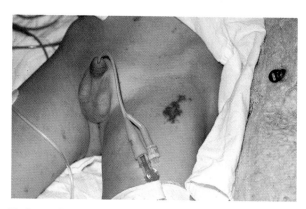

D. Irregular confluent ecchymoses and petechiae in a critically ill 6-year-old with meningococcemia, who recovered fully. See Chapter 3.

Introduction

CHAPTER DIVISIONS: THE SCREENING AND THE EXTENDED EXAMINATION

Approach

The chapters in this book are divided into two sections: the screening examination and the extended examination. The screening examination section is designed to teach the beginning student how to acquire assessment skills prior to learning about clinical medicine or medical problem solving. The extended examination section is directed to the advanced learner and focuses on the body of skills that are essential as the student progresses in experience and medical responsibility. This latter section is also appropriate as a review for the practicing clinician facing an unusual or seldom-encountered assessment problem.

Content

The division of content between the screening and extended examination sections must, to some degree, be arbitrary although carefully considered in every case. Overall, the goal of the divisions is to help distinguish between what must be known and used in every case and what must be known and used in special circumstances.

The screening examination section relates to the complete medical history and physical examination. To determine the content of screening examination sections we asked the following questions: Given the knowledge base limitations inherent in the traditional learning sequence, what is the appropriate extent of clinical skill we can reasonably expect a student to master during the first 2 years of medical education? What can this student do in terms of collecting a primary database that can be used, in turn, in clinical problem solving?

We expect the student who successfully masters this competency-based curricular material to be able to

1. Demonstrate the ability to listen attentively and guide a patient effectively through the process of a complete medical history, designated as the screening interview
2. Conduct a full screening physical examination in a rational, thorough, and accurate fashion with efficiency and with minimal discomfort to the patient
3. Transmit the acquired data, in writing and verbally, in an organized fashion and with complete accuracy in terms of observations (not diagnoses)
4. Become sufficiently familiar with normality and innocuous variants to recognize deviations from normal, though not necessarily fully understand or diagnose them

There is no universally accepted canon for the data set comprising the screening physical examination, and no two clinicians will agree precisely and consistently about what information is essential to it. For the purposes of this text, however, the authors needed to define their own content boundaries for the examination to be conducted by a second-year medical student. We recognize that individual teachers may choose to abbreviate or delete certain parts of the examination or to add others.

The extended examination section provides deeper exploration of selected and focused medical problems. The examination techniques presented here are more sophisticated than those of the screening examination and could not practically be completed on a routine screening examination. They are generally called for by information uncovered in the medical history or by abnormalities detected during the screening physical examination. This section of each chapter is designed to help advanced students grow in knowledge and to provide clinicians with a reference on special maneuvers and their interpretations.

An example of a special maneuver would be squatting for the purpose of seeking mitral valve prolapse. This is the type of maneuver that a clinical clerk must master while working with patients and learning the pathophysiology of mitral prolapse and its symptoms and signs. We would not do cardiac auscultation with the patient squatting unless there was an indicator of possible mitral prolapse, e.g., atypical chest pain or a systolic murmur and/or click found while listening to the supine patient. If such a specialized maneuver is taught in a knowledge and experience vacuum, it cannot be effectively incorporated into the student's clinical armamentarium. Its inclusion at that point might even dilute and obscure the transmission of the core curriculum. Squatting for the purpose of seeking mitral prolapse also exemplifies the kind of maneuver that the practicing general surgeon may need to review if, while doing a preoperative patient evaluation, it is suspected from the history or screening examination that the patient has the abnormality.

SCOPE OF BOOK

We designed this text to meet finite objectives. These are

1. To provide, for the beginning student of clinical assessment, a defined body of information and a programmed methodology for acquiring the skills necessary to conduct and record the results of a comprehensive screening assessment, contained within the *screening examination* section of each chapter
2. To provide, for the more advanced clinician, a reference source for special maneuvers, their indications, and the interpretation of findings elicited by these maneuvers, contained within the *extended examination* section of each chapter
3. To provide, for all clinicians, suggestions for handling unusual but difficult clinical situations or settings that demand special approaches or modification of standard interviewing or physical examination procedures, contained both in Chapter 16 entitled Special Challenges and, where pertinent, in other chapters.

The scope of the book is purposely sharply limited to acquiring, recording, and verbally transmitting medical history and physical examination information. It makes no pretense of serving as a miniature textbook of disease or of medicine, of clinical problem-solving, or of laboratory or radiographic diagnosis.

When the student reaches a stage wherein medical problem-solving incorporating paraclinical data (laboratory, imaging) is indicated, the student will need systemic or specialized textbooks of disease or of medicine or one of the extant textbooks on differential diagnosis or clinical problem-solving to use in concert with our book. Neither supplants the other; rather, they are complementary.

For example, when the clinical clerk finds that the squatting cardiac auscultation alters the position of the click in the systolic interval, it will be necessary to go to a medicine or cardiology textbook or to a preceptor to learn the therapeutic and prognostic implications of this discovery. When the general surgeon determines that a preoperative patient has squatting auscultatory findings consistent with mitral valve prolapse, then it is time to go to the cardiology textbooks or to the cardiologist for a refresher on the implications of that anomaly for intraoperative and postoperative care. The physician who is unsure how to interpret a CT scan also must utilize sources other than this book. This textbook focuses strictly on primary bedside assessment.

METHOD OF PRESENTATION

We have chosen narrative description with summary tables for a number of reasons. We recognize that the intense time demands made on all persons in medicine present a compelling argument for tabular construct; however, there are so many nuances in the skills to be learned that narrative description is indispensable. Its deletion cannot adequately be made up in shorthand, no matter how skillfully constructed. Thus we employ tables as forms of reiteration and convenient summary of the content of selected text. The user is welcome to employ the book in whatever way best meets individual needs, e.g., to consult the tables as freestanding summaries for review or overview and return to the narrative only when questions arise or explication is indicated. On the few occasions when tables are presented in lieu of narrative, this is clearly stated in the text.

Regional Approach to the Physical Examination

The authors have chosen to organize the material by *anatomic regions* rather than strictly by physiologic systems. This preference makes sense pedagogically as well as practically, since this is the way clinicians routinely conduct screening examinations. It provides the student with a structure that is based on the way data are acquired and examinations conducted rather than on the way physiologic systems operate. Since it is logical and efficient to palpate the dorsalis pedis pulse while doing the examination of the legs rather than as a part of a systemic arterial examination, the material is organized regionally. The user who is looking for peripheral vascular maneuvers need only remember to seek the topic under the pertinent anatomic region (arm, leg, groin, etc.) rather than by its system designation (vascular). We provide such systemic and systematic organization by way of the index and, when indicated, with textual cross-reference by chapter.

Organization of Age-Specific Special Maneuvers

Pediatric assessment is treated separately from adult assessment because of its very different approach to the history and sequencing of the physical examination, which are age specific until the child approaches adolescence. Pediatric assessment has its own chapter in this book, with subdivisions to indicate the process and content changes required as the newborn becomes a toddler, the toddler a preschooler, and so on. The content of the screening examination and that of the extended examination are separated within each developmental stage.

On the other hand, assessment of the pregnant woman and the older person are treated as variants in process, content, and interpretation of findings of the adult regional assessment. Since the standard technical approach to assessment of all adults is the same, separate sections or chapters for these two subsets are unnecessary. Where alterations in technique or interpretation are needed because of pregnancy or advanced age, the material is incorporated into the various subsections of each regional chapter: Technique and Normal and Common Variants, or Conducting the Extended Examination and Interpreting the Findings.

Note on the Use of Third-Person Pronouns

As there is yet no gender-neutral third-person singular pronoun in the English language, we deal with this problem as follows. Unless dictated by gender-specific content (such as the menstrual history or the gynecologic examination), the patient is usually referred to with the masculine pronouns. The clinician is referred to by the feminine pronouns. And where photographs accompany text, the third-person singular pronoun choice is dictated by the gender of the individual(s) in the illustration.

Definitions of Selected Terms as They Are Used in This Book

Because the authors have chosen a format that may be unfamiliar to readers of older texts, some terms chosen for classification of material have been defined for the reader's ease of access:

- *Examination.* This term encompasses both the medical history and the physical examination elements of the primary database. It does not imply, in this context, the clinical decision-making process in which the Weed system uses the *A* to equal the assessment portion of the SOAP format. It means nothing more or less than the H&P (history and physical examination) findings without interpretation of their diagnostic or therapeutic significance.
- *Medical interview.* This term delineates the *process* by which the medical history data are obtained. It i s an integral part of the medical history.
- *Medical history.* The medical history is the composite of subjective information (content) supplied by the patient and/or the patient's informants about symptoms and the narrative of their development. The medical history is defined as the content of the patient's story obtained by means of the medical interview.
- *Physical examination.* This consists of the process by which the clinician observes, palpates, percusses, and auscultates the patient's physical being and the findings (signs) elicited by this process.
- *Screening or comprehensive examination.* This designation is applied to the "complete" medical history and physical examination, the type of evaluation made on the undifferentiated patient, on the patient newly admitted to the hospital or ambulatory practice, and on the patient who comes in for a "complete" or general assessment with or without chief complaint. This is the examination that all physicians have had to perform at some time and that many of us perform often in our practices. This is also the basic assessment we expect beginning students to master as the foundation of their clinical skills.
- *Extended or problem-focused examination.* This designation means an extension of the screening process, wherein the health professional follows leads suggested by specific symptoms or the elicitation of abnormal physical findings. The problem-focused examination is a subset of the extended assessment, in that it confines itself to a system (or systems) or to a region that declares itself as the basis for a specific chief complaint or cluster of signs and symptoms. This is the type of assessment that commonly occurs when a patient presents to an emergency department or office with a narrowly confined complaint that may necessitate the use of special maneuvers to clarify the problem.

Abbreviations used in the text and common abbreviations used in medical record keeping are defined in Appendix A. Samples recordings of written and oral presentation screening and extended examinations are available in Appendices B–D.

1

Two Tiers of Investigation: The Screening and Extended Examinations

SCREENING OR COMPREHENSIVE EXAMINATION

ADULT SCREENING MEDICAL HISTORY

Most clues leading to solution of any individual patient's diagnostic mystery are gathered from the medical history taken during the medical interview. During this encounter, the clinician and the patient establish their working relationship. Impressions are created, guidelines are worked out, and critical data are collected. Because this is usually the first meeting of the two individuals involved, the conduct and the process of the interview are as important as the content of the history.

This section on primary data gathering begins with a discussion of the clinician-patient relationship and of the interviewing skills most likely to result in a mutually beneficial outcome. The content of the medical history and its structure are then defined in detail, with strategies for obtaining the patient's health history and/or illness narrative even if the interviewer possesses relatively little medical knowledge. It is feasible to obtain and organize an accurate, relatively complete medical history without knowing much about the pathologic basis of the symptoms being described and certainly without any clear diagnosis in mind.

This chapter is written for the preclinical student and presumes no ability to formulate diagnostic hypotheses. The latter process grows with experience and a broader knowledge base than students at this level generally command. The more the clinician knows about disease, the greater the hazard of misguiding the patient or arriving at a diagnostic closure prematurely. We encourage learners to capitalize on their knowledge limitations in order to concentrate on hearing—attentively listening to—what the patient has to say. The experienced practitioner's eye sometimes loses this freshness in attempting to fit the square peg of the patient's words into the round hole of a diagnosis.

The Medical Interview

Preparation for a successful medical interview begins before the encounter. The interviewer must assume a professional role that requires special decorum and appropriate dress. The student must accept that she has the right to enter a patient's room and private life. The patient, in turn, should know precisely where the student fits into the complex medical hierarchy. The patient has usually given permission for a student to visit and ask questions. Such preliminary courtesy is the responsibility of the faculty supervisor. Even when these preparatory steps have been taken, the interviewer needs to establish the patient's understanding of the interaction before proceeding to the medical history (Table 1.1).

Table 1.1
Beginning the Interview

Introductions	Physical arrangements
Clarify names	Negotiate with third parties
Greet with a handshake	Ensure privacy
Clarify role	Ensure quiet
Define task(s)	Settle in to listen

INTRODUCTIONS

The encounter should begin with the formal introductions that precede any conversation between strangers. You, as interviewer, state your own name and indicate that you are the student who has come to take a medical history. The patient's last name is used, and if there is uncertainty as to its pronunciation, he is asked to pronounce it as he prefers. It is inappropriate, except when interviewing a child, to use the patient's first name. Your patient deserves the respect of being addressed as Mr., Mrs., Ms., or by any professional title the patient uses, unless a less formal address is requested. A handshake on introduction constitutes good manners and may, incidentally, provide important information about the patient (see Chapter 3, General Appearance).

ENVIRONMENT

Once you have completed these preliminaries, make the physical arrangements necessary for a successful interview. If there are visitors in the room, do not begin the interview until you and the patient have agreed on the level of privacy needed. A close family member sometimes asks to remain in the room. If the patient prefers this arrangement, you may choose to allow it. The presence of a third party presents a challenge to your interviewing skills; i.e., you must assume sufficient authority to guarantee that the conversation remains primarily between you and the person from whom you wish to obtain information. For the beginner it is often more comfortable to be alone with the patient, and you are free to request this if you wish; e.g., "I need to speak with your father alone. May I ask you to wait in the family room until I'm done—probably in about 30 minutes? I'll let you know when I'm finished."

A quiet environment is essential for concentration on the task at hand. Radios and televisions should be turned off; bed curtains, if there is another patient in the room, should be pulled shut; and doors should be closed. Since the interview may take as long as an hour, both you and the patient should be comfortably positioned such that vocal and eye contact can be easily maintained. There is no shame in discontinuing the interview temporarily, especially if the patient is very ill or elderly and tires easily. Acknowledge the patient's need to pause, and return after a brief rest.

INTERVIEWING STRATEGIES

Before discussing skills specific to the medical history, we review some generic strategies to facilitate any interview. These include both nonverbal and verbal behaviors (Table 1.2).

Nonverbal Behaviors

Body language. Body language is a term used to describe the way an interviewer positions herself and uses her body to communicate. A relaxed (but not slovenly) posture conveys interest and concern. The interviewer should face the

Table 1.2
Interviewer Nonverbal and Verbal Behaviors

Nonverbal behaviors	Verbal behaviors
"Body language"	Question type
Distance	Open questions
Relative position	Closed questions
"Habits"	Jargon
Eye contact	Duplication of questions
Nonverbal cuing	Positive verbal reinforcement
Encouragement	Use of silence
Showing interest	Pacing
Physical contact	
Empathetic modes	

patient directly or at a minimal angle from face to face. The distance between the two persons should be sufficient to allow movement but not to give the impression of avoidance or repugnance. The interviewer remains near enough to the patient that touching him is possible, should this be desirable during the course of the conversation, e.g., to convey emotional support. Awareness of your own movement habits, such as twirling a pencil or tugging at an earlobe, is important. Such "nervous" repetitive motions are distracting and should be suppressed. Several excellent articles detail the fine points of "body language" as it relates to formal interviews.

Eye contact. Effective eye contact displays the interviewer's interest in and concentration on the patient's story most powerfully. Intense, unbroken eye contact is disconcerting, so one relieves the contact by brief, slight eye movement—something we do quite naturally in informal conversation. On the other hand, avoidance of eye contact conveys discomfort with the situation. A frequently observed avoidance technique is the use of pencil and paper as a barrier. For this reason, note-taking should be brief, and its necessity should be explained to the patient such that it interferes minimally with the primary goal of *hearing* what the patient has to say.

Nonverbal cuing. Several methods of encouragement enhance rapport and reinforce continuity of conversation. The interviewer may nod the head slightly from time to time to indicate comprehension and desire to hear more. Leaning forward also shows interest. On occasion, physical contact, such as a touch, tells the patient that a particularly painful or distressing symptom has been heard and acknowledged for its affective component as well as its intellectual content. Simplicity and good humor, conveyed by a smile or an empathetic laugh, have their place in the medical interview. Stay in mental and emotional "touch" with the patient while you hear his story—much as you would for a friend—and the exchange will usually flow comfortably.

Verbal Behaviors

A few of the more significant verbal nuances in the interview setting are reviewed here.

Types of questions. There are two types of questions: closed and open. The closed question is one that demands a brief answer, usually "yes" or "no." The open question invites the patient to emphasize what seems most important to him in the narrative. Both types have their place in the medical interview. Think of the history of the present illness as a triangle. By beginning at the broad base with an open question, the interviewer allows the patient to find a starting place that reflects his own agenda. As the arena of discussion is defined, the interviewer begins to "close" the questions in order to obtain specific data, moving toward the apex of the triangle. Specific applications of open and closed questions are subsequently illustrated.

Certain question types predictably flaw the accuracy of the information. A sequential list of questions results in constricted, incomplete answers. For example, if you ask the patient three questions in one—"Did you experience blurred vision, double vision, or eye pain?"—the answer may relate only to the last of the list. The patient may respond, "No. My eyes are never painful," but fail to mention blurring as a positive element in the sequence. Leading questions will often yield a compliant rather than an accurate answer. Questions having a built-in answer or an implied value judgment tend to create the same problem. For example, if the interviewer asks, "You've not had fever with this, have you?" the patient is prompted to answer in the negative, perhaps in contradistinction to the actual experience he has had. To avoid this complication, always ask closed questions neutrally: "Have you had fever during this time?"

Jargon. Medical jargon is a language of power and special privilege. It may lead to confusion and is sometimes used as a weapon to imply superior knowledge or sophistication. It has no place in the medical interview. As a beginner, you may have little problem with jargon, since the paucity of your medical vocabulary resembles that of the patient. As medical expertise grows, however, the use of jargon can creep in. Determine the educational, linguistic, and medical sophistication of the patient. It is safer to use lay terms with the patient to obviate misunderstanding in either direction. Summarize periodically to be sure that you are both talking about the same thing. Some of the miscommunication resulting from use of jargon is illustrated below.

Duplication of questions. To ask the same question twice vividly announces that you have not been listening. There is a place for repetition to clarify, provided the patient knows you are aware this question has already been discussed. For example, you might say, "You mentioned that your urine seemed darker than usual this week. Could you describe its color in more detail?"

Positive verbal reinforcement. Positive verbal reinforcement complements nonverbal encouragement. If the patient describes a particularly distressing situation, don't be reluctant to say that you are sorry or that you recognize his difficulty in speaking about a painful event. When the patient describes a success, such as smoking cessation, demonstrate support with a verbal affirmation. Failure to acknowledge affective content as it flows from the patient's narrative sends a message of unconcern, emotional ineptitude, or even of negative feelings about the patient or the events. These subtle messages play a significant part in the completeness and the candor with which the patient will give information.

Use of silence. The effective use of silence in an interview is a powerful tool. If you need time to collect your thoughts or to organize mentally what has been said, say so. There is no shame in admitting that you need to think. The patient would prefer this admission to an awkward pause or fumbling to buy time. Patients also may need quiet time to think about a question you have asked or to regain equanimity after a particularly emotional disclosure. Remain sensitive to these needs. If you ask a question that is not promptly answered, give the patient a chance to formulate an answer before adding questions or clues to answers. Silence that is pregnant with thought, deliberate, and purposeful enhances information transfer and the development of the clinician-patient relationship.

Pacing. Pacing refers to the tempo with which the interview is conducted. Some of the briefest and most productive interviews are those that seem the most leisurely. Patients open up best if you give the impression of being in no hurry, to the extent that time is not being wasted. Open-ended questions—usually the most productive—support the sense of a leisurely pace. A rapid-fire questioning style breaks down by producing flawed data. Give the patient time to answer your queries, but redirect his attention if he begins to ramble. A well-balanced pace requires confidence and should be sought consciously from the student's first medical interviewing efforts. Effective pacing grows with practice and specific application.

These are some elements of an effective interview technique. The student develops these while learning the conduct and content of the medical history, and becomes a far more efficient and effective data collector, thus taking a large step on the road to becoming a healer.

Content Components of Screening Medical History
OVERVIEW

The medical history is the story of illness, functional disability, or deviation from normality as defined by the patient. It is also the story of behaviors related to the maintenance of health. Story means narrative, the unfolding of the symptom or symptoms as they develop and change over time. Deviation from normality is a value judgment that the patient makes in the context of his own life and his own culture. Because of the variability in interpretation of what is normal, the medical history needs to be considered first in terms of the patient's perception. If the patient believes that what is happening to him is illness, his definition is of primary importance. If you as interpreter of the science of medicine disagree with the patient's interpretation, resolution of differences will have to be negotiated later. For the moment, however, you as historian allow the patient to tell his story. The medical interviewer's role is to guide the teller through the details of health and illness without subverting the "facts" as the patient presents them.

To help the interviewer assist the patient, a formal structure for the medical history is provided (Table 1.3). The beginner is well served by learning and using this structure to ensure that essential information is obtained. Flexibility within the formal structure is advantageous and becomes more natural as the student gains experience. For example, there are occasions when the pattern of the formal structure should be broken to follow leads offered by the patient. However, the presence of structure enables the interviewer to maintain a framework within which the large volume of information to be required may be placed.

First, we define the components of the formal medical history, then suggest methods for acquiring the necessary information. Finally, some common problems are described along with strategies for overcoming them.

FORMAL STRUCTURE OF THE MEDICAL HISTORY

By convention, the formal medical history has six segments, which together address present and significant past health issues comprehensively. These segments are: chief complaint (CC), history of present illness (HPI), past medical history (PMH), patient profile (PP), family (medical) history (FH), and review of systems (ROS). Although it is seldom necessary or feasible to obtain all of this information in a single clinical encounter, this chapter provides details of how to acquire a complete medical history. Sound decisions about how much information must be collected on any given occasion can only be made with experience. The learner must master the totality first. The following description, then, provides a comprehensive, nonselective approach to the database.

Table 1.3
Content Components of the Medical History

Chief complaint (CC)	**Patient profile** (PP)
History of present illness (HPI)	Educational level
Onset	Occupational history
Temporal sequence or chronology	Current living situation
Quality of symptom(s)	Family structure and support systems
Quantity of symptom(s)	Health habits
Aggravating factors	Diet and nutrition
Alleviating factors	Exercise
Associated symptoms	Tobacco, alcohol, and drug use
Contemporaneous medical problems	Hobbies and special interests
Past medical history (PMH)	Sexual activity and concerns
Surgical procedures	Daily routine
Other hospitalizations	**Family (medical) history** (FH)
Major trauma	**Review of systems** (ROS)
Medications	
Allergies	
Childhood illnesses	
Immunization status	
Significant past medical illnesses	
Pregnancy and delivery history	

Chief Complaint

The CC is the **patient's description** of the symptom that precipitated the decision to seek medical attention. The CC is also the entry point into the HPI. It provides both patient and interviewer with a place to start the narrative.

History of Present Illness

The HPI is the story of the current problem(s). It can be simple, short, and straightforward, as in the case of acute infection or a new injury, or it may be long, convoluted, and multidimensional. In either case, it should evolve such that it has a beginning, a middle, and an end—the end being the current status. There may be many concurrent or overlapping tales within the HPI. Each must be attended to as a separate narrative. For example, a patient's CC is "pain in the foot." While developing the temporal sequence of this symptom, he mentions that he is being treated for a flare-up of asthma. After obtaining the story of the foot pain, the interviewer will then return to the asthma and develop its history. Since both problems are current, though apparently unrelated, each has its own narrative, its own HPI.

To clarify the details—the **dimensions or parameters**—of the patient's current problems or symptoms, the clinician obtains the following information about each of them:

- *Onset:* When did the patient first notice the symptom? What was he doing at the time?
- *Temporal sequence:* What has happened to the symptom since it was first noted? Has it gotten better or worse or remained the same? Has it become more or less frequent? How is it today compared with yesterday, or last week, or the time it first occurred? Has anything like this ever happened in the past? Are there any family members, co-workers, or friends with the same condition? (This is the framework of the narrative of the symptom.

Effective methods for establishing this framework are detailed in the next section.)

- *Quality of the symptom:* What is it? Where in the body is it located? Does it move or radiate? How does it feel, or look, or smell, or sound?
- *Quantity of the symptom:* How bad or how extensive is the symptom? What words would the patient use to describe its quantity? On a scale of 1 (minimal) to 10 (agonizing), where would the patient place it?
- *Aggravating factors:* What, if anything, has been observed that will bring on the symptom or make it worse?
- *Alleviating factors:* What, if anything, has lessened the symptom or made it disappear? What has failed to do so? Has professional medical care been employed for this problem? What was done? Did it help? Have other remedies or treatments been attempted, such as over-the-counter drugs or nontraditional therapies?
- *Associated symptoms:* Has there been anything else different noticed by the patient or his associates? (This question is key to establishing symptom complexes or concurrent illness. When the patient's attention has been focused on a single symptom, there is commonly failure to mention others without specific prompting.) If the patient does have other symptoms, then connections between them are explored after each is characterized individually.

Although other **ongoing medical problems** are not a formal parameter of the HPI, at this point in the interview many clinicians choose to ask questions about concurrent medical conditions that might be affecting the present problem. Are there other medical conditions? Is the patient taking medication now for any other problem? Ask specifically about common adult illnesses such as high blood pressure, diabetes, ischemic heart disease, arthritis. Each concurrent condition is assessed for its dimensions and temporal sequence.

Past Medical History

The PMH is a catalog of significant past health problems. Significance represents a value judgment, so the assessment of what constitutes significant problems will vary from setting to setting and practitioner to practitioner. Problems the interviewer should always ask about include:

- *Long-term past medical illnesses,* i.e., illnesses that have receded with treatment or on their own but that have the potential for recurrence or late sequelae. Tuberculosis, certain malignancies (lymphoma or acute lymphocytic leukemia), hepatitis B, alcoholism, and severe depression, for example, fall into this category.
- *Surgical procedures,* i.e., any operation the patient has ever had, including the date of the operation, the symptoms that led to the procedure, the nature of the procedure, the final diagnosis, any adverse reactions to anesthesia (especially if additional surgery is contemplated), and any sequelae of the procedure.
- *Other hospitalizations,* i.e., the dates of, reasons for, and outcomes of the hospitalizations.
- *Major trauma not previously covered,* i.e., the nature of the trauma, treatment rendered, and any resultant disability.
- *Medications,* i.e., all medications that are currently being taken or have been taken with any regularity in the past, including over-the-counter medications such as laxatives, aspirin, antihistamines, and vitamins, as patients seldom consider these nonprescription formulations as "medications" or "drugs" and therefore do not volunteer their use.

- *Allergies:* Seasonal, environmental, or food allergies with their manifestations and treatments are documented. By far the most critical of these is any history of **medication allergies.** If a history of allergic reaction to any drug or agent used in diagnosis or treatment is obtained, the details of the reaction as well as the name of the substance involved should be ascertained. It is important to differentiate between true allergic reactions (e.g., skin rashes; histamine reactions such as facial and oral edema; allergic interstitial nephritis or anaphylactic shock) and nonallergic side effects such as nausea or loose stools. Because of the ubiquity of penicillin derivatives and the frequency of significant allergy to them, it is wise to ask specifically about penicillin reaction. An economical means of covering the ground is to ask, "Have you ever had an allergic reaction to penicillin or any other medicine?"
- *Childhood illnesses:* This information carries more import in the history of a younger person than from an elder. When the history is indicated, elements to be included are common viral infections—mumps, rubella (German measles), rubeola (regular measles), chickenpox—and rheumatic fever.
- *Immunization status:* Essential data change with the age of the patient. All children and young adults should have a full immunization record for the chart, including immunization for measles, mumps, and rubella (MMR), hepatitis B, polio, diphtheria, pertussis, and tetanus (DPT, in children), and *Haemophilus influenzae* type B (HiB). Older adults and chronically ill patients of all ages require annual influenza vaccine and immunization against pneumococcus once every 6 years. The date of the last tetanus shot should be ascertained.
- *Pregnancy and delivery history,* i.e., determination of the number of pregnancies, live births, and spontaneous or induced abortions, as well as documentation of types of delivery (vaginal or cesarean section) and any complications of pregnancies or deliveries.

Patient Profile

The PP is an inventory of medically relevant lifestyle. It is intended to give the interviewer a sense of the patient as a member of society and of family and as a person who lives, works, and plays. The PP includes at a minimum:

- *Educational level,* the highest attained.
- *Employment history,* current and past, with details of possible exposure to hazardous materials if relevant (see Chapter 16, Environmental Health History, for the more extensive occupational history required when a medically significant exposure is suspected).
- *Current living situation,* including where and with whom.
- *Family structure and social support systems.*
- *Health habits,* including: *Diet:* number, content, and regularity of daily meals; food fads or special diets such as vegetarianism or unusual weight control diets. (Chapter 16, Dietary and Nutritional History, provides the more extensive nutritional history that may be indicated when irregularities are found during the basic screening dietary history.) *Exercise:* frequency and type of regular exercise. *Tobacco use:* intensity of smoking is usually quantified as the number of packs of cigarettes smoked daily, multiplied by the number of years of smoking, expressed as pack-years. If the patient no longer smokes, the same information is acquired, and the date of cessation is recorded. Pipe and cigar smoking require parallel documentation, as does the use of "smokeless" tobacco. *Alcohol use:* type, amount, duration, and complications. *Recreational drug use,* such as cocaine, marijuana, or heroin: type, frequency, duration, and complications.

- *Hobbies and special interests:* Modes of relaxation as well as clues to physical hazards or risks.
- *Sexual activity and/or concerns:* Extent and method of query are situation dependent and are discussed in greater detail later in this chapter.
- *Daily routine,* if not already ascertained.

Family (Medical) History

The FH is a survey of the health of the patient's relatives and should include three generations: parents, siblings, and offspring, for the adult patient; and grandparents, parents, and siblings, for the child patient. For the elderly, inquiry about grandchildren yields more insight than questions about ancestors. The age and present state of health, including any significant disease, or age at death and cause of death should be ascertained for each pertinent family member. A secondary review is then made of any other history of potentially familial health problems, such as adult-onset diabetes mellitus, premature coronary heart disease or sudden unexpected death, cancer, high blood pressure, and Alzheimer's dementia.

Review of Systems

The ROS is a checklist usually reserved for the end of the interview and is designed as a final search for missed issues. An experienced clinician takes pride in "an empty ROS," which indicates that major issues have already been ferreted out. However, this final check may bring to the surface a new and important problem. The list is a long series of closed questions. There are many variations on the content of the ROS available. One such list follows.

- *General:* Current weight and any recent change; fatigue; fever; energy level.
- *Endocrine:* History of thyroid disease; history of high blood sugar; recent intolerance to heat or cold; excessive thirst, hunger, or volume of urine output.
- *Hematologic:* History of anemia; easy bruising or difficulty controlling bleeding; history of blood transfusions including dates, reactions to blood products; history of blood clots or anticoagulation.
- *Psychiatric:* History of treatment for psychiatric or emotional problems; nervousness; anxiety; undue sadness; sleep disturbance; death wishes or suicidal thoughts.
- *Skin:* Recent changes in texture or appearance of hair, skin, or nails; new rashes, lumps, sores; history of treatment for skin condition.
- *Eyes:* Recent change in vision; blurring of vision; double vision; red or painful eyes; history of glaucoma or cataracts; most recent eye examination and results.
- *Ears:* Recent change in hearing; pain in or drainage from ears; ringing in the ears; dizziness with or without changes in head position.
- *Nose and sinuses:* Increase in frequency of colds or nasal drainage; nosebleeds; history of sinus infections.
- *Mouth, throat, teeth:* Sores of tongue or mouth; dental problems and dental care history; bleeding of gums; hoarseness or voice change.
- *Neck:* Stiffness or injury; new lumps or swelling.
- *Breasts:* Tenderness; lumps; nipple discharge; history of self-examination; last physician examination and/or mammogram; any prior aspiration or biopsy.
- *Cardiorespiratory:* History of asthma, bronchitis, pneumonia, pleurisy, tuberculosis; new cough, sputum, coughing blood, wheezing or shortness of breath. History of high blood pressure; heart disease; heart murmur; palpitations; chest pain; shortness of breath on exertion or while lying down; ankle swelling; history of electrocardiogram, chest x-ray, or other diagnostic tests.

- *Blood vessels:* Pain in legs with walking (how far); sensitivity or color change in fingers or toes with cold temperatures; varicose veins or history of phlebitis.
- *Gastrointestinal:* Difficulty swallowing, change in appetite; nausea, vomiting; diarrhea; abdominal pain, vomiting blood, or blood in stool; constipation or recent change in bowel habits or appearance of stool; history of jaundice, liver, or gallbladder problems; indigestion or new food intolerance.
- *Urinary:* Change in frequency of urination, volume of urine, or nature of stream; burning on urination; blood in urine; hesitancy; urgency; incontinence; history of urinary infections or stones; nocturia.
- *Male genitoreproductive:* History of hernia; venereal diseases; sores on penis; pain in testicle; frequency of testicular self-examination; sexual preference, function, satisfaction, or concerns if not raised and covered adequately in earlier portions of the history.
- *Female genitoreproductive:* Menstrual history, including age of menarche, cycle length, pain with menses, change in duration, amount, or frequency of menses (may be omitted in the postmenopausal woman). For the older woman, history of age and any difficulty with menopause such as hot flashes, irregular bleeding; history of hormone therapy, postmenopausal vaginal bleeding. For all postmenarcheal women, history of venereal disease, vaginal discharge, painful sexual intercourse, vulvar itching, or unexpected vaginal bleeding. Sexual preference, activity, satisfaction, and concerns if they have not been discussed during other portions of the history. If not obtained earlier, the history of pregnancy and delivery, birth control method(s), and concerns about reproductive health may be asked at this time.
- *Musculoskeletal:* Muscle weakness, pain, tenderness, or stiffness; pain or swelling in joints; history of arthritis, gout, or back pain.
- *Neurologic:* History of headaches; seizures; blackouts; paralysis; numbness or tingling; trembling or weakness; difficulty speaking; memory loss or difficulty concentrating.

This completes the definition and core content of the formal comprehensive medical history. The HPI is, by virtue of its centrality to the encounter, both the most critical and the most flexible of the components. It also happens to be, not coincidentally, the hardest to organize. The remainder of the history develops supportive data and identifies ancillary issues; it is obtained in a more formulaic manner. Each component requires a slightly different strategy on the part of the interviewer.

How does the beginner wade into this quagmire of required data and emerge with cogent information? The next section delineates approaches that yield the most information without requiring extensive knowledge about disease. Special attention is directed to the HPI, since it is the most pressing and by its very nature the least predictably structured of the components.

Acquisition of the Screening Medical History
OVERVIEW

After studying the formal content requirements for each segment of the medical history, the student considers how best to direct the interview so as to acquire the requisite information. As a general principle, the HPI should remain as open and controlled by the patient as possible, whereas most of the remainder of the history can be structured and largely closed and compartmentalized by the interviewer. The degree of structure applied to the PP will vary from patient to patient. Following are methods of gaining information effectively in each of the six components of the medical history. As in any dynamic human interaction, no single formula can be applied universally. The interviewer must remain alert and be prepared to change approaches when the situation so dictates (Table 1.4).

QUESTIONS TO ASK

Chief Complaint

Most patients have formulated their reasons for seeking medical attention. Hence they readily respond to an opening such as, "What brings you to the clinic today?" "Why were you admitted to the hospital?" "What problem is bothering you most now?" Hear, and make a mental note of, the patient's precise response to your opening question. Regardless of the ultimate medical conclusions about the patient's most compelling problem, the CC should reflect the issue identified by the patient as such. The patient's response to the initial question guides the entry into the HPI.

History of Present Illness

The HPI flows from the CC. Whenever feasible, the next question should be fully open, such as: "Tell me more about your chest pain." "Take me back to the first time you passed out and tell me everything you can about the attacks." "Describe as best you can what you mean by dizziness." Once the interviewer has a sense of the symptom that the patient has identified as the CC, she can begin to explore its dimensions.

Temporal sequence and descriptive parameters. In the instance of an acute problem, one obtains the highest yield by asking the patient to start at the beginning and tell everything that has been noticed since the symptom began. "As I hear you, the first thing you noticed was belly pain yesterday afternoon. Start at the beginning and tell me everything that has happened in the past 24 hours." The observant and articulate patient usually responds by providing most, if not all, required dimensions of the symptom without further prompting. The interviewer listens to the account, mentally checking off each parameter. She reserves closed questions that add or confirm detail until after the narrative has been reeled out by the patient. This is a quick and accurate way to obtain the history. Missing details can be filled in by direct questioning immediately afterward, such

---

Table 1.4
Conducting the Adult Medical History

Encouraging the narrative development	Effective closure of the interview
Effective balance of open and closed	Questions?
questions	Other concerns?
Chronologic approach	Additions or corrections?
Summarization	Explain next step or finalize interaction
For accuracy	
For acquiring additional information	
Transition statements	
Question types related to content area	
HPI: from open to closed	
PMH: closed and directive	
PP: from open to closed	
FH: closed	
ROS: closed and directive	

as "What have you found makes the pain better?" if this has not surfaced in the spontaneous narrative.

With chronic or longstanding recurrent symptoms, the fully open "tell me all about it" may lead to rambling or irrelevant detail. When the story does not seem to be evolving in sequence or needed data are being circumvented, the interviewer may find it necessary to interrupt (politely) and redirect the patient with more closed questions. "I am interested in these concerns about what your husband would do if you need to be hospitalized, but we need just now to get details about your shortness of breath. What seems to make it worse?" Sometimes, such a concrete question alerts the patient to what is being sought; necessary details may follow. Another helpful approach is to ask the patient to recall the last time he felt well and to begin the narrative of his illness from that point. Sometimes you must ask a series of direct questions about sequence, alleviating factors, duration, quality, or quantity to obtain the information required. The open approach should always be attempted first. Turning to direct or closed questions if it fails is a simple example of flexibility in the conduct of the interview.

Once satisfied with the temporal sequence and the descriptive parameters of the primary symptom, the interviewer asks about other symptoms. If there are others, each is pursued in the same fashion until there is a story for each problem, and a handle on their interconnections. Finally, inquiries are made about any other ongoing medical problems. If these exist, each one is developed until the assessment of the patient's current health status is complete.

Summary. Now it is time to **summarize**. Verbal summary by the interviewer of what she has heard serves two critical functions: (1) it permits her to reconstruct the narrative(s) just revealed for purposes of recall and understanding, and (2) it provides the patient with the opportunity to confirm, correct, or add information that was left out or that has been misunderstood or missed. The summary of the HPI should be prefaced by a brief explanation to the patient of its purpose, with instructions to the patient to correct, add, or delete as needed: "Let us see now if I have everything straight. I am going to tell your story. Please correct me if there are errors, or if there is anything you would like to add." The interviewer then shares her version with the patient, acknowledging any corrections or additions he makes. Close this segment by asking, "Is there anything else I should know about this?" If the interviewer and the patient have agreed about the comprehensiveness and accuracy of the current problem(s), a shift is made into the other components of the medical history.

Transition. The interviewer now uses the first formal **transition statement**. When the interviewer moves from the patient's presenting complaint and current concerns to the more remote and potentially less compelling (from the patient's perspective) portions of the history, an explanation is helpful. The interviewer selects any of the remaining segments of the history to turn to next. Whichever is chosen, an explanation for the change of direction will reorient the patient and justify the movement away from the patient's declared primary agenda. Some standard transition statements include: "Now that I have a sense of your major concerns, I would like to explore your past medical history for any information that might bear on your medical care." Or, "Let's pause a moment, and let me learn more about you [patient profile]." "Sometimes, learning about the family helps us to understand medical problems better [family history]."

Past Medical History

The PMH is discussed next, not because there is any dictum that says it must be obtained after the HPI but in order to parallel the content format presented above. For the most part, the PMH is easily structured and usually less personally intrusive than the PP. It may present a welcome break for patient and interviewer alike, especially if the HPI has been emotion laden. Most of the questions follow the format outlined above under Content and are clear and straightforward. Of most use to the patient is a definition of terms and expectations: "If you have ever had surgery, I would like to know about it." Since surgery is a memorable event in anyone's life story, the information is usually forthcoming. Let the patient know what you wish to learn: dates, procedures, reasons for procedures, diagnosis, outcome. (This is one point in the PMH in which note-taking may be indicated, especially if there are multiple events to be chronicled.) The same principles hold for other hospitalizations, long-term medical illnesses requiring extended treatment, and the history of major trauma.

Medications and nonprescription drug use. Although the history of contemporaneous medication use should have come out in the HPI, it is important to check again about any drugs the patient may be taking. Also, obtain here the history of long-term or regular use of medicines and the symptoms for which they were recommended.

Most persons use nonprescription drugs on occasion without considering them as "drugs." Aspirin or acetaminophen can be found on almost everyone's shelf for use with fever or minor aches and pains. Because these medications may either cause or confound medical problems or interact with other drugs, it is important to document their use. This question must be specific: clues jog the patient's memory. Queries are made about pain medications, laxatives, antacids, cold remedies, or sleeping preparations, since any one of these may complicate the medical history or future therapeutic plans. For example, common over-the-counter cold formulas can impair bladder emptying in the elderly.

Immunization status. As noted above, questions about childhood diseases and immunizations are variable and age-dictated. In the elderly patient, you may bypass most viral diseases as being remote and irrelevant. A question about rheumatic fever remains important. For details of the history of immunizations in the child, see Chapter 15, Pediatrics. All patients should be queried about their last tetanus toxoid injection (now recommended to be given every 10 years) and whether or not they have received influenza vaccine or antipneumococcal vaccination (PneumoVax). There is increasing impetus to encourage hepatitis B vaccine for all persons in the health care professions; inquire about this, if pertinent. Measles immunization is recommended for all young adults who were either never immunized or were immunized before 1970. All adult women of childbearing age should have had documented rubella (German measles), immunization against this virus, or proven protective serum antibody titers. Polio immunization is important in adults as well as in children. The interviewer should document these immunization details to the extent that the patient is able to provide the information.

Pregnancies. The history of pregnancies and deliveries may be obtained at this time or may be reserved for the ROS. The questions are simple: "Have you ever been pregnant?" "How many times?" "How many babies have you had?" "Were there any miscarriages?" "Any abortions?" "Were there any problems with your pregnancies or deliveries?" If the answer to this last question is affirmative, ask the patient to expand on the problems.

Patient Profile

Unlike the PMH, the PP has the potential for introducing very personal and sensitive issues that the patient is not in the habit of discussing with strangers. For this reason, a clear explanation as to its relevance to the medical history must be made. In some situations, this portion of the interview is perceived by the patient as an emblem of interest in him as a person; in others, it may appear to be an intrusion into privacy. If the interviewer has not yet arrived at a conclusion about the patient's level of trust, she should be cautious about the method of introducing this segment of the history and how far it is pursued.

If in doubt about the patient's comfort, you may introduce the PP with a neutral statement such as, "I would like to learn more about you and your life, to understand how your present difficulties affect the rest of your activities." If the patient is amenable to this line of questioning, one gathers the data in a formal manner, explaining the reason for each question in turn. More commonly, the patient is relieved to see an interest in what he does and the implicit permission to discuss these socially private matters. One open-ended inquiry can start, "Tell me what you think I should know about you, your family and friends, and how you spend your time." Whatever the response of the patient to this plan to ask "personal" questions, the interviewer must have strategies for obtaining the data that defines the content of the PP. Some question options are noted.

Educational level. As a rule, this is nonthreatening to the patient and should be asked directly.

Occupational history. Most people like to talk about their jobs. Ask the patient to describe all the types of work he has done. If he indicates that he is currently unemployed, inquire how he feels about this and about his plans. Should there be an indication of occupational hazard, a more detailed work history will be required (Chapter 16).

Current living situation. This piece of information may be important to treatment plans or suggestions for lifestyle changes. At the very least, the clinician needs to learn where the patient lives (apartment, own home, extended-care facility, etc.) and who shares the space with him. Are there other persons living in the space who might provide help or support? Is there physical access compatible with the patient's level of function? Can he get to and from the facilities necessary for basic needs, such as shopping for food, transportation to medical care, physical therapy? The detail and extent of such questioning are dictated by perceived patient needs.

Family structure and support systems. If there is any indication of present or future need for help, it is important to assess the patient's resources. Who is available that might be called in times of need? Is there someone to "fetch and carry" if necessary? In the case of the vital young patient with an acute illness and loved ones clustered around, these questions are superfluous and thus are omitted. If, on the other hand, the patient is alone or is obviously disabled, such information is critical to planning.

Health habits. An assessment of the patient's health habits helps to define both risk factors as indicators of potential disease, and the level at which immediate intervention is necessary. These are not questions of idle curiosity. Rather, they are important to a full understanding of the patient's health practices. Explain this as you seek the following data.

Diet. "Tell me about your diet" may give all the information needed. If the patient proceeds to describe a regular, balanced diet and interest in good nutrition, there is seldom need to go further. On the other hand, if there is a clue that the patient eats irregularly or is following an unusual dietary pattern, more detail is sought. A second-level question might be, "Could you recall what you ate at each meal yesterday?" If there is still uncertainty, refer to Chapter 16, under Nutritional History, for a more detailed type of dietary history.

Exercise. "Do you engage in any regular exercise or physical fitness program?" If the answer is "yes," obtain details about the type and frequency of the exercise pattern. If the answer is "no," you must determine whether further questioning is important. A 30-year-old business executive who denies any physical exercise might be a candidate for further risk assessment. A 95-year-old bed-bound woman obviously does not need to be questioned about exercise. Common sense prevails in determining the extent to which details of exercise need to be acquired.

Tobacco use. "Are you a smoker?" is the best opening question. It is non-judgmental and thus allows the patient to answer honestly. If the answer is "yes," inquire about the type of smoking (cigarettes, pipe, cigars, or, in some instances, snuff), duration, and amount. When the patient started using tobacco and how much he uses on a daily basis allows quantification of consumption. The standard for quantification is in pack-years, i.e., the number of packs of cigarettes the patient has smoked per day, multiplied by the number of years he has smoked. For example, the 40-year-old man who began smoking at age 20 and estimates that he smokes 1 pack of cigarettes each day, has a 20 pack-year smoking history (20 years × 1 package/day = 20 pack-years). Pipes, cigars, and snuff are more difficult to quantitate, but a sense of frequency and duration is important should these habits be described.

Alcohol use. The best opening question is, "How much alcohol do you drink?" It is better to assume that alcohol consumption is present than to give the patient the impression that he is expected to deny drinking. The nonjudgmental nature of this opening question usually encourages the patient to be honest about alcohol. If the patient contends that he does not use alcohol when the question is posed in this manner, this should end the query. When the patient supplies an estimate of alcohol consumption, narrow the question in order to quantify. The patient may be assisted in answering the question by the provision of a guide such as, "How many drinks do you have each day, or each week?" Once the number of drinks is established, inquire about the type of alcohol, such as beer, wine, or whiskey, since the alcohol content per unit volume of each is quite different. If the answers to the questions suggest a problem, actual or potential, with alcohol, refer to Chapter 16, under Extended Substance Use History, for the more detailed questions dictated by a concern about excessive consumption, e.g., the CAGE questions.

Illicit drug use. The terminology for introduction into this area is often difficult. Some patients know what is meant by "drugs"; others just look puzzled. Yet, alternative descriptors for marijuana, cocaine, heroin, etc. have built-in value judgments. "Do you use any drugs such as marijuana or cocaine?" seems as neutral as one can get. Ask the question of everyone—young, old, or in-between. A business suit does not mean the wearer doesn't "shoot up." If the response is "yes," request more details as to what, how often, what form, and questions about complications or concerns.

Hobbies and special interests. Questions about what the patient does "for fun" are often very productive. You may, for instance, uncover toxic exposure in the patient's pursuit of a hobby. Special interests may indicate a healthy concern with pleasure and relaxation or a series of risk factors such as with the "type A" marathon fanatic. It is not the interviewer's role to judge, but merely to ask and record.

Sexual history. The patient's sexual history can reside in the PP or elsewhere. Detailed questions about sexual activity may be required in the HPI if the presenting complaint is in any way related to sexual behavior. Questions about sexuality may naturally surface during a discussion of pregnancy history, menstrual history, or the history of current medications (such as antihypertensives, which often lead to impotence). They may be introduced directly at any point by the patient. It is important to remember that sexuality is a significant part of most people's lives and that concerns about it may arise at any point during the formal medical history.

If the patient's sexual history has not been mentioned, acquisition of the PP is a logical time to let him know that the interviewer is aware of and open to any discussion of concerns. A good opening question is, "Are you sexually active?" A "no" answer should induce at least one further question: "Is this a problem for you?" If the answer is again "no," further questioning is not necessary. The patient knows that the interviewer is amenable to further discussion if desired. Otherwise, the topic is allowed to drop.

If the patient acknowledges sexual activity, you might ask the patient, "Do you have any concerns or questions?" or "Is your sex life presenting any problems you would like to discuss with me?" A negative answer to the above questions is a cue to move on. A positive answer necessitates an open-ended response such as, "Tell me more about your concerns." From this point forward, treat any sexual worry as if it were like any other medical question. Ask for the information needed, modulated by what the patient is willing to share. If there is indication here or in any other part of the interview that more detailed and specific questions about sexual problems or issues need to be addressed, the student, if not versed in the extended conduct of such an interview, may decide to defer to a more experienced colleague. A detailed discussion of the complexities of this important area is presented in Chapter 16, Extended Sexual History.

Daily routine. If a clear picture of the patient's lifestyle has not emerged, it is sometimes useful to ask him to describe a typical day in his life. By fully opening the question, the interviewer encourages the patient to talk freely about himself and the way he lives. Some clinicians use this as entry into the PP. Try it. If it works, you may choose to use this as a primary mode for acquiring lifestyle data from patients.

Family History

There are two components to the FH: (1) a **genogram,** which produces a "family tree" of health and disease, and (2) a search for common, **recurring familial patterns.** Together, the student and the patient can construct a genogram that charts the health history of the patient's family (Fig. 1.1). The genogram is usually a three-generation tabulation. The cross-check is a survey of disease patterns.

Explain the FH portion of the medical history before beginning the tabulation. If given the proper instructions, the patient will usually be able to follow the pattern easily. "I would like to learn about the health and the health problems of close members of your family. Starting with your parents, please tell me their ages if living, ages of death if deceased, and any major health problems they have had." Follow the parental generation with that of siblings, again asking for the same information. The third level is that of the patient's children, if any. A resultant genogram is illustrated in Figure 1.1. After the formal genogram has been constructed, review the FH for any other evidence of diseases that tend to run in families. For example, if the genogram shows that there is breast cancer in a mother or sister, cross-check to see if the patient knows of any cases of breast cancer in daughters, aunts, or grandmothers. If premature heart attack has appeared in the genogram more than once, it is helpful to ask about other cardiac difficulties or sudden death in grandparents, aunts, and uncles. If the patient has a history of potentially familial disease, inquire as to other family members with similar or identical problems.

Review of Systems

The ROS segment of the medical history is best treated as a last checklist to retrieve any potentially important problems that were missed previously. For conducting the ROS it is helpful for the interviewer to explain its purpose and

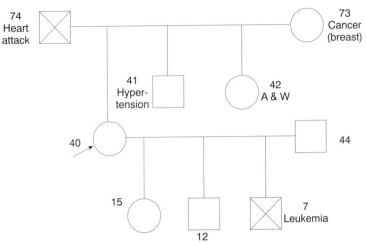

Figure 1.1   A sample genogram. *Arrow* points to patient whose interview is recorded. *Central Xs* indicate deceased persons. *Squares* indicate males; *circles,* females.

its process. The historian is concerned with "medically significant" problems and may avert trivia by laying down guidelines: "Now, I am going to ask a series of questions about other problems you might have. If you have any of the symptoms I inquire about, we will spend some time determining their importance to your current health." It is incumbent on the interviewer to have paid sufficient attention to the preceding portions of the history that she will not repeat questions already answered. For example, if the CC and HPI fully covered important gastrointestinal symptoms, the routine questions included under "gastrointestinal ROS" are not repeated. If while eliciting the PMH she has already obtained details of the patient's frequency, urgency, and decreased urinary stream that was cured by prostatic surgery, there is no need to go into this again.

Sometimes, there are "leftovers" that should be picked up during the ROS. For example, if there has been no prior indication of difficulty with the menstrual cycle in a currently menstruating woman, this is the time to get the details of the menstrual history, such as age of onset of menses, regularity of periods and length of cycle, duration of each menstrual period and presence of pain or other symptoms, and any changes that the patient has noted. In general, the ROS moves quickly with the use of closed questions.

CLOSURE

At this point, the formal medical history is complete. The student should make certain that she has

- Covered all six segments of the history.
- Verbally summarized the HPI to the patient and made any additions, corrections, or deletions.
- Attended to the patient's agendas as well as to her own.

Before leaving the patient, the student should carry out the following tasks of closure:

- Ask the patient if there is anything else that he would like to add or to ask.
- Thank the patient for cooperating.
- Ascertain that any expectations on the part of the patient have been clarified and attended to.

- Return the room to its pre-interview state, if the history took place in the patient's space, or direct the patient to his destination, if the patient has visited the interviewer's space.
- Notify any visitors that the interview is completed.

Recording the Medical History

If the medical history is not to be followed by a physical examination—as in a course on history taking—the student should make the necessary notes or do the medical history write-up as soon as possible after the interview. Samples of conventional formal recording of a medical history are provided in Appendix B. Formats vary from institution to institution, but the basic structure is standard.

If the medical history is to be followed by a physical examination, the two are best done as an unbroken continuum. The history portion of the encounter has established the relationship. The physical examination consists of a logical sequence that is discussed in the following chapters.

Troublesome Interviews

Up to this point we have presented medical history content and process as though everything progresses according to the best-laid plans. In real life, this is seldom the case. Several things can go wrong with the interview. Some common difficulties are mentioned here (Table 1.5); other problems are dealt with in detail in Chapter 16.

PROBLEMS CREATED BY BEING SICK

Sick people are not always on their best behavior. Illness or worry about potential illness elicits all sorts of responses and behaviors that differ from everyday actions. Consider, when interviewing people in this unique situation, that what they do and say may be dictated or, at least, affected by any of the factors that follow.

Pain

Pain changes behavior. How nice were you the last time you experienced a headache, a toothache, or a painful injury? Be tolerant of the patient in pain, and recognize that behavior deteriorates in its presence.

Table 1.5
Troublesome Interviews

Problems created by being sick	Problems created by situation or topic
Effect of pain	Sensitive content
Effect of fear	Interruptions and interference
Distrust and sense of vulnerability	Third-party interviews
Anger and frustration	
Denial	
Problems created by behavioral styles	
Lying, malingering, withholding	
Manipulation	
Controlling the interview	
Garrulous, wandering, vague	
Demented, delirious, drugged	
Language and culture as barriers	

Fear

Persons with unpleasant symptoms or diagnoses are often afraid—afraid of outcomes, afraid of tests, afraid of the unknown. Fear, like pain, alters behavior. There is also a widespread fear of doctors and medical interactions in our society—a fear that often plagues the healthy and may explain otherwise apparently irrational behavior.

Distrust and Vulnerability

The sick person often has considerable reason to distrust the environment into which he has been thrust. It may be new or, if not new, at least threatening. Sickness creates a realistic sense of vulnerability and of loss of control that is vexing and disorienting. Again, the attitudes and behaviors of the sick person are colored by the loss of control and the acute awareness of that loss.

Anger and Frustration

The sick and vulnerable patient may show clear signs of anger and frustration, which can be displayed only by acting out against the personnel encountered in an environment he links with what he is feeling. It is difficult for the patient to know how and where to direct anger. It may be directed at the interviewer, not because of anything she has done, but simply because she is there, because she reminds the patient that he is in an uncomfortable sick role, or because the student is the "low person on the totem pole" of medicine and therefore a safe target.

Denial

Rarely do patients deliberately tell lies about themselves and their symptoms. However, they very often deny because they are not ready to accept that all is not well. If what is observed or already known about the patient does not correlate with the story that he tells, consider the possibility of denial. The interviewer may not be able to overcome this barrier but needs to learn to recognize it.

Recently, one of us observed a first-year medical student interview a 28-year-old man who had just lost both legs in an accident. The man spoke cheerfully and confidently about his plans to climb the Matterhorn this summer. His new pitons were on his bedside table. This man was not trying to fool the student. Rather, he wanted and needed to believe that he would be able to climb again. The student listened carefully to the patient's plans, neither affirming nor contradicting. Suddenly, the patient shouted at the student, "You don't believe me, do you? You don't think I'll ever climb the mountain." The student didn't answer, just reached out and took the young man's hand. Together they cried. After the interview was finished, the patient handed the pitons to the student and asked her if she could find someone who might be able to use them. She received them and acknowledged that she knew climbers. The patient had crossed his first barrier to acceptance, assisted by the quiet compassion of a very sensitive novice interviewer.

If the interviewer approaches each patient with the realization that no one can be consistently cooperative, affable, and congenial, she will avoid personalizing affronts. Most of the traps into which interviewers fall result from forgetting the extent to which behaviors are affected by the foreign situations—unfamiliar or treacherous behavior of the body, new and threatening environments—in which patients find themselves.

BEHAVIORAL STYLES AS PROBLEMS

Situations in which the interaction with the patient is flawed by other behaviors or circumstances are reviewed briefly here.

Lying, Malingering, or Withholding

Incorrect information may result from denial, from true memory loss, from drugs, or from distraction by pain. Much less often, it represents the patient's deliberate attempt to gain control. If a patient refuses to answer a question or provides an answer that is clearly absurd, don't argue or cajole. Leave the question, with or without an observation that silence isn't assent, depending on the particulars of the interaction. You may decide to return to it later or may have to simply indicate in the case write-up that the answer is not reliable.

Attempts at Manipulation

An occasional patient, on perceiving that the student is the most inexperienced member of the team, may try to manipulate her, often prefacing the requests with exaggerated, unearned, or unduly personal praise. Should the patient ask the student to do something or obtain something for him that seems inappropriate, the student may suggest that he ask his own doctor or nurse. If the interviewer remains firm and reiterates that her role is simply that of history taker, most attempts at manipulation will cease.

Control of the Interview

In the best of all possible worlds, the medical interview is conducted by mutuality of control. Occasionally, the patient will attempt to wrest total control, disabling the interviewer's mission. Attempt to redirect if the patient attempts to take the interview on useless tangents. Explain why it is important to alter the line of discussion. Don't be discouraged by failure. The beginner gets better with this uncommon challenge as she gains both experience and confidence.

Garrulous, Wandering, or Vague Style

Like the controlling patient, the patient who is garrulous, wandering, or vague can be very frustrating to the interviewer. Unlike the controlling patient, the vague patient has no ulterior motive and usually responds to firm, polite redirection. If the interview seems to be drifting far afield, don't be afraid to interrupt the wanderer with a reminder of the task at hand. "Your wife's travels in Europe are fascinating, but I really need to learn more about your chest pain. Please describe what happened to you this morning."

Demented, Delirious, or Drugged Patient

Gaining reliable and cogent information may be impossible (a) when the patient is disoriented or truly demented or (b) when mental processes are affected by intoxication or other acute brain dysfunction. On these occasions, there is no recourse but to look to third parties, i.e., family members, companions, or caregivers for information.

Language and Cultural Barriers

Significant difficulties can be created by differences in native language or cultural practices between interviewer and patient. The risk for misunderstanding or misinterpreting information rises when these differences exist. The interviewer should remain aware of this potential, which is not abated by a skilled interpreter. Chapter 16 addresses this problem in more detail.

TOPICAL AND SITUATIONAL PROBLEMS

In addition to the specific interactional categories noted above, certain topical and situational problems can arise.

Topical deterrents to a successful interview include sensitive data areas such as drug and alcohol use, family violence, or sexual difficulties. Because these topics come up frequently and are often particularly important in medical interviewing, strategies for approaching them are developed more fully in Chapter 16.

Situational problems are defined here as those that involve interruptions, third-party interviews, or interference in the interview.

Interruptions

In today's hospital environment, interruptions are the rule rather than the exception. Frustrating as it can be to the student interviewer, some patient care procedures must have priority over training in interviewing. Administration of timed medications, measurements of vital signs, and trips to radiology or physical therapy will often break up the continuity of an interview. Try to be graceful about having your patient whisked away; if possible, ascertain from the nurse when the patient is expected to return to his room and try to plan a return visit or to accompany the patient if allowed. In the outpatient setting, the pressure will come from other providers waiting to use a room or from a bus schedule that the patient must meet. Unfortunately, these events are often beyond the control of the student and even of the system. They are not the patient's fault any more than they are the interviewer's. Accept the hindrance; tomorrow will be better.

Third-Party Interviews

Third-party interviews—those in which data are obtained from someone other than the patient himself—are common in pediatrics. They are further discussed in Chapters 15 and 16. On occasion, in adult medicine, the interview is conducted with a friend, family member, or professional companion serving as proxy for an incompetent or aphasic person. The student must remain aware of the differences in perception between patient and observer, no matter how intimate the relationship may be, and of the divergent history that inevitably follows. Clearly identify the data source if it is anyone other than the patient when communicating this information to a colleague or to the patient record. If the patient gives the history but seems unreliable for whatever reason, record that too.

Interference

If you must obtain information from a patient with another party participating, define the ground rules carefully. Insofar as possible, the interaction should be primarily between interviewer and patient. If the third party is interrupting or dominating the conversation or is answering questions for the patient (usually with the best of intentions of facilitating or of "protecting" the patient), don't hesitate to ask that the patient be allowed to speak for himself. The interviewer positions herself such that dialogue flows most easily between her and the patient. She remains polite but firm about whose story she wants to hear. It is an old axiom of geriatrics that there are often two CCs: that of the patient and that of the family. Both are important, but the latter shouldn't be mistaken for the former!

To the Beginner: Words of Encouragement

ADVANTAGES

There are distinct advantages to being a novice in medical interviewing. Some of these advantages are described below.

Apprentice Status

There is no expectation that you are responsible for solving the patient's problems. As long as your role has been specified, you serve as an interested party but not one whose knowledge or expertise can be challenged. Most patients enjoy the idea of helping students to learn, respect you for your goals, and teach you what they can.

Time to Listen

Your relatively leisurely interview is often a welcome relief to the patient, compared to the harried dashing in and out of tired interns and pressured consultants. It is nice to have someone come in, sit down, stay a while, and listen attentively. Unless the patient is plagued with pain, worry, or anxiety that overrides the need for attention, he will generally be happy for the diversion and the legitimate sense of his importance that this encounter provides.

Absence of Jargon

Your absence of jargon and your willingness to let the patient tell his story in his own words also make you, as a learner, especially appealing to a patient who may have been silently poked, prodded, and nodded over by technically expert but humanly inept persons. You may be one of the few professionals he has encountered who appears to value his opinions on the matter of his illness.

Asking for Help

If you run into difficulty, you can always, without losing face, call for help. Don't be embarrassed to admit that you have reached an impasse. The patient will understand, and your teachers should too.

DISADVANTAGES

There are also disadvantages to not being an expert. Although they cannot be ignored, they are temporary and manageable. Discussion of some of these disadvantages follows.

Sense of Inadequacy

Try as you may, you cannot always overcome feelings of nervousness and inadequacy as you work through the first few interviews. It is futile and arrogant to pretend you are what you are not. On the other hand, there is never a need to apologize for your learner status. If you don't know something or if you don't know quite how to proceed with the interview, be honest with yourself and with the patient. If you must consult your notes or your preceptor, there is no shame in admitting a need for such help.

Lack of Expertise

Do not attempt to answer medical questions, to second-guess doctors, or to provide opinions. Your personal comfort about saying "I don't know" is especially important at this level. It is the most underused phrase in the doctor's vocabulary, although it shouldn't be. No doctor ever knows the answers to all of the questions she is asked. Since you may appear to the patient to be the most interested and concerned of the staff he has yet met, he may press you for information you do not possess. Even if you do possess it, it may not be your place to respond. If the patient asks you for an opinion, refer him back to his primary caretakers or offer to find someone who can provide the best answer.

Feeling of "Using" the Patient

A common concern of the preclinical student is the feeling of "using" the patient. Since you do not participate on the primary health care team, you may feel that your presence is an intrusion without benefit to the patient. Practically speaking, this perception may be entirely true, but it is indispensable to the care of future patients. Medicine is not learnable in a vacuum, and the calling to medicine is fundamentally one of service. Thus the issue is realistic only if the patient feels used.

If the patient's permission for your visit has been properly obtained and you have stated your role clearly, the patient's agreement to proceed is your passport to the encounter. Do not be reluctant if the patient is not reluctant: Let the patient give, too, and receive graciously. Remember that as a novice you have explicit permission to make mistakes and to ask for help. The training period is designed for you to learn. Use the problems you encounter to your advantage and get advice from your preceptor as to how you might better handle specific problems the next time they arise. Have fun learning to take a medical history! Even more than dissecting the cadaver, it represents a threshold crossed between a classroom student and a beginning healer.

ADULT SCREENING PHYSICAL EXAMINATION: A REGIONAL APPROACH

Overview

The learner of basic physical assessment faces a complex task. She must not only master the techniques and use of new instruments but must also deal simultaneously with the human dimension of the encounter while learning to be efficient and competent in differentiating normal from abnormal. By providing the learner with a rational sequence, a set of skills, and methods for keeping the patient comfortable, we will enable her to gain the most from the experience. Before the novice can begin to think about pathology and differential diagnosis, she must master technique and feel confident with examination of the physically normal person.

This chapter describes what is needed for conducting a physical examination, including the instruments and setting required, the positioning of the examiner and of the patient, and a logical regional sequence in which to conduct a basic (symptom-independent) physical examination. Once the student has become facile with the structure and content of this examination and has committed its sequence to memory, she may concentrate on the abnormal and on the formulation of diagnostic hypotheses as she works through the steps of the physical examination.

The regional approach to performing the physical examination makes sense because of its efficiency, its comfort, and its utility as a system for recall of steps. The examination is, however, recorded (written) predominantly in an organ-system modality rather than by region. In thinking about patients' problems, we very often think systemically rather than regionally. There are obviously situations in which physiologic systems must be examined as nonregional units; these will be considered in the sections of those chapters in which the extended or focused physical examination is discussed.

For the moment, we assume that the examiner is here to learn the steps—the mechanical procedures—essential to basic physical examination. Where regional overlaps or system crossovers are necessary, these problems will be made clear, and solutions will be provided. This issue is most strikingly relevant to examination of the skin, the lymph nodes, the central and peripheral nervous system, and certain parts of the cardiovascular system. As details of the regional examination are developed in subsequent chapters, the student will come to reconcile discrepancies between the "regional" approach and the "systems" approach quite automatically and, eventually, without effort.

The **four basic modes** applied to the physical examination are *inspection, palpation, percussion, and auscultation*. Each is used to varying degrees, depending on the body region being examined. The modes are defined as follows:

- *Inspection:* Informed and critical use of the examiner's eyes. The inspection of the patient begins with general observation during the medical interview and is the primary mode of the physical examination.
- *Palpation:* Touching and feeling mode. Light palpation is used to assess skin and superficial structures, variations in surface temperature, moisture, or dryness. Deep palpation is applied to deep visceral organs such as those of the abdomen.
- *Percussion:* Use of sound to define structure density and content. The classical percussion method is to create vibration by tapping against the body surface, listening and feeling for differences in sound wave conduction.
- *Auscultation:* Use of the stethoscope to judge the movement of gases, fluids, or organs in body compartments.

Preparing for the Examination

Efficient performance of the physical examination (Table 1.6) is greatly facilitated by attentive preparation, which obviates surprises and fumbles. Proper space, adequate time, and the availability of all necessary tools are indispensable for effective examination. This section describes the details of "getting ready" to do a full, regionally organized examination.

SPACE

The examining area should contain a piece of furniture that the patient can sit on with legs dangling, and it should be accessible from sides and front and back. The patient must be able to lie supine for some parts of the examination. There should be walking space for assessment of motion.

The patient requires proper privacy, covering, and basic elements of comfort such as room warmth. The patient must be supplied with gown and sheet or appropriate substitutes so that the body can be exposed as needed without undue nudity or physical or psychic discomfort.

Table 1.6
Keys to an Effective Examination

Preparing for the examination
    Adequate and efficient space
    Adequate time and concentration
    Adequate and operational equipment and supplies
Orchestrating the examination
    Arrangement of equipment
    Positioning of patient
    Positioning of examiner
Sequencing the examination
    For efficiency
    For patient comfort
    For examiner comfort

The examiner requires a place for instruments and supplies, the space to maneuver for the various segments of the examination, adequate lighting to make essential observations, and a place to dispose of used supplies.

Hand-washing facilities must be available.

TIME

The learner usually requires 1 hour to conduct a full physical examination. One goal of the novice is to become efficient enough to complete the procedure, including the pelvic examination, in 30 minutes. At first the student needs the luxury of unlimited time. With increasing experience, the time required must constrict to realistic limits. The patient should be informed in advance that an hour of his time will be required for examination.

INSTRUMENTS AND SUPPLIES

The instruments and supplies listed here include everything used in doing the complete general examination (Table 1.7). The equipment of various specialists and subspecialists is not included. Each student should assess which items from the list will be available routinely in the rooms where the work is to be done. The student should achieve comfort with personal instruments and to avoid time-consuming dependence on another examiner's materials that may be unavailable, locked up, or defective. Faculty preceptors or course directors can provide a list of instruments and supplies that the student must own as well as guidelines for locating and purchasing them. Local preferences may override our generic advice to the student about purchases.

The most valuable instruments that the student brings to the physical examination are sharp eyes, ears, fingers, and mind, a basic knowledge of the anatomy and physiology of the human body, and a healthy curiosity. The mechanical devices and other materials extend these primary tools.

Table 1.7
Instruments and Supplies

Instruments	Supplies
Examining table	Examination gown
Thermometer	Half-sheet for draping
Sphygmomanometer	Disposable gloves
Stethoscope	Tongue blades
Ophthalmoscope	Paper cups
Otoscope	Cotton-tipped swabs
Penlight	Tape measure
Tuning fork(s)	Visual acuity chart of Snellen[a]
Percussion (reflex) hammer	Visual acuity chart, pocket
Nasal speculum or attachment	Gauze squares
Cloth measuring tape	Water-based lubricant gel
Paper and pencil	Stool occult-blood measurement cards and
Wristwatch with sweep hand	developer
Skin-marking pencil	For pelvic examination:
Equipment for measuring weight and height[a]	Labeled glass slides
Goose-neck lamp or other light source[a]	Papanicolaou devices for collecting cervi-
Vaginal speculum with light source	cal and endocervical cells
	Fixative for slides

[a]Usually available in most clinical settings.

Sphygmomanometer

The basic blood pressure cuff is either a mercury or an aneroid device. The former is more accurate but bulkier than the latter. Cuffs come in several widths for the range of arm circumferences encountered. The standard adult cuff width and bladder length are discussed more fully in Chapter 2. For many adults, a large-arm cuff is ideal. Infants, children, and extremely thin adults require different cuffs. A wider cuff with longer bladder is necessary for obese arms and for measuring leg pressures. Improper cuffs cause false readings (see Chapter 2 for indications for selecting alternative cuff sizes).

Stethoscope

The range of available selections for this emblematic instrument is overwhelming. The student is advised to purchase a good quality instrument with both a bell and a diaphragm. The decision to invest in a more complex, multiheaded stethoscope may be deferred, but one learns best on a stethoscope that is not a "throwaway," just as beginning artists are advised to invest in good watercolors. A tubing length of 30–40 cm is best, and well-fitting earpieces are important.

The "Diagnostic Kit": Ophthalmoscope and Otoscope

In general, these two instruments are sold together, and they represent the largest single financial investment the student must make in physical diagnosis equipment. However, they are built for longevity and, if well cared for, will likely never need to be replaced. Again, the range of selections is large. The basic requirements for each are:

- *Ophthalmoscope:* light source (bulb and batteries), lens systems with a diopter range from –20 to about +20, and a rechargeable-battery handle. Most manufacturers equip their most basic instrument with these, and usually more, options. Halogen lights are now standard on most scopes and are preferable. Probably the most critical variation is in handle size. The examiner needs to be able to grip and hold the scope comfortably, and to turn the rheostat and the lens wheel easily.
- *Otoscope:* light source (usually the same rechargeable-battery handle as the ophthalmoscope with interchangeable heads) and a variety of speculum sizes. Most otoscopes are provided with a pneumatic bulb for air insufflation, a useful device in assessing the mobility of children's eardrums.

Reflex (or Percussion) Hammer

The simple, hard rubber triangle with metal handle is standard and sufficient for eliciting all muscle stretch reflexes.

Tuning Fork(s)

The high frequency (512 Hz) tuning fork is recommended for testing hearing, whereas the lower frequency (128 Hz) is the most useful for determining vibratory sense. If only one tuning fork is obtained, the 128 Hz is more versatile and easier to use.

Miscellaneous Equipment

Although the otoscope light may be used for oral cavity examination and pupillary reflexes, it is more convenient to carry a pocket **penlight.** The examiner will need a 15-cm pocket ruler and a more versatile cloth **tape measure** for accurate recording of the dimensions of organs and of lesions. A **wristwatch** with a sweep second hand is essential. **Visual acuity charts** are available in pocket size for determination of near vision. The familiar large wall chart (Snellen) should be available in any clinic setting. It is used for the assessment of longer-distance vision and demands a 7-meter distance for accurate measurement. Each student should be able to use and read an ordinary **mercury thermometer.** Many clinics now provide electronic devices for temperature recording, but occasions will repeatedly arise that call for the more pedestrian version. Disposable thermometers are readily available, and the student should obtain a few of these, which come individually wrapped.

Supplies

Disposable (nonsterile) **gloves** are necessary for palpating the oral cavity, rectum, genitalia, and open skin lesions. Glove sizes range from small (6) to large (8½). A good fit is necessary for optimal tactile assessment. Gloves are required for protection of patient and/or examiner at various points in the examination. The indications for gloving are noted as regions are discussed in detail.

Nonsterile wooden **tongue blades** are sometimes necessary for oral and pharyngeal examination, as are large **gauze squares** (for tongue manipulation). A **paper cup** with a small volume of water is helpful in assessing swallowing. **Cotton-tipped applicators** are useful for light sensation ("light touch") testing, and with the wooden handle snapped, for testing pain sensation.

It is not appropriate to use a pin for pain sensation; if the examiner needs steel points, each should be discarded after one examination in order to avoid the theoretical hazard of transmitting blood-borne infection from patient to patient.

For the rectal examination and the pelvic examination, special supplies and equipment include **vaginal specula, lubricant gel, devices for obtaining cytologic specimens and cultures, 95% ethanol or a spray to use as a Papanicolaou fixative, and stool occult-blood-testing cards and developing solution.** These are discussed in detail with the relevant regional examinations.

Finally, the student should have a **writing instrument and paper** handy for the recording of notes and measurements. Accuracy for transmission to the patient's permanent record demands that some data be noted during the course of the examination rather than be entrusted to later recall. (See Table 1.7 for a quick checklist of instruments and supplies.)

Orchestrating the Regional Adult Physical Examination

As the student learns each of the steps of the physical examination, "orchestration" may be divided conveniently into manageable segments. Eventually, however, the student needs to put the entire examination together and conduct it as a single event. To appreciate the place of each portion of the examination in its relationship to the whole, and to begin thinking about a rational and efficient system, the student may benefit from a preview of the final product. Orchestration in this context refers to the movements of both patient and examiner as the two cooperate in expeditious completion of the potentially overwhelming task at hand.

The physical examination should begin after a history has been obtained. By the end of the history, the effective clinician will have established sufficient rapport with the patient that the initiation of physical examination is a comfortable and natural transition. Levels of concern and anxiety on the part of the patient should have been assessed and considered in preparation for examination. A general explanation of the content and time required for the physical examination is provided before commencing, and expectations of the parties are shared. The patient is appropriately gowned and draped so that there will be no struggles with clothing to impair examination. **All equipment and supplies for the exami-**

nation will be present, within easy reach, and ready for use. Examination is preceded by careful hand-washing by the examiner, preferably within sight of the patient.

POSITIONING OF EXAMINER AND PATIENT

The positioning and comfort of both examiner and patient are essential to conducting the examination properly. Close attention to minimizing position changes for both participants is a prime factor in sequencing the procedure. The healthy and agile patient may bound up and down easily, but the examiner needs to establish a protocol that minimizes unnecessary repositioning on behalf of the numerous acutely sick or chronically disabled patients encountered in daily practice. Efficiency and recall are well served by development of a reproducible system for examination.

SEQUENCE AND CONTENT OF THE EXAMINATION

There is no consensus among practitioners as to what constitutes a "complete" physical examination. The following sequence and content list represents a composite, drawn from the teaching of basic physical examination to second-year medical students by faculty at a single medical school and from the authors' combined personal experience. Each may have a unique core list of examination maneuvers. Overriding the specific items included on our list are the concepts of reproducibility, system, efficiency, and comfort for both the patient and examiner. Each student can adapt our model to local and personal preferences, retaining a system that achieves the objectives stated above (see Table 1.8 for content and sequencing of the examination).

In utilizing the regional sequence of the examination, the student must recognize the physiologic systems crossovers, especially as they apply to the skin, the lymph nodes, and the neurologic examination. In performing a regional examination, for example, the skin, cranial nerves, and lymph nodes of the head and neck are assessed with the more purely regional head and neck structures, even though the former represent only portions of systems. The skin is anatomically considered an organ system unto itself, yet it makes no sense to examine the skin separately rather than as it is exposed regionally. The utility of the regional approach resides in its efficiency and in the potential for committing to memory all portions of the total basic examination.

Recording the Findings

By convention, the written record of the physical examination is structured by systems rather than by regions. With experience, the student will find that the translation of data gathered by body regions into data recorded by organ systems becomes second nature. For a sample record of a screening physical examination see Appendix B.

EXTENDED OR PROBLEM-FOCUSED EXAMINATION

The extended or problem-focused medical history and physical examination (assessment) of the patient is the mode that most characterizes the practice of medicine. Unlike the screening history and physical examination, this problem-directed encounter is utilized to investigate the most pressing symptoms and

Table 1.8
Examination Sequence

Positions	Examination Maneuver	Equipment

Patient: seated
Examiner:
   facing patient
	Inspect general appearance
	Inspect hands
	Palpate hands
	Assess grip strength
	Palpate radial pulse
	Count radial pulse
	Take blood pressure
		
		Wristwatch
		Sphygmomanometer,
		   stethoscope

	Inspect scalp Inspect face Assess facial mobility and sensation Inspect conjunctiva Inspect sclera Assess ocular movement Assess visual fields Assess hearing Assess pupillary reflexes Fundoscopic examination Ear examination Inspect nose Inspect oral cavity	 Cotton swab Penlight Ophthalmoscope Otoscope, speculum Light, speculum Light, gauze, glove, tongue blade
	Assess deglutition Assess neck range of motion Assess shoulder shrug, neck turning Palpate head and neck lymph nodes Inspect and palpate thyroid Palpate carotid arteries	Cup of water
Patient: seated Examiner: behind patient	Observe thorax and spine, posteriorly Percuss spine for tenderness Percuss costovertebral angle for tenderness Test tactile fremitus, posterior lungs Percuss posterior lungs Auscult posterior lungs	 Stethoscope
Patient: seated Examiner: facing patient	Auscult anterior and lateral lungs Percuss anterior and lateral lungs Inspect breasts Palpate axillae	Stethoscope

Patient: supine
Examiner: to
   patient's right
   side
	Palpate breasts
	Auscult precordium
	Auscult carotid arteries
	Inspect cervical veins
	Observe abdomen
	Auscult abdomen
	Percuss abdomen
	Palpate liver
	Palpate spleen
	Palpate abdomen
	Palpate inguinal lymph nodes
	Palpate and auscult femoral arteries
		
		Stethoscope
		Stethoscope
		
		Stethoscope
		
		Stethoscope

Table 1.8 *(continued)*

Positions	Examination Maneuver	Equipment
	Inspect and palpate legs and feet	
	Palpate leg and foot arteries	
	Test hip range of motion	
Patient: seated		
Examiner: facing patient	Test shoulder, elbow, knee, ankle range of motion	
	Test upper and lower limb muscle strength	
	Test muscle stretch reflexes	Percussion hammer
	Test plantar reflexes	Broken swab stick
	Test cerebellar function with rapid alternating motion and heel-to-shin tests	
	Test pain and light touch	Broken swab stick, cotton wisp
	Test vibratory sense, lower limbs	Tuning fork
	Test proprioceptive sense, lower limbs	
Patient: standing	Measure orthostatic pulse and blood pressure	Sphygmomanometer, stethoscope
Patient: standing	Test back mobility	
Examiner: variable	Test Romberg maneuver	
	Observe gait and transfers	
	Male genital and hernia examinations	Gloves
	Male rectal and prostate examinations[a]	Gloves
Patient: lithotomy	Female pelvic and rectal examination[a]	See Table 1.7

[a]Patients of either sex may be examined in left lateral decubitus position.

signs and to begin the process of diagnosing their cause(s) and approaching their management. Because accurate and timely focusing demands a greater knowledge base in pathologic anatomy and disordered physiology, as well as more highly developed medical problem-solving skills, the teaching of the problem-directed assessment usually follows completion of a comprehensive screening approach. The expectation is that the student's fund of knowledge and problem-solving skills have grown apace.

ADULT EXTENDED (PROBLEM-FOCUSED) MEDICAL HISTORY

The adult extended (problem-focused) medical history is defined as a medical history concentrated exclusively on the immediate problem (present illness) and those elements from the other five segments of the screening history essential to understanding this single problem. Taking such a focused history requires a sound understanding of basic pathophysiology, hypothesis formulation, and information sorting, grounded in a knowledge of disease processes.

The expediency of providing care and the appropriate prioritization of patient needs are major demands dictating use of such a problem-directed assessment. Typical settings calling for the extended or problem-focused medical history are emergency rooms, immediate-care centers, and ambulatory care sites.

The process of obtaining a problem-focused medical history differs from that utilized in the screening interview. The clinician selects elements of the history essential to the solution, based on the nature and urgency of the problem at hand. The history is obtained in a modified order as well as in this abbreviated format.

Hypothesis Formulation

The content of the history is usually suggested by the presenting symptom or CC. The chronology of the major symptom(s) is obtained, as are full dimensions, i.e., circumstances of onset, quality and quantity, aggravating and alleviating factors, associated symptoms, etc. As the story unfolds, the clinician formulates hypotheses about which organ systems are disordered, in part to dictate which components of the PMH, FH, PP, and ROS need consideration. She deliberately and selectively omits all elements of the screening medical history that are expected to add nothing to the solution of the focused problem.

Data Gathering and Hypothesis Testing

Once the HPI is clearly defined and the clinician has formulated a hypothesis as to the organ systems implicated, specific items from the ROS are obtained. Further information about the organ systems suspected of being abnormal is gathered by direct, and often directive, questioning. Positive responses are incorporated, and pertinent negatives are noted.

A **"pertinent negative"** is defined as the **absence** of a symptom or historical datum that would implicate involvement of the organ system in question. For example, if a patient presents with a story of increasing shortness of breath, the cardiovascular and the respiratory systems are primary etiologic contenders. Thus, a check of other symptoms relevant to these systems or organs would include inquiries about exertional dyspnea, orthopnea, and paroxysmal nocturnal dyspnea, about chest pain, palpitations, and ankle swelling, or about cough, wheezing, hemoptysis, sputum production, and fever. Is there is a history of asthma or other pulmonary disease? Positive responses are clustered and placed in the chronology as appropriate. Negative responses become grouped in the clinician's thinking.

Hypotheses are modulated by responses to ROS items that have been subsumed into the focused HPI. It is evident that the processes of data gathering and hypothesis testing become inextricably intertwined in such an interview. The construction, testing, and modification of hypotheses in real time call for much *activity* in the interviewer's brain. The exercise challenges and delights the clinician, whose cognitive and integrative faculties produce a *performance* of history taking.

Role of Past Medical History

PMH is obtained to the extent expected to illuminate the present problem or to aid in further refinement of diagnostic hypotheses. Have there been illnesses or operations in the past that affect the organ systems under current consideration? Has the patient ever experienced the symptom or constellation of symptoms before? If so, what were the circumstances, the diagnosis (not to be taken at face value, but only as one more datum), and the outcome? Routine questions from the traditional PMH are not pursued unless the interviewer believes they will help solve the current problem. Exceptions to this rule are drugs (prescription, over-the-counter, and illicit), allergies, and the possibility of pregnancy, which deserve inquiry in every patient.

The clinician must decide what, if any, questions about FH will be useful. This decision is determined strictly by the interviewer's diagnostic hypotheses.

Role of Patient Profile

The same premise holds true in part for the PP. For example, our patient presenting with shortness of breath may have a cigarette-smoking history or a history of exposure to toxins, which will add significant data, whether positive or negative.

The "universal" PP data—to be sought in every encounter—are age, occupation, living situation, and recent psychologic or physical stressors. Information on alcohol, tobacco, and drug use is also frequently necessary.

On completion of the extended medical history, the clinician is empowered to make rational selection of the elements of the physical examination necessary to develop the diagnostic possibilities formulated from the history.

ADULT EXTENDED (PROBLEM-FOCUSED) PHYSICAL EXAMINATION

The content and comprehensiveness of the problem-directed physical examination rely on the interviewer's diagnostic and functional impressions from the history. The focused "physical" is as narrowly focused as the diagnostic hypotheses will permit, yet retains enough latitude to exclude lesser possibilities while supporting or proving diagnosis. The sequence of the examination addresses the problems under consideration. It often differs from the sequence within a comprehensive examination, yet it always remains logical, i.e., efficient about patient positioning.

Questions Raised by the Problem-Focused Examination

The questions to be addressed by this examination are those raised by the history. The questions to be asked are: What organs and physiologic systems are most likely to be involved in creating the symptoms presented? Within these systems, what pathologic process or processes could account for the patient's complaints?

Further Considerations

Answers, possibly incomplete, to the above questions have come out of the history. Based on those answers, you need to ask: What physical examination abnormalities should be sought? What, if any, special maneuvers might augment the probability of locating the abnormality? What other system(s) or organ(s) must be assessed to guard against the hazard of premature closure? That is, what realistic diagnostic possibilities can be excluded by physical examination, and which others will become more probable?

From this framework, the clinician determines the extent of examination to be conducted, remaining flexible in the event of encountering unexpected findings that may alter the hypotheses, uncover new or unrelated issues, and potentially redirect the examination. However, the problem-focused physical examination relatively infrequently provides *surprising* new information when a specific set of symptoms is being assessed. Note that *every* patient physical examination should include a pulse rate, respiratory rate, blood pressure, and temperature, regardless of the nature of the presenting problem.

The approach to this form of extended medical history and examination becomes case specific (individualized) beyond the very basic formula outlined. An example of a flexible, nonstatic, problem-directed assessment illustrating application of these principles follows.

Case Study: A Sample Extended (Problem-Focused) Examination

A 32-year-old man is brought to the emergency department with a chief complaint of 2 hours of severe abdominal pain. He is observed to move restlessly about, frequently changing positions or getting up from the examining table to pace. Initial supine vital signs taken by the nursing staff are recorded as oral temperature 37.5°C (99.5°F), blood pressure 140/88 in each arm, pulse 110/minute and regular, and respirations 18/minute; neither pulse nor blood pressure changes when he stands upright.

The history of present illness is obtained by asking the patient to describe exactly what he had noticed since the pain began 2 hours earlier.

"The first thing I felt was a sort of gripping discomfort deep in here [indicating the right paraumbilical area] and in my back on the right side. At first it wasn't too bad, and I went on with patching my bike tire. But then, it got worse, and it moved down here [indicating the right lower quadrant and right hemiscrotum]. In a while it was so bad that I couldn't finish what I was doing, and I went in the house to lie down. But that didn't help. The pain got worse and worse, and I got scared and asked my wife to bring me here."

Following this general description of the events since the symptom began, the present illness is refined by addressing the dimensions of the problem. A further question about the nature of the pain yields:

"As I said, it was sort of grabbing and mild at first, then it became intense, steady—almost tearing—all down the right side of my belly. And I feel it in my testicle, too. It is the worst pain I've ever felt!"

The patient is asked exactly what he was doing when the pain started and what, if anything, he had done in the hours preceding the symptom.

"I had competed, earlier in the day, in a 40-km bicycle race, during which I had a flat tire, which I changed on the road. When I got home I decided to patch the tube and that was what I was doing when the pain started. I wasn't in any contorted body position." He volunteers that he has never experienced anything like this before and is frightened about what it might be.

What, if anything, has he noticed that changes the intensity or character of the pain?

"Nothing seems to make any difference. Lying down doesn't help, moving around is just the same. There is no position I can get into that relieves it. I drank plenty of Gatorade and one beer after the race. I took two aspirins about 15 minutes ago, before coming here. No effect—yet, anyway."

Is there anything else he has tried to do?

"Well, I had a bowel movement an hour ago. It was normal and didn't change the pain. This thing seems to have a mind of its own."

Has anything seemed to make the pain more intense?

"Nothing specific. It has just gotten progressively worse on its own. Walking in here from the parking lot had no effect."

To seek possible warning signs or antecedents, the patient is asked about his health and activities in the hours and days prior to the onset of the pain.

"I've been feeling great! My time in the race was the best I've ever clocked. I'm a very healthy person. I just don't understand what is happening to me!"

The patient is asked about anything else he might have noticed about himself preceding or since the onset of the pain.

"Well, I have felt like I had to urinate several times during these 2 hours but can only pass a few drops at a time. I think it's just nervousness. I always feel like I have to pee when I'm scared. The urine didn't burn when it came out."

Was it abnormal in color?

"A little dark, but no more so than after other races."

Was there any penile pain or discharge today, or has anything been different in his sex life in recent weeks?

"Not a bit. Stable situation, no new practices, and we're both faithful."

With this basic sense of the patient's story, the clinician may begin to formulate hypotheses in order to acquire pertinent past historical information, family history information, lifestyle questions, and organ system-specific data. The sudden onset of well-localized abdominal and testicular pain in a previously healthy

young man presents a narrow spectrum of likely sources of the problem: the midgut (distal ileum, appendix, cecum, and ascending colon), the kidney and/or ureter, the testicle–spermatic cord–epididymis complex. The pancreas, foregut, hindgut, biliary tree, and the great vessels of the abdomen are all remote alternatives. From the past medical history, it is important to learn about prior episodes of like character, prior abdominal trauma or especially surgery, chronic medications, or prior abdominal organ diagnoses.

"I had my appendix out when I was 6 years old. That's the only time I was ever operated on, or in the hospital for that matter. I broke an arm several years ago, but that's the only injury I've ever had. I take Motrin [a brand of ibuprofen] for 24 hours before a long ride because one knee sometimes bothers me and the medicine keeps it under control. Since the Motrin bothers my stomach, I take it with one of those little bottles of Maalox, but I only do this about once a month when I'm going to compete. Otherwise, I'm perfectly healthy. Haven't seen a doctor since—oh, probably, the last time was when I had a sports physical in college—I played baseball then." When asked more about the symptom associated with ibuprofen use, the patient relates that a vague burning associated with the drug is relieved completely and promptly by antacid, and occurs at no other time. "I even tried one of those little Maalox bottles as we started over here. It hasn't made a bit of difference."

The family history of possible significance to the immediate problem is limited to that of gout and renal stones.

"Well, my dad used to suffer with joint pain, which he was told was from gout. He took medication for it, I remember, at least while I was living at home. I never heard anyone mention kidney stones."

An alcohol history is obtained. How much and how often does the patient consume alcohol? This is helpful generically, and in this case it also bears on the remote possibility of acute pancreatitis.

"Maybe once or twice a week, my wife and I will split a bottle of wine with dinner. And, I like a couple of beers after a softball game or a bike ride—probably adding up to a six-pack a week. No drugs and no butts, though—you doctors always ask those, too."

Now, the important review of systems questions may be focused as they relate to the systems potentially involved. Gastrointestinal: Has there been any nausea or vomiting (nonspecific for gastrointestinal disease, but placed here for convenience)? Diarrhea or constipation? Black, tarry stools or bloody stools? Change in appetite? Any history of suspected or diagnosed bowel disorder in the recent past? Each query is made individually.

The patient's answer to each of the questions is "no."

Specific inquiries relative to the renal-urinary system are made: Has there been a history of kidney or bladder infection? Renal stone? Blood in the urine? Frequency? Urgency? Incontinence? Fever or flank pain?

Again, the patient indicates that he has suffered none of the above symptoms.

Questions about sexual activity and function, i.e., possible exposure to sexually transmitted diseases, dysuria, or penile "drip" (discharge), are included despite the prior preemptive response, as is an inquiry about perineal pressure or low back pain that could point to possible prostatitis or epididymitis.

"My wife and I have both been monogamous for the 5 years of our marriage. I have never had any of those symptoms."

The above answers are recorded as pertinent negatives.

In the setting of this very acute onset of discrete abdominal, flank, and testicular pain in a man with a limited history of prior medical problems, further detailed questioning at this time will be nonproductive. After summarizing the history for the patient and asking for any additions or corrections in the story, the physical examination is conducted.

This particular background leads to hypotheses that direct the clinician to abdominal examination, since the vital signs have already been obtained. The abdomen is observed for distension, skin discoloration, or abnormal contour. The presence and nature of bowel sounds are determined by auscultation, and attention is paid to vascular sounds. Before percussion and palpation are undertaken, the patient is asked to indicate with a hand the precise location of the pain. The potentially uncomfortable modalities in a case of abdominal pain (touching, pressing, and tapping) begin in a remote quadrant. This sequence serves both kindness and diagnostic efficacy: The patient is kept comfortable as long as possible and responds favorably to considerate behavior. Moreover, the clinician avoids trying to obtain data from "neutral areas" in the presence of the involuntary tensing that would follow major discomfort. The clinician is wondering: Are there signs of peritoneal irritation or bowel obstruction? Are the kidneys enlarged or tender? Is there a palpable mass?

The examination of this patient's abdomen reveals normal contour and skin color, with a well-healed McBurney's incision (appendectomy) scar. The bowel sounds are normally active, and there are no bruits or rubs. Light palpation meets no resistance and does not intensify the pain. There is no rebound tenderness nor referred pain on deep palpation. In short, no peritoneal signs are present. Deep palpation yields only very slight additional discomfort in the right lower quadrant. There is no suprapubic tenderness. Neither kidney is palpable, and a nontender liver edge is barely felt at the costal margin. There is no suprapubic or flank tenderness and no tenderness to percussion of the costovertebral angles. The femoral pulses are full and symmetrical to palpation.

Because acute abdominal pain can result from genital pathology, a complete genital examination is required.

The scrotal contents are nontender and of normal size and consistency. Each testicle is mobile and in its proper position. The epididymides and cords are unremarkable. There are no penile lesions, and the urethra is nontender on palpation of the whole length of the penile shaft. There is no expressible urethral discharge.

A rectal examination is indicated in any presentation of abdominal pain, to examine the lower abdomen transrectally, to test stool for occult blood, and to seek intrinsic problems in the anorectum and prostate.

This patient's rectum contains scant, soft brown stool, and no masses are palpable. Occult-blood reaction is negative. The prostate gland is of normal shape, size, and consistency, without fluctuance, and is nontender.

The essentials of the focused medical history and physical examination have been completed. The initial hypotheses have been tested to the extent that this portion of the clinical bedside assessment allows.

With the information obtained from this problem-directed history and physical examination, rupture or obstruction of a hollow viscus may be excluded with confidence. Vascular occlusion as cause for the pain is eliminated because of the presence of normal pulses and normal bowel sounds, the absence of tenderness to abdominal palpation, and the lack of even microscopic blood in the stool. There is no evidence to support torsion of the testis, epididymitis, or orchitis. Intraperitoneal organs appear to be normal. The urinary tract remains the most likely organ system. The kidneys are hard to assess clinically but have been not implicated by anything uncovered. There is strong evidence against acute urethral pathology. Nothing points to the bladder. A ureteral stone would best explain the symptoms and the absence of abdominal signs. It is now time to turn to the laboratory for further exploration of this hypothesis.

The patient voids a stone with dramatic relief, providing diagnosis and resolution at the same time. Long-term workup and management will be entirely separate issues.

The problem-solving approach to a specific presenting complaint is the hallmark of experienced clinicians in practice. The masterful, case-specific use of the method is a goal of every serious student of physical diagnosis, from the early learner to the experienced practitioner. It is the cornerstone of both effective medical practice and the pleasure of the clinician in her work.

RECOMMENDED READINGS

Baldwin JG Jr. The healing touch. Am J Med 1986;80:1.

Block MR, Coulehan JL. Teaching the difficult interview in a required course on medical interviewing. J Med Educ 1987;62:35–40.

Fitzgerald FT, Tierney LM Jr. The bedside Sherlock Holmes. West J Med 1982;137:169–175.

Grady MJ. Teaching physical diagnosis in the nursing home. Am J Med 1990;88:519–521.

Hardison JE. Whatever happened to the chief complaint? JAMA 1981;245:1942.

Holbrook J, Schneiderman H. Honing physical diagnostic skills. Patient Care 1990;24:123–141.

Hooper PL, Hooper EM, Stehr DE. Guidelines for interviewing. Ann Intern Med 1981;95:238.

Lazare A. Shame and humiliation in the medical encounter. Arch Intern Med 1987;147:1653–1658.

MacKenzie TB. The initial patient interview: identifying when psychosocial factors are at work. Postgrad Med 1983;74:259–265.

Milhorn HT Jr. The genogram: a structured approach to the family history. J Miss State Med Assoc 1981;22:250–252.

Novack DH. Therapeutic aspects of the clinical encounter. J Gen Intern Med 1987;2:346–354.

Paton A, Saunders JB. ABC of alcohol: asking the right questions. Br Med J 1981;283:1458–1459.

Riegelman RK. The dogged physical examination in the era of the C.A.T. Primary Care 1980;7:625–635.

Schneiderman H. The review of systems. Postgrad Med 1982;71:151–158.

Steel K. History taking from elderly patients. Hosp Prac 1985;20(5A):70–71.

2

General Appearance and Vital Signs

APPROACH AND ANATOMICAL REVIEW
Introduction
GENERAL APPEARANCE

The **general appearance** of the patient provides tremendous help to the clinician, who may know within seconds in the clinical encounter that, for example, the patient is gravely ill. This part of the physical examination is often performed in passing, rather than being allocated a separate place in the examiner's routine. It is the least taught, least quantitatively studied portion and is commonly absent from case write-ups, all of which is a paradox considering its utility for functional assessment, for prognosis, and sometimes for specific diagnosis. This chapter gives the topic its full due.

VITAL SIGNS

The **vital signs** are pulse, respiration, temperature, and blood pressure. All should be measured in every complete examination and in many briefer encounters. They are *vital* because they constitute quantitative clinical measurements of enormous value. As with general appearance, they provide inestimable help in global assessment of a patient and can yield specific diagnoses such as hypertension. The irony about vital signs is not their *omission* but their *relegation* to the least educated and experienced members of the health care team. Considering the importance and uniqueness of these data, they deserve measurement by knowledgeable and senior persons. As a result of poor measurements, clinicians lose the insight gained from early awareness of, for example, tachypnea (rapid breathing). If physicians plan to remeasure selectively when readings by other personnel suggest a problem, they will systematically miss false-negative measurements.

Vital Statistics

Vital statistics, namely, **height and weight,** are used widely in clinical medicine. Weight varies somewhat from hour to hour in response to extracellular fluid volume status, whereas height changes over years or decades in adults. Neither is capable of the minute-to-minute changes that can be seen with the *vital signs.*

Anatomy and Physiology
PULSE

The **pulse** is a peripheral reflection of cardiac action and of the propagation of a wave from proximally (the aortic root) to distally. It is felt as an expansile upward-outward pressure at any of the points listed in Table 2.1. The pulse wave

Table 2.1
Principal Palpable Pulses in Most Healthy Adults,[a] from Head to Toe

Superficial temporal artery anterior to ear
Superior orbital artery, near 12 o'clock position on orbital rim[a]
Common carotid artery in mid to upper lateral neck
Subclavian artery behind junction of middle and medial thirds of clavicle[a]
Aortic arch inferoposterior to sternal notch[a]
Cardiac apex[a]
Brachial artery under biceps tendon
Radial artery at wrist
Ulnar artery[a]
Digital arteries on ulnar aspects of fingers, especially second, third, and fourth fingers at or
    about proximal interphalangeal joints[a]
Abdominal aorta in epigastrium or just below[a]
Femoral artery at inguinal ligament
Popliteal artery in popliteal fossa[a]
Dorsalis pedis artery at some point(s) between extensor retinaculum of foot and hallux-
    second toe interspace[a]
Posterior tibial artery, 1 fingerbreadth behind medial malleolus

[a]Indicates pulsation palpable only in about one-half of normal adults.

does not coincide with blood flow but propagates faster. It is perceptible during midsystole, while cardiac contraction and ejection of intracardiac blood are ongoing. The speed of pulse propagation falls in some diseases of heart, blood, or blood vessels but rises in others. Stiffening of the arterial wall with aging and atherosclerosis *accelerates* the pulse wave.

The *intensity* of the pulse relates both to characteristics of the blood vessel and to the *pulse pressure* (see below). Normal pulse rates in healthy adults range from 50 to 100 beats/minute.

RESPIRATION

Respiratory rate and pattern are controlled by chemosensors and the brain. For normal persons, increased blood concentrations of carbon dioxide and hydrogen ion stimulate an increase of ventilation, whereas hypoxemia does so less powerfully. A normal respiratory rate does *not* mean that oxygenation is adequate. Chronic obstructive pulmonary disease and narcotic drugs can impair both chemosensing and response. Anxiety speeds up respiration, as do other behavioral and psychologic stimuli. The examiner must beware of the *involuntary increased respiratory rate* often produced when a subject realizes that his respiration is under study. For this reason, counting of respiratory rate is surreptitious. Normal respiratory rate is 12–18/minute in adults.

TEMPERATURE

Mammalian enzyme systems operate best within a narrow temperature range. Human core body temperature therefore stays rather constant. Temperature homeostasis is achieved in an environment of wide temperature swings by thermoregulatory mechanisms including (*a*) thyroid thermogenesis to generate more heat, (*b*) peripheral vasoconstriction to conserve heat, (*c*) peripheral vasodilatation for cooling, and (*d*) sweating, which cools by water evaporation. Thus the internal temperature gradient between core and periphery must vary. Inconstancy relative to the key datum, **core temperature,** makes random measurement of **skin temperature** useless clinically.

Fever

Fever represents a resetting of core temperature in response to endogenous pyrogen or other factors. Fever seems to help rid the body of certain infections, and there is research evidence of superior antiviral action both in vivo and in vitro when the temperature rises from the mean physiologic level in humans of 37°C (98.6°F) to 38°C (100.4°F). This gain is achieved at the price of accelerated metabolism, increased work of the heart, and increased oxygen demand. In the absence of environmental cold, the sensation of a chill means that the thermal set point has risen and the body temperature has not yet caught up with it.

There are many gravely ill persons without fever and many febrile persons who are not very sick. Among the host of influences on body temperature besides infection are age, renal function, and metabolic state. The very old and the very young are more prone to accidental *hypo*thermia. Chronic renal failure blunts the febrile response. Hypothyroidism tends to down-set the thermostat, whereas hyperthyroidism may raise it.

BLOOD PRESSURE

Blood pressure (BP) is measured in **torr,** short for torricelli, the unit of pressure formerly known as millimeters of mercury. Since many measuring systems no longer use mercury, the change in terminology is appropriate, although almost no one specifies the unit of measurement. Normal blood pressure in most healthy adults ranges from 90/50 to 140/90.

The standard blood pressure cuff readings do not precisely match those obtained with intra-arterial measurements. However, conclusions about normality, disease, and change are consistent and reliable.

Pulse Pressure

The **pulse pressure** is the palpable force of pulsation. It relates not to the absolute value of the *systolic pressure (the higher number)* or of the *diastolic pressure (the lower number),* but to the **difference between the systolic and the diastolic pressure.** Thus with severe high blood pressure but a narrow pulse pressure, e.g., 190/150, the pulse could actually feel weaker than with a desperately low blood pressure of 60/0, because the pulse pressure is less. Normal pulse pressure in healthy adults ranges from 30 to 70 torr.

TECHNIQUE
GENERAL APPEARANCE

The general appearance is what one sees by looking directly at the patient or out of the corner of one's eye—literally and figuratively. The old dictum, "we see only what we know," applies to this component, as do common sense and the use of "nonclinical" life experiences. With increased formal experience and knowledge the examiner can gain more from looking, if skill has been cultivated.

OVERVIEW FUNCTION

A checklist of elements in the general appearance is inimical to its function as an *overview of the whole person,* not a detailed investigation of any particular system. With assessment of the general appearance at the outset of the clinical encounter or while taking the history, the clinician "looks for the forest, not the trees." Delineation of some "forest" issues is in order for the learner and practitioner of this art.

ACUITY OF ILLNESS

The first and most vital question is, "Is the patient acutely ill?" An appearance of severe acute illness, also called a *toxic* appearance, is rather insensitive for delineating acuity and flawed for delineating specificity. The patient may appear to be having *trouble breathing,* as manifested by gasping, noisy breathing, or striking rapid or deep breaths or by pausing for breath or losing voice during the interview. The *voice quality* can be identified at this point as normal, hoarse, gurgling, or whispered.

DEFORMITY AND LESIONS AT A GLANCE

Other general observations include skin color, major visible skin lesions, gross bodily deformities or injuries, and bruises. Gather an impression of *asymmetries* in face or body and of swelling in any body parts.

DISTRESS: PHYSICAL AND PSYCHIC

Look for evidence of pain (a grimace on the face, a hand or fist pressed against a part, or a body part kept unduly still) or of other discomfort. Sometimes a patient is clearly in agony, yet the clinician can't tell whether the source is *physical or psychologic.* For the general appearance, it is enough to observe and respond to the severity of the problem. Moaning, visible malaise, agitation, or "disconnection" from the examiner can all result from either physical symptoms or mental troubles.

MOBILITY: GLOBAL AND REGIONAL

Another critical component is *mobility* and *body position:* the patient lying stock still in bed presents a very different set of diagnostic possibilities from one who continually hops around the room. Watch, too, for any *focal limitation* or *absence of movement.*

NUTRITION AND HYDRATION

Next is a search for state of *hydration:* Does the patient look or feel bone dry? A look in the mouth may help, as may palpation of the axilla for sweat; orthostatic vital signs (in the section on the extended examination) further the search. At the same time, secure an impression of *nutritional state,* at least subdividing into a broad range of normal, malnourished and obese, with the terms *cachectic* and *morbidly obese* reserved for the far ends of the spectrum.

Developmental appropriateness is a related issue: Does the skinny, short adult look growth-retarded or just small?

SPECIAL ASPECTS OF GENERAL APPEARANCE

Although this subtitle may sound oxymoronic, it refers to two specific skills, diagnosis by smell and examination of material that is not part of the patient's body.

Olfactory Diagnosis

Olfactory diagnosis consists of paying attention to the sense of smell. *Odors,* such as the smell of urine on person or clothing, offer clues to mental, physical, or social dysfunction.

Extracorporeal Diagnosis

Good observers make diagnostic use not only of what they see of the patient's body but also of anything else that crosses the field of view, such as nicotine stains on the fingernails. Clothing, shoes, jewelry, and makeup can also be clues. Friends at the bedside have diagnostic meaning, and so does a stuffed toy clutched by an adult. A book of calculus on the bedside table suggests deep concentration or that the patient is putting on a show. A hospital room crammed with flowers and get-well cards bespeaks an emotional context quite different from that of a bare room. Chocolates on a diabetic's table may be for the grandson or may reveal noncompliance.

Body products. Bodily products and fluids can alert the attuned clinician, as well as the patient or family member. Bloody urine stains on underclothing or in the toilet bowl, or sputum that looks like pus, can change a diagnosis.

Vital Signs
PULSE

Pulses are palpable at many bodily sites (Table 2.1). The radial pulse is the one most commonly checked, but at times the carotid gives more information, and the apical is more likely to reflect every ventricular contraction.

Radial Pulse

The radial pulse is felt at the radial artery, on the radial aspect of the bone, 2–4 cm proximal to the crease of a wrist that has been extended but not hyperextended. The examiner has the patient remove any watch or bracelet in the vicinity and unbutton or roll up long sleeves. Then she curls the tips or anterior pads of her dominant index and middle fingers with light to moderate force against the radius, perpendicular to the long axis of the bone. If you don't feel a radial pulse, try the maneuvers in Table 2.2.

A common error of the learner is to seek the pulse on the inner (ulnar) aspect of the radius rather than on the radial or outer aspect. Every patient has cardiac action, and almost all have a radial pulse, except the desperately ill.

Carotid Pulse

If a radial pulse cannot be found, the carotid pulse is a backup. For this purpose, *gently* touch the Adam's apple (laryngeal cartilage) with the same two fingertips, then point them posterolaterally and move to the edge of the cartilage. Just beyond, and in a somewhat more posteriorly directed groove, a pulsation is felt. *Gentle* pressure is essential to avoid causing harm here, particularly in the aged.

Peripheral Pulse Characteristics

Once you have found a pulse at whatever site, "park" there to assess regularity, intensity, and character. Besides counting the pulse when you feel it, assess for regularity of both timing and force. Regularity is assessed in a timesaving fashion during a minute of the interview that is not too emotionally charged (Fig. 2.1). If irregularities are detected, however, you will want to concentrate on the pulse,

Table 2.2
Measures to Find the Radial Pulse

Try the other side
Try *passively* flexing the wrist a few degrees
Try moving a bit proximally
Move a bit distally
Lighten the pressure
Intensify the pressure if lightening the pressure fails

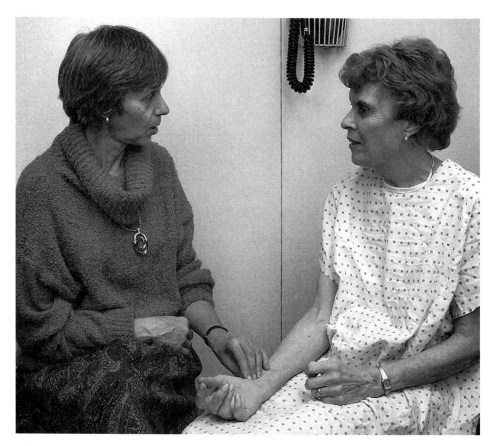

Figure 2.1   Pulse quality and regularity can often be assessed during the interview, typically with both parties seated and without breaking eye contact with the patient. This means that pulse *counting,* which requires looking at a stopwatch, is unsuitable for completion during the interview.

which requires repeating the maneuver free of the competing demands of history taking.

Measurement of Heart Rate

If the pulse is absolutely regular, count the number of pulsations in a 15-second period, multiply by 4, and you have the pulse rate, which is always expressed as beats per minute. Most normal adults have a regular pulse between 50 and 100 beats/minute. For this purpose, a watch with a sweep second hand is indispensable. There is no need for a fancy watch or stopwatch. Large legible numbers help, as do markings to indicate each second, and water resistance for hand washing.

If the pulse is irregular, i.e., the pulse speeds up slightly with inspiration and slows slightly with expiration, you may be observing sinus arrhythmia (see below). If there is any other irregularity in the pulse, including extra beats or skipped beats, count the pulse for 30 seconds and multiply by 2.

Apical Pulse

The heart's rate can be assessed directly by finding the apical pulse rate. This is done by auscultation. It calls for use of the stethoscope.

Stethoscope. The stethoscope consists of two earpieces, tubing, and one or more heads that are applied to the body of the patient. The earpieces fit perpendicularly into the examiner's ear canals or are directed slightly forward. If they are directed somewhat backward, then the stethoscope is on backwards and should be reversed. The earpieces should not be uncomfortable in your ears. If they cause discomfort or you remain aware of them for more than a few minutes, get new ones, or softer ones, or a different size. The earpieces should fill most of the external auditory meatus and block out much of the ambient "room" noise while you have them in. Many stethoscopes have two heads. The large flat one is the *diaphragm, and it picks up high-pitched (high-frequency) sounds.* The smaller hemispheric recessed one is the *bell.* When applied lightly to the skin, the bell transmits *low-pitched sounds.* When pressed firmly against the skin, the bell stretches the skin, converts the skin to a diaphragm, and then filters out low-pitched sounds and reveals only high-pitched sounds. The apical pulse consists principally of *high-frequency heart sound,* so it is logical to use the diaphragm. The bell may be used if pressed firmly.

Locale to auscultate for apical pulse. If the apical pulse is measured outside the context of the cardiac examination, the patient may be clothed but have the upper one or two shirt buttons opened. The stethoscope head is applied firmly at the second intercostal space, just to the left of the sternum. The second intercostal space is readily detected by sliding a finger *lightly* down the anterior midline from the jugular notch. Within a few centimeters a substantial bump is felt. The bump is the junction of the manubrium sterni and the corpus sterni. Called the **angle of Louis,** it is at the level of the second rib. Moving the finger leftward and down a centimeter or so leads to an area devoid of bone, bounded above by the second rib and its cartilage and below by the third. This **second left intercostal space at the left sternal border,** also known as the **pulmonic valve focus,** can be auscultated to determine the apical pulse with minimal intrusion on the modesty of the patient. (The apex of the heart is actually at the fifth intercostal space in the midclavicular line and is accessible in the patient who is disrobed for examination. However, this site is no more reliable than the second left intercostal space for counting the heart rate.)

RESPIRATORY RATE AND RHYTHM

Respiratory rate and rhythm are assessed without the patient's awareness in order to minimize the **Heisenberg effect,** whereby measurement alters the variable. The most reliable method is to walk behind the patient and observe the chest cage while out of the patient's view, under pretense of studying the skin of the back. Alternatively, leave the firmly applied bell of the stethoscope over the upper sternum (Fig. 2.2) or the diaphragm over any large airway with audible sound on each expiration, and count from there. Fifteen seconds is the usual duration of counting, and the number of breaths counted is multiplied by 4. Normal respiratory rates vary from 12 to 18/minute in healthy adults and a bit faster in healthy aged persons. Counting proceeds longer if there is marked irregularity or very slow breathing. If the stethoscope is pressed directly on the trachea, it may produce a choking sensation, which can stimulate more rapid or deeper breathing. Hence the trachea is not the place to park for this test.

TEMPERATURE

The attempted assessment of core body temperature by touching the body surface is both insensitive and nonspecific for detection of fever. Cutaneous temperature reflects blood flow as well as core temperature. To confirm this, feel the scalp of a healthy newborn baby and then of an adult. A substantial difference is apparent, yet core temperatures are the same—37°C for the healthy human, give or take 0.5°C. Feel your own forehead and then your feet after sitting barefoot for an hour. The inequality of peripheral temperatures will be striking despite what must be a unitary core temperature.

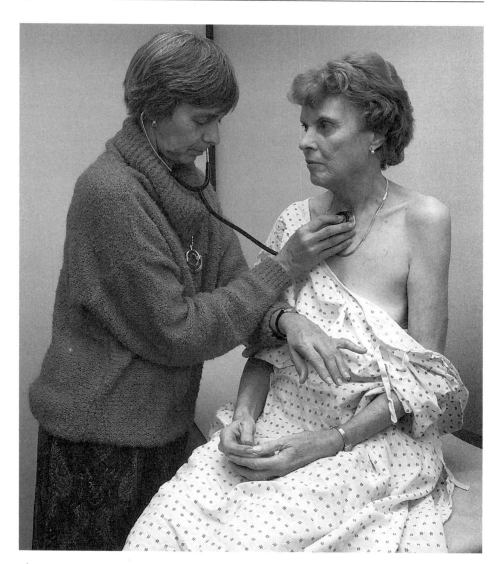

Figure 2.2 Respirations may be counted surreptitiously from the back or while auscultating a large airway and putatively concentrating on something else (heart or breath sounds, heart rate).

Instrumentation: Thermometers

We need to assess with an instrument and to sample an area reflective of the interior of the body. Thermometry, whether by *oral (blue-tipped) or rectal (red-tipped) instrument,* serves this need. The most difficult issue with a glass mercury thermometer is to turn it just right so that the silver-colored column within is magnified, opacifying the lumen to the left of the meniscus and leaving it transparent to the right. Inspect a thermometer that has not been used in a patient that day. It may record a temperature anywhere from 34.5°C (94°F) to 39°C (102.2°F). The reading usually far exceeds ambient air temperature. Thermometers have to be *shaken down* to 35°C (95°F) or below before use. This is done by *firmly* grasping at the end with the top of the temperature scale and offering a series of short sharp shakes. Centrifugal force moves the mercury column down, part of a degree with each shake. Once the reading is low enough, the procedure varies depending on thermometer type. All the instructions to follow are suitable for older children or adults. Small children can break the glass and be harmed, as can adults with abnormal involuntary movements and those prone to violent biting or rolling around. For them, alternative methods are preferred.

Oral thermometers. An oral thermometer is inserted bulb first (i.e., with the low-reading end) under the tongue, to lie nearly parallel to the floor of the mouth, with most of the instrument protruding between the lips. The lips are sealed around it, but the teeth are not clenched on it, to avoid breakage. After 4 minutes it is removed and inspected (*without* shaking down). The column should have risen from the baseline level. Even though the column height might remain stable longer, the temperature must be read at once after removal. If fever is suspected but not recorded, the thermometer can be returned to the mouth for another 3 minutes. Unfortunately, we don't know how long a thermometer needs to be left in place to record accurately the core temperature. Textbooks and package inserts vary widely, with some suggesting up to 7 minutes, which is impractical. After each use, the thermometer is cleaned according to manufacturer's directions.

Rectal thermometers. When a rectal thermometer is used, a *small* amount of Vaseline may be applied over the bulb (low-reading) end of the instrument and smeared about one-third of the way up the outside of the thermometer. Then the patient assumes a lateral decubitus position, preferably with the upper thigh flexed on the abdomen, the lower thigh extended, and the pelvis tilted toward the table. These maneuvers ease visualization of the anus. Now the clinician, wearing plastic gloves, retracts the buttocks from the anus. The thermometer is *never* to be inserted except under direct vision. The tip is placed at the anal verge for a second or two. A brief involuntary anal spasm may occur and will then ease. The thermometer is gently inserted some 4 cm, in a direction *aimed at the patient's navel,* and is left in this position for 4 minutes. Thereafter, the procedure is completed just as explained for oral thermometry above.

Sources of false readings. It is most important to know common sources of error in thermometry. Rapid breathing lowers oral temperatures, as does mouth breathing, which is common in general and commoner still if the nose is stuffed. The drinking of hot liquids (including soup) can produce false elevations, and conversely, cold liquids can lower the reading compared with core temperature. Ideally, the patient should neither eat nor drink for half an hour before an oral temperature is taken. If there is any suspicion of intentional falsification of temperature, continuous observation during measurement is essential. Rectal thermometry avoids many of these pitfalls but has its own, including *very rarely* laceration of the rectum. *Gentleness* is the essential attribute to prevent this. Rectal temperatures are normally about 0.5°C higher than oral temperatures. Many specialists define fever as a rectal temperature of 37.8°C (100°F) or more.

Other thermometers. *Axillary* temperatures are sometimes taken in the uncooperative patient. The thermometer is placed vertically or horizontally on the chest wall, and the ipsilateral arm is adducted and immobilized to cover the thermometer for 4 minutes. Axillary readings often run 0.5°C *below* oral measurements. They are less accurate than either oral or rectal ones.

Electronic thermometers require a shorter period for each measurement. Many employ a disposable sheath that reduces cleaning work. Most are sublingual, with liquid-crystal numeric displays. Electronic thermometers have been shown to take particularly inaccurate axillary temperatures.

Ear probes, relying on still different methodology, are used in many offices and emergency departments. They work rapidly but may be distressing and, if the patient has otitis or a perforated eardrum, should probably be avoided.

BLOOD PRESSURE

The taking of a blood pressure with a sphygmomanometer is a complex orchestration. As illustrated in Figure 2.3, the test employs three senses—sight to inspect the gauge, hearing for special Korotkoff sounds (see below), and touch for localization of the brachial artery pulse. One hand supports the patient's arm while the other inflates and deflates the cuff, and two instruments are used at once—the stethoscope and the sphygmomanometer. Each of these elements is addressed in turn.

Instrumentation

The **sphygmomanometer** is an instrument used to apply controlled pressure to the limb and thus to the artery within it (Figs. 2.4 and 2.5). It consists of a bulb connected to rubber tubing (*T*). The tubing is attached to a bladder enclosed by a cuff (*C*). The tubing goes to a manometer or gauge. The cuff and bladder encircle the limb. There is usually Velcro or other fastening material to facilitate closing the circle around the arm. When the pressure in the bladder is raised, the gauge displays this pressure. Because of poorly understood acoustic phenomena, sounds (**Korotkoff sounds**) are heard when a stethoscope is applied to an artery distal to the bladder and cuff when blood flow to that artery is restricted to systole. This takes place when the pressure applied by the bladder exceeds the diastolic blood pressure in the artery but lies below the systolic pressure in the artery (Fig. 2.6). The pressure in the instrument is raised high at the outset (see below) and then *slowly* lowered with the release valve (*R*) until Korotkoff sounds are heard, marking the systolic blood pressure (SBP). With further slow release,

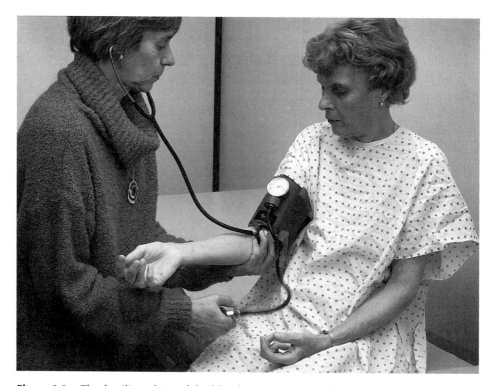

Figure 2.3   The familiar taking of the blood pressure is actually a very complex orchestration of eyes, ears, both hands, and two instruments. The examiner depicted will actually obtain a slight spurious elevation compared with the true intra-arterial pressure. Why? (Review the answer printed at the end of this chapter.)

sounds continue to be heard with each cardiac cycle. Eventually, a point is reached at which the sounds muffle or disappear permanently. One of these latter two levels is the diastolic blood pressure.

Sources of error. An immense array of variables impacts on the accuracy of this measurement. Instrument specifications vary from one model and manufacturer to another. Statements herein apply to many popular brands. Variations and correctives are found in the very useful booklet of the American Heart Association (AHA), *Recommendations for Human Blood Pressure Determination by Sphygmomanometers* (1987), which belongs in every clinician's library.

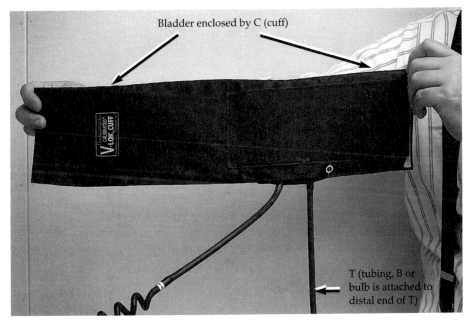

Figure 2.4 Front of cuff of popular sphygmomanometer.

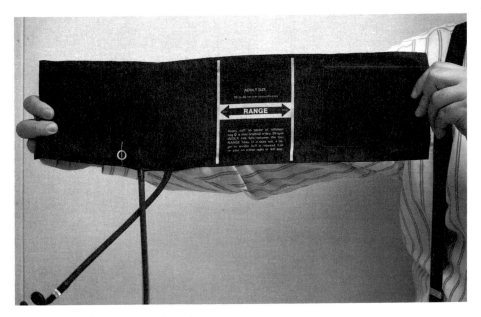

Figure 2.5 Back side of popular sphygmomanometer.

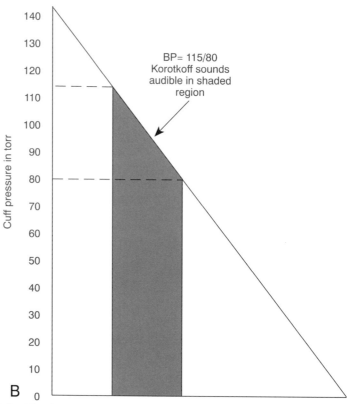

Figure 2.6   If the blood pressure is 115/80, as the cuff is slowly deflated from a starting pressure of 140 torr, Korotkoff sounds are audible, as illustrated, only from the level of 115 to that of 80 and not below or above this level.

Handling the cuff. A common concern is whether to wrap the cuff clockwise or counterclockwise (Figs. 2.7 and 2.8). Erroneous wrapping will cause the cuff to inflate poorly and eventually pop off rather than apply pressure inwardly on the artery. This difficulty is avoided by those sphygmomanometers that have an aneroid manometer attached directly to the outer surface of the cuff. If the gauge is in view, such a cuff has been applied correctly (see Fig. 2.10).

Details of technique. Preparation of the patient includes removal of any garment that covers or constricts the upper arm and having the patient, if possible, *sit quietly* in a room with comfortable ambient temperature for 5 minutes. Then the **brachial pulse** is palpated. This pulse is tricky to find (Fig. 2.9). It is located **just proximal to** (up the arm from) **the antecubital fossa.** In many persons it seems faint or absent. For these persons, the biceps tendon and the most distal portion of the biceps muscle must be pushed or retracted laterally, and the palpating fingertip must be slid a bit laterally under the site to find the pulse. After the pulse has been located, the sphygmomanometer is applied so that the distal edge of the cuff lies 1.5 cm proximal to the pulse. If the cuff has a dial on it, this must be out of the way but within sight. The release valve is locked closed. The *radial* pulse—or, less commonly, the brachial pulse—is then palpated continuously while the cuff is inflated at a moderate pace by squeezing the bulb.

Problems and solutions. If the pressure on the dial refuses to rise even after eight squeezes on the bulb, one of three problems is likely. The valve may have been left open and should be closed by screwing it down clockwise as far as can

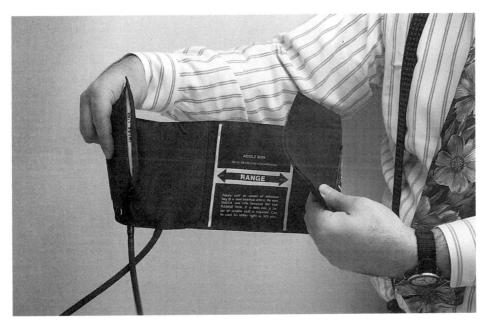

Figure 2.7 One direction of wrapping the cuff around the patient's arm.

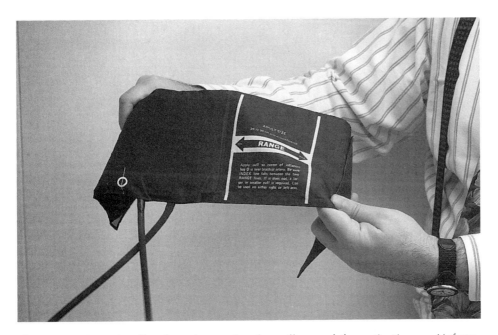

Figure 2.8 Opposite direction of wrapping the cuff around the patient's arm. Unfortunately, manufacturers have imposed no uniformity, so the correct direction with one instrument will be wrong with another.

be done comfortably. If the valve is *leaky*, there will be a transient rise in dial reading after each squeeze followed by a decline, often with some hissing as air escapes the system. Finally, if the cuff has been placed on backwards (inside out), the pressure will rise poorly or not at all, and the bladder will expand grotesquely (Figs. 2.10 and 2.11), making a balloon-like enlargement of the cuff that will pull open the Velcro attachments.

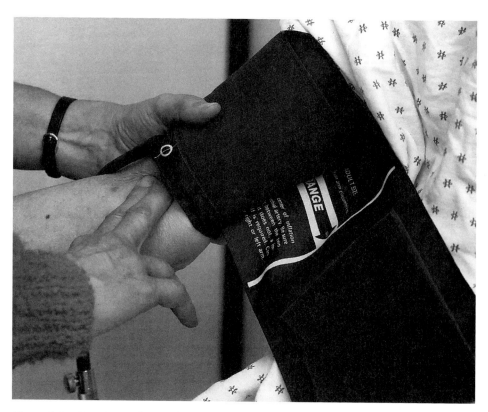

Figure 2.9   Examiner palpates the brachial pulse before applying the cuff to the arm, slipping the fingers proximal to the edge of the cuff. The "artery marker" on the cuff is to overlie the proximal end of the pulsation. More importantly, the stethoscope must be applied just distal to this point, i.e., just beyond the bottom of the cuff.

Systolic and diastolic pressure detection. The pulsation will become faint, then impalpable, as the dial reading rises. This is the SBP or very close to it. If the valve is opened *a little* at this point, the pressure will drop at a controlled rate. A fall of 3 torr/second is ideal. Soon the pulsation becomes palpable again, confirming that the pressure in the cuff has fallen below the SBP. Blood flow through the segments under the cuff and beyond has resumed, thus restoring propagation of the pulse wave. Now you have an estimation of SBP by palpation. Deflate the cuff completely and wait 15 seconds. Utilize this time to place the diaphragm of the stethoscope directly on the *brachial* pulse site. Then close the valve tightly and reinflate to 20 torr above the point where the radial pulsation disappeared. Start listening through the stethoscope. Now open the valve a bit, so that the pressure drops by 3 torr/second or 10 torr every 3 seconds. Within a few seconds, a faint tapping will be heard. The first point at which you hear this Korotkoff sound is the SBP. The intensity of the Korotkoff sounds will increase either gradually or abruptly as the cuff pressure falls, then will continue at a loud level.

As the pressure falls further, the sounds become abruptly muffled, defining phase IV, and then disappear, defining phase V in the blood pressure measurement. In adults, phase V is the diastolic blood pressure.

Further pointers on optimizing technique. Most clinicians find the diaphragm easier to use routinely for blood pressure checks, even though some experts recommend the trickier bell.

Besides correct cuff placement (Fig. 2.10), accurate measurement requires that the site assessed be at *heart level* in order to avoid gravitational artifact. The limb

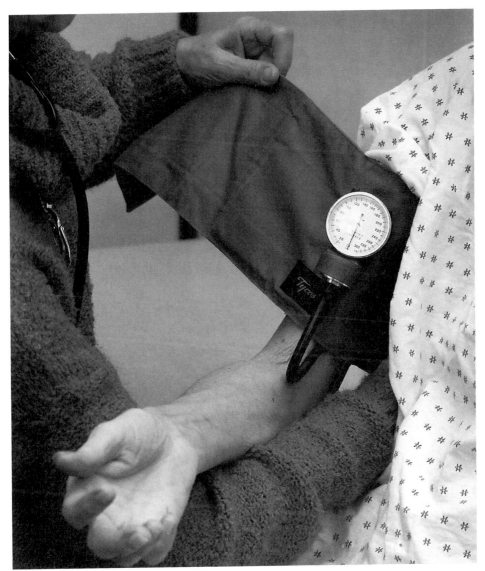

Figure 2.10 With this model of cuff, the presence of the gauge on the outside ensures correct placement and precludes what occurs in the next figure

must be *passively* supported to avoid artifactual elevation from muscular contraction. The patient has to stay still, because movements will cause errors. The cuff must be the right size with a bladder *length* at least 80% of arm circumference. Smaller cuffs often overestimate blood pressure, resulting in *spurious hypertension of the obese,* and larger cuffs may underestimate the pressure. The examiner has to have adequate hearing to perceive Korotkoff sounds and good enough vision to assess the dial of an aneroid model or the height of the meniscus on a mercury instrument at some distance if it is wall mounted (Fig. 2.13).

Vital Statistics

Weight. Standard clinical scales are used to measure the patient's weight. The weight quantifies the impression of state of nutrition and development at which the examiner has made a first pass during assessment of the general appearance. It also may *alter* this impression. Research has shown various sys-

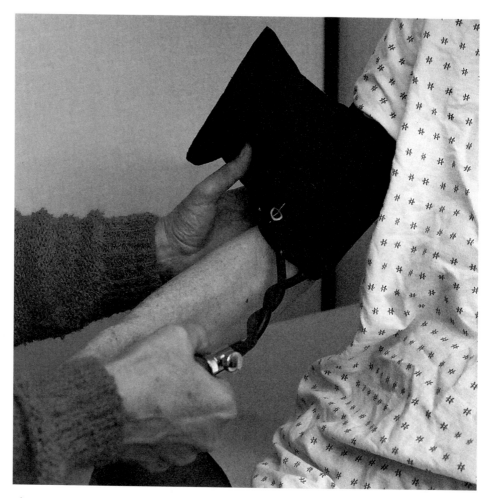

Figure 2.11   On inflation, this misapplied and tangled device puffs up rather than increasing the pressure exerted on the artery. Everybody is embarrassed, and no useful data emerge.

tematic biases in global assessment of obesity, malnutrition, and normality. Quantitative measurement permits detection of trends and changes too subtle to be assessed from general appearance.

Height. In adults, total height can be estimated by general appearance. Quantitative measurement using the instrument mounted on a scale is useful. Besides endocrine and developmental disorders associated with short stature, reduced stature is usually a functional correlate of loss of vertebral bone height resulting from osteopenic anterior vertebral compression fractures.

NORMAL AND COMMON VARIANTS
General Appearance
TOXIC APPEARANCE

The full-blown toxic appearance is of a flushed, hypervigilant, sweating, febrile patient whose pulse is rapid and thready and who is somewhat hungry for air. This appearance can be seen not only in bacterial *septicemia*, where it is most familiar, but in a host of other conditions, e.g., psychotic decompensation, adverse drug reactions including some salicylate intoxications, thyroid storm,

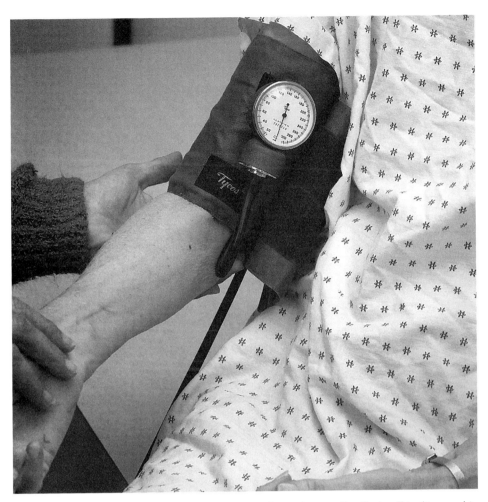

Figure 2.12   The examiner has the cuff on properly, with a small tail of cuff trailing, and is about to straighten the patient's elbow, and to support the cuff at heart level, to optimize the quality of data obtained.

other acute infections, and after severe environmental stress such as heat stroke. Although some patients may be terribly ill without these features, any patient with this appearance needs immediate diagnostic and therapeutic measures.

LOOKING OLDER THAN STATED AGE

The patient who appears *substantially* older than his stated age may have a mis-recorded or misreported birth year, i.e., may be as old as he looks rather than as old as he (or his chart) says he is. In our youth-worshiping society, some persons intentionally edge their birth year forward. If this is not the case, excessive skin wrinkling, thinning, and aging most commonly result from *cigarette smoking* and from *unprotected sun exposure*. Patients who are very *underweight* can look older than they are, although mild underweight is sometimes associated with a youth-ful look. Those who have had severe or incapacitating *chronic illness* often look prematurely old. This assessment may, in part, reflect a misinterpretation of face and posture suggesting physical and psychic *weariness*, neither of which always accompanies aging. Persons with widespread vascular disease may be judged to look older than they are, often because of an implicit sense that, for instance, a man who has had a heart attack and a leg amputation for gangrene is epidemio-

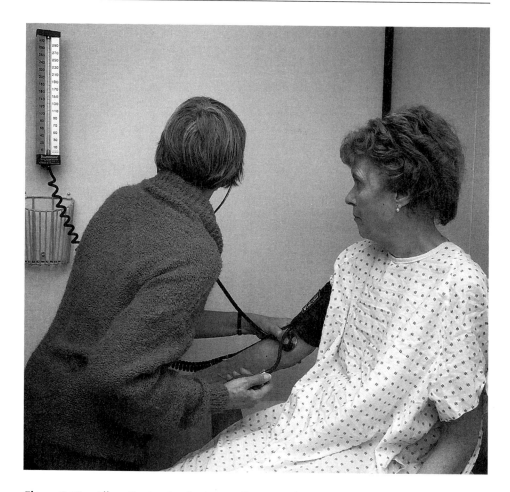

Figure 2.13   All parties tend to look at wall-mounted units, although the patient obviously can only guess at the pressure in the absence of hearing Korotkoff sounds. Patients usually take enormous comfort in having the blood pressure measured.

logically more likely to be 74 than 44. **Progeria** is an extreme rarity in which biologic aging outpaces chronologic age.

LOOKING YOUNGER THAN STATED AGE

Intentional misreport or error is likely when a patient appears unexpectedly youthful. Cosmetics can play a role, including wrinkle-reducing agents such as topical retinoids, collagen injections, and cosmetic surgery to hide the honorable physical signs of aging.

Reduction of facial skin wrinkling plays a role in the few medical disorders associated with youthful appearance. Among these are obesity, which tends to flatten out wrinkles; local facial edema; systemic sclerosis (scleroderma); and leprosy, apparently from expansion of the dermis. Sometimes, systemic corticosteroid therapy reduces wrinkling. *Persistent adolescent-like appearance* is seen in some patients with anorexia nervosa, in immunosuppressed persons such as organ-transplant recipients (Gary Coleman being a public figure so affected), and in persons with endocrine disorders of developmental arrest or retardation.

CHRONIC VERSUS ACUTE ILLNESS

The chronically ill lack toxic features, except for those with superimposed acute illness. *Listlessness* may be part of either acute or chronic illness, whereas *flushing* suggests acuity. Prototypes from everyday life include the patient in the first or second day of a bad "flu" who looks acutely ill and somewhat toxic. As the symptoms recede and the person looks "washed out" before recovering fully, the appearance mimics that of chronic illness—even to reactive psychologic depression.

APPREHENSION AND AGITATION

Apprehension and agitation indicate psychologic reactions to physical or mental stimuli and reflect not only the intensity of the stimuli but also the coping style of the host. A visibly upset, anxious person may have pain, great mental anguish, both, *or neither*. A calm demeanor, on the other hand, does not exclude massive intrapsychic or physical stress.

PALLOR

Although often cited as a prime feature in general appearance, pallor as a sign has only fair positive predictive value for anemia and no useful negative predictive value. Research has produced a listing of elements that can mask or mimic "anemic" pallor; emotional upset ranks high. Pallor has little utility in determining acuity of illness, notwithstanding being frequently adduced in this regard. The logical connector between pallor and acuity, cutaneous vasoconstriction from catecholamine release, is clearly not the whole story.

HABITUS

Obesity is familiar to all in industrialized countries, where the prevalence may exceed a quarter of the adult population. *Morbid obesity* is defined as a weight more than 100% above ideal and is suspected in anybody whose size stands out from the pot-bellied crowd. The importance of this diagnosis is its medical and prognostic implication. Abnormal *thinness* is more difficult to define, since societal standards advocate an extreme below the level associated with optimal group health; this is most clearly embodied in the phrase from a popular advertisement, "You can never be too rich or too thin." Deaths from self-starvation in anorexia nervosa testify to the falseness of this ideal. Sunken cheeks are now fashionable, and visible ribs have become an emblem not of need but of fashion. If malnourishment comes to mind when assessing the general appearance, follow-up is called for. Unfortunately, many self-starvers also binge, and their net weight and general appearance may be deceptively normal.

IMMOBILITY

Immobility may be *voluntary* or *involuntary, local* or *generalized, partial* or *absolute, painless* or *painful.* Reduced movement is common but not inevitable with abdominal pain in acute peritonitis. The patient who arises easily from a chair, walks over and shakes the examiner's hand, but braces his leg only while seated has good mobility. The malingerer may give away his cover-up in just such a fashion.

RESPIRATORY DISTRESS

The observation of labored or unduly deep breathing on general appearance has two implications. *Etiologically,* it suggests cardiac dysfunction, respiratory disease, acidosis, or some mixture of anxiety and panic. *Therapeutically,* it mandates rapid assessment and intervention, since some causes rapidly progress to death. More subtle respiratory distress is only detected by counting respiratory rate or by other means.

SPECIAL COMPONENTS OF THE GENERAL APPEARANCE
Olfactory Diagnosis

The commonest cause of *offensive body odor* is failure to wash either one's self or one's clothing. *Incontinence and caregiver neglect* amplify the problem and usually add a smell of urine or even feces to that of stale sweat. Acromegaly, hyperhidrosis, and the disturbed sweating of hidradenitis suppurativa can cause strong body odors despite frequent washing and hygiene. A *urinary odor* is common with poor care and in such context cannot be taken as evidence of urinary incontinence. If the body and clothing do *not* have this odor but the breath does, the question of *uremia* arises. Tiny beads of white matter—crystallized urea—on the skin over sweat glands will support this impression.

The odors of *alcohol* and *tobacco* on the breath or person offer important correctives when a patient has lied about using these. Cigarette smell may cling after passive exposure, but given the toxicity of passive smoking, noting such an odor, even in a nonsmoker, can be of help.

Foul breath (halitosis) usually means poor oral hygiene producing marked anaerobic infection of the gingiva. Other causes are decomposing foreign bodies such as an inhaled pea or, rarely, intrapulmonary suppurative infection *with necrosis.*

Extracorporeal Diagnosis

Outlandish attire, hypersexual costumes, and worn-out and ill-fitting clothes all suggest particular social environs, *depending on local group norms,* as well as possible financial or medical issues. Shoes are the most medically illuminating garb. A shoe that is worn down on one side (lateral or medial) is typical of abnormal stance or gait, whereas wear on one shoe of a pair is seen when a limb is "favored" either with an *antalgic* gait resulting from pain or because of reduced range of motion, absent proprioception, or decreased power.

Tinted spectacles (sunglasses, "shades") worn indoors have been cited as bespeaking mental disorders, but research has not borne this out. Clearly, thresholds for this adornment as for others vary within populations.

Body products. *Effluvia* offer opportunities for diagnosis. *Very dark urine* is seen with maximal tubular concentration in depletion of extracellular fluid volume, as well as with obstructive jaundice and other conditions. Visible *fresh blood in the stool* is an extracorporeal feature recognized by everybody.

Vital Signs

Marked deviation of any vital sign from normal range calls for prompt assessment and, often, intervention. Unfortunately, the opposite is not true: normal vital signs ensure neither health nor the absence of acute disease.

PULSE
A Variant of Normal

Sinus arrhythmia is a physiologic (normal) phenomenon in which the pulse speeds up (accelerates) on inspiration and decelerates on expiration. Often most prominent in healthy children and young adults, this should not be confused with dysrhythmia. It also should not be confused with variation in pulse *amplitude* through the respiratory cycle, a phenomenon known as pulsus paradoxus that is characterized under Vital Signs in the section entitled Conducting the Extended Examination.

Rapidity

Sinus tachycardia refers to a regular heart rate over 100 beats/minute in an adult. Its causes are legion and include fever, exercise, intravascular volume depletion, cardiac disease of any type, anxiety, and any physical or psychologic strain.

Irregularity

Extra beats feel as though they have come too soon after the preceding beat. Often, they are followed by a compensatory pause that is longer than a normal cardiac cycle. Extra beats are common, and associated compensatory pauses cause the sensation of *skipped heartbeats,* of which the patient is usually aware even if the premature contraction itself was asymptomatic. The commonest causes of extra beats are premature atrial contractions (PACs) and premature ventricular contractions (PVCs), both of which may occur in normal persons, particularly those with bradycardia (see below), as well as in various cardiac and metabolic disturbances. The cardiac chamber of origin of a premature contraction cannot be determined by pulse palpation. The chief diagnostic difficulty lies in the case of very frequent premature contractions, which may mimic an absolute irregularity. If every other beat is premature, the condition is called **bigeminy,** and it may be difficult to distinguish from something called pulsus alternans (see under Vital Signs in the section entitled Conducting the Extended Examination).

Irregularity in pulse rate (and sometimes in force of the pulse) is classified into *regularly recurring irregularity,* as when every fourth beat is dropped, and *absolute irregularity,* as in the *irregularly irregular pulse of atrial fibrillation.* Regular irregularity is seen with **trigeminy** and with Mobitz type I (Wenckebach) second-degree atrioventricular block. A regular background on which are superimposed numerous premature contractions may seem absolutely irregular. In atrial fibrillation, the stroke volume and pulse pressure are usually larger after longer pauses, so that the pulse feels fuller ("stronger") on beats that are long in coming.

Slowness

A regular pulse under 50 beats/minute is **sinus bradycardia** and is normal in trained athletes. A slow regular pulse is also produced with a lower intrinsic pacemaker, for example, in idioventricular rhythm ("slow ventricular tachycardia"). It is common in intrinsic disease of the conduction system, such as sick sinus syndrome. Frequently, medications slow the heart rate to this level. *Digoxin* and related compounds can be responsible, as can β-*blocking agents.*

Intensity

With regard to pulse *force,* a *wide pulse pressure* as appreciated by pulse palpation (or confirmed by sphygmomanometry) is commonest with inelastic atherosclerotic vessels and a high systolic but normal diastolic pressure. It is also common with *increased cardiac output* as is seen in anemia, thyrotoxicosis, and pregnancy. Finally, it is seen in states with unduly low diastolic blood pressure, classically in severe aortic valve insufficiency.

An apparently *narrow pulse pressure* is seen when the systolic pressure is selectively reduced. Atherosclerotic peripheral vascular disease is one cause, and severe aortic valvular stenosis is another. States of low cardiac output such as end-stage heart failure offer another setting.

RESPIRATION

Rapidity

Tachypnea refers to unduly rapid breathing, usually 22 breaths/minute or more, without reference to depth of respiration. Tachypnea with shallow breaths is characteristic of pain. Tachypnea with breaths of any depth may be seen with anxiety and in most forms of cardiac disease. In respiratory disease, tachypnea may be a hallmark of stiff lungs, but as adequacy of gas exchange falls, tachypnea will develop even in lung disorders not characterized by stiffness. **Acidosis** causes tachypnea *even in the setting of normal cardiac and respiratory function.* The last is an important differential diagnosis to bear in mind when physical findings in the chest seem normal despite tachypnea. (Others include anxiety and *Pneumocystis carinii* pneumonia.) **Kussmaul breaths** are excessive in depth as well as rapid and are the classical pattern in diabetic ketoacidosis and other acidemias.

Excess Depth

Hyperpnea is unduly prominent breathing, usually both deep and rapid as in Kussmaul breathing but at times limited to excessive depth with normal rate. This pattern may occur in most of the settings mentioned above and is sometimes seen during recovery from "oxygen debt" after strenuous activity, as well as in *panic attacks* and other anxiety states.

Periods without Breaths

Apnea is failure to draw a breath for a period of perhaps 20 seconds or more while awake or 30 seconds while asleep. Short periods of apnea may occur in normal adults during sleep and perhaps in extreme old age. Apnea in neurologic disorders and sleep disorders has great significance, and even a 10-second waking period without a breath should prompt attention. The corresponding figure for duration of apnea in sleep is obscure. Depending on context, apneic periods may be anything from innocuous to grave.

Slowness

Bradypnea is unduly slow breathing, 10 breaths/minute or less. It is seen in persons with slowed metabolism, after overdoses of street drugs and prescription medicines that suppress respiratory drive, e.g., heroin, morphine, and as a physiologic adaptation in obstructive airway disease, both asthma and chronic bronchitis with emphysema. With reduced airflow, slowing the breaths per minute lowers the work of breathing and promotes more effective gas exchange—to a point.

TEMPERATURE

Fever

Fever has neither high sensitivity nor good specificity for infection. Many local infections such as skin abscess and viral gastroenteritis seldom produce fever, nor do some systemic infections, particularly in the very old or in those with renal insufficiency. Even bacterial endocarditis, the prototype of life-threatening infection, may be associated with normal body temperature.

Infection. Nevertheless, fever may be a useful marker. It occurs commonly in a host of infectious disorders ranging from the trivial common cold to fatal meningitis. It can also be a persistent "thermostat resetting" after prolonged febrile illness, the other manifestations of which have cleared. (A recommendation for families troubled by persistent fever in this setting is to stop measuring the temperature!) Such cases account for some of the "febricula" ("little fever") category in older studies, i.e., patients with persistently elevated body temperature, usually of low grade (38°C or less) and no cause demonstrable on study and long-term observation.

Noninfectious causes. The list of noninfectious causes associated with fever is immense. *Ovulation* is one, along with the *luteal phase* of the menstrual cycle and *pregnancy.* Although recording of daily temperatures with a vaginal thermometer has been used for ovulation monitoring, utilizing a 1° rise from baseline as an indicator, this method is unreliable regardless of the site or method of thermometry. *Drug effects, environmental warming, and thyroid storm* are among the other noninfectious causes of fever. To this list some persons would add *psychologic stress, dehydration* (intravascular volume depletion), and *fecal impaction,* although evidence for these is not conclusive.

Iatrogenic fever. Iatrogenic fever is common. Antimuscarinic (anticholinergic) drugs such as the tricyclic antidepressants decrease sweating and can produce fever and even heat stroke. Nearly half of patients develop fever *even without infection* after major surgery, perhaps in response to release of tissue constituents into the bloodstream. Akin to the luteal phase temperature rise, exogenous *progesterone* may elevate the temperature. Many biologic therapeutics also cause fever, whether from impurities that stimulate pyrogen release or as an intrinsic pharmacologic property. *Interleukin*-2 and *interferon*-α can both produce fever.

Hypothermia

A temperature below 35°C (95°F) defines hypothermia. To make this diagnosis, the thermometer scale must extend low enough, and the examiner must shake down the instrument as described above, or the measurement will overrepresent core temperature. Finally, the examiner must interpret the low reading as accurate, not as an instrument malfunction. Hypothermia can result from environmental heat deprivation in *accidental hypothermia.* The aged are particularly prone to this condition, which occurs not only on mountainsides and outdoors on skid row but also in underheated homes, particularly when drafty or with broken windows. *Vasodilating drugs* may also cause excessive heat loss. Diminished thermogenesis in *hypothyroidism* lowers body temperature. Most ominously, hypothermia resulting from septicemia augurs a very high mortality rate.

BLOOD PRESSURE

Normality

The normal range of blood pressure in the adult is alluded to above but cannot be conclusively defined. Some healthy small women have blood pressures that constantly run as low as 80/50. Blood pressure is dynamic from minute to minute and across a wide range of values in any individual, healthy or not. Continuous 24-hour ambulatory blood pressure monitoring has shown that in normal people the sleeping blood pressure often falls below a level ordinarily associated with clinical shock without adverse effect. At the other end of the scale, with intense activity and emotion—prototypically during orgasm—a normal person may transiently have a blood pressure exceeding 200/120. Independent of physical activity, there are diurnal and circadian variations, some perhaps relating to the release of cortisol or vasoactive substances. Emotion exerts a substantial influence, as does any stimulus to release of catecholamines. There are also characteristic patterns of change postprandially. Diseases and medicines may exaggerate, inhibit, obliterate, or have no effect at all on variations.

Hypertension

Hypertension in adults is defined as blood pressure consistently over 140/90 on three readings taken a week or more apart. To be diagnostic, the blood pressure must be taken with appropriate timing and technique to avoid artifactual or transient elevation from, for example, a cold room or mental anguish. Elevation of either component (systolic or diastolic) justifies the diagnosis. When only the SBP is elevated, e.g., 160/85, it is known as *isolated systolic hypertension*. Isolated *diastolic* hypertension is very rare. The more typical scenario is elevation of both systolic and diastolic. Patients and families often react with panic to any hypertensive value, and they need to know that the pressure over months to years is what matters, not today's or next week's, unless it is extreme.

Hypotension

An unintended drop of 40 torr from previous readings is hypotensive, but so are many other values. A syndrome of the extreme is **shock.** This syndrome consists of low blood pressure along with acute illness, often with features of reactive catecholamine release, i.e., cold, clammy, sweaty limbs with pallor, marked tachycardia, and altered mental status.

Comparison with previous blood pressure readings is important in establishing an individual's pattern. Someone who has had a blood pressure of 130/85 on each of six prior visits and who now shows 100/60 is hypotensive relative to baseline. The same pressure found every week in another patient is not. True hypotension needs to be managed promptly. The commonest causes are intravascular volume depletion (hypovolemia), hemorrhage, overuse of antihypertensive medicines and the adverse effects of all types of medicines, cardiac disease, adrenal insufficiency, and excessive vasodilation as in heat stroke and septic shock.

RECORDING THE FINDINGS
Pitfalls

There are four pitfalls to avoid:

1. Don't write "afebrile," since this does not distinguish normal temperature from hypothermia. A quantitative datum has been generated. Recording it requires less ink than writing out a qualifier that applies to the dead as well as the quick!
2. Don't use the cliché, "Well-developed, well-nourished white male in no acute distress." Make the record of the general appearance provide meaningful first-pass information about the patient's global health and individual characteristics. Describe this clearly enough so that the reader could pick out the patient from others in the ward.
3. Don't provide a *conclusion* in place of data. Least of all, don't record unsupported conclusions. Often an admission physical examination will say "VSS (vital signs stable)." This statement is usually wrong. How narrow a limit exists? Is a pulse that increases from 70 to 79 beats/minute stable, and is it unstable at 80? This statement misses the opportunity to share data and to leave conclusions where they belong, in the assessment. And it is often ludicrous. If recent prior measurements are not extant, how can first data be *stable?*
4. Don't feel impelled to include race. Unless germane to the medical issues, it is inappropriate.

Sample Write-up

General appearance: Ms. S. is a warmly conversational, aged woman who appears a bit younger than her stated 88 years. Overtly concerned about her leg ulcer but not fixated, and evinces no pain as she moves spryly from waiting room to chair to examining table. Quite thin, well hydrated, neatly dressed in worn but clean clothing and sneakers; sports immense earrings.

Vital signs:
Pulse, 68/minute and regular
Respirations, 14 and unlabored
Temperature, 36.2°C PO
BP, 102/58 right arm sitting

Vital statistics:
Weight, 46 kg
Height, 132 cm

Impression: Basically healthy, aged woman, with stable low weight and BP. Leg ulcer has not hampered gait, general function, cognition, affect, GA or vital signs.

EXTENDED EXAMINATION FOR GENERAL APPEARANCE AND VITAL SIGNS

INDICATIONS

The concept of an extended examination applies less here than to an anatomic region or body system. Every full physical examination calls for a check of pulse, respirations, temperature, and blood pressure. These are also checked at least daily, and often more frequently, in every acute-hospital patient. Many situations call for *frequent monitoring* of vital signs. Special bedside investigations of general appearance and each vital sign are called for in diverse situations.

Acute Illness, Baseline, and Long-term Trends

In monitoring acute problems and highly unstable situations, the vital signs are measured very frequently. No study has ever defined how much monitoring is enough for any given situation. At the other end of the scale of acuity, many thousands of nursing home residents have vital signs measured once monthly, but there is no research demonstrating whether this produces earlier or better diagnosis, let alone superior outcome. Vital signs are often taken unnecessarily, as well as omitted inappropriately.

Cardiorespiratory Disease

The pulse, respiratory rate, and blood pressure are monitored with any acute cardiac or respiratory problem. The patient with *arrhythmias* will have a *longer* (up to 1 minute) initial pulse count, as described earlier under Vital Signs in the section entitled Technique. There will also be many repeat measurements. Tachycardia is sought in *coronary artery disease* both as a marker of effort and as a treatable exacerbating condition. Tachycardia can be the first manifestation of *congestive heart failure,* and the patient who has been treated for heart failure has the pulse counted frequently. In addition to patients with primary lung or airway problems such as *asthma,* those with neurogenic respiratory suppression—classically *drug overdose*—require frequent counting of respiratory rate.

Orthostatic Pulse and Blood Pressure

The impact of venous pooling in the upright posture on pulse and blood pressure is assessed with *orthostatic checks* (see Conducting the Extended Examination). This is the commonest extended examination of vital signs. Assessment of **volume status** is the usual indicator, i.e., the amount of extracellular intravascular fluid relative to normal. Abnormal orthostatic measurements are frequently found in the setting of volume depletion (hypovolemia), which is difficult to detect by other means. Orthostatic pulse and blood pressure checks are also performed to assess for *autonomic dysfunction.*

Patients are likely to have a check for orthostatic hypotension if they have light-headedness on rising, dizziness, falls, or syncope. The settings in which volume depletion is suspected include substantial bleeding, inadequate oral intake (Table 2.3), or excessive obligate fluid loss as with marked emesis, diarrhea, or sweating (Table 2.4).

CONDUCTING THE EXTENDED EXAMINATION

Serial observation and the detection of *trends* are key to the extended examination. As with routine vital signs, these special techniques are sometimes repeated more frequently than other portions of the physical examination.

Special Components of the General Appearance

One can explore the surroundings of the patient. A *house call* can enhance observations on the *total environment.* When a patient arrives in coma and without family, a check for a *Medic Alert bracelet* is routine. A *search of the wallet* is performed with a *security officer* to protect all parties. A formal *search of the room* of a patient suspected of producing *factitious disease* requires authorization by administrator and the law. The discovery of unprescribed syringes, for example, provides diagnostic help and also a means to show the patient that his practices have been discovered. Visual inspection of *urine, feces, sputum, or vomitus* by the clinician is a portion of extracorporeal examination.

Vital Statistics

SERIAL MEASUREMENT

Daily weight measurements aid assessment of fluid balance in the patient with *acute renal failure or congestive heart failure.* Weigh-ins are highly charged for the obese or anorectic patient and for patients with human immunodeficiency virus (HIV) infection or cancer. The examiner weighs such patients less often than "biologically" indicated, judging their course by other parameters, such as general appearance, function, intake, and activity.

Table 2.3
Causes of Decreased Oral Intake

Anorexia	Lack of food	Odynophagia
Malaise	Environmental water deprivation	Nausea
	Hypodipsia	Oral pain

Table 2.4
Causes of Increased Fluid Loss

Excess diuretic medication
Increased insensible loss with fever or diaphoresis
Blood donation
Vomiting
Diarrhea
Loss into an internal wound or other third-space collection
External drainage

IMMOBILE PATIENTS

The office scale requires that the patient step up and stand still. This is impossible for some persons with movement disorders and for the wheelchair-bound person. There are scales with broad platforms onto which a wheelchair and its occupant can be pushed and weighed. The empty wheelchair is then weighed separately, and this figure is subtracted from the combined weights. For the *bed-bound patient*, there are *bed scales* onto which the patient is transferred. These usually have a 0 reading that incorporates the weight of the instrument.

Vital Signs

PULSE

If the apical pulse is counted, and the peripheral pulse is subtracted from it, a **pulse deficit** is calculated. If all heartbeats are perceptible in the periphery, the pulse deficit will be 0.

To assess *consistency* of pulse intensity, the pulse must be regular. The examiner must not vary the palpating pressure on the radial artery and must concentrate on the *force* rather than on *regularity*. **Pulsus paradoxus** is an exaggeration of the normally slight (0–8 torr) physiologic decrease in SBP, and thus in pulse pressure, on inspiration. When you can feel the pulse weaken on inspiration, the drop must be 20 torr or more. Slow, quiet breathing is essential to render a pulsus paradoxus perceptible (Fig. 2.14).

For **pulsus alternans** (mechanical alternans), focus on *equally spaced* beats that run strong-weak-strong-weak. Pulsus alternans can be brought out by dangling the legs or standing: these maneuvers decrease venous return.

It would be hard to diagnose these two abnormalities together. The examiner might confirm pulsus alternans by having the patient hold his breath during the pulse taking, to temporarily exclude paradoxus.

RESPIRATION

Cheyne-Stokes respiration, also called **periodic breathing,** consists of alternating episodes of **apnea** or **hypopnea**—extremely shallow and infrequent breaths—terminated by rapid deep breaths, i.e., marked **hyperpnea** (hyperventilation). If the pattern shifts from one phase to the other during observation, Cheyne-Stokes is confirmed.

TEMPERATURE

The examiner can construct a fever curve (temperature chart) by plotting temperature on the ordinate and time on the abscissa. In the absence of antipyretic therapy, this will show higher temperatures in the afternoon and evening than in the morning, both in normal persons and in many persons with febrile illnesses.

Use of a special *low-registering thermometer* permits detection of *hypothermia* and is indicated when a patient feels very cold to the touch or when a conventional thermometer has not budged from its bottom number.

In the suspected fever-fabricator, as well as in the patient unable to cooperate, measurement of temperature of a freshly voided (under direct observation) urine specimen provides a reliable datum. The temperature should be the same as that measured rectally.

BLOOD PRESSURE

The sphygmomanometer is the object of innumerable misuses. The list that follows is necessarily incomplete.

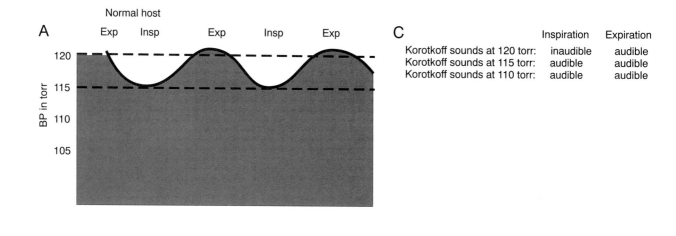

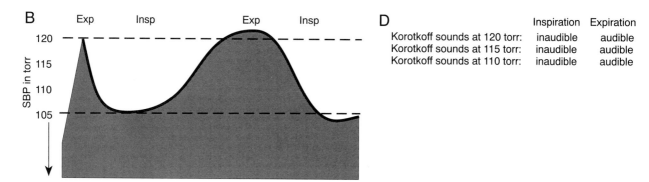

Figure 2.14   Pulsus paradoxus illustrated. **A.** In the normal host, the SBP, graphed on the ordinate, is between 0 and 8 torr higher in expiration than in inspiration. This tracing might have been made with an intra-arterial manometer. **B.** In the patient with an abnormal pulsus paradoxus, often miscalled "a patient with pulsus," the inspiratory drop is exaggerated. In this instance, it measures 14 torr, so that the expiratory SBP is 120 torr and the inspiratory SBP is 106 torr. **C.** As a result, if the sphygmomanometer is locked at the levels given, Korotkoff sounds are audible only in expiration at 120 torr in the normal and throughout the respiratory cycle only at 115 or below. **D.** In this individual with an abnormality, the Korotkoff sounds are not heard throughout the respiratory cycle until 106 torr.

Pitfalls and Correctives

Numerous sources of error are described under Vital Signs in the section entitled Technique or in the AHA booklet. Others require mention here, along with correctives and preventives (Tables 2.5 and 2.6).

Instruments. If the *stethoscope* is not adequately positioned in the examiner's ears, the effects mimic *hearing loss,* i.e., failure to appreciate the first and last soft Korotkoff sounds. Hence the SBP will be underestimated, and the diastolic pressure will be overestimated.

The *sphygmomanometer* is subject to a host of problems, as detailed in Tables 2.5 and 2.6.

With *all* sphygmomanometers, a bladder or cuff that is off-size will lead to erroneous blood pressure readings. The *large adult cuff* (15 cm wide) works well *on all adults* except those with notably thin or extremely large arms.

Any cuff applied inside-out will "explode," embarrassing all parties.

Table 2.5
Causes of Artifacts in Blood Pressure Measurement

Artifacts due to equipment
   Inadequately tested or calibrated systems
   Mercury/gravity or aneroid sphygmomanometer defects: clogged air vent; improper cali-
      bration; incompletely deflated bladder; faulty tubing, inflation system, or exhaust valve;
      insufficient mercury in reservoir; failure to "zero" indicator
   Cuff size/arm size disparity. Limb circumference-to-cuff width ratio of greater than 2.5
      produces falsely high indirect pressure readings

Artifacts due to examiner technique
   Unsupported arm gives falsely higher pressure
   Examiner positions instrument at level above or below heart or presses stethoscope too
      firmly over vessel
   Examiner has preference for even-numbered digits, etc.
   Cold hands of examiner or cold equipment raises blood pressure
   Subject-examiner interaction affects pressure reading
   Acoustic monitoring system is impaired.

Table 2.6
Common Sources of Variation in Blood Pressure Measurement

Instrument Source	Cause	Effect	Method to Reduce
Manometer	Loss of mercury	Reading impaired	Have medical equip ment dealer add mercury to 0 mark
	Clogged air vent at top of manometer tube	Mercury column will respond sluggishly to pressure	Clean or replace air vent
	Loose air vent nut	Mercury column will bounce	Tighten knurled nut at top of column
Bladder	Too narrow	High reading	Determine bladder and cuff size
	Too wide	Low reading	Determine bladder and cuff size
	Not centered over artery	High reading	Use proper technique
Cuff	Loose application	High reading	Use proper technique
	Applied over clothing	Reading impaired	Use proper technique
	Too narrow	High reading	Use large adult cuff
	Too wide	Low reading	Use pediatric cuff
Tubing	Pressure leaks	Reading impaired	Check for leaks and replace
Stethoscope	Eartips not forward	Auditory impairment; low systolic, high diastolic	Use proper technique

If tubing *leaks*, producing a fall of 1 torr/second or more when the valve is "locked," accurate reading is impaired. This problem is detected if the examiner locks and waits just a moment before beginning deflation: If there is a leak, the dial or mercury column begins to fall. If a leak is found, tighten the tubing connections by hand or seek servicing or replacement.

Sensory and technique problems. Eliminate extraneous sound while auscultating: Turn off the television, close the door, turn off buzzing and bleeping monitors, and request interruption of all nearby speech. In an unavoidably *noisy* environment, *palpation* gives the best estimate of SBP.

If the clinician has *low vision,* false readings of dial or column can hamper measurements. Clinician *motor deficits* such as hemiparesis or tremor may impair or prevent measurement of blood pressure.

Positioning errors hamper readings. If the cuff or the stethoscope is not centered over the brachial artery, Korotkoff sounds are heard poorly, recreating the hearing impairment errors. The brachial artery segment auscultated needs to lie at the level of the heart, i.e., the anterior fourth intercostal space. If the arm is *drooping,* the pressure reading will be erroneously elevated. Arm support at heart level must be achieved *passively,* because muscular contraction to maintain position falsely elevates the blood pressure in the limb.

Discrepant Side-to-Side Readings

If there is a known discrepancy between blood pressures in the arms, the *arm with the higher reading is used.* If the arms are unavailable and the leg must be used (see below), the examiner must recall that SBP usually runs 20–30 torr higher in the leg than in the arm of the normal adult, whereas diastolic blood pressure may be unaffected. Thus the interpretation of pulse pressure and set points for hypertension and hypotension are changed in the leg.

Clinician Behavior, Patient Affect

The *interpersonal manner of the clinician* and the *patient's outlook* affect this clinical encounter. An adversarial interaction will raise blood pressure, as will *anxiety, cold hands, or cold equipment.*

Measurement over clothing produces acoustic and manometric artifact (Fig. 2.15). Working around tangled instruments wastes time and promotes measurement errors (Fig. 2.16).

Inflation and deflation problems. *Too-high inflation* may cause pain and amplify the "white-coat effect" that produces a higher blood pressure. *Too-slow inflation* can result in venous pooling, akin to the effect of repeating the blood pressure measurement without allowing time for venous emptying: A beet-red forearm and hand are dead giveaways.

Unduly slow deflation may cause an **auscultatory gap,** i.e., a zone between systolic and diastolic in which Korotkoff sounds are absent (Fig. 2.17). How can erroneous readings based on an auscultatory gap be avoided? If the SBP has been estimated by palpation, you will not misconstrue the low end of the gap as the SBP. Rather, you may hear disappearance of Korotkoff sounds at the high end of the gap and thus overestimate the diastolic blood pressure. The corrective is to *keep listening* for another 30 torr or more below the last Korotkoff sound. If further Korotkoff sounds appear, you have crossed an auscultatory gap, and the diastolic blood pressure is redefined by the (new) last sound. Unduly *rapid deflation* renders assessment of both SBP and diastolic blood pressure inaccurate, with both underestimation and overestimation occurring.

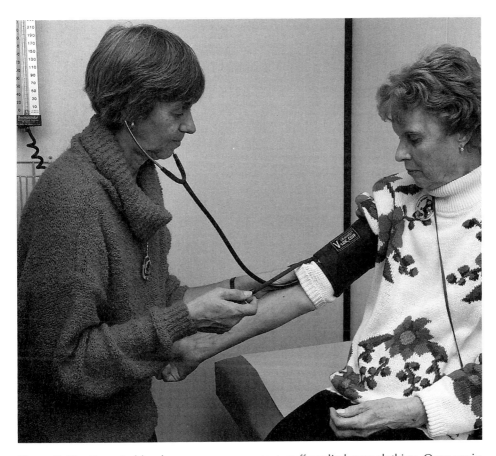

Figure 2.15   Errors in blood pressure measurement: cuff applied over clothing. Once again the shortcut of not having the patient disrobe results in generation of meaningless data. Rolling up the sleeve would be a barely acceptable alternative; proper use of a hospital gown or instructing the patient to wear short sleeves would be far better.

Individual Patient Characteristics

Physical and psychic discomfort both tend to raise the blood pressure, as do many other factors (Table 2.7). Some factors lower the pressure (Table 2.8). Spending time with the patient to obtain the history and offering the patient the opportunity to use the toilet will alleviate most of the conditions cited.

Arrhythmia hinders measurement: SBP varies with cardiac filling and thus with cycle length. Occasional extra beats are ignored even if they mimic a "mini-auscultatory gap." In atrial fibrillation, multiple readings are necessary.

There are several relative contraindications to using an arm for blood pressure measurement (Table 2.9). Cuff inflation might lead to calamitous thrombosis of a fistula or cellulitis in an arm with defective drainage. If both arms are inappropriate, a leg is used. Concern about altered neurogenic vasomotor tone has led to avoiding measuring blood pressure on the side of a hemiplegia, but the difference is probably not clinically significant. The rare true bruit in the brachial artery precludes use of the limb for blood pressure measurement. In any of these situations, state in the clinical notes and orders which side must be used and why it must be used.

The patient with a known *auscultatory gap*, even when proper technique is employed, is at risk for gross underestimation of systolic pressure and overestimation of diastolic pressure. Here a chart label, "Patient has auscultatory gap,"

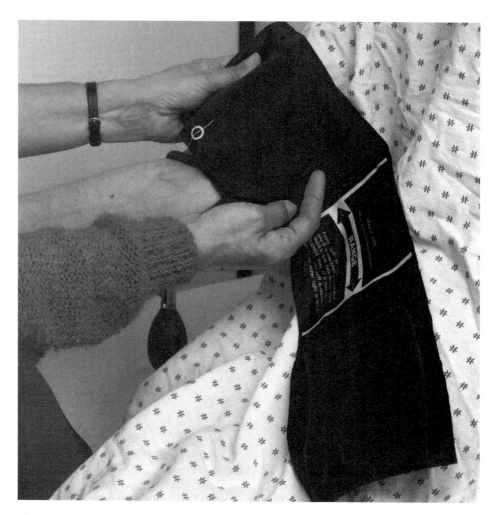

Figure 2.16 Further errors in application: tangled cords and a bladder running over them will vitiate this measurement even if the direction of winding is correct—which it does not appear to be.

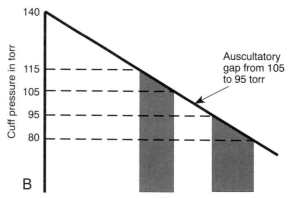

Figure 2.17 An auscultatory gap is a point above true diastolic blood pressure and below SBP at which, counterintuitively, no Korotkoff sounds are heard. It is graphically illustrated in this instance, which is parallel to the normal situation illustrated in Figure 2.6.

Table 2.7
Some Patient Characteristics That Falsely Elevate Blood Pressure

Pain	Recent exercise	Chilling
Full bladder or rectum	Sleeplessness	Recent smoking
Auscultatory gap		

Table 2.8
Some Patient Characteristics That Falsely Reduce Blood Pressure

Recent eating
Volume depletion
Auscultatory gap (lower end misconstrued as SBP)

Table 2.9
Contraindications to Using a Limb for Blood Pressure Measurement

Intravenous line in place	Local thrombophlebitis
Arteriovenous fistula for hemodialysis	Recent fracture or trauma to the limb
Mastectomy or axillary dissection on this side	Brachial artery bruit
Local lymphedema	

may alert even a hurried clinician to interpret correctly.

In some patients the Korotkoff sounds muffle (phase IV) but never disappear completely (phase V). This phenomenon is more common and prominent in high-output states such as aortic valve insufficiency and thyrotoxicosis. Therefore, record the phase IV reading—the point of muffling—as the diastolic blood pressure, and note this in the chart. The quickest shorthand is to record phases I, IV, and V together—a practice otherwise unnecessary—as, for instance, 130/75/0.

Orthostatic Checks

The technique for orthostatic checks is simple (Fig. 2.18). Count the radial pulse and measure the blood pressure with the patient supine (Fig. 2.19). Deflate the cuff but do not remove it. Then have the patient sit up with legs dangling and remeasure the pulse and blood pressure. If neither has changed, have the patient stand up; and then repeat the measurements immediately or at 1 minute (Figs. 2.20 and 2.21) and 3 minutes if need be.

Caveats. **If abnormalities are demonstrated on the supine-to-seated portion, there is no diagnostic gain in proceeding with a seated-to-standing portion, and there is a risk of precipitating syncope. And if the test produces chest pain or a sense of impending syncope ("brownout"), the test is terminated,** and the patient is returned to the supine position. Reproduction of dizziness and minor faintness *if tolerable* do not require termination until immediately after a first postsymptom measurement. This sequence will conclusively demonstrate whether the symptom correlates with orthostatic changes or not.

If symptoms occur on arising from a chair, omit the supine measurement and proceed directly from seated to standing.

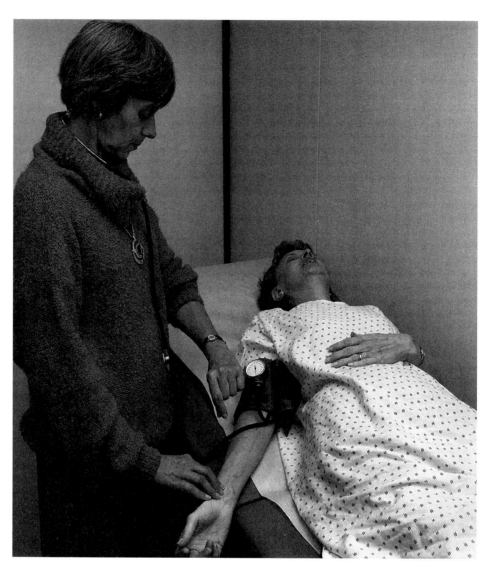

Figure 2.18 The most common and important extended vital sign evaluation is the checking of orthostatic pulses and blood pressures.

Deconditioning. The mild exertion of sitting up or arising will increase heart rate a bit, particularly for the sedentary and deconditioned and those with reduced cardiac reserve. Purposeful delay in measurement for a minute after transfer minimizes false-positive results. For the patient who has difficulty standing, offer a hand to hold, a cane, or a walker or have the patient lean his backside against an examining table for support throughout the upright part of the test. Only upright posture and venous pooling are essential.

Blood Pressure in the Legs

If the arms are unavailable, the legs provide an alternative site, subject to the above caveats about higher SBP. Detection of obstructive lesions of the aorta beyond the left subclavian artery ostium or in the femoropopliteal system requires comparing blood pressure in the legs to that in the arms.

Blood pressure in the thigh is measured with the patient *prone;* a large *thigh cuff* whose width is 80% of thigh circumference is used. The knee is passively

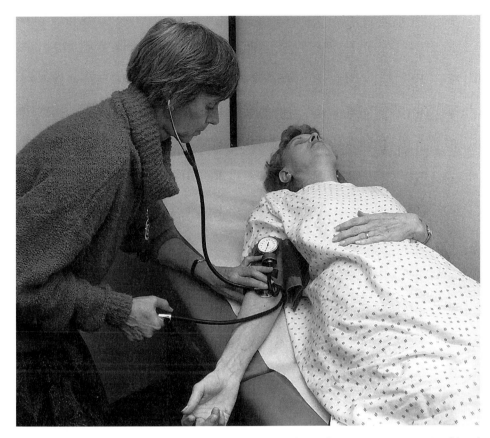

Figure 2.19 This examiner has obtained the supine pulse and now is getting a supine blood pressure. Having one of these baseline measures without the other virtually ensures that no safe inference can be drawn from values obtained with the patient seated or standing.

flexed, and the popliteal space is auscultated, either over the popliteal pulse, if one can be found (see Chapter 10, Extended Examination of the Limbs), or blindly over midfossa.

If this method is impractical or unsuccessful, a *calf blood pressure* is measured. Depending on the size of the patient, the thigh cuff or a large adult arm cuff is used. It is placed low on the calf (a good fit may prove impossible). Auscultation of the site of the dorsalis pedis pulse often reveals no Korotkoff sounds, but palpation will give the SBP.

Pulsus Paradoxus

Pulsus paradoxus is better identified with a sphygmomanometer than by palpation. Pulsus paradoxus is a SBP on inspiration that is 10 torr or more below the SBP on expiration.

Detailed techniques. Three techniques are in use.

1. Take the blood pressure in the usual way and then deflate the cuff completely for 30 seconds. Thereafter, reinflate the cuff to 20 torr above SBP, and lower it slowly, listening for the very first tap of a Korotkoff sound during expiration *only*, expecting silence during inspiration if the cuff is then locked. This is the **expiratory SBP.** The cuff is then deflated 10 torr and relocked. If Korotkoff sounds are still audible only in expiration, there is an abnormal pulsus paradoxus (often referred to simply as a pulsus paradoxus!). If, however, Korotkoff sounds are heard throughout the respiratory cycle, you are

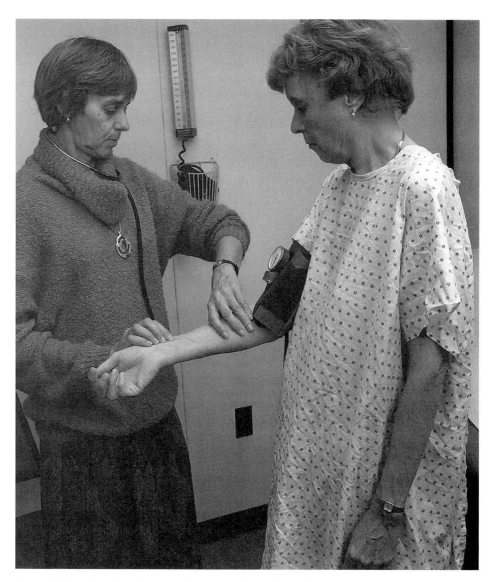

Figure 2.20   Counting the pulse in the upright position. Note that the sphygmomanometer has been left in place, although deflated. This saves extra work and ensures comparability of measurements.

clearly at or below the **inspiratory SBP,** and the difference between the two is within normal range; i.e., the patient does *not* have an abnormal pulsus paradoxus.

2. Proceed as previously, through delineation of the expiratory SBP. Then deflate the cuff *very slowly* (1 torr/second or so) until Korotkoff sounds are heard throughout the respiratory cycle. This is the inspiratory SBP, and the difference between the two figures is recorded (Fig. 2.14).

3. A hybrid method serves when bradycardia renders assessment difficult: Drop the cuff 3 torr from a starting point and relock, then listen through a couple of cardiac and respiratory cycles before dropping the cuff down another 3 torr.

Limitations and practice method. These methods depend on finding a point at which Korotkoff sounds are audible only in expiration, which is not feasible in every patient. For some patients the "paradoxus" is 0 torr.

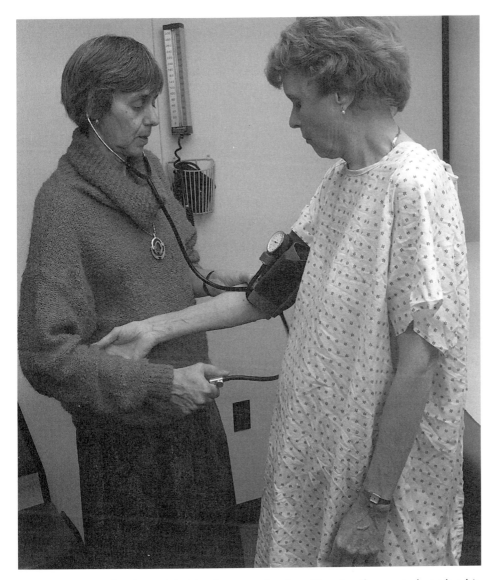

Figure 2.21 Finally, the upright blood pressure is taken. Elevating the arm to heart level is needed when counting the *pulse rate* with the patient in the upright position.

Everybody gets confused trying to keep cardiac and respiratory cycles straight. Practice alleviates this confusion. To produce an abnormal paradoxus in a normal subject for teaching, the subject breathes through a cardboard cylinder taken from the center of a roll of paper towels. With the far end crimped, an abnormal inspiratory resistance and a "paradox" are produced.

Valsalva Maneuver

The SBP can be altered in a way that is useful for identifying left heart failure, by the **Valsalva maneuver:** expiration against a closed glottis. Instruct the patient to bear down as though trying to breathe out, but with the airway closed so that no air can escape; i.e., "Push out your stomach as far as you can." The SBP can be measured at rest, just before straining (phase I), after 10 seconds of continued straining (phase II), immediately upon release of straining, and in the period of overshoot 30 seconds later (phase IV). The sphygmomanometer is inflated 15 torr above the prestrain SBP, which will obliterate Korotkoff sounds, and locked. Listen at the start of straining (phase I), 10 seconds later (phase II), and 30 seconds after release (phase IV), recording at whatever points Korotkoff sounds are found. Successful completion of the test requires auditory and cognitive capacity, regular heart rhythm, and cardiorespiratory function and abdominal musculature sufficient to sustain the effort.

Osler's Sign

Osler's sign is a maneuver employed to assess for arteriosclerosis. The radial pulse is palpated at rest, with the fingers left on it as the sphygmomanometer is inflated to just above the SBP. If the radial artery remains palpable when it then becomes *nonpulsatile,* the test is abnormal. A normal artery is not distinct from the surrounding tissues at this point. The test is performed just after auscultatory measurement of blood pressure, by repalpating the radial pulse site after deflation, waiting a few seconds, and then reinflating above the SBP just measured.

Rumpel-Leede Sign

The sphygmomanometer is employed in a nonspecific but useful test for increased bleeding risk–the Rumpel-Leede sign. A circle 2.5 cm across is drawn on the patient's forearm. The sphygmomanometer is inflated above the diastolic blood pressure but below the SBP and is locked. The circled area is observed for development of petechiae. Ten petechiae or more constitute a positive result. As soon as these develop, or after 5 minutes, the test is stopped. (If the cuff is left on for 5 minutes unattended, confluent purple ecchymoses can develop over the forearm.)

Minor and Discredited Signs

Hill's sign consists of measuring the popliteal artery SBP and the conventional brachial artery SBP and then finding the difference. This has been used in assessment of aortic insufficiency but seems to involve misinterpreting a normal phenomenon. Further investigation is needed.

Mayne's sign, a fall in the diastolic blood pressure greater than 20 torr when the patient raises the arm over the head, has been discredited. The "rollover test" for hypertension in pregnancy is also not accurate.

INTERPRETING THE FINDINGS
General Appearance
MORE ON THE TOXIC APPEARANCE

A special form of an acute *toxic* appearance is called the **typhoid state,** although it is not specific for infection with *Salmonella.* It is characterized by muttering, vigilant *delirium* (see below), often with muscular activity, and classically with picking at the bedclothes. The constellation carries a grave prognosis.

CEREBRAL AND AFFECTIVE STATE

The patient whose brain is not working well, as evidenced by intellectual and communicative failure and poor establishment of interpersonal contact with the clinician, suggests one of five broad classes of differential diagnosis at the level of general appearance:

Delirium

Delirium is an acute deficit of attention with normal level of consciousness, i.e., no coma or stupor. Medication toxicity is a major etiology, especially in the aged. Noncerebral disorders such as fracture, urinary tract infection, and bladder distension can also be responsible, as can alcohol intoxication or alcohol withdrawal. The Hollywood image of delirium as a wild-eyed state must be consciously replaced by that of a patient with sudden, nonpsychogenic deterioration of brain function. This includes the patient who is quiet as much as the one who grows rambunctious.

Dementia

Dementia is a slowly progressive loss of intellectual function, stable from day to day and from minute to minute. Inappropriate word choices and lack of concern for social failure may mimic psychologic disorders at first-pass assessment.

Mental Retardation

For mental retardation, the history augments the assessment of general appearance. A lifetime deficit suggests Down syndrome or other genetic or congenital causes.

Psychiatric Disorders

Depression is familiar when the patient is dysphoric and sluggish, less so when agitated or manic. Cognitive dysfunction rather than affective problems may predominate in a variant sometimes labeled *pseudodementia.*

Schizophrenia is suspected if the flight of ideas and tangential thinking are especially bizarre. It can mask or mimic organic brain dysfunction.

Communicative Deficits

Wernicke's (receptive) aphasia may be misconstrued, particularly on first look, as dementia or psychiatric disease. Uncorrected *hearing loss* must be identified early in the encounter, so that verbal and communicative failures are not mislabeled as brain processing problems.

POOR CARE

Signs of *self-neglect* or *caregiver failure* can be overlooked from the human tendency to avoid unpleasantness. Environmental deficits such as extreme poverty can produce these signs. So can intentional mistreatment or the defective self-care of mental illness and dementia.

Foul odor, filthy clothing, and lack of grooming are striking, as are grossly *ill-fitting* garments *inappropriate to the season.* Other signs include *food remnants on face and clothing* and substantial urinary or fecal remnants on person or clothing.

A PAIR OF INAPPROPRIATE DESIGNATIONS

Those uncomfortable with the care of incapacitated persons in a late stage of dementia and disability may refer to the "O" sign and "Q" sign. These "signs" refer to the shape of the mouth hanging slackly open (O), with the person being asleep or noncommunicative. When the person's tongue hangs to the left and down, the "O" sign becomes a "Q" sign. We mention this to emphasize the discomfort of the observer, a real factor in clinical diagnosis.

MOVEMENT: DECREASED AND ABERRANT

Hemiplegia is usually apparent on general appearance, although as with any motor deficit, assessment is refined by neurologic examination. *Paraplegia,* i.e., paralysis below the waist, is obvious in most cases. Motor losses of lesser severity, *hemiparesis, paraparesis, monoplegia, and monoparesis,* are less noticeable.

Slowing and reduced movement are seen in local disorders of muscle and power; with local pain; and with central lesions, notably *Parkinsonism.* The latter is also one cause of *abnormal involuntary movements*. Others include *essential tremor, drug toxicities* and *cerebellar disease*. Abnormal involuntary movements are easy to miss. They may come out only during the history or only with maneuvers undertaken for another reason.

"WALK-IN" DIAGNOSES

Some conditions are better recognized as the "forest"—global impression—than by the individual "trees"—their signs and symptoms. *Depression* belongs in such a listing, as do *hypothyroidism, hyperthyroidism, acromegaly, and scleroderma*.

Thyroid Disease

The patient with hypothyroidism may seem to have all functions turned down, with slow movement, coarse skin and hair, hoarse slow speech, decreased mental acuity, or so much reduction in subtlety and abstraction that the examiner infers depression. The patient with *hyper*thyroidism may also appear psychiatrically rather than physically ill, with a rapid heart rate and speech that suggest the manic phase of bipolar disorder. Although many patients with thyroid dysfunction present neither picture, the ensembles must be recognized lest these treatable conditions progress unheeded.

Acromegaly

The patient with excess growth hormone has either gigantism or acromegaly: exceptional stature belongs to gigantism, while facial deformity and spade-like hands are more characteristic of adult onset, i.e., acromegaly. Any very tall and especially skinny patient should raise a differential diagnosis that also includes Marfan's syndrome.

Systemic Sclerosis

Some patients with scleroderma are recognizable at first glance by tight, shiny facial skin, fingers that look shrink-wrapped in their skin and that may have ulcers on the digital pulp, and perhaps cutaneous calcium nodules and telangiectases about the lips and elsewhere. In the advanced stages of this disorder, the diagnosis is first suggested by the general appearance.

SPECIAL COMPONENTS OF GENERAL APPEARANCE
Olfactory Diagnosis

Foul-smelling pus is characteristic of anaerobic infections, not coliforms or mycobacteria. Necrotic tissue also smells awful, if perhaps less feculent. The diagnostic difficulty is that aerobic suppuration may produce malodor from necrosis, mimicking anaerobic infection. Staphylococcal infections, the prototype of yellow purulent inflammation, do *not* produce a characteristic odor. Pseudomonal infections at times yield a sickly fruity-sweet smell. Patients with *typhoid fever* are said to smell like freshly baked bread.

Breath that smells of *cloves, peppermint, or Clorets* may reflect a habit or may bespeak intentional olfactory cover-up, usually of alcohol or tobacco. The slightly fruity, acetone breath of *diabetic ketoacidosis* may speed diagnosis of the unlabeled patient in delirium or coma in the emergency department. Unfortunately, *hypo*glycemia gives no clue on general appearance unless a Medic Alert bracelet "announces" underlying diabetes.

Researchers have detected a substance that makes some *schizophrenics* smell different from controls.

Extracorporeal Diagnosis

Nobody can replicate the superlative listing and discussion of extracorporeal signs found in Faith Fitzgerald's splendid article, "The Bedside Sherlock Holmes," of 1982. However, a few representative examples follow.

Stools that are *red* but give a *negative stain for occult blood* may reflect *beets* or other ingested matter (the same holds true for red urine). *Black stools with negative fecal blood tests* can come from *iron supplements and bismuth preparations.*

Red urine and *orange urine* routinely follow use of Pyridium for cystitis and the urethral syndrome. Again, tests for blood are negative. *Rifampin* can turn all body effluvia red, including tears and sweat. Patients often fear that bleeding is the cause.

A patient who wears regular clothing in preference to the hospital gown almost always feels great improvement. This sign is uncommon, however, because patients usually await permission from hospital staff before resuming normal garb. Rarely, the wearing of "street clothes" means planned departure against medical advice.

A jar of sourballs at the bedside may be a clue to oral dryness from the sicca syndrome.

Vital Signs

PULSE

Character

A *shallow pulse* is found with narrow pulse pressure and in *shock*. The simplest methods used to investigate a shallow pulse are to check the general appearance and to measure the blood pressure. *Pulsus alternans* is found almost exclusively in left-heart failure, with or without other signs. It may occur rarely during and just after arrhythmia in the absence of heart failure. Pulsus alternans may be associated with reduced SBP on the weaker beats and is thus a potential source of confusion with *pulsus paradoxus* if the examiner does not pay close attention to the factor associated with weakness—inspiratory phase versus alternate beat. Bigeminy can also mimic pulsus alternans. It is not possible at the bedside to be sure which of the latter two is present.

Pulsus paradoxus. Pulsus paradoxus exceeding 10 torr is seen in, among other conditions, *obstructive airway disease* including both stable chronic bronchitis with emphysema ("COPD") and acute asthma. Any cause of *heart failure* can produce this sign, as can *severe cardiomyopathy*. It is usually present in *cardiac tamponade*. Confusingly, pulsus paradoxus is less frequent in *pericardial constriction*, which shares several physiologic features with cardiac tamponade. The sign is present in *shock* but is never essential to that diagnosis. The interpretation of an elevated paradox is more functional than etiologic. In an asthmatic, "paradox" signifies severity and supports hospital admission. After recent heart surgery, the development of an elevated paradox mandates urgent evaluation for tamponade resulting from pericardial bleeding. The PARADOX of this phenomenon is that in the extreme case the peripheral pulse can disappear on inspiration while, *paradoxically*, heart tones remain audible during the "missed" beat.

A *reversed pulsus paradoxus*, with an *expiratory* fall in SBP, has been described in some patients receiving continuous airway pressure on a mechanical ventilator (respirator).

Pulse Rate

Pulse deficit. A pulse deficit, in comparing radial to apical pulse rate, is seen in atrial fibrillation, which is recognized by the absolute irregularity of heartbeats. A pulse deficit develops in *pulsus alternans* if weak beats are so feeble that they cannot be felt at the radial artery. A pulse deficit is also present in extreme *pulsus paradoxus,* as implied above. In both the latter situations, the remaining heartbeats are regular, and severely impaired breathing is obvious.

Tachycardia and fever. Tachycardia carries a long differential diagnosis that includes most cardiorespiratory and pericardial disorders and many others. One key cause is *fever,* which may be missed if not thought of. Tachycardia has been called the "poor man's thermometry" because it is detectable qualitatively even in the home, without equipment. The appreciation of the heart rate-fever link can result in thermometry for quick confirmation or refutation of fever as a cause. The presence of both abnormal vital signs does not prove that fever is *the* cause of the particular tachycardia.

Uncoupling of the two. When tachycardia is *absent* in the presence of fever, this *uncoupling* of temperature from heart rate suggests, depending on context: *Legionella* infection; ornithosis; salmonellosis, especially typhoid fever; drug fever, i.e., an adverse drug reaction that includes pyrexia (fever); sinoatrial node dysfunction as with digitoxicity and primary disease of the conduction system, e.g., sick sinus syndrome; the toxic effect of extreme hyperbilirubinemia on the sinoatrial node; and factitious fever.

RESPIRATION

Respiratory Pattern

Cheyne-Stokes respiration has most frequently been linked to heart failure and remits with successful therapy for this disorder. Brainstem disorders, perhaps in the respiratory center in the medulla, can produce Cheyne-Stokes breathing without heart failure. Severe respiratory disease may also produce a final common medullary neuronal hypoxia. Interpretation centers on prognosis rather than on detailed etiopathogenesis. After realizing that the pattern is not hyperventilation due to panic—when the hypopneic component becomes recognized—many observers regard Cheyne-Stokes respiration as a harbinger of impending death.

Noisy Breathing

Noisy breathing is encountered in airway dysfunction more than in pure restrictive lung disease. It may relate to turbulent, nonlaminar air flow at the larynx, trachea, and major bronchi. It is a surprisingly common and little-used correlate of exacerbations in asthma and one that may be reported by patient or spouse in the history, as well as detected by observation.

TEMPERATURE

A Distinction

Diaphoresis (sweating) and fever are separate entities with some overlap. The patient who is markedly *diaphoretic* may be in the midst of defervescence, or may be responding to environmental stimuli such as a hot day, sustained muscular exertion, etc. Diaphoresis is not fever, and some medical conditions produce one without the other; for example, severe angina pectoris verging on acute myocardial infarction often creates diaphoresis as does shock. Core body temperature in the setting of diaphoresis may be normal, elevated ("warm shock," heat stroke), or depressed.

Fever

Fever of unknown origin (FUO). FUO signifies a febrile condition whose etiology is not readily apparent. A stricter definition is "an illness characterized by daily fever of 38°C or more for 3 weeks or longer, without identified cause," a definition that varies with basal diurnal temperature curve of the individual—something very rarely recorded in advance. In adults, the most frequent causes of FUO are infections. Worldwide, malaria with its characteristic every-other-day "tertian fevers" and every-third-day quartan fevers, is a major etiology. Infection causing FUO may be localized, e.g., an abscess, or systemic, as in malaria. HIV is a major addition to the list. More traditional elements include tuberculosis, intra-abdominal abscesses, osteomyelitis, biliary tract infection, occult urinary tract infection and perinephric abscess, infective endocarditis, fungal infections by *Candida* species, and histoplasmosis. *Malignancies* can be found on such lists, with *renal cell carcinoma and malignant lymphomas* being most likely, and leukemias and hepatomas less so. *Hepatic metastases* from any primary cancer can produce fever. *Hodgkin's lymphoma* rarely produces a pattern of 3–10-day cycles of fever alternating with normal temperatures, the Pel-Ebstein fever.

Drug fever. Drug fever is an *allergic* cause of both ordinary fever and FUO and is suspected when the pulse is too low or the patient "looks too good" for the temperature elevation. Rash and eosinophilia support drug fever, but their absence does not militate against it. Antimuscarinic drugs may predispose to fever *pharmacologically,* by reducing mechanisms of heat dissipation.

Noninfectious fevers. Numerous noninfectious *inflammatory diseases and autoimmune ("collagen") disorders* can cause fever. The vasculitides include systemic lupus erythematosus, hypersensitivity vasculitis, polyarteritis nodosa, and giant cell arteritis—in both its temporal arteritis and polymyalgia rheumatica variants. Inflammatory bowel disease (Crohn's and ulcerative colitis) can cause fever, in which one could postulate inflammation from either the disease itself or a breached mucosal barrier. Granulomatous hepatitis, a catchall of unclear etiologies, can be found on the list, as can sarcoidosis.

Central fever. Central fever resulting from hypothalamic thermoregulatory instability can complicate several neurologic conditions. The patient who has suffered major *anoxic brain injury* after cardiac arrest may develop this problem. The examiner must step back to recognize central fever amid the other differential diagnoses of *fever in the critical care unit* (Table 2.10).

Vascular disorders. It was long believed that careful perioperative temperature charts show a "bump" with development of *deep venous thrombosis,* but the method is unacceptably insensitive and nonspecific. Some deep venous thrombi cause fever, as do some *pulmonary emboli,* with or without associated pulmonary infarction. Pulmonary emboli are generally thought of in relation to low-grade fever, but a reliable small series shows fever exceeding 39°C from this cause. Fever with deep venous thrombosis and pulmonary embolism may reflect local and systemic inflammation that can follow thrombosis and that is more pronounced with tissue *infarction* or *necrosis.* Fever was an old confirmatory sign a

Table 2.10
Fever in the Critical Care Unit

Infection	Tissue necrosis
Pneumonia	Myocardial infarction
Septicemia and infections associated	Hepatic infarct
with foreign bodies such as	Multiorgan failure
intravascular catheters	
	Central fever
Other	Blood transfusion reaction
Drug fever	Venous thrombosis and pulmonary embolism

day or more after *myocardial infarction.* Fever occurs in many patients recovering from myocardial infarction. Workup for other causes, if not obvious on history and examination, is usually unrewarding. A hard look for infection seems rational only with signs, symptoms, or a peak temperature of 39°C or above.

Endocrine rarities. *Adrenocortical insufficiency* (Addison's disease) can produce a febrile illness. This differential and *hyperthyroidism* are considered whenever a case of fever does not "add up."

Factitious fever. This term refers to fever produced intentionally. It should be considered early in the differential diagnosis of FUO. Medical, nursing, and laboratory personnel have fever of factitious origin most commonly, with women outnumbering men and young adults seen most often. Among the least self-destructive means used to produce this is heating a thermometer or taking hot liquid in the mouth before thermometry. At the other extreme, some persons inject fragments of feces into the bloodstream to produce fever! Polyspecies bacteremia suggests either enterovascular fistulization, widespread denuding of the mucosal barrier, or some such extraordinary behavioral aberration.

Extreme pyrexia. This term refers to fevers, in adults, exceeding 40.5°C (104.9°F). Infection remains a leading cause, but autonomic failure, at both hypothalamic and midbrain levels, assumes a large role, as do two disorders of central thermoregulation, peripheral muscular thermogenesis, and heat dissipation: *neuroleptic malignant syndrome* and *malignant hyperthermia.* Both share the propensity for temperature elevations up to 42°C (107.6°F). *Neuroleptic malignant syndrome* entails autonomic failure with profuse sweating and tachycardia. It occasionally lacks high fever. It is caused by neuroleptics (major tranquilizers) including all the *phenothiazines*—even those used for nonpsychiatric indications. *Malignant hyperthermia* results when any of a group of *anesthetics* is administered to susceptible persons. Hallmarks are muscular contraction with excess thermogenesis. A positive family history increases the risk of malignant hyperthermia, whereas a personal history of uneventful exposure to the general anesthetic in question is reassuring. Intraoperative temperature monitoring helps delineate an early and treatable phase.

Deceptively normal temperature. Patients with azotemia and, in particular, patients with uremia can have normal temperature coexisting with systemic inflammation. There may also be a transition from fever to hypothermia as tissue perfusion falls. Potent anti-inflammatory drugs, roughly in proportion to efficacy, including *phenylbutazone, indomethacin, and systemic corticosteroids,* and any *nonsteroidal anti-inflammatory drug (NSAID)* including *aspirin* can normalize temperature measurement. The saw that "important fever breaks through acetaminophen suppression" is not true. Suppressibility does *not* shed light.

Hypothermia

Low body temperatures are seen in *accidental (environmental) hypothermia,* some cases of *septicemia* and other forms of *vasodilatory shock,* and *hypothyroidism* and other hypometabolic states. Rarely, hypothermia occurs in end-stage cardiac disease with superimposed peripheral arterial disease. More often, the patient who feels glacial to the touch has a normal core temperature but an increased temperature gradient from core to periphery. The examiner must test this speculation by measurement of core temperature.

BLOOD PRESSURE
Common Orthostatic Patterns

Normal. The normal adult shows a stable heart rate or a rise of 10 beats/minute or less when measured 1 minute after *orthostatic shifts* (lying to sitting or sitting to standing). In normal persons the SBP may decrease by as much as 10 or 15 torr, but the diastolic pressure may stay the same, may rise, or may even fall by some 5 torr. There is considerable individual variation.

Orthostatic tachycardia. In the person with good vascular tone and reflexes, intravascular volume depletion is often compensated by *orthostatic tachycardia,* i.e., maintenance of blood pressure at the expense of increasing the heart rate considerably. The significance of pure orthostatic tachycardia is the same as that of orthostatic hypotension, i.e., hypovolemia. Intravascular volume depletion occurs commonly in three principal settings: (1) major hemorrhage, (2) decreased oral intake, and (3) increased fluid loss.

Orthostatic hypotension. When not further specified, this term refers to orthostatic shifts that produce (1) pulse rise exceeding 10 beats/minute, (2) a fall in SBP, usually 10 torr or more, and (3) a fall in diastolic blood pressure of 5 torr or more. The changes may be demonstrable in the standing position only and, occasionally, only on maintaining that position for 3 minutes.

Three critical points to keep in mind are:

1. Orthostatic blood pressure checks without orthostatic pulse checks are meaningless (see below).
2. If the seated patient demonstrates orthostatic hypotension, the test is not extended to the upright position except under very rare special circumstances.
3. **If frank (supine) hypotension is present, orthostatic checks are contraindicated and dangerous.**

Orthostatic hypotension is common in old age, particularly among hypertensives, and in mineralocorticoid deficiency. Most antihypertensive medicines can produce orthostatic hypotension. Numerous other medicines including phenothiazines and tricyclic antidepressants also belong in the differential diagnosis.

Dysjunction: blood pressure drop without pulse rate rise. If orthostatic hypotension is present but the pulse does *not* rise, or rises only very slightly, there is **autonomic dysfunction.** This finding is common in *diabetic neuropathy, B$_{12}$ deficiency,* and occasionally in isolation. Iatrogenic autonomic interference, typically β-*blockade,* can produce this pattern. **When autonomic dysfunction is present, it is impossible to assess for hypovolemia via orthostatic checks.**

Corollaries. Some corollaries concerning orthostatic hypotension follow:

1. If orthostatic hypotension is found, but the pulse has not been counted in both positions, the examiner cannot discriminate between hypovolemia and autonomic dysfunction.
2. Check pulse and blood pressure in two positions in a well-patient checkup. If autonomic dysfunction is found at baseline, no time will be wasted attempting to assess volume status with orthostatic checks when the patient presents acutely ill.

Three caveats about orthostatic interpretations are:

1. The SBP varies with some *arrhythmias,* and by definition so does the heart rate. Caution is needed in interpreting orthostatic checks in patients with arrhythmias. In atrial fibrillation, repeated measurements may help confirm that an apparent orthostatic change is, for instance, real, not artifactual.
2. In the patient with a clear clinical picture of hypovolemia, the examiner must not demand orthostatic hypotension to confirm the diagnosis. Conversely, in the patient who appears euvolemic, orthostatic hypotension should suggest other considerations also. In *selected* instances, repeat orthostatic checks after intravenous infusion of a quantity of sodium chloride solution may help determine if hypothermia was the cause and has been corrected.

3. The examiner must not interpret *extravascular volume overload* (edema at the ankles, lung crackles, etc.) as evidence against *intravascular hypovolemia.* There are many settings in which these apparently contradictory phenomena can coexist. Edema does not exclude hypovolemic orthostatic hypotension; orthostatic checks must still be made if clinically indicated.

Problem-solving. Examine Figures 2.22–2.30, each of which depicts a set of orthostatic checks. *Write down* an interpretation that can be checked against the answers printed at the end of the chapter.

Severe and Malignant Hypertension

Any systolic pressure of 180 or more or any diastolic pressure of 110 or more requires prompt attention but not necessarily a change in therapy.

The term *malignant hypertension* is applied to an accelerated form of hypertension. It is associated with rapid impairment of renal function, heart failure, acute brain dysfunction, retinal hemorrhages, and sometimes permanent damage to brain, eyes, heart, and kidneys. There is no specific blood pressure at which the diagnosis of this medical emergency is made. Some persons lack the syndrome at 220/160, whereas others have it at 180/120. The blood pressure is interpreted in context.

Valsalva Maneuver

Adequacy of the Valsalva maneuver is confirmed by observing reddening of the face, prominence of jugular and forehead veins, and effort without audible or visible air exchange, grunting, or speech. At the *outset* of straining, Korotkoff sounds normally become audible with the sphygmomanometer locked 15 torr above the

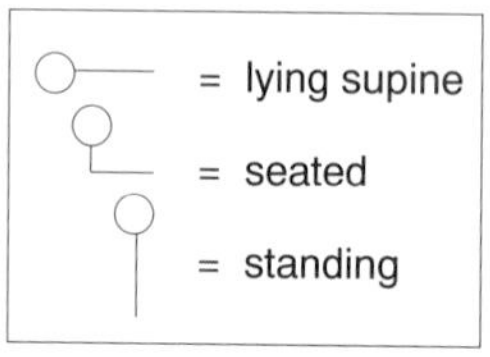

= lying supine

= seated

= standing

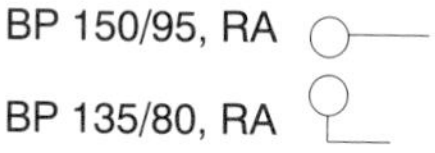

BP 150/95, RA

BP 135/80, RA

Figure 2.22

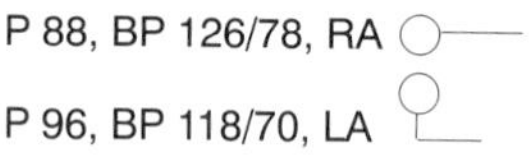

P 88, BP 126/78, RA

P 96, BP 118/70, LA

Figure 2.23

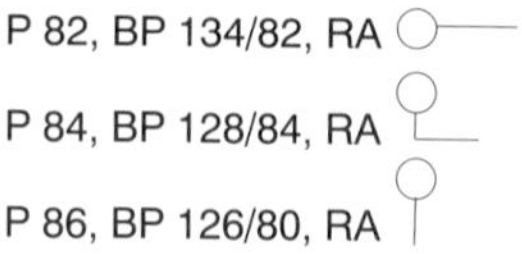

P 82, BP 134/82, RA

P 84, BP 128/84, RA

P 86, BP 126/80, RA

Figure 2.24

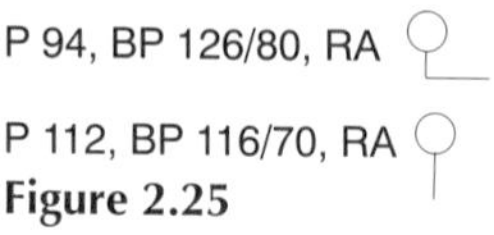

P 94, BP 126/80, RA

P 112, BP 116/70, RA

Figure 2.25

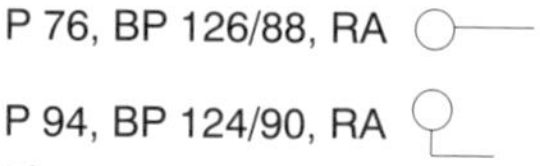

P 76, BP 126/88, RA

P 94, BP 124/90, RA

Figure 2.26

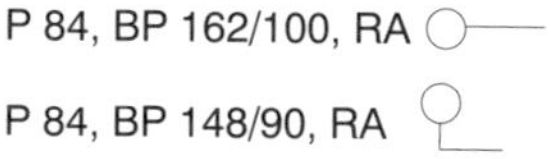

P 84, BP 162/100, RA

P 84, BP 148/90, RA

Figure 2.27

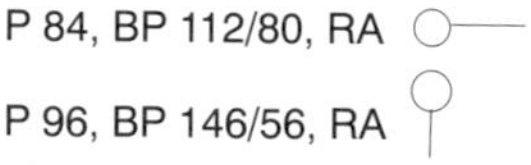

P 84, BP 112/80, RA

P 96, BP 146/56, RA

Figure 2.28

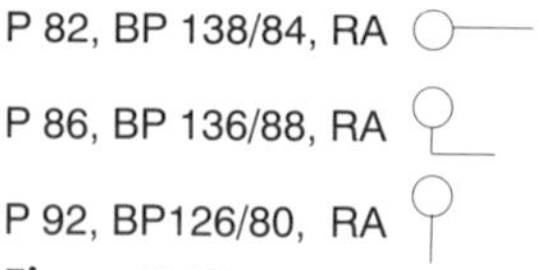

P 82, BP 138/84, RA

P 86, BP 136/88, RA

P 92, BP126/80, RA

Figure 2.29

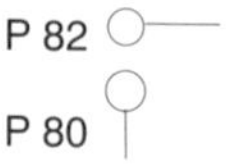

P 82

P 80

Figure 2.30

prior systolic pressure. After 10 seconds of straining, persistently audible Korotkoff sounds mean a *square-wave blood pressure pattern,* the pattern most highly correlated with left ventricular dysfunction. (Korotkoff sounds should be *inaudible* 30 seconds after release of the Valsalva maneuver in this setting.) If Korotkoff sounds are inaudible after 10 seconds of straining, straining is then stopped with release of breath and resumption of normal breathing. Thirty seconds later—making sure that the cuff pressure remains at the original level—Korotkoff sounds should be *audible* in normal persons and *absent* in patients with *the absent overshoot response.* This last pattern is also correlated with left ventricular dysfunction (Table 2.11).

Trousseau's Sign

The application and tightening of the blood pressure cuff can produce spasm of the wrist flexors and finger extensors, *Trousseau's sign,* which is most characteristic in the neuromuscular irritability of *hypocalcemic tetany.* There is no standardization of this test. Data on predictive value and comparisons with other signs are scant. If this *carpal spasm* is seen during blood pressure measurement or any sphygmomanometric variant, blood measurements of calcium, magnesium, and phosphate are indicated. Results of the Trousseau test lack sufficient predictive value to preempt bloodwork.

Osler's Sign

A positive test indicates arteriosclerosis. In epidemiologic studies, patients with a positive Osler's sign are more likely to have *pseudohypertension:* The blood pressure measured by sphygmomanometry overestimates true intraluminal pressure. Unfortunately, Osler's sign does not have sufficient positive predictive value *in an individual* to correct a cuff reading that might exceed the true pressure by, for instance, 20 torr. The examiner *cannot* redefine the threshold for hypertension in a pseudohypertensive as, for example, 160/110.

Rumpel-Leede Sign

A positive test does not distinguish among four causes of excessive extravasation: (1) elevated capillary pressure, (2) defective or deficient blood coagulation proteins, intrinsic or iatrogenic (as with anticoagulant therapy), (3) capillary fragility as in scurvy, and (4) thrombocytopenia.

Hill's Sign

A popliteal SBP 20 torr above the brachial SBP has been suggested as a mark of aortic insufficiency. This difference is also reported as normal. Definitive interpretation awaits further research.

Table 2.11
Valsalva Test Results[a]

Phase	Normal Sinusoidal	Absent Overshoot	Square Wave
Before test	K–	K–	K–
I. Start straining	K+	K+	K+
II. Continue straining 10 seconds	K–	K–	K+
IV. 30 seconds after release	K+	K–	K–

[a]K–, Korotkoff sounds absent at this level; and K+, Korotkoff sounds present with sphygmomanometer locked 15 torr above casual SBP.

Ankle/Arm Systolic Blood Pressure Ratio

The ratio of dorsalis pedis SBP to conventional brachial SBP has been used to assess arterial obstruction between the proximal aorta and the large vessels. The ratio normally exceeds 1.0. (A **palpable** difference in pulse intensity is not reliable.) Reduced ratios of 0.5 or less signify atherosclerosis obliterans of the aorta or the femoral or popliteal artery, coarctation of the aorta, which will usually produce additional signs also, or dissecting hematoma of the aorta.

RECORDING THE FINDINGS
Sample Write-up

G. R. is a 26-year-old man with advanced cardiomyopathy, seen because he felt faint and short of breath. Has received diuretics. On restricted sodium and water intake.

General appearance: Chronically ill-appearing, thin but not cyanotic. Adequately groomed and dressed, clean but loose clothing. Looks very dry, skin puckered. Uncomfortable. Speech production, content, and comprehension intact. Affect appropriate: anxious, depressed, interactive, able to be encouraged. Moves all limbs readily.

Vital signs:
Supine: pulse, 84, regular; BP right arm, 102/64.
Seated: pulse, 98, regular; BP right arm, 94/52.
Respirations, 22, slightly labored.
Temperature, 37.4°C.
No pulsus alternans. Paradox 6 torr. Unable to sustain Valsalva maneuver due to dyspnea.

Assessment: Baseline BP low due to poor cardiac output and medications. Superimposed orthostatic hypotension, probable intravascular volume depletion. Minimal fever likely environmental. No clear decompensation, but marked dyspnea and slight hyperpnea even with hypovolemia—worrisome. Thinness and loose-fitting clothes—weight loss from severe heart disease (cardiac cachexia). Needs hospital admission with close observation.

BEYOND THE PHYSICAL EXAMINATION
General Appearance

No laboratory indicators or imaging studies refine or duplicate the *overall clinical impressions* of the general appearance. There is little correlative research to show which impressions have the greatest prognostic or diagnostic power. Close investigation and observation over time remain valuable follow-ups for a striking general appearance.

Vital Signs

Repetition furthers investigation of abnormalities. Serial measurement may be done not only by the clinician but also by the patient, a family member or caregiver, other health personnel, home machine, or equipment of ever-increasing cost and sophistication.

PULSE

Self-measurement is frequent. Simple machines count pulse rate based on oscillometric techniques at baseline or after medication or exercise.

The *electrocardiogram (ECG)* in the form of a *rhythm strip* is used to clarify arrhythmias. *Ambulatory electrocardiographic monitoring* with a *Holter monitor* applied for 24 hours has greater accuracy than a rhythm strip because many thousands of beats are analyzed by computer. A *symptom diary* explores whether arrhythmia corresponds to symptoms. *Transtelephonic monitoring devices* assay rhythm after being patient-activated because of symptoms. *Cardiac monitors* are used in critical care units and telemetry suites in hospitals to detect life-threatening irregularities of heartbeat. *Electrophysiologic studies (EPS)* are the most advanced means of studying the pulse.

Very *slow pulses* are also studied by bloodwork to exclude hypothyroidism.

Pulsus paradoxus commonly leads to *echocardiography* in search of *pericardial effusion*. Pulsus paradoxus can be read directly from continuous *arterial catheter* manometric tracings. *Pulsus alternans* may lead to *chest radiography, echocardiography* for assessment of ejection fraction and regional myocardial function, *nuclear cardiology* studies of perfusion, or even *cardiac catheterization* in search of coronary arterial or valvular causes of heart failure.

RESPIRATION

When *hyperpnea or tachypnea* is found, there should be a search for abnormalities of oxygenation, of carbon dioxide excretion, and of hydrogen ion homeostasis. Sometimes this entails *arterial blood gas* measurements. Alterations in diffusion and air movement are explored with *pulmonary function tests* and occasionally with *respiratory flow-volume loops*. Underlying structural changes are sought by *chest radiographs* and other imaging modalities.

Persons with suspected abnormalities of nighttime breathing may have *sleep (apnea) studies (polysomnography)*. Measurements of airflow, ECG, and other variables are correlated with direct observation and electroencephalogram (EEG) monitoring.

Unexpectedly slow or scant respiration leads to evaluation for neurologic deficit, to assessment of arterial blood gases, and to a search for narcotic respiratory depressants by blood or urine toxicologic studies.

TEMPERATURE

Urinary thermometry helps check core temperature. Inserting a temperature probe into the center of a freshly defecated stool can achieve the same. Central temperature can be measured with a thermistor attached to a central vascular catheter.

Fever evaluation includes history, review of medication list, exploration for new symptoms, physical examination, and *cultures* from sites of suspected infection. Blood cultures, throat swabs, and urine cultures are frequent. Chest radiographs are commonly performed in search of pneumonia.

Among studies to assess marked hypothermia are, again, blood tests of thyroid function.

BLOOD PRESSURE

There are small *instruments* for measuring pulse and blood pressure in a single finger. These have not yet been widely validated. Many patients perform *home monitoring* with an ordinary sphygmomanometer and stethoscope. The contortion required to check this on one's self is considerable. If a family member can perform the measurements, the data will be more dependable. *Electronic blood pressure measuring machines* work with an arm cuff and seem reliable.

Ambulatory blood pressure monitoring employs a variant of the preceding attached to a recording device. The machine has an arm cuff that inflates (and deflates) several times each hour for 24 hours. A computer generates a listing of readings. The technique helps assess mean arterial pressure in patients with *labile hypertension* or *"white coat hypertension."* Intra-arterial catheters with manometers work directly, continuously, and instantaneously. They are expensive and invasive.

Assessment of stable moderate *hypertension* is controversial. For *refractory hypertension,* most authorities advocate seeking remediable secondary causes including: blood studies for elevated levels of cortisol, thyroid hormones, aldosterone, and epinephrine; imaging or functional studies for renal artery stenosis; and a chest radiograph in a search for coarctation of the aorta.

Hypotension in a person who is not acutely ill leads to a search for hypothyroidism and adrenohypocorticism (Addison's disease). In the acutely ill patient, hypotension prompts seeking septicemia, via complete blood count with differential count and blood cultures, and a cardiac calamity with ECG, cardiac enzymes, and echocardiogram.

When blood pressure cannot be determined with a sphygmomanometer because of *inaudible Korotkoff sounds,* as in shock or distal arterial disease, *Doppler ultrasound* can be used for blood pressure determination. This is easier than palpating faint pulsations and thus is widely used for determination of ankle/arm SBP ratios.

Innumerable studies can investigate *orthostatic hypotension* that is not merely hypovolemic. One is the *tilt table test* whereby effects of gravity and body position on several variables are assessed.

RECOMMENDED READINGS

Screening Examination for General Appearance and Vital Signs

Crawford MH. Inspection and palpation of venous and arterial pulses. Dallas: American Heart Association, 1990.

Felts JH. From cold feet to hot hands. N C Med J 1982;43:590.

Fitzgerald FT, Tierney LM Jr. The bedside Sherlock Holmes. West J Med 1982;137:169–175.

Frohlich ED. Recommendations for blood pressure determination by sphygmomanometry. Ann Intern Med 1988;109:612.

Frohlich ED, Grim C, Labarthe DR, Maxwell MH, Perloff D, Weidman WH. Recommendations for human blood pressure determination by sphygmomanometers. 5th ed. Dallas: American Heart Association, 1987:1–34.

Hayden GF. Olfactory diagnosis in medicine. Postgrad Med 1980;67:110–118.

Howell TH. Oral temperature range in old age. Gerontol Clin 1975;17:133–136.

McFadden JP, Price RC, Eastwood HD, Briggs RS. Raised respiratory rate in elderly patients: a valuable physical sign. Br Med J 1982;284:626–627.

Tandberg D, Sklar D. Effect of tachypnea on the estimation of body temperature by an oral thermometer. N Engl J Med 1983;308:945–946.

Verghese A. The "typhoid state" revisited. Am J Med 1985;79:370–372.

Extended Examination for General Appearance and Vital Signs

Abbas F, Sapira JD. Mayne's sign is not pathognomonic of aortic insufficiency. South Med J 1987;80:1051–1052.

Feussner JR, Blessing-Feussner CL, Linfors EW. Blood pressure measurement: getting the right cuff. N C Med J 1983;44:241.

Howard RJWM, Valori RM. Hospital patients who wear tinted spectacles—physical sign of psychoneurosis?: a controlled study. J R Soc Med 1989;82:606–608.

Meissner H-H, Franklin C. Extreme hypercapnia in a fully alert patient. Chest 1992;102:1298–1299.

Moss AJ. Criteria for diastolic pressure: revolution, counterrevolution, and now a compromise. Pediatrics 1983;71:854–855.

Murray HW, Tuazon CU, Guerrero IC, Claudio MS, Alling DW, Sheagren JN. Urinary temperature: a clue to early diagnosis of factitious fever. N Engl J Med 1977;296:23–24.

Pines A, Levo Y. Straight or oblique? J Am Geriatr Soc 1989;37:1004.

Rebuck AS, Pengelly LD. Development of pulsus paradoxus in the presence of airways obstruction. N Engl J Med 1973;288:66–69.

Sapira JD, Kirkpatrick MB. On pulsus paradoxus. South Med J 1983;76:1163–1164.

Soffer A. Smokers' faces: who are the smokers? Chest 1986;89:622.

ANSWERS TO FIGURE PROBLEMS

Figure 2.3 Answer   The point of measurement is below heart level, and so a hydrostatic component will be added.

Figure 2.22 Answer   Orthostatic hypotension. Cause? No pulse measurements have been recorded; therefore, one cannot differentiate between hypovolemia and autonomic dysfunction.

Figure 2.23 Answer   Inconclusive blood pressure difference may represent side-to-side difference. One cannot get a "two-for-one" shortcut and compare two sides and two positions this way (and the pulse rise alone is inconclusive).

Figure 2.24 Answer   Probably normal. The pulse rise is minimal, the systolic drop is within the normal range, and the trivial diastolic drop should not be given undue attention.

Figure 2.25 Answer   Classic orthostatic hypotension. There is both orthostatic tachycardia and a fall in SBP of 10 torr, with a comparable fall in diastolic pressure.

Figure 2.26 Answer   Orthostatic hypotension manifest as orthostatic tachycardia alone. Although the diastolic blood pressure has actually climbed and the SBP is stable, this is done at the expense of an 18-point pulse rise, and it is likely that hypovolemia is present.

Figure 2.27 Answer   Autonomic dysfunction. Note that although the SBP and diastolic blood pressure have both fallen, there is no appropriate compensatory rise in the pulse rate.

Figure 2.28 Answer   Probably erroneous measurement. The numbers are not sensible, and the measurement ought to be repeated. If the SBP has risen and the diastolic blood pressure has fallen, it is hard to figure out and appears contrary to reason.

Figure 2.29 Answer   Orthostatic hypotension, only brought out by the "extreme" position shift that unmasks significant pulse rise, SBP fall, and diastolic blood pressure fall.

Figure 2.30 Answer   Indeterminate. If the blood pressure was measured in both positions, the examiner could distinguish between normal findings and the isolated blood pressure changes without pulse changes found in autonomic neuropathy.

3

Skin

SCREENING EXAMINATION OF THE SKIN

APPROACH AND ANATOMICAL REVIEW

Approach

The skin is the largest organ in the human body. It, with its extensions, the mucous membranes, covers the surface of all body parts. Examination of the skin is a prime example of the distinction between the regional and the organ system approach to physical examination. The clinician gains an *overall impression* of the general characteristics of each patient's skin, just as she notes other items of general appearance and behavior; however, the *details* of skin inspection and palpation are carried out as each body *region* is examined.

Explicit terminology and specific descriptive terms are used to assess and record the details of the skin examination. The approach to skin lesions requires a systematic set of questions and observations. The modes of the examination are **inspection** and **palpation.** The skin includes the covering of the surface of the body; **hair** and **nails,** which are appendages of the skin; and a specific set of **glands,** which lubricate and help control body temperature.

Elements of the medical history relevant to the skin are those of observed **change**—change in color or texture, change in the characteristics of the nails or the distribution or appearance of the hair, change in the function of the glands, and the appearance of new skin markings or alteration in preexisting lesions. Pruritus is another major skin symptom and may bespeak a systemic disorder with secondary skin manifestations. If a patient mentions or the clinician elicits a history of such change, the patient is asked to describe what he has noticed and to point out the area of concern during the course of the physical examination.

Anatomical Review

The skin is composed of two layers overlying the subcutaneous fat, the dermis and the epidermis. The thickness of each layer varies with body site and with age. See Figure 3.1 for schematic cross-sectional drawings of the skin and its appendages and glands.

Epidermis. The epidermis is the most superficial layer of skin, and its outermost part is composed largely of keratinized cells that are being constantly shed and replenished from deeper strata. The epidermis is avascular, and its nutrition is provided by diffusion from the vascular dermis.

Dermis. The dermis contains vessels, sensory nerve endings, and autonomic nerve fibers that supply the vessels and glands.

Hypodermis. Deep to the dermis lies a layer of connective tissue, sometimes referred to as the hypodermis, and fat that connects the dermis to underlying structures.

From within the skin and its subcutaneous understructure arise specialized glands and the follicles from which hair growth occurs. These glands and appendages include the following:

Sebaceous glands prevent the skin and hair from drying by means of the production of sebum, are intimately associated with hairs including subvisible (vellus) hairs, and are most numerous in oily areas such as the alae nasi.

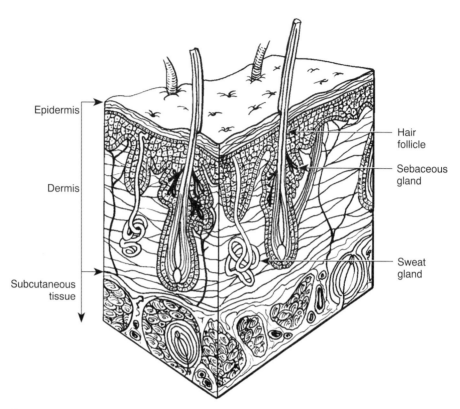

Epidermis

Dermis

Subcutaneous tissue

Hair follicle

Sebaceous gland

Sweat gland

Figure 3.1   Cross-sectional view of the skin and its appendages and glands.

- **Eccrine or sweat glands** open onto most of the body surface and are responsible for secreting water and salt in response to changes in internal body temperature and environmental temperature variations, to enhance thermal homeostasis. They are widely distributed but are most heavily concentrated where humans sweat most, i.e., the axillae and groin.
- **Apocrine glands** secrete a complex fluid. They are found only in the axillae and anogenital areas, and they respond to emotional stimuli.
- **Hair** is a dermal product arising from pilosebaceous follicles. Its color, like that of the skin itself, is determined by melanocytes—in the case of hair, by those that reside in the shaft.
- **Nails,** another skin appendage, are composed of uniquely keratinized epidermal cells that arise from a vascular growth plate at their proximal base. The fold of skin covering the base of the nail is known as the **eponychium,** and the soft tissue surrounding the nail is known as the **paronychium.**

TECHNIQUE

Inspection of the skin requires good light, an alert observer, and, on occasion, a magnifying glass. The most important instruments for the examination are the examiner's eyes and brain, a ruler or tape for measurement of lesion size, and sensitive fingers for the assessment of texture, temperature, and the contour of lesions in relationship to the surrounding skin surface and subcutaneous tissue underlying them. The area of skin being examined must be fully exposed to the light and to the eye and the hand of the examiner.

General Examination of the Skin

General examination of the skin should include observations regarding its color, its turgor, and the distribution and integrity of appendages.

- **Color** of normal skin is both genetically and environmentally determined and is a reflection of melanin quantity and distribution and melanocyte activity. The examiner notes variations in color from area to area as the examination proceeds. Special attention should be paid to the color of the lips, fingers and toes, earlobes, and beds of the nails.
- **Turgor** of the skin in the healthy, well-hydrated young adult is plump and elastic. If the skin surface is "pinched up" ever so slightly from the subcutaneous tissue, it will immediately return to its smooth, preelevation state when tension is released. As the skin and subcutaneous tissue lose some of their resiliency with aging, the skin may "tent" when pinched so that the test loses its specificity for extravascular fluid volume depletion.
- **Texture** of the skin varies with hydration, cosmetic care, and sun exposure. The texture of the skin surface, determined by touching or stroking lightly with the fingerpads, is a part of the regional observation that the clinician makes continuously while conducting the physical examination.
- **Temperature** of the skin is crudely assessed by touch. It is unproductive to attempt to quantitate core body temperature by tactile means, but variations from region to region or gross deviations from normal can be determined. Common descriptors include cool and dry, cool and moist (or clammy), hot and dry, hot and moist. In particular, areas of rubor (redness or erythema), swelling, or tenderness are studied for temperature deviation from the remaining regional surface, and distal limbs are palpated for unusual coolness suggestive of decreased arterial and/or capillary perfusion.

Examination of Skin Lesions

SYSTEM

The examination of discrete **skin lesions** proceeds systematically with observations of the following:

Dimensions (always measured for accuracy), including height if there is any elevation

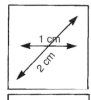

Configuration

Elevation

or

Depression

Palpable characteristics, if any, e.g., **smoothness, induration, tenderness**

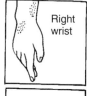

Color(s)

Body location(s)

Right wrist

Pattern of distribution

TERMINOLOGY

In addition to a sound system of skin examination, a working knowledge of standard descriptive terminology of skin lesions is critical to recognition and communication of findings. An accurate description of a skin finding, even if the examiner has no idea what diagnosis to attach to it, enables follow-up for any changes that might occur and occasionally permits diagnosis by a more experienced clinician. Skin findings may be conveniently classified by using mutually exclusive terms describing their relationship to surrounding skin (in addition to the individual characteristics noted above): flat (nonpalpable) lesions; raised, solid (palpable) lesions; raised, cystic (palpable) lesions; and depressed lesions.

Flat (Nonpalpable) Lesions

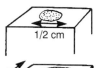

Macule: a flat, circumscribed discoloration less than 1 cm in largest dimension

1/2 cm

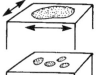

Patch: a flat lesion larger than 1 cm

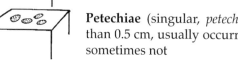

Petechiae (singular, *petechia*): purple to red spots, each less than 0.5 cm, usually occurring in groups; sometimes palpable, sometimes not

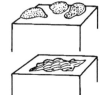

Purpura: purple to red discolorations less than 0.5 cm each (may be faintly palpable)

Ecchymoses (bruises): purple to red zones of discoloration under an intact epithelial surface

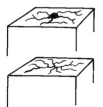

Spider angioma: red spot with radiating "legs" that blanches with central pressure and fills from the center

Venous "spider": superficial collection of tiny veins in stellate configuration; empties with pressure and fills slowly from the periphery

Raised, Solid (Palpable) Lesions

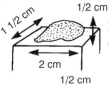

Papule: raised lesion less than 1 cm in diameter (variable height)

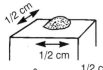

Plaque: raised lesion greater than 1 cm in diameter but confined to the superficial dermis

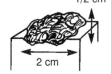

Nodule: raised lesion greater than 1 cm in diameter, deeper in the dermis than a plaque and/or extending for a greater distance upward from the skin surface

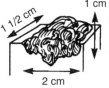

Tumor: a nodule that is poorly demarcated or about which the examiner suspects a neoplastic origin; or a nodule that is larger than 2 cm in greatest dimension

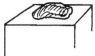

Wheal: pink to very pale, slightly elevated and circumscribed area of skin edema

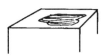

Scale: a flaky heap of keratinized cells that exfoliate with scraping (can occur at the surface of a plaque or patch or entirely by itself)

Crust: elevated dried exudate of blood, serum, and/or pus (usually on surface of a lesion, although it may be seen on its own)

Raised, Cystic (Palpable) Lesions

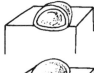

Vesicle: a surface elevation filled with clear serous fluid, less than 1 cm in diameter

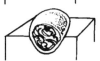

Pustule: a vesicle-like structure filled with purulent (yellow, viscous to solid) content

Bulla: same as a vesicle but measuring greater than 1 cm in diameter

 Cyst: an encapsulated fluid-filled (rather than solid) mass

Depressed Lesions

 Atrophy: an area of loss of skin markings and loss of full skin thickness, often with a pale, shiny surface

 Erosion: an area, often but not inevitably moist, of superficial loss of epidermis

 Ulcer: area of loss of epidermis and dermis forming a crater of any dimension (this may be depressed, flat, or elevated, depending on context, origin, and extent of associated inflammation and hemorrhage)

 Fissure: a narrow, linear (but not necessarily straight) crack in the epidermis with exposure of the dermis

DISTRIBUTION AND PATTERN

If skin lesions are multiple, note their surface distribution and pattern.

Distribution

Where on the body surface do the lesions appear: **generalized** over all parts of the body or **localized** to one or more of the following areas?

- **Palms and/or soles** (or excepting palms and soles)
- **Intertriginous areas** (in moist skin folds such as under the breasts, in the groin)
- **Extensor surfaces only**
- **Trunk only**
- **Face and neck, or malar area only**
- **Dermatomal distribution**
- **Pressure areas**, as where tight clothing chafes or where the sacrococcyx, heels, shoulder blades, or hips bear the weight of the bed-bound patient
- **Any combination** of the above

Pattern

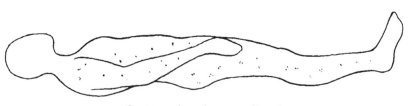

Scattered and generalized

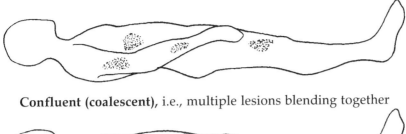

Confluent (coalescent), i.e., multiple lesions blending together

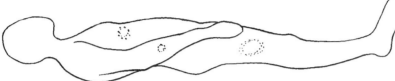

Annular, i.e., in ring formation(s)

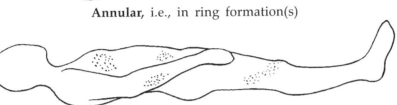

Clustered, occurring in a group or groups different from any of the prior patterns

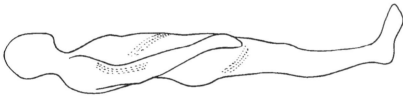

Linear, i.e., occurring in streaks

Any combination of the above

Examination of Skin Appendages

The **fingernails** may be examined in the initial inspection of the hands, usually carried out just before or after the vital signs are taken. Inspect the nails for their color, their shape, the condition of the eponychium and paronychium, and evidence of surface variations. Note their care, often a clue to the emotional state of the patient. Are they bitten with ragged edges? Have they been cleaned of ordinary collected dirt (keeping in mind that there are certain occupations, such as engine repair, that obviate perfect cleanliness under the nails)? Are the nails unduly long?

The **toenails** are most efficiently inspected during the course of the lower limb examination. The observations are the same as those for the fingernails.

The **hair** of the head (scalp) and body is examined with each region, e.g., scalp hair with the head and neck examination, pubic hair with the abdominal and genital examinations, and axillary hair with the lymph nodes and breasts. The hair is inspected for its quantity and distribution and is sometimes palpated for thickness and texture. Don't forget that eyebrows and eyelashes are skin appendages easily studied as part of the examination of the face and the external eye.

NORMAL AND COMMON VARIANTS

The range of normal in skin characteristics is almost as wide as the number of persons being examined. The combinations of possible normal variants are vast, and it is the combinations that give each person a part of his unique biologic identity.

Normal skin **color** ranges from ebony to brown to yellow to near porcelain white—with every imaginable variation in between. The color is often a few shades darker in the folds or intertriginous areas and on the male genital and perianal skin and areolae in both sexes, as well as following sun exposure. Dark-skinned persons often have a bluish tinge to the lips and nailbeds. Heat, excitement, or embarrassment may flush the skin of the face and upper torso a dull to bright red, as may the hormonally controlled vascular instability of peri-menopausal "hot flashes."

Pregnancy and use of hormones for birth control purposes may create darkening of the skin of the forehead and around the eyes. This reversible change in color is known as the "mask of pregnancy" or chloasma; it usually reverts when the hormonal status returns to baseline. Pregnancy may also produce white striae over the taut skin of the distended abdominal wall, a result of dermal stretching. These same linear markings may appear with nongestational deposition of adipose tissue on the thighs and abdomen in both sexes.

Skin **turgor** varies with hydration and especially with age. Turgor may be diminished as a result of severe systemic dehydration. As the skin ages, the elastin in the dermis is altered, and the "loosened" skin pulls into folds more readily, often retaining a tented appearance for some time unless smoothed deliberately.

Skin **texture** is also highly variable in normal persons. Skin of the sun-exposed areas, unless artificially oiled, becomes drier and somewhat coarser than the protected surfaces. Aging skin is thinner, sometimes almost transparent, with increased visibility of the superficial venous networks. "Dry skin" is a common complaint sometimes signifying roughening rather than loss of moisture. When does "dry" mean pathologic? This subtle and difficult assessment sometimes requires a dramatic change from normal baseline.

Skin **temperature** varies with both ambient (room) and core body temperature, as well as with emotional (autonomic) responses to the environment. Some normal persons have hands and feet that feel cool to the touch. Regional variations in the examiner's tactile perception of skin temperature must be considered in the full context of the patient's clinical condition.

Skin "Lesions" as Normal Variants and Common Minor Problems

Almost every adult human skin surface is marked with visible discolorations or palpable variations in its smoothness. A few commonly noted variations are described here.

FLAT LESIONS

"**Birthmarks**" are the flat or slightly raised, usually irregular discolorations with which many persons are born. They may occur anywhere on the body and range from very dark brown, through red or blue, to fawn-colored. To be considered as true birthmarks, the lesions should have been known from parents' accounts to have been present at birth and unchanged for as long as the patient can recall. Scattered tan to brown macules, especially in the sun-exposed areas (commonly designated as **freckles**) are individual normal characteristics. They may appear first in childhood but generally remain unchanged after adolescence, except to lighten or disappear with old age.

Café-au-lait spots are flat, pale tan irregular patches usually present from birth or childhood. Although most commonly a normal variant, they may be associated with other neuroectodermal abnormalities in neurofibromatosis, particularly if six or more, each greater than 1.5 cm in maximum dimension, are present and most especially if they are accompanied by axillary freckles.

Vitiligo, the patchy complete loss of melanin pigmentation, is an acquired condition of unknown cause. It may be considered a normal, if sometimes cosmetically distressing, variant. Some cases are associated with endocrinopathies including diabetes and autoimmune polyendocrine syndromes.

Aging of the skin is accompanied by increasing varieties of discolorations and lesions. **Venous "spiders"** become more evident and widespread, especially in the lower limbs, as venous stasis increases and the skin thins. **Telangiectases,** or dilation of superficial capillaries, may become evident on the face, especially over the nose and malar eminences. **Bruising** and traumatic or spontaneous **purpura** are more common in the thin and vulnerable skin of the elderly. **Lentigines** ("age spots," "liver spots") are the brownish macules seen on the hands, arms, and face of older persons.

RAISED LESIONS

Occasionally, a dark **nevus** will be present from birth (congenital nevus). Often it contains long, dark hair (congenital hairy nevus). More frequently, the number of nevi increases around puberty, but new nevi are uncommon after age 30. There seems to be a hereditary pattern for multiple nevi. The usual benign nevus is of a single shade of brown, sharply circumscribed, and, once apparent, unchanging in size and configuration over time. Benign nevi may be flat or, uncommonly, palpably raised above the surface of the surrounding skin.

Cherry hemangiomas are small, bright red papules, usually perfectly round and sharply circumscribed, that are progressively acquired with maturity of the skin. They occur most commonly on the trunk, although they may be seen anywhere. They are completely harmless.

Hyperkeratinization or **lichenification,** the thickening and elevation of the skin caused by recurrent trauma such as scratching or abrasive rubbing, is common enough in the absence of underlying skin disease to be considered a normal variant.

Corns and **calluses** secondary to pressure trauma are seen as occupational side effects, such as those on the tip of the middle finger of a seamstress or the side of the pen finger of some writers and students. Most commonly, these areas of heaped-up keratin are found on the feet and reflect poor shoe fit or underlying bone changes that subject the surface skin to chronic or recurrent pressure injury.

Dermatographism is a histamine response to minor trauma in sensitive skin and presents as transient linear wheals, usually caused by scratching.

Common benign **nodules** of the skin include **sebaceous cysts** and **lipomas.** The former represent dilated sebaceous epithelial lining containing an accumulation of sebum beneath the epidermis. They occur most commonly on the face, neck, and upper trunk. Lipomas, benign fatty neoplasms of the subcutis, are soft and slow-growing and may become quite large and unsightly. Some cases tend to be familial and multiple. They are of cosmetic importance only, unless a more ominous differential diagnosis is being considered. **Skin tags** are small, usually multiple, fleshy, smooth, and partially pedunculated projections increasing in frequency with age. Attempts to link them to colonic polyps have been inconclusive. **Seborrheic keratoses,** also more common in aging skin, are raised, rough, greasy brown-to-black lesions on the face and trunk. They are benign and of cosmetic concern only, except in the rare instances when they mimic melanoma.

Keloid is the term used to define unusually exuberant scar formation wherein a scar from surgery or other trauma is broader and thicker and has more surface irregularity than expected. The formation of a keloid is a variant of tissue response to trauma and tends to repeat itself in any given person with each new assault on the skin. Blacks are more susceptible to keloid formation than Caucasians.

Common warts, the skin response to an ubiquitous virus, are extraordinarily common. They may appear on any part of the body but are most usual on hands or feet. Warts may grow to greater than 1 cm in lateral dimension and often arise in clusters. They are usually raised and painless, although the **plantar** wart of the sole of the foot may be flat and tender to deep pressure, including that resulting from weight bearing (standing or walking). Warts commonly regress spontaneously. Genital warts have entirely different characteristics and significance (see the Extended Examination section of this chapter).

Solar (senile, actinic) keratosis presents as a slightly raised, erythematous or brownish, rough (sandpapery), and irregular lesion on sun-exposed surfaces. It is a direct result of chronic sun damage. This keratosis is noted here because of its frequency and its low-grade malignant potential. When discovered, it requires careful observation and, if change occurs, biopsy or cryoablation.

Acne is a common occurrence in adolescence and young adulthood. The changing nature of secretions, under the influence of sex hormones, leads to an increased oiliness of the skin with plugging of glandular exits on the skin of the face, neck, shoulders, and upper trunk. Comedones (singular: comedo, the oxidized plugs of secretions), pustules (the secondarily infected skin around these plugged glandular openings), and tiny abscesses are among the physical manifestations of acne.

COMMON VARIATIONS OF THE NAILS

Nail **color** varies with the general pigmentation of the bed of skin underlying the nail itself. In dark-skinned persons, heavily pigmented bands may be visible. **Longitudinal ridging and shallow pitting** are normal variants. Heavy smokers may have yellow to brown nicotine stains of the nails of the fingers with which the cigarette is held. **Anonychia** is the rare congenital absence of nails. Boggy, swollen, inflamed paronychia at the distal corners of the great toenails signals ingrowth of a deeply trimmed nail into the surrounding soft tissue ("ingrown toenail"). A blow or heavy pressure as from firm boots on the surface of the nail may result in blue-black discoloration secondary to hemorrhage beneath the nail (**subungual hematoma**).

COMMON VARIANTS OF HAIR DISTRIBUTION

Male pattern baldness is a progressive loss of scalp hair at the forehead hairline and on the crown of the head. This recession of the hairline may begin at any age and follows familial patterns. Uncommonly, a similar loss of scalp hair may occur in aging women; the cause in this instance is unclear and cannot be related to aberrant sexual endocrinology.

The thickness and texture of hair varies genetically. The significance of any variant lies in its presentation as a change from the prior status. Distribution of body hair is genetic and gender-determined. Some normal females develop thick, dark hair around the nipples and in the lower abdominal midline at puberty; unless accompanied by other evidence of androgen excess (clitoral hypertrophy, undue acne, voice and somatic changes), this may be considered a normal variant. If it becomes more marked after full development of other secondary sex characteristics have stabilized, workup may be indicated. Normal axillary hair varies from a long, thick, exuberant growth to scant, fine hair; again, stability of pattern is the key to normalcy. In the aged, axillary hair is frequently, and pubic hair is sometimes, lost without disease.

Eyebrows also may be very thin and light or heavy and dark. Only if the patient notes a change in the distribution of brow or lash hair should the clinician consider a pathologic basis.

With aging of the skin, the hair tends to become finer in texture and more scant. This normal change applies to body as well as to scalp hair. Only if the hair seems to be falling in perceptible clumps should consideration be given to systemic problems as a basis for hair thinning with aging.

RECORDING THE FINDINGS

The skin examination may be recorded in one of two ways: generalized findings, such as color or texture characteristics or a notable distribution of hair, can be recorded after the VITAL SIGNS, and the general look can be recorded under the categorical designation SKIN. Local findings, such as a surgical scar, single nevus, or clusters of warts, may be recorded regionally unless they are considered manifestations or parts of a systemic condition.

When lesions are described, each is characterized as to its size, shape, margins, palpability, color, body location, distribution, and other distinguishing characteristics, such as blanching with pressure. A sketch is particularly helpful in recording skin findings. A typical physical examination write-up of SKIN might read as follows:

Skin: Fair in color, cool and dry. No cyanosis nor icterus. Hair distribution consistent with age; normal male pattern balding with generalized thinning over remainder of scalp. Multiple flat lentigines over dorsa of hands, forearms, and on posterior neck. Several raised, dark brown, sharply circumscribed papules on anterior chest, all less than 5 mm across. A few cherry angiomata present on trunk.

Abdomen: Bilateral, well-healed herniorrhaphy scars. Normal color.

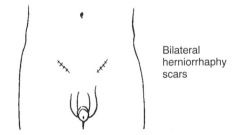

Bilateral
herniorrhaphy
scars

Limbs: Large, symmetrical calluses on ball of each foot. Skin of toes cool, but color, hair growth, and nailbed filling normal. Black, markedly raised irregular lesion is noted on the lateral calf of the left leg, mobile, not fixed. Surface not ulcerated, no "spillage" of pigment around it, and minimal variegation (red, blue) on its knobby, dry surface.

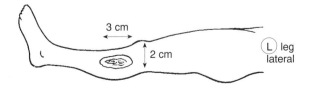

3 cm

2 cm

(L) leg
lateral

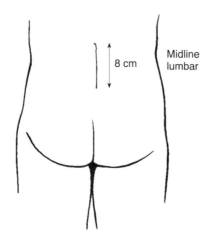

Lower back: Midline surgical scar from level of L2 to L5, with some keloid formation.

EXTENDED EXAMINATION OF THE SKIN

INDICATIONS

The skin has a number of special features not shared by other organ systems. It is highly and continuously accessible, provided we take the trouble to have the patient disrobe. Second, it is not confined to one anatomic region, and in that sense it powerfully illustrates the principle, "Examine regionally, think systemically," a statement that applies equally well to examinations of the lymph nodes, of the neurologic system, and of endocrine function. Many skin lesions have no systemic significance, but the examiner must think systemically at least for a moment in every case. For example, a wound that heals slowly and with exuberant granulation tissue might relate not only to poor local blood supply or regional infection but also to a systemic problem such as diabetes. Several other special principles apply.

History

The history can be relatively limited, although symptoms sometimes direct the inquiry and provide the diagnosis. For example, a history of itchy feet and ankles and a rash that developed just after switching soaps used for washing socks strongly suggests contact dermatitis regardless of what the skin looks like. If the skin appears absolutely normal in a 65-year-old who complains of 1 day of burning and pain in the left T6 dermatome, the probable diagnosis is herpes zoster (shingles). However, the more usual situation is incomplete illumination from the history, so that the examiner often relies predominantly on details of the physical examination. In this respect the skin has much in common with the eye.

SYMPTOMS

Cardinal symptoms of skin disorders include skin pain, pruritus, visible rash, or palpable mass. Any of these symptoms may arise from primarily extracutaneous disorders as well as from the skin itself.

SETTING

There is an extraordinary range of normal appearances of skin that spans changes related to age, race, degrees of solar damage, and other factors. In parallel, there is an immense prevalence of insignificant abnormal findings such as minor photoaging and seborrheic keratoses. So the examiner must discriminate normal from trivial within the epidemiologic group to which the patient belongs, or she won't separate major from minor or distinguish background from foreground.

A SPECIAL DISTINCTION

Physical signs in the skin are of two types: **pathophysiologic** and **symbolic** (or semiotic). In the former group, there exists understanding—not necessarily complete—of why the particular sign occurs in the disorder. A simple example is erythema at a fresh burn site, which reflects the vasodilation of acute inflammation. The other type of sign, the semiotic, bespeaks a condition, either local or systemic, but merely in the role of signpost: There is no known *mechanism* connecting illness and sign, but the association is recognized and exploited. One example of this is the red nail lunula in heart failure. We have no rational connection between the sign and the disease it speaks for. Of course, with the development of scientific insight, individual signs may move from one group to the other. The importance of recognizing whether a sign is physiologic or semiotic lies in being able to reason about its context and to place it within the total perspective of a patient's problems rather than to memorize lists of associations without insight.

In common with some other organs, the skin is capable of only a limited number of reaction patterns after *injury*. Therefore, the cutaneous manifestations of various diverse processes share common features. The lack of perfect specificity is shared by other parts of the history and the physical examination but is particularly striking with regard to the skin.

CONDUCTING THE EXTENDED EXAMINATION

Magnification

Magnification is a simple and powerful technique to determine the character of skin lesions. Although many lesions display an obvious and diagnostic character without any such effort, details of uniformity of pigmentation, for example, may call for the use of a good-quality magnifying glass.

Diascopy

Diascopy consists of pressing a flat transparent lens or other object against a lesion. It helps the examiner assess how much of a red or purple lesion represents *intravascular* blood. If the lesion consists principally of vascular congestion, it will blanch. The higher pressure to which the capillaries are passively subjected drives the red cells into adjacent vessels that have lower pressure. Failure to blanch or incomplete blanching suggests either that many red cells are extravasated or that the vasculature containing them is abnormal and does not permit free passage of cells. Thus a reddened hand on which you have sat while reading the past three paragraphs should blanch on diascopy, while a bruise should not. Kaposi's sarcoma includes both aberrant neoplastic vessels and extravasated erythrocytes, and therefore it does not blanch. Try diascopy of a simple capillary hemangioma (almost all adults have a few). You may be surprised by the result. Some masks and mimics of skin hemorrhage are listed in Table 3.1.

Examination in Better Light and in Daylight

Examination in better light and examination in daylight, which are two low-tech, high-touch, and unglamorous methods, are strikingly underutilized. Often a better look under the lights in an operating room changes or reinforces the preoperative diagnosis. For assessment of jaundice, daylight is indispensable. Fluorescent

Table 3.1
Red Rashes That Might Mimic or Mask Skin Hemorrhage

Condition	Comments or Caveats
Seborrheic dermatitis	Greasy yellow component, location on face usually distinguishes it
Erysipelas	Setting characteristic, with accompanying fever, sharp delineation, brilliant red rather than "venous" red-purple of ecchymoses
Kaposi's sarcoma	Variety of hues, shapes, and depths; in patient known to harbor HIV, consider even with apparent bruise (ecchymosis); may occasionally have surrounding yellow-brown breakdown just like ordinary ecchymosis
Trauma	Diffuse erythema may render it difficult to assess widespread erosion versus substantive extravasation
Acne rosacea	Location on face and nose, pustular component
Exfoliative erythroderma (exfoliative dermatitis)	Whole-body extent helps distinguish it

lighting is better than incandescent, but both produce more false-positive and false-negative results than inspection in daylight.

Palpation

The value of *touching* skin lesions deserves special emphasis. Disposable plastic gloves are mandatory for touching *any* lesion that might be infective or whose nature is completely mysterious in any patient regardless of HIV status. However, it is important and safe to use ungloved fingers to touch the *unbroken* skin of patients with AIDS to help reduce their devastating emotional sense of intentional isolation.

Gloves are vital for palpation of genitalia or oral mucosa. In these settings the gloves provide microbial protection. For genitalia, they also serve a critical psychosocial "distancing" function.

A special subset of *palpation* consists in determining whether a lump is intracutaneous or subcutaneous. If the skin can be slid over it, the mass is clearly subcutaneous; if the skin moves with it, it is either intracutaneous or, much less likely, tethered to the skin.

Wood's Light

The Wood's light, an ultraviolet light source, highlights certain features indistinguishable in ambient light. As long as the examiner lets it warm up long enough, darkens the room, and attends to proper precautions for its use, it can solve several kinds of bedside puzzles. Details appear in Table 3.2.

INTERPRETING THE FINDINGS
Rationale for Aggregation of Data by Region

In considering where to proceed beyond the basics with skin examination, one is struck by the contrast between a paucity of examination techniques and an intimidating plethora of content areas and signs. We attempt to make the body of information more accessible by presenting key conditions, each in its most common region of presentation. There are pitfalls, however: Any condition may develop at sites other than where it is here assigned. Thus the reader should be wary of using this chapter as a short handbook or list.

Table 3.2
Wood's Light Findings[a-c]

Process	Color under Wood's Light
Vitiligo	Bright white, sometimes with blue tinge
Postinflammatory hyperpigmentation	Purplish brown
Pseudomonas infection	Blue-green to blue
Erythrasma	Coral pink-red
Tinea versicolor	Yellow to golden-orange

[a]False-negative errors can result from washing within the previous 24 hours. Inadequate darkening of the room can also produce false-negatives, as can holding the source more than 10 cm from the area to be checked.
[b]Topical products can create false-positives.
[c]The light should not be shined on the cornea.

Generalized Skin Abnormalities
EXFOLIATIVE ERYTHRODERMA

Exfoliative erythroderma is a prototypical condition of involvement of the entire skin surface. It produces reddening of the whole body and can result (*a*) from psoriasis; (*b*) from an adverse drug reaction, sometimes of an allergic nature; (*c*) as a paraneoplastic phenomenon with internal cancer, especially malignant lymphoma; or (*d*) from direct infiltration of the skin with malignant lymphocytes in the variants of cutaneous T-cell lymphoma. The appearance is so striking that it can hardly be mistaken for anything else. When the pattern is mixed with typical silvery scales and crusts, it is recognized as psoriatic. If there is lymphadenopathy, lymphoma rises in the differential diagnosis, although exfoliative erythroderma itself frequently produces reactive lymph node enlargement (dermatopathic lymphadenopathy). If skip areas of normal-colored skin form islands amid the red, the condition is pityriasis rubra pilaris, a variant of psoriasis. In at least half the cases of exfoliative erythroderma no specific etiology can be found.

MEASLES

The rash of **classic measles (morbilli, rubeola)** begins at the hairline and spreads downward so that it eventually afflicts the whole skin surface. The innumerable tiny macules and papules may become confluent. The pattern is characteristic but nonspecific. Thus, many other rashes are also described as morbilliform (measles-like), which refers to the features of constituent lesions and to a tendency to involve the whole body. The term *morbilliform* does *not* mean that the rash in question spread down from the scalp edge.

Atypical measles can result from incomplete protection with killed-virus immunization and is therefore becoming rare. The rash of atypical measles is not as predictable as that of classic measles and may start at the wrists or elsewhere instead. It can also be hemorrhagic and can be confused with that of meningococcemia (see Atlas Plate IV*D*) or even that of dengue fever, a rarity in the United States but a condition with a high prevalence elsewhere on the globe.

OTHER EXANTHEMS AND ENANTHEMS

Distinction between one childhood viral infection and another has been made for many years on the basis of the pattern of purely cutaneous lesions (the classic viral **exanthems**) or combined skin and mucous membrane lesions (the **enanthems**). A few details about hemorrhagic rashes and lesions in febrile hosts are presented in Table 3.3. Many textbooks describe the constellations of signs and

Table 3.3
Hemorrhagic Rashes and Lesions in Febrile Patients

Condition and Classification	Comments or Caveats
Infectious Diseases	
Bacterial	
Meningococcemia	Petechiae may coalesce into large ecchymoses
Gonococcemia	Pustules often prominent; skin lesions may be scant
Staphylococcal bacteremia	Skin involvement variable, Janeway/Osler's
Bacterial endocarditis	nodes (metastatic and/or immune skin lesions?) and seek Roth spots
Pseudomonal bacteremia	Usually part of ecthyma gangrenosum
Subbacterial, e.g., rickettsial	
Rocky Mountain spotted fever	Predilection for wrists, ankles
Typhus	
Viral	
Enteroviremias, e.g., Coxsackie A virus	Skin involvement not classical, can have pustules, vesicles
Hemorrhagic measles	Mechanism of variant unclear
Immune Disorders	
Systemic lupus erythematosus	Petechiae may reflect vasculitis, thrombocytopenia, or both
Drug hypersensitivity reactions	Usually leukocytoclastic angiitis, the pathologic counterpart of hypersensitivity vasculitis, also seen with other causes
Purpura fulminans	Particularly rapid, malevolent variant, often with DIC[a]
Other	
Fat embolism syndrome	Petechiae; neurologic, respiratory compromise usually seen

[a]DIC, disseminated intravascular coagulation.

features that constitute the best-known syndromes, but this lies outside the scope of the present work. Individual signs in the exanthems and enanthems, such as Koplik's spots, have fallen somewhat in predictive value, particularly the predictive value of a negative test, as variants grow more numerous.

Localized Skin Problems

FOREHEAD AND/OR HEAD

The scalp is very commonly dry and flaky with dandruff, which is familiar to every nonmedical person. When unusually severe scalp flaking is associated with a greasy red-yellow discoloration and scale over the upper face, nose, and perioral zone, the process is **seborrheic dermatitis,** an extremely common condition, and one that is more prevalent and sometimes more pernicious in patients with neurologic disorders such as Parkinson's disease and in patients with AIDS.

Battle's sign consists of ecchymosis over the mastoid process. It is an insensitive sign of fracture of the base of the skull with hemorrhage into the middle cranial fossa. Its appearance is usually delayed some days after the fracture, diminishing its utility. Nevertheless, its high *specificity* renders it extremely useful when found. It also introduces the idea that certain specific locales and kinds of ecchymoses have more specific diagnostic value in assessing internal injury than the ordinary bruises and black-and-blue marks familiar to us all.

MALAR LESIONS AND FACIAL LESIONS

The facial and other lesions of **acne** are well known. They are primarily papular, cystic, and pustular, often partially ulcerated. They have physical features predictable from the acute inflammation that is part of their histology: erythema, edema, and tenderness. Besides the face, acne lesions are sometimes seen on the neck, upper back (see Atlas Plate III*D*) and even midback. When they occur outside the familiar setting of postpuberty through the early 20s, they can, but do not always, bespeak a hormonal imbalance such as corticosteroid excess or relative androgen excess. Thus in a less familiar *context* they become a hallmark of internal derangement (or of iatrogenic change!).

Loss of the lateral third of the eyebrows that occurs spontaneously rather than as a result of conscious cosmetic grooming—something determined from the history—may reflect **hypothyroidism.** It also occurs in normal aging, so that the predictive value of this **Queen Anne's sign** is slight. The sign deserves attention anyway because of the high prevalence, substantial morbidity, and easy treatment of the condition being sought.

When the eyes are surrounded by ecchymosis, the resulting appearance mimics a raccoon's mask and is therefore called the **raccoon eyes sign.** This is a less reliable indicator than Battle's sign but is employed in the search for evidence of skull fracture. The development of a raccoon eyes sign without major trauma, e.g., after placement in the Trendelenburg position, suggests vascular fragility and has assisted in the diagnosis of conditions with fragile vessels, such as amyloidosis and scurvy.

In the upper eyelids, the appearance of a purple color not due to makeup is the **heliotrope sign,** which is most highly associated with dermatomyositis. Perhaps it relates in some manner to the thinness of upper-lid skin, the most delicate in the body.

Two generations ago, malar erythema was often associated with severe mitral stenosis, and the look that it imparted to the face was described as a "mitral facies." Now this sign is vanishingly rare, and malar rashes, when not eczematous or seborrheic, are most often due to systemic lupus erythematosus. However, a study from a lupus clinic has shown that even among patients in a lupus center, most malar rashes are *not* lupus-related.

Darkening and reddening of the cheek areas are common in pregnancy, and constitute **melasma** and **chloasma,** respectively. These changes pose no threat to life or function and are nonprogressive, usually disappearing after delivery.

Patients with Immunosuppression or Leukopenia

Patients with immunosuppression or leukopenia are subject to a special set of skin problems in addition to the more common ones. Invasive fungal disease of the face and sinuses is one such condition, a devastating opportunistic infection that may present with nasal stuffiness and erythema of the skin overlying the maxillary antra, with or without palpable *fluctuance* there, generalized *facial edema, purulent nasal discharge,* or severe local tenderness. Although previously seen predominantly with mucormycosis, this syndrome is now increasingly reported with invasive aspergillosis also.

Patients with Bullous Disorders

Patients with bullous disorders commonly present with facial as well as intraoral lesions. The most important bullous diseases are bullous pemphigoid, which displays large intact bullae (see Atlas Plate IV*A*), and the more lethal pemphigus vulgaris, in which intact bullae are nowhere to be found so that the examiner discovers instead ruptured, flaccid bullae that may be mistaken for simple erosions (see Atlas Plate I*A*). Other conditions associated with bullae or their lesser cousins, vesicles, are listed in Table 3.4.

NOSE

The nose contains a high concentration of sebaceous glands, so that sebaceous disorders are often worst here. For example, there is an adult condition resembling acne plus telangiectases that is known as **rosacea.** This is due to improperly regulated cutaneous vascular dilation, with eventual structural consequences. It reaches its most severe form with hypertrophy of nasal soft tissues, **rhinophyma.** While alcoholism is sometimes suspected on the basis of these conditions, and

Table 3.4
Vesicular and Bullous Lesions and Rashes

Condition	Comments or Caveats
Infectious Diseases	
Viral	
Herpes simplex virus	Localized, vesicular, intensely painful
Herpes genitalis	Variant of herpes simplex occurring in perineal zone
Herpes zoster virus	
Chickenpox (varicella)	Generalized; crops of erupting vesicles, fever
Shingles	Typically dermatomal vesicles; often more widespread in patients with HIV coinfection
Molluscum contagiosum	Umbilicated lesions in which vesiculation is less conspicuous
Bacterial	
With erysipelas	Usually a minor component: erythema, skin edema predominate
With impetigo (transient)	Usually far less conspicuous than the purulent ulcerations
Direct Trauma	
Overlying fractures	Associated with extensive skin hemorrhage, "blood blisters"
Common blisters	Bullae, usually on feet, associated with marked exercise or trauma or with ill-fitting garments or weight-bearing straps
Associated with barbiturate overdose	One of several patterns of injury associated with these agents
With pressure ulcers	Setting usually makes nature of these bullae obvious
Immune Injury	
Drug hypersensitivity reactions	Long list of medicines may produce these
Eczematous contact dermatitis	Vesicles among erosions, scale, erythema
Dyshidrotic eczema (pompholyx)	Same, with history of frequent immersion, often on hand(s)
Primary Bullous Disorders	
Dermatitis herpetiformis	Associated with celiac disease; extensor surfaces, papules and vesicles
Bullous pemphigoid	Intact large bullae usually readily found
Pemphigus vulgaris	Intact bullae rare, usually shaggy surfaces of ruptured or flaccid bullae are found
Epidermolysis bullosa	Usually lifetime history; many variants

while alcohol can exacerbate the underlying vasodilation, many teetotalers develop the same problem.

A most devastating condition can start on the tip of the nose: HIV-associated *Kaposi's sarcoma.* The blue-purple to brown-red to bright-red lesions of this malignant neoplasm usually disrupt the pattern of the overlying epithelium even when they do not actually breach it. Kaposi's sarcoma presents an enormous spectrum of appearances, from one that resembles a simple bruise (Atlas Plate II*A*) or a plain capillary hemangioma, to a blackness recalling malignant melanoma. Its masks and mimics are legion. Thus the examiner must consider this diagnosis in virtually any purple, red, or dark skin lesion in a patient seropositive for HIV or at high risk of having HIV.

EXTENSOR SURFACES

The clinician may encounter extravasated red cells anywhere. The dorsum of the forearm is frequently affected, and bland ecchymosis here may reflect loss of skin turgor with aging, so-called **senile purpura.** Persons receiving substantial corticosteroid therapy are prone to morphologically similar lesions that are termed **steroid purpura.**

Psoriasis

Psoriasis is a very common dermatosis that may present anywhere on the body but has a special predilection for two extensor surfaces: elbows and knees. The lesions are so characteristic that diagnosis is usually unequivocal. Psoriatic lesions are sharply delimited, have silver scaly surfaces, and show a glossy erythema under the scale or, in some instances, near the scales. There are many variations of psoriasis; some lesions resemble classic lesions, e.g., those of pustular psoriasis. Others, such as purely red and unscaly vulvar lesions, do not look psoriatic except to the dermatologist, yet their psoriatic nature on biopsy is histopathologically clear-cut.

Xanthomas

Xanthomas are papules and nodules that reflect disordered lipoprotein metabolism. They occur in diverse settings and with diverse appearances, with the extensor tendon areas being one common locale. All form palpable three-dimensional lesions; a few show epidermal involvement and even ulceration, while more show only deep dermal or subcutaneous localization.

FLEXOR SURFACES

Many processes can localize to flexor surfaces. The various *eczemas* are the best known conditions that have a predisposition to flexor skin.

The antecubital fossa is frequently inspected for skin signs of *intravenous drug abuse,* such as noniatrogenic needle tracks and puncture marks. Unexplained skin punctures may be found anywhere as the addict progressively destroys more familiar sites for self-injection and with desperate ingenuity seeks new ones. No area is exempt. Darkened veins are usually seen, often with macroscopic white scars over parts of their surfaces. Fibrous remnants of skin infection, often with postinflammatory hyperpigmentation, commonly mark consequences of prior nonsterile needle punctures.

SUN-EXPOSED SKIN

Photoaging is covered under Screening Examination of the Skin. Lesions highly associated with solar toxicity and seen most frequently on the head, face, and hands include the following:

- *Actinic keratoses*, squamous cell *precancers* that are recognized by their reddish to light-brown color and sandpapery rough feel
- *Basal cell carcinomas*, which form pearly-colored and -textured exophytic masses on the surfaces of which telangiectases are often visible
- *Solar elastosis*, which often produces a crosshatched area of deep indentations on the back of a reddened neck (see below)
- *Malignant melanoma*, the most dangerous of all skin lesions

Pigmented Lesions: Melanoma

Malignant melanoma is extremely curable if recognized and treated early in its natural history but is highly lethal otherwise. It is an exemplar of an entity for which the examiner needs to screen carefully and to make the diagnosis from physical findings before any symptoms have developed. This is because the prognosis is usually dreadful by the time symptoms such as ulceration or itching have developed.

Part of the problem with melanoma is the *plethora of innocent pigmented lesions* that can mimic or mask this process. These are so numerous that it is impracticable to undertake excisional biopsy for diagnosis and simultaneous eradication of all pigmented lesions. The clinician needs to recognize features that suggest possible early malignancy. Start with a substantial index of suspicion, since the incidence of this malignancy has risen rapidly in recent decades. Be most attuned in lighter-skinned persons of whatever race. With regard to the *history,* bear in mind that the incidence doubles with every $10°$ of latitude closer to the equator and rises steeply in persons with a personal or family history of melanoma. It is also doubled in people who have had even one severe sunburn in the teen years.

The *life history of melanomas* is well characterized. Melanomas begin as macules and follow a prolonged period of scant growth or lateral growth only, before entering a vertical phase that ultimately provides access to lymphatics and blood vessels, leading to metastasis. What this means for the examiner is that *flatness—*a macular character—*does not exclude melanoma.* It is precisely in the flat phase that recognition by way of physical diagnosis followed by biopsy has the best chance of saving the patient's life (and without mutilatingly extensive surgery). Four physical examination criteria figure prominently in suspecting melanoma. These form the ABCD acronym or mnemonic (see also Table 3.5):

Asymmetry: Benign lesions tend to be symmetric about a reasonably easily seen axis, whereas melanomas may **not** be **symmetric.** As with the other criteria, this one displays imperfect sensitivity and specificity. On biopsy, some asymmetric lesions turn out to be benign nevi, and some proven melanomas are absolutely symmetric.

Borders: **Edges** that are **irregular** rather than smooth raise suspicion. Scalloped edges, *notches,* pseudopods or *"satellite" foci of pigment* discontinuous with a given lesion are of concern.

Color: **Very deeply pigmented** lesions, i.e., the truly black, are suspect. Even more worrisome are lesions with **highly variable pigmentation,** either within

Table 3.5

Characteristics Suspicious for Malignant Melanoma, the ABCD Schema

---

Asymmetry

Borders irregular

Color is very deep brown, black, highly variegated, red-white-and-blue, or there are areas of depigmentation

Diameter over 6 mm in greatest dimension

---

the lesion or in and about it (Atlas Plate III*B*). Dark brown plus white is not a combination one ignores or feels reassured about. Zones of depigmentation strongly suggest melanoma. Combinations of *red, white, and blue* call for definitive diagnosis, which is to say histologic evaluation.

Diameter: Lesions **larger than 6 mm** across, the size of a pencil eraser, are more likely than smaller lesions to be melanomas.

Other Pigmented Lesions

What other lesions may be confused with melanoma? They include a variety of melanocytic lesions, such as *ephelides* (singular, *ephelis*) and *lentigines* (singular, *lentigo*) which are mere freckles; and *melanocytic nevi,* which are benign neoplasms found in numbers on the skin of every adult except the very darkest. *Seborrheic keratoses* are another differential; they are "stuck-on", warty-looking, and *greasy-feeling* lesions that are extremely common in older persons. The shared histologic characteristic among all these is an excess of melanocytes or more uniform dispersion of melanin pigment, which accounts for the dark color that all may show. The color of some nonmelanocytic entities may fool the clinician into thinking that melanin is at work. These include occasional *dermatofibromas*—also known as sclerosing hemangiomas—as well as a few ordinary *capillary hemangiomas* and some instances of HIV-associated *Kaposi's sarcoma* in dark-skinned persons. In these cases, there may be excess melanin production or better dispersion in association with a nonmelanocytic lesion, which is the mechanism of darkening of seborrheic keratoses.

One bedside test to distinguish dark dermatofibroma from melanocytic lesions is the **dimple sign:** Lateral compression makes a dermatofibroma pucker inward but will "extrude" a nevus or a melanoma upward. Unfortunately, the test *does not discriminate between benign nevus and melanoma.*

Dysplastic Nevus Syndrome

Dysplastic nevi represent an increasingly recognized and very important substrate on which melanomas develop much more frequently than in age-matched controls. They have a number of characteristics on history and physical examination that differ from ordinary nevi, including a frequent familial inheritance, continued appearance of new lesions past age 30 (a rarity with ordinary nevi), extraordinarily numerous lesions in some instances, larger size, more occurrence on non-sun-exposed skin and on atypical areas, and a greater prevalence of lesional features associated with suspicion of melanoma, as detailed above.

It is crucial to remember that while solar damage predisposes to melanoma, malignant neoplasia can occur on any surface. In fact, melanomas of the soles carry a particularly adverse prognosis. Thus **the search for suspect pigmented lesions must encompass the entire body.**

NECK

The skin of the front of the neck is shaded by the head. Thus solar lesions are uncommon, whereas the back of the neck develops them with regularity. Deep furrows in this skin represent **solar elastosis,** a condition of no import except for those who find it cosmetically undesirable. However, the neck serves as a dosimeter for solar damage, so that marked solar elastosis should lead to enhanced surveillance for more threatening sun damage.

Skin tags, simple soft polyps of normal-looking and normal-feeling skin, are very common about the base of the neck, upper chest, and axillae (see Atlas Plate III**C**). They carry no systemic import in unselected patients. Thus searches for polyps by endoscopy or barium enema are not necessary in these patients, although some researchers have claimed that the incidence of polyps is higher in persons with skin tags—an unproven and semiotic rather than mechanistic hypothesis.

BREASTS AND AXILLAE

The commonest cutaneous physical finding of the breasts and axillae is *inframammary dermatitis,* typically caused by superficial mycosis in the moist zone beneath a pendulous breast. The condition presents an erythematous, tender, and often eroded zone, usually without frank purulence and almost always without edema. Long-ignored cases can produce some pustules, however. Associated hyperpigmentation (so-called postinflammatory hyperpigmentation) is common; the examiner also frequently encounters tiny damp white flakes of debris from skin cells, microbes, and inflammation.

Similar irritation and infection can occur in any other area subjected to the same moisture-retaining conditions, e.g., under a roll of abdominal adipose tissue or in the groin. All of these *intertriginous areas* are subject to superficial infection.

The overarching concern in examining the skin of the breast, as in examining the breast parenchyma, is *breast cancer.* Actual ulceration of the skin from breast cancer is uncommon except where treatment is not sought until very late in the natural history of the disease (see Atlas Plate ID). Tethering of the skin by the dense stroma elaborated in relation to a cancer is relatively common; it can sometimes be brought out by the maneuvers described in Chapter 6 when not seen on unaugmented inspection.

A special form of breast cancer with cutaneous signs is **Paget's disease of the breast,** an adenocarcinoma that grows outward in one or more lactiferous ducts. This carcinoma presents clinically as *apparent eczema or irritation of nipple and areola,* with a surface that is reddened, often superficially eroded and sometimes moist. There may or may not be a palpable mass beneath it. Because of this condition, every apparent irritation of the nipple-areolar complex outside the lactational period must be investigated for cancer.

Prominent veins of the breast are seen frequently as a physiologic change in pregnancy. At any other time, localized prominence of veins is considered a sign of probable cancer. When a mammary vein undergoes thrombosis, the condition is referred to as *Mondor's disease,* which may mimic cancer by producing a cord that feels like a mass or an area of postobstructive edema that resembles a cancer, perhaps with *peau d'orange* character, but is more tender than most cancers.

Hidradenitis suppurativa is a recurrent infection of sweat glands in the axilla, groin, or both. It produces all the cardinal features of acute inflammation (redness, swelling, tenderness, heat, and often expressible pus). Later, healing with scarring may mat the tissues together and deform them. The diagnosis is often obvious from the history and striking on the physical examination. It shouldn't resemble malignant axillary lymphadenopathy from breast cancer or lymphoma, which will produce nontender and uninflamed nodes that are usually palpably distinct from the overlying skin.

Freckles in the axillae are reported only in neurofibromatosis, for which they constitute **Crowe's sign,** which is allegedly pathognomonic. Surely a brown dot in an axilla might be a nevus instead. Do not put too much faith in *any* one-disease-with-one-sign connection.

Skin tags are also common in the armpits.

SUPERIOR VENA CAVAL DISTRIBUTION

Obstruction of the superior vena cava causes selective cutaneous cyanosis and plethora, venodilation, and edema constituting the **superior vena cava syn-**

drome. In the authors' experience, variations of the syndrome outnumber full-blown cases, so that one may find only a single arm or an arm plus the neck affected; variations are not always explicable on the basis of venous anatomy.

So-called **spider angiomata** also occur preferentially in the superior caval drainage and are a common and rather specific sign of *chronic* liver disease. They do not discriminate between chronic alcoholic damage and other etiologies. The mechanism for preferential occurrence in the superior caval distribution is obscure.

Spider angiomata are distinguished from simple clustered telangiectases by a pattern of "arms" or "spider legs" emanating more or less radially from a central point. Pressing this center will cause the "spider's legs" to disappear: When the central arteriole from which the peripheral components are filled is blocked, they soon empty.

ABDOMEN

The abdominal skin is infrequently involved with the ailments that cause the "acute abdomen," although occasional cases of appendicitis and peridiverticular abscess have "pointed" with erythema and surface signs over the intraperitoneal pathology.

Among the abdominal cutaneous signs of internal pathology are two variant ecchymoses, reflecting *flank discoloration* (Grey Turner's sign) and *periumbilical blueness* (Cullen's sign). They may be seen with blood extravasation and dissection, classically in pancreatitis wherein the release of enzymes facilitates tracking of the leaked blood across usual fascial barriers. They have also been reported in peritonitis from peritoneal dialysis, in splenic rupture from infectious mononucleosis, and in ruptured ectopic pregnancy, among many other conditions. Their detection always calls for prompt workup, since some of the causes can be rapidly fatal. The signs are perhaps more valuable for assessing *severity* (functional impact) than etiologic diagnosis.

The skin of the abdomen is sometimes the first site affected by morbilliform drug rashes of *medication (drug) allergy.* Drug rashes can assume almost any appearance on physical examination and can produce almost any physical finding. Often they are nonspecific-looking and nonspecific-feeling maculopapular rashes (see Atlas Plate III*A* and in the background of Plate II*A*). Sometimes, **palpable purpura** is present. This finding, in which the fingers perceive a *third dimension* in many or most of the petechiae, is a hallmark of capillaritis (vasculitis) and is not typical of thrombocytopenia alone. The specific pathoanatomic basis is leukocytoclastic vasculitis, the pathologic counterpart of *hypersensitivity vasculitis,* which may reflect an adverse drug reaction or any of a host of other stimuli. The nature of drug eruptions is suspected primarily from the history and secondarily from the rash pattern (with or without concomitant fever) and by blood and urinary indicators.

Scars on the abdomen are often abnormal in character in the patient with defective healing. Diabetics often show poor scar formation and widened scars. In several *inborn* immune deficiencies, exuberant hypertrophic scar (keloid) is typically formed after any skin damage. Curiously, this pattern is not described in AIDS.

Excess pigmentation of a surgical scar could reflect *postinflammatory hyperpigmentation* or an abnormality of the pituitary-adrenal axis, particularly hypoadrenalism. If the anterior pituitary is overproducing adrenocorticotropic hormone (ACTH) in response to primary adrenal insufficiency, there is likely a spillover effect with excess melanocyte-stimulating hormone (MSH). This leads to unduly dark pigmentation of *new* epithelium and subepithelium, i.e., darker-than-expected scars. If a patient has adrenocortical insufficiency on the basis of pituitary deficits, there is likely to be scant MSH, and unusually pale scars are then expected.

DERMATOMAL DISTRIBUTION

The best-recognized dermatomally distributed skin lesion is that of herpes zoster virus (HZV) infection. Unilaterality, dermatomal distribution—including any branch of the trigeminal nerve—and vesicles confirm the diagnosis. Patients with HIV infection often develop more severe zoster than others, with lesions that do not follow the rules: They may be bilateral and may traverse multiple dermatomes. Chickenpox, a different disease, although also caused by HZV, produces a generalized and nondermatomal rash.

PRESSURE ZONES

Pressure sores, also known as *pressure ulcers, decubitus ulcers,* and *bedsores,* are found at any point where skin and soft tissue are compressed against bony prominences. Typically, the host is immobile.

The most usual sites are the *sacrococcyx and intergluteal fold.* Other areas at risk correspond to all bony prominences of the body: greater trochanters, elbows, shoulder blades, lower ribs, ankles, heels, occiput and sides of the feet in the bedbound patient; lower back, buttocks, and ischial tuberosities in the chair-bound patient.

The classification of these very serious lesions follows Shea's schema, which depends on physical examination characteristics (Table 3.6) for insight about extent and prognosis:

- **Stage I lesions,** which include microscopic necrosis, show a *nonblanchable* erythema. The importance of diagnosis at this early stage lies with prevention of progression and, when treatment begins at this point, with the vastly superior therapeutic results.
- **Stage II pressure ulcers** show visible ulceration of the skin, but the base is recognizably in or about the dermis, i.e., has the white color of dermal collagen, insofar as the examiner can judge amid accompanying erythema and exudate.
- **Stage III bedsores** breach the full thickness of the skin, so that yellow fat is visible in the base and the visible depth is greater than that of a stage II lesion.
- **Stage IV decubitus ulcers,** the very worst, extend down to red muscle, white periosteum (see Atlas Plate IV), tendon, or viscera. They always look deep and horrifying. Often they show significant margins of black necrotic debris and eschar. Purulence and foul odor are often prominent also. There may be lesser degrees of ulceration, e.g., a stage II zone at one part of their rim concentrically about them.

Table 3.6
Shea Classification of Pressure Ulcers

Grade	Characteristics
1	Nonblanchable erythema, characteristically in pressure area
2	Frank ulceration, confined to the skin
3	Ulceration extending into subcutaneous fat
4	Ulceration extending to muscle, bone, or viscus

BACK

Pilonidal cysts often show a dimple overlying a prominent fold of skin and tissue at mid-lower back. Sometimes, there is a central pore through which purulent-looking and often foul matter is visible or otherwise detectable. Host characteristics help exclude the differential diagnoses, such as atypically deep and narrow pressure ulcer. In an ambulatory 25-year-old, there is no trouble deciding which is present. However, in a bedridden centenarian, the examiner might discover a pilonidal sinus and cyst even when the setting is ripe for pressure ulcers also.

Large **collateral arteries** may be seen over the shoulder blades and in between them in some cases of **coarctation** of the aorta. However, this sign is not sensitive enough or early enough to be a useful screen for coarctation in unselected hypertensive patients.

PERIANAL AREA

External hemorrhoids present as small gray-blue to flesh-colored masses near the anal verge. They can undergo thrombosis. When they do, the degree of accompanying inflammation, ulceration, and trauma determines the extent of erythema, white fibrinous surface exudate, and tenderness on examination. The characteristic symptom is *continuous pain,* not merely pain on defecation.

Exquisitely tender linear breaks in the perianal skin are likely to be **fissures in ano.** The unwary examiner may regard the patient as exaggerating the discomfort associated with them, since many are minuscule. These do tend to hurt only when touched or with defecation or wiping.

Larger, more ragged and inflamed defects in the perianal skin may represent the cutaneous exit points of **fistulae in ano,** which occur most frequently in Crohn's disease, and may exit perianally, on the labia of the vulva, or anyplace in or about the perineum.

A few of the many other skin disorders in this area are discussed in Chapters 13 and 14.

GENITALIA

A host of skin lesions of great importance may occur in the genital region. Several are described in Chapters 13 and 14 rather than here.

Genital herpes simplex virus infection is recognized by tiny vesicles on erythematous bases. Its key attribute is severe pain that frequently precedes the development of the physical signs.

Genital warts (**condylomata acuminata**) result from infection with specific strains of human papilloma virus (HPV) that differ from those that cause common warts of hands, feet, and other nongenital sites. The importance of these lesions is not only cosmetic and local but also systemic: Some strains cause cancers of the vulva, penis, and uterine cervix. Genital warts classically appear as papillomatous masses (warty, with fronds), usually quite small, typically white-pink, and sometimes clustered on the penis, vulva, perineum, scrotum, or anal region.

Vulvar dystrophies are a heterogeneous group of discolorations, usually macular or patch-like rather than raised, that can occur in women of any age. They are found most commonly in the later reproductive years or beyond. Some are associated with increased cancer risk. Most produce white or pink zones with loss of skin markings, sometimes with overt skin atrophy—thinned, shiny skin or, in a variant, very fine wrinkling that has been compared to the texture of cigarette paper. They seldom cause frank or macroscopic ulceration, which is more typical of syphilis (see below) and Behçet's vasculitis. The principal differential diagnosis of the vulvar dystrophies is **atrophic vulvovaginitis.** One major distinguishing criterion is diffuseness: If widespread, it is likely to be atrophic vulvovaginitis.

The old prototype genital lesion in both sexes is the shallow painless ulcer of primary syphilitic infection, the **chancre.** This is typically solitary and may occur under the foreskin, on the glans or shaft, or anywhere in the lower female genital tract (including on the cervix, in which case it can be noticed only on speculum examination). Other genital ulcers, typically more painful, include the lesions of bacterial **chancroid,** which is relatively uncommon in the United States but highly prevalent in some other countries.

Fordyce spots are small red hemangiomas of the scrotal skin. They are a normal if sometimes overinterpreted finding in adults, particularly men of middle age and older. When they occur in boys, they are associated with the storage disorder, **Fabry's disease.**

With rupture of or leakage from the lower aorta, the examiner may rarely find the **blue scrotum sign of Bryant.** To produce this, extravasated blood tracks down and discolors the scrotum or even the penis. The importance of this sign lies not only in pointing to the life-threatening underlying condition but also in reminding us of the continuity between peritoneal space and intrascrotal space, which leads to *scrotal swelling in tense ascites.*

HANDS

Dermatitis—skin irritation—of the hands is extremely common. It presents with roughening of the dorsum of the hand, more rarely with palmar flaking and soreness, and sometimes with maceration and vesicles in the webs between fingers and on the lateral surfaces of the fingers. The last-named pattern is most typical of **dyshidrotic eczema** (pompholyx), while the others may be seen in **contact dermatitis** of both allergic and irritant varieties. **Occupational skin disease** is prototypically manifested by dermatitis, and the hands are the prime locale, since they are so commonly exposed to toxic substances, heat, prolonged immersion, and endless noxious stimuli from which one instinctively averts the face and eyes.

Clubbing represents a final common pathway for a variety of abnormalities ranging from bronchiectasis and lung cancer to cirrhosis of the liver and cyanotic congenital cardiac malformations. Despite a century of intensive investigation, the mechanisms of its production and the reasons why its "penetrance" is so variable have eluded detection. The fundamental abnormality is an overgrowth of soft tissues beneath the nail (and toenails may be affected as well as fingernails). Many persons have prominent terminal phalanges without clubbing. The three most reliable markers of genuine clubbing are

1. **Loss of the hyponychial angle** (see Atlas Plate IIC). Examine your own left index finger from the medial side. Note that the hyponychial angle made by the very base of the nail and the adjacent proximal skin is slightly less than 180°. In the person with clubbing, it will be slightly more. Be sure to measure the angle made with the proximal part of the nail, not the main axis of the nail, which produces many false-positive readings.
2. **Ballotability of the nailbed.** Unfortunately, this marker is also found in some very old people who do not have clubbing. Outside of that group, it is a reliable sign. Press on the skin just proximal to nail and see if it springs back up at once. If so, there is clubbing.

   To learn the difference between normal and abnormal, do the following: With your right index finger, press on the soft tissue immediately proximal to your left index fingernail. There will be no bounce-back. Then place tension on that same left index nail by pulling its free edge downward with the terminal pulp of your *left* thumb. Upon then indenting the nailbed just proximal to the nail with your right index finger, you will appreciate a very different sensation.

3. **Schamroth's sign.** This sign is loss of the "window" normally created by apposition of the terminal phalanges of paired digits. Schamroth was a physician who developed recurrent clubbing during three bouts of bacterial endocarditis.

Fingertip ulcers are seen with vasospastic *Raynaud's phenomenon* in its gravest setting, systemic sclerosis (see Atlas Plate IIC). Periungual blackening, by contrast, occurs with small digital infarctions in *small vessel vasculitis* from extreme rheumatoid disease or from systemic lupus erythematosus.

The fingernails and toenails offer a host of clues to disease on examination. Two pertinent examples are (*a*) discoloration with cancer chemotherapeutic agents including zidovudine (AZT) for HIV infection and (*b*) onycholysis—ragged dissolution of the distalmost part of the nail, with separation from the underlying skin tissue—in Graves' hyperthyroidism.

SHINS

Venous ulcers produce shallow epithelial defects, sometimes complicated by infection of the ulcer bed or by a surrounding cellulitis. They characteristically occur about the medial malleolus. Chronic venous insufficiency will usually have produced frequent small extravasations with hemosiderin residues that make numerous tiny to confluent rust-colored macules in the background skin of the region.

There are no reliable skin markers for **deep venous thrombosis.** Swelling of the limb and several other features may raise the clinician's index of suspicion. Erythema and local venodilation, as well as warmth, are so common in primary acute infection of the skin and subcutis (*cellulitis*) without venous obstruction as to be useless in furthering the differential diagnosis.

Diabetic shin spots are **sunken** brownish spots over the anterior shins and related zones. They are not pathognomonic, also being seen with chronic immune suppression in kidney transplant patients as a part of their poor wound healing. A more dramatic and uncommon diabetic finding is **necrobiosis lipoidica diabeticorum,** whereby a large sunken and partially ulcerated area assumes a yellow-white sickly hue. This is seen even in younger diabetics without clinical vascular disease.

Erythema nodosum consists of nodules deep in the subcutaneous fat, with or without overlying erythema and slight heat. It is seen without known cause in some hosts, as an adverse medication reaction in others, and as a manifestation of an underlying condition, especially *inflammatory bowel disease* (particularly Crohn's colitis), *sarcoidosis* or *tuberculosis,* in still others. The more common skin manifestation of **ulcerative colitis,** by contrast, is a deep purulent ulcer of the calf or elsewhere called **pyoderma gangrenosum.** This is not infected, but looks it. It too can occur as an isolated condition or, less commonly, secondary to other systemic inflammatory disorders.

FEET

Diabetic foot ulcers present variously sharp to ragged defects on the sole, often over bony prominences proximal to the metatarsal heads. They may appear clean or purulent and shaggy. Depending on whether blood flow suffices to support inflammation and depending on the hygienic and nursing care to which they have been subjected, they may look as serious as they are or more so or (commonly) less so. Their locale on the sole is distinct from the toes and dorsa of the feet, which are more usual sites for purely ischemic lesions; diabetic neuropathy with repetitive unrecognized trauma may play a role in this selective localization. The ominous interpretation of this lesion is covered in Chapter 10.

Tinea pedis is a superficial fungal infection better known as **athlete's foot.** It is frequent in the moist web spaces between the toes, as well as on the sole. It produces varying degrees of pruritus, tenderness, and desquamation of white epithelium with scant exudate. The value of recognizing and treating this condition lies partly in restoring the integrity of the epithelial barrier and thus preventing the access of bacteria such as streptococci that can cause cellulitis.

Gangrene of the toes most commonly complicates severe arterial insufficiency. Two forms are recognized: **dry gangrene,** which represents coagulative necrosis of skin, with or without infarction of deeper tissue (see Atlas Plate IVC); and **wet gangrene,** which is usually a complication of dry gangrene whereby ulceration, infection, and purulent to seropurulent exudate supervene.

SKIN FINDINGS OF SYSTEMIC (OR INTERNAL) DISEASE

Skin findings of systemic (or internal) disease form a large topic unto themselves. The reader is referred to the Recommended Readings for definitive information in this vast and fascinating sphere.

For our purpose, let a single example suffice: the **sign of Leser-Trélat,** in which the sudden and explosive development of numerous seborrheic keratoses may reflect a visceral, noncutaneous malignancy. The importance of such signs resides in the opportunity for early diagnosis of the internal disorder, before it would be detectable otherwise, with superior therapeutic results. Whereas many such signs remain purely semiotic, the pathophysiology of the Leser-Trélat sign has recently been studied. It appears to involve paraneoplastic production of an epithelial growth factor-like substance. A few skin signs of internal *cancer* are mentioned in Table 3.7.

RECORDING THE FINDINGS

Sample Write-up

Examination: 18-year-old medium-complected woman with family history of melanoma in two first-degree relatives. Little solar damage seen on back of neck or elsewhere. However, has 18 brown macules and patches scattered on the head, neck, shoulders and superior aspects of breasts. These range from 0.3 to 1.9 cm across; some have irregular borders; none black, ulcerated, or highly variably pigmented.

Impression: Possible dysplastic nevus syndrome (familial?). Will need regular physician reexamination, self-examination, serial photography for monitoring, and solar protection.

BEYOND THE PHYSICAL EXAMINATION

The investigation of skin lesions embodies limited technology, since the organ in question is so accessible to direct inspection and palpation. The principal method of laboratory analysis is *microscopic examination of scrapings or exudate,* often with *specimen treatment with potassium hydroxide and heat* to render the keratin content of squamous cells transparent and so permit the causative fungal organisms to be visualized. Although *Gram stains* of skin material are feasible, interpretation can be clouded by the large resident flora of the region; demonstration of a single bac-

Table 3.7
Skin Signs of Internal Malignancy[a]

Name of Sign	Nature of Sign	Commonest Site/ Type of Cancer
Sign of Leser-Trélat	Eruptive development of numerous seborrheic keratoses; exaggerates normal phenomena	Adenocarcinomas, but not uniform
Acanthosis nigricans	Velvety brown-black lesions in axillae, neck, sometimes groin	Carcinoma of stomach
Tylosis palmaris et plantaris	Hard white keratosis of palms and soles, not related to trauma or occupation	Squamous carcinoma of esophagus
Necrolytic migratory erythema	Coalescent patches of erythema with vesicles and bullae	Glucagonoma (a rare pancreatic islet cell neoplasm)
Dermatomyositis	Most commonly symmetric heliotrope (purple) rash of eyelid(s), especially upper lids, and Gottron's papules; violaceous plaques over knuckles (metacarpophalangeal joints) and other finger joints	Any internal cancer
Exfoliative erythroderma	Bright red discoloration and some-times shedding and scale, often over whole body	Most typically malignant lymphoma
Herpes zoster infection (shingles)	Usually painful vesicles in dermatomal (or polydermatomal) distribution	Disproven as marker for cancer; predicts more aggressive progression to AIDS in patients with HIV seropositivity
Sweet's syndrome (acute febrile neutrophilic dermatosis)	Ulcerated, purulent-based nodules, especially on hands	Leukemias, sometimes solid tumors

[a]None of these is independent proof of an internal cancer; each carries with it some differential diagnoses. For example, acanthosis nigricans is also seen with some endocrinopathies, with obesity, and as a benign familial condition.

terial morphology may help, however. The technique works very well on pus, exudate of any kind, or material aspirated from the leading edge of what on physical examination appears to be an advancing *cellulitis.*

The other major investigation of cutaneous problems is by **skin biopsy.** This extends the diagnostic reach in cases that are not diagnosable by history and physical examination alone. Skin biopsy is widely used by many expert derma-tologists. It is a quick, simple, and cheap procedure devoid of significant morbid-ity. Biopsy is useful not only in studying neoplasms but in characterizing a vast array of inflammatory and reactive disorders, as well as in diverse situations ranging from amyloidosis to inborn errors of metabolism.

RECOMMENDED READINGS

Boyce JA, Bernhard JD. Routine total skin examination to detect malignant melanoma. J Gen Intern Med 1987;2:59–61.

Callen JP, Jorizzo J, Greer KE, Penneys N, Piette W, Zone JJ. Dermatological signs of internal disease. Philadelphia: WB Saunders, 1988.

Cwach NL, Driscoll CE. Wood's light examination. Patient Care 1990;24:153–154, 156.

Fallon TJ, Abell E, Kingsley L, et al. Telangiectasias of the anterior chest in homosexual men. Ann Intern Med 1986;105:679–682.

Fitzpatrick TB, Gilchrest BA. Dimple sign to differentiate benign from malignant pigmented cutaneous lesions. N Engl J Med 1977;296:1518.

Friedman RJ, Rigel DS, Kopf AW. Early detection of malignant melanoma: the role of physician examination and self-examination of the skin. CA 1985;35:130–151.

Kelly JW, Crutcher WA, Sagebiel RW. Clinical diagnosis of dysplastic melanocytic nevi: a clinicopathologic correlation. J Am Acad Dermatol 1986;14:1044–1052.

Martin L, Khalil H. How much reduced hemoglobin is necessary to generate central cyanosis? Chest 1990;97:182–185.

Strobach RS, Anderson SK, Doll DC, Ringenberg QS. The value of the physical examination in the diagnosis of anemia: correlation of the physical findings and the hemoglobin concentration. Arch Intern Med 1988;148:831–832.

Witkowski JA, Parish LC. The touching question. Int J Dermatol 1981;20:426.

4

Head, Eyes, Ears, Nose, Oral Cavity, and Throat

SCREENING EXAMINATION OF THE HEAD, EYES, EARS, NOSE, ORAL CAVITY, AND THROAT

APPROACH AND ANATOMICAL REVIEW

Since this book follows a regional approach to physical examination, some orientation is indicated here. The head, eyes, ears, nose, oral cavity, and throat (HEENT) examination incorporates many structures of the head, including special sensory organs and several cranial nerves, rendering this examination highly complex in terms of systems and detail. However, the efficiency of inspection, palpation, and the neurologic assessment of all structures of the head that are in anatomical proximity justifies this use of *topographic* rather than systemic data acquisition. It is then the examiner's job to arrange these data both anatomically and by organ system—neurologic localization included—both mentally and in the case write-up. See Table 4.1 for a review of a logical sequencing of this regional examination and Table 4.2 for a listing of the cranial nerves studied here. The numerous instruments and supplies required for HEENT examination are listed in Table 4.3.

This portion of the examination is conducted with the patient seated, eyes level with the examiner's. The examiner faces the patient and is free to move from side to side, avoiding time-wasting changes of patient position. Likewise, for efficiency, changes of instruments are minimized; thus neurologic assessment is interwoven with other maneuvers. (Note that because of the number of structures to be included in this chapter, the anatomical review will be presented with each subsection.)

TECHNIQUE

Head and Scalp

INSPECTION

The head is inspected for its contour, size, and general shape (Fig. 4.1*A* and *B* for landmarks). The amount and distribution of scalp hair are noted. Careful inspection of the scalp calls for lifting sections of hair, separating them to reveal underlying skin at several sites. Is the skin normal, without lesions? Is the hair evenly distributed?

PALPATION

While raising strands of hair to inspect the scalp, note the texture of the hair. Is it unusually dry or coarse? Does it come out when gently tugged? Palpate the contour of the cranium for protrusions or depressions. It should be symmetrical and generally smooth except for the normal mastoid prominence behind and inferior to each ear. If there are other protuberances or depressions, they should be characterized and their location and dimensions should be measured and recorded. If skin lesions have been noted on inspection, they should be palpated and their characteristics should be noted (see Chapter 3).

Table 4.1
Sequence of the Screening HEENT Examination[a]

Head and scalp
Face
    CN VII: facial mobility
    CN V
        Sensory to skin of face and cornea
        Motor to muscles of mastication
Eyes and periorbital structures
    CN III, IV, and VI: extraocular muscle movement
    CN II
        Visual acuity
        Visual fields
    CNs II and III: pupillary reflexes
    CNs V and VII: corneal reflexes
    Ophthalmoscopic examination
Ears
    External ears (auricles)
    CN VIII
        Hearing acuity
        Vestibular function
    Otoscopic examination
        Auditory canals
        Tympanic membranes
Nose and nasal cavity
Oral cavity and contents
    CN X: palatal elevation
    CN XII: tongue protrusion
Oropharynx
    CNs IX and X: pharyngeal contraction ("gag")

[a]CN, cranial nerve.

Table 4.2
Cranial Nerves[a]

"On Old Olympus' Towering Top
A Finn and German Viewed Some Hops."
Old Clinician's Mnemonic

CN I ("On")—**Olfactory:** sense of smell
    TESTS
        See Extended Examination section
CN II ("Old")—**Optic:** visual acuity
    TESTS
        Snellen chart for distance vision
        Printed card for near vision
        Visual fields (by confrontation technique)
        Component of direct and consensual pupillary light reaction
CN III ("Olympus")—**Oculomotor:** motor nerve to five extrinsic eye muscles, superior rectus, inferior rectus, medial rectus, inferior oblique, and palpebrae superioris the outermost fibers of the third cranial nerve innervate pupillary constriction.
    TESTS
        Extraocular eye movements, excluding conjugate motion
        Pupillary response to light (direct and consensual) and accommodation

Table 4.2 (*continued*)

CN IV ("Towering")—**Trochlear:** motor nerve to superior oblique extrinsic eye muscle (downward and inward movement of eye)
> TESTS
>> Extraocular eye movement

CN V ("Top")—**Trigeminal**
A. Sensory to skin of face and cornea
> TESTS
>> All sensation for facial skin representing three divisions of nerve (V1, V2, V3)
>> Corneal reflex component

B. Motor to muscles of mastication
> TESTS
>> Bite and bulk of masseter muscle

CN VI ("A")—**Abducens:** motor to the lateral rectus muscles of eyes (lateral movement)
> TESTS
>> Lateral (abducent) extraocular movement of each eye

CN VII ("Finn")—**Facial**
A. Motor to muscles of face
> TESTS
>> Smile—symmetry of lower facial muscle movement
>> Frown—symmetry of forehead movement, tight eyelid closure

B. Sensory for taste, anterior two-thirds of tongue
> TESTS
>> See Extended Examination section

CN VIII ("And")—**Acoustic:** sensory
A. Cochlear branch: hearing acuity
> TESTS
>> Watch ticking, fingers rubbing, measured audible distance of whisper for symmetry

B. Vestibular branch: balance
> TESTS
>> Nystagmus on lateral gaze (Romberg test, visible tremor, past pointing,
>> abnormal results on "cerebellar" tests)

CN IX ("German")—**Glossopharyngeal**
A. Motor (elevation) of posterior pharynx; laryngeal musculature
> TESTS
>> Gag reflex, deglutition, invoice quality, water swallowing

B. Sensory: taste to posterior one-third of tongue
> TESTS
>> See Extended Examination section

CN X ("Viewed")—**Vagus:**
A. Motor: deglutition, elevation of palate, laryngeal musculature
> TESTS
>> Say "haaat"—symmetrical elevation of palate; voice quality; water swallowing

B. Sensory: pharynx and larynx
> TESTS
>> "Gag" reflex—afferent loop

CN XI ("Some")—**Spinal accessory:** motor to trapezius and sternomastoid muscles
> TESTS
>> A. Rotating the head against force
>> B. Shrugging the shoulders against force

CN XII ("Hops")—**Hypoglossal:** motor to the tongue
> TESTS
>> Protruding the tongue in the midline
>> Protruding the tongue into each cheek

---

[a]CN, cranial nerve.

Table 4.3
Equipment and Supplies for the HEENT Examination

Bright light source (penlight, lamp, or diagnostic kit light)
Prepared brain, eyes, ears, fingers
Wristwatch or other mobile sound source
Visual acuity chart(s)
Ophthalmoscope
Otoscope with disposable specula
Light source (penlight, flashlight) with nasal speculum
Tongue blades
Disposable (nonsterile) gloves
Cotton swab or wisp for light-touch stimulus
Broken swab stick for "sharp" pain stimulus
2×2 gauze squares

Face

INSPECTION

Is the face symmetrical? If asymmetry of structures is found, the nature of the differences should be assessed. For example, is one orbit smaller than the other? Does the nose deviate to one side? Is the smile or mouth movement crooked? Is the chin too large for the remainder of the face (**prognathia: protuberant jaw;** macrognathia: enlarged jaw), or is the jaw tiny and recessed (micrognathia)? Do both sides of the face move evenly when the patient talks or laughs?

CRANIAL NERVE VII: MOTOR BRANCH TO THE FACIAL MUSCLES

Each seventh cranial nerve (CN) innervates the ipsilateral muscles of the forehead, the eyelid, the cheek, and perioral area (Fig. 4.2). Function of the bilateral nerves in concert is assessed as follows (Fig. 4.3):

1A. Ask the patient to frown or wrinkle the brow; observe for symmetry of the motion from side to side.

or

1B. Ask the patient to close both eyelids and resist the examiner's attempt to lift them open.

2A. Ask the patient to smile; observe for symmetrical elevation of the corners of the mouth.

or

2B. Ask the patient to puff out both cheeks; observe for symmetrical contour of the puffed cheeks.

CRANIAL NERVE V

Sensory to the Skin of the Face

1. *Light touch:* Pick up a cotton swab and tug out a few strands to make a fluff. Ask the patient to close his eyes. Instruct the patient that you will be touching him on various portions of the face. He is to indicate when he feels the cotton fluff and where he perceives the contact. Recall that CN V has three divisions on each side of the face that should be checked (see Fig. 4.4 for dermatomes of the three divisions of the trigeminal: the forehead is served by the first division (ophthalmic); the cheek, by the second division (maxillary); and the jaw, by the third division (mandibular)). Touch each skin area on each side, in random fashion, asking the patient to respond to the touch as directed above.

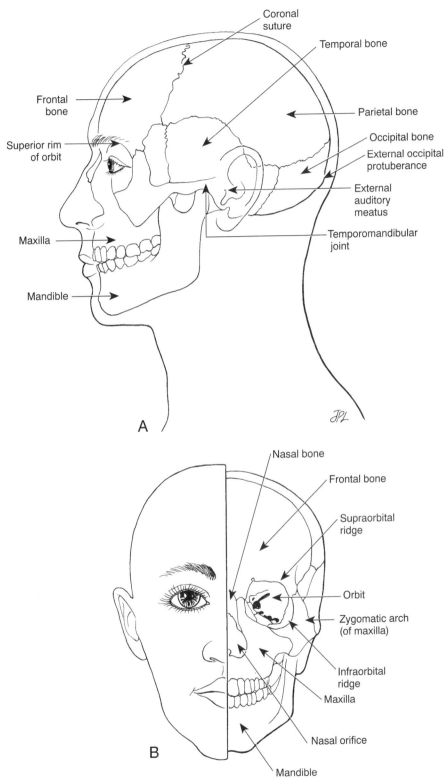

Coronal
suture

Temporal bone

Frontal
bone

Parietal bone

Superior rim
of orbit

Occipital bone

External occipital
protuberance

External
auditory
meatus

Maxilla

Temporomandibular
joint

Mandible

A

Nasal bone

Frontal bone

Supraorbital
ridge

Orbit

Zygomatic arch
(of maxilla)

Infraorbital
ridge

Maxilla

Nasal orifice

B

Mandible

Figure 4.1 **A.** Bony structure and landmarks of the head, left lateral view. **B.** Bony structure
and landmarks of the head, frontal view.

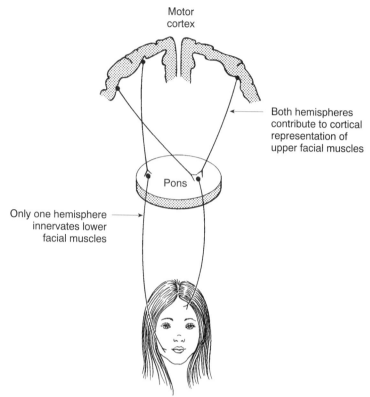

Figure 4.2   Schematic representation of CN VII, from its cortical sources to its peripheral projections.

2. *Pain:* An alternative to light touch perception is that of pain in the same three divisions of CN V. Using a broken swab-stick—not a pin or needle—and a firm cotton swab, ask the patient to discriminate between *sharp* and *dull.* Instructions to the patient include closure of the eyes to avoid visual cuing and a response that includes the sensation perceived—sharp or dull—and the area where the stimulus is felt, e.g., "right cheek" or "left forehead."

Motor to Muscles of Mastication

The masseter muscles are palpated bilaterally simultaneously as the patient is instructed to "bite down hard." Upon clenching the jaws, both masseter muscles should become equally firm and bulky. Asymmetry in bulk or tension of the two muscles should be noted and recorded.

Eyes and Periorbital Structures

INSPECTION

Structures about the eye to be inspected include the brows and lashes, bony orbits, lids, conjunctivae and corneae, sclerae, irides, and pupils (Fig. 4.5).

The **brows** and **lashes,** although dermal appendages, are most efficiently inspected as parts of the face. The brows are noted for symmetry and contour. Lashes, like brows, vary widely in their range of normal appearance but should be present and symmetrical.

The **eyelids** are protective structures composed of skin, conjunctiva on their tarsal linings, and muscle. Ask the patient to close his lids gently, and then look at them for symmetry of closure and presence or absence of swelling, nodularity,

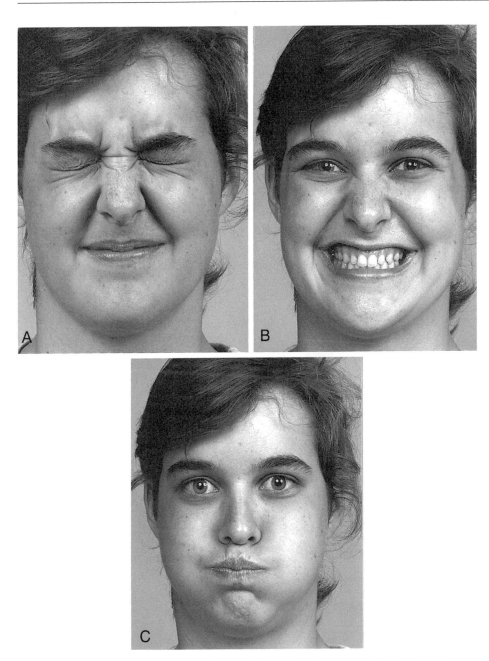

Figure 4.3   Testing the function of CN VII. **A.** Volitional closure of both eyelids (upper divisions). **B.** Exaggerated smile (lower divisions). **C.** Puffed cheeks, alternate test for lower divisions.

or tremor. With the lids open, note the symmetry of exposure of the iris and surrounding sclera. In the open position, the upper lid should extend slightly below the superior rim of the iris, and the lower lid usually allows exposure of a small rim of sclera beyond the limbus (junction of iris and sclera). The tarsal conjunctiva should not be separately visible.

   With thumbs immediately under the lower lashes, pull the lower lids downward to view the inferior recess of the **conjunctiva;** observe for exudate, erythema, or nodularity. For the technique of inspecting additional conjunctiva, look at Conducting the Extended Examination section of this chapter.

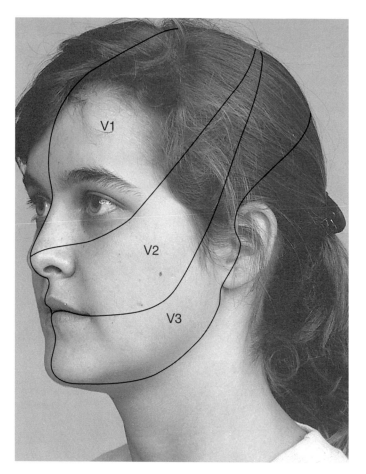

Figure 4.4 Facial distribution of the three divisions of CN V. *V1,* ophthalmic; *V2,* maxillary; and *V3,* mandibular.

The **sclera** makes up the "white" of the eye. Inspect for increased vascularity—"redness"—or other discoloration and for exposure relative to the eyelids. The **cornea** is a transparent extension of the conjunctiva that overlies the iris and thus ends at the limbus. If normal, the cornea cannot be perceived as a separate structure. The **iris,** the visible colored disc of the eye, is a pigmented muscular diaphragm whose central aperture (the pupil) enlarges and contracts to control admission of light to the sensitive retinal structures. Inspect the irides for sharp borders and for consistency of size and of color. The **pupil** is the black circle residing within the iris, the size of which is altered by contraction of the iris. Normal pupils are perfectly round with sharp margins, black, and symmetrical in size under equal light stimulation. Observe for any deviation from this normal configuration.

PALPATION

Ask the patient to close his eyes. The **orbits** may now be palpated for bony symmetry and smoothness. Palpation of the globes (eyeballs) should be reserved for special indications (see the Extended Examination section of this chapter). If swelling or asymmetry of any periorbital structure has been noted on inspection, palpate the area in question. If tenderness or nodularity is found in any periorbital structure, note its location, characteristics of color and consistency, dimensions, and presence or absence of tenderness to manipulation.

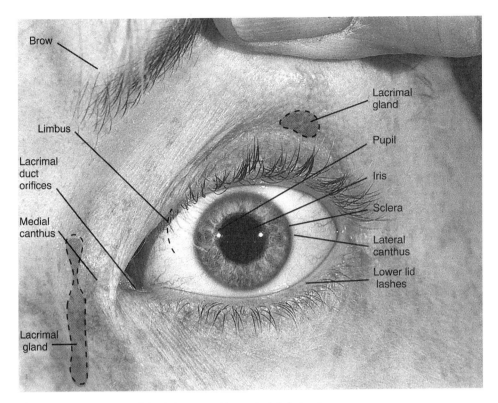

Figure 4.5   Anatomy of the left eye and its periorbital structures.

CRANIAL NERVES III, IV, AND VI: EXTRAOCULAR MUSCLE MOVEMENT

The symmetrical tracking of the eyes that permits focused binocular vision is controlled by a well-matched and integrated set of muscles regulated by three cranial nerves (Fig. 4.6C1 and C2). Basic functional testing of these muscles and nerves is accomplished in the following manner:

1. The examiner faces the patient directly, at eye level, and at approximately 30-cm distance.
2. Using a finger or other object as focal point, the examiner asks the patient to follow with his eyes the movement of the object without moving his head.
3. The examiner moves the object systematically through six directions of motion (Fig. 4.6B2–B7) while noting the symmetry of the patient's eye movement. Any unilateral deviation of eyeball motion or patient complaint of double vision should be noted and recorded.

CRANIAL NERVE II

Visual Acuity

Acuity of vision is a test of CN II, specifically central visual discrimination. Distance vision is estimated by means of the Snellen or "E" chart. This measurement requires a wall chart and a 6-meter distance; ideally, it is done as a part of the preliminary screening of any new patient and thus is discussed in Chapter 2. At this point in the regional examination, near vision may be estimated by use of a near-vision pocket card (such as the Rosenbaum model). The card is held 35 cm from the patient's eyes (or at whatever distance is specified on the instructions), and he is asked to read the smallest line clearly visible.

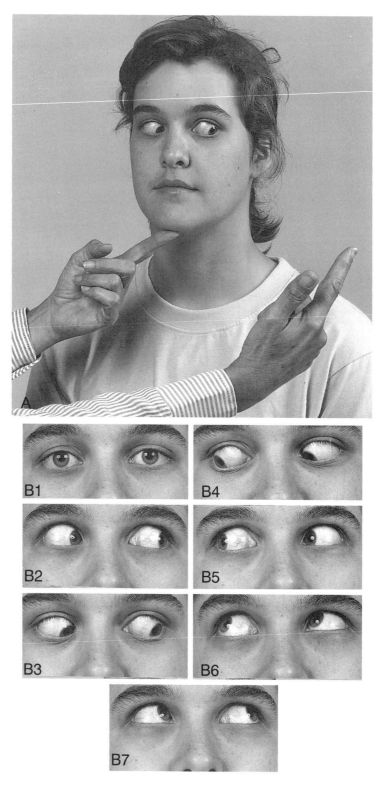

Figure 4.6 Testing of extraocular movements (CNs III, IV, and VI). **A.** Proper positioning of patient and examiner. **B1.** Normal, resting position. **B2.** Conjugate left lateral gaze. **B3.** Left down and lateral gaze. **B4.** Right down and lateral gaze. **B5.** Conjugate right lateral gaze. **B6.** Right up and lateral gaze. **B7.** Left up and lateral gaze. **C1.** Schematic summary of muscles controlling eye movements. **C2.** Tabular summary of nerves controlling eye movements.

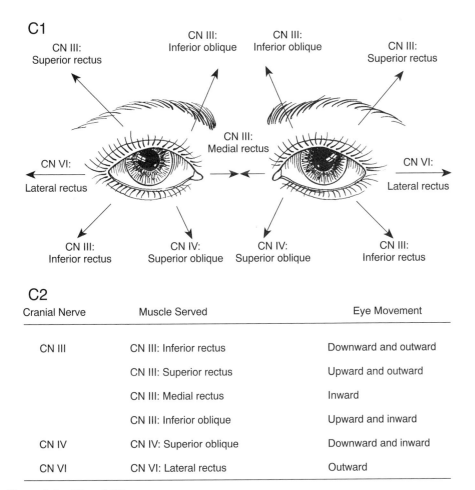

C2

Cranial Nerve	Muscle Served	Eye Movement
CN III	CN III: Inferior rectus	Downward and outward
	CN III: Superior rectus	Upward and outward
	CN III: Medial rectus	Inward
	CN III: Inferior oblique	Upward and inward
CN IV	CN IV: Superior oblique	Downward and inward
CN VI	CN VI: Lateral rectus	Outward

Figure 4.6   C1 and C2.

Visual Fields by Confrontation

The estimation of the integrity of peripheral vision, a measure of optic nerve, chiasm, calcarine radiation, and occipital lobe function, is conveniently made by means of the confrontation test. **Major** compromise of portions of the optic disc, the optic chiasm, the retrobulbar optic nerves or their posterior connections may be detected by this screening. The test is conducted as follows:

1. The examiner and the patient must be face to face, at eye level with one another, and approximately 1 meter apart.
2. The patient is asked to cover one eye, and the examiner covers her mirror image eye; the patient is instructed to look right at the examiner's open eye in order to conduct the test of peripheral vision only.
3. In this position, the examiner systematically places her free hand equidistant from the opposing faces and sequentially at the lateral (temporal), inferior, superior, and medial (nasal) extremities of arm reach. Moving her fingers or carrying an object such as pen or colored card, the examiner moves her hand toward center, asking the patient to indicate when he first sees the hand or object. This initial entry into the visual field defines the boundary of the periphery being tested. The examiner's field of vision is the control, and any discrepancy between her limits and those of the patient is noted.

4. Normal peripheral fields should approximate 90° temporally, 50° nasally, 50° superiorly, and 70° inferiorly. Marked deviation from this estimate or a constriction compared with the normal (examiner) control indicates the need for laboratory evaluation, i.e., formal perimetry.

CRANIAL NERVES II AND III: PUPILLARY REFLEXES

Pupillary responses to light and accommodation require light perception by the retina, conduction of the afferent sensory impulse through the optic nerve (CN II), and an intact efferent nerve (CN III) to the constrictor muscles of the pupil (Fig. 4.7).

Light reflex is tested as follows:

1. Lights in the room are dimmed such that the pupils dilate slightly.
2. The patient is instructed to fixate on the far wall (to avoid inadvertent accommodation)
3. A bright light source (penlight or beam from the otoscopic head) is shone directly into the right pupil. This pupil is observed for prompt and symmetrical constriction (direct pupillary response).
4. The light source is removed such that the pupil dilates again.
5. The light is shone again into the right pupil, and the left pupil is observed for prompt and symmetrical constriction (consensual pupillary response).
6. The same procedures are repeated, illuminating the *left* pupil and observing both direct (left) and consensual (right) pupillary responses.

Accommodation response is tested as follows:

1. The patient is asked to focus on the examiner's finger held at 30 cm from the patient's nose, then to follow the finger as it moves toward the nose.
2. The two pupils are observed for progressive and symmetrical constriction as the focal point moves closer to the eyes.

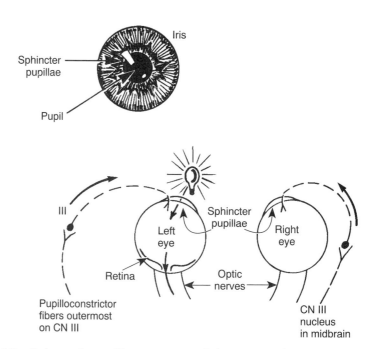

Figure 4.7   Pathways for pupillary response to light (CNs II and III).

CRANIAL NERVES V AND VII: CORNEAL SENSITIVITY

The eye normally responds to noxious stimulation of the cornea by a protective blink. This response requires intact sensory fibers of CN V and motor fibers of CN VII to the orbicularis oculi muscles. The test is conducted as follows:

1. Pull out a fine cotton wisp from the tip of a swab
2. Ask the patient to focus on a spot past the examiner's shoulder
3. Without its entering the patient's field of vision (a bit of a trick!) the swab is touched lightly to the cornea. The eyes should blink reflexly. Each cornea is tested separately (Fig. 4.8).

OPHTHALMOSCOPIC EXAMINATION

An adequate funduscopic examination requires the use of the ophthalmoscope. With this instrument, the anterior chamber, the lens, the retina with its vessels, the optic nerve head, and the macula may be inspected. The examination is conducted as follows (Fig. 4.9):

1. The patient is seated at approximately eye level with the examiner. The lights in the room are dimmed to facilitate pupillary dilatation and to reduce distracting reflections. Before beginning the examination, the examiner explains to the patient that a bright light will be used and that he is free to blink or ask for a respite if the examination becomes uncomfortable. The patient should be instructed to maintain his focus on a distant and specifically designated point until instructed otherwise.
2. The anterior chambers are inspected first, casting the light beam from the side and observing for cloudiness or irregularity.
3. For examination of the lens, retina, and attendant structures of the patient's right eye, the examiner holds the instrument in her right hand and uses her right eye; to inspect the patient's left eye, the examiner uses her left hand and eye.

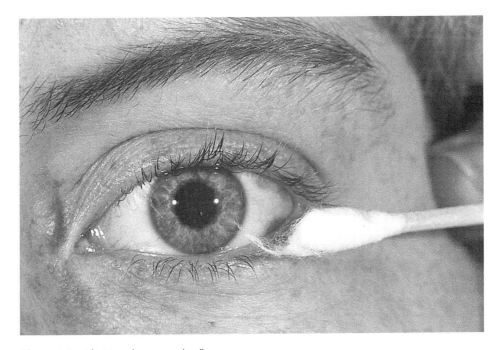

Figure 4.8   Eliciting the corneal reflex.

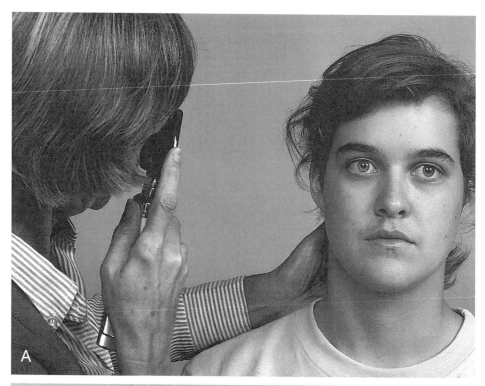

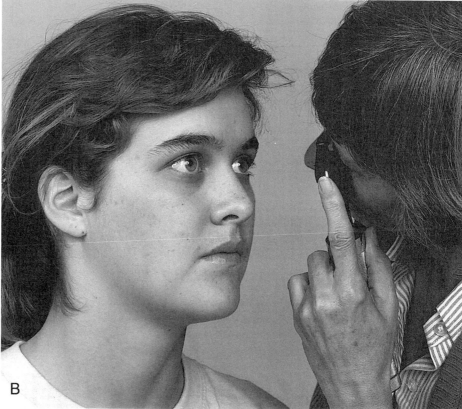

Figure 4.9 Conducting the funduscopic examination. **A.** Approaching the patient's right eye with the examiner's right eye peering through the ophthalmoscope. **B.** Last few centimeters of ophthalmoscopic approach to the patient's left eye.

4. The examination is begun with the instrument held 30 cm from the patient, the diopter indicator at +10, and the light source set by rheostat at a moderate to high intensity. The examiner moves the light gradually toward the patient's eye while observing for black dots, which are lens opacities, and seeking the "red reflex," which is the pink-orange reflection of the beam from the retina. Downturns in lens diopters are made as the retina comes into view until sharp focus on vessels is possible—usually to 0 or –2. The retina is systematically observed by quadrants.

- *Arteries and veins:* The vessels of the retina emerge from the optic disc and spread into quadrantic pairs over the retina. Each pair of vessels should be traced from its central emergence as far peripherally as possible, while observing for the relative sizes of artery and vein, crossings, and irregularities (e.g., focal constrictions) in the course of the vessels (see Normal and Common Variants). After each pair is assessed, move into an adjacent quadrant and repeat the process. Careful observation will often reveal slight pulsation of the retinal veins in normal subjects, usually best seen just over the disc.

- *Retina:* As you study the quadrants, observe the background of the retina for uniformity of pigmentation and presence of discoloration or lesions (see the Extended Examination section of this chapter).

- *Optic disc:* Returning to the butter-yellow, slightly elliptical optic nerve head from which the vessels have emerged, observe its margins, its color, and its focus relative to that of the vessels. The margins should be sharp; slight nasal blurring is seen in some normal persons. The color of the disc usually resembles the yellow of butter, although some variation is found individually and racially. The disc margins and the vessels should be in focus at the same diopter setting.

- *Macula:* Central vision is concentrated in the macula or in the fovea, which is a more darkly pigmented area, approximately one-fourth the size of the optic disc, located temporally at about two disc widths from the temporal margin of the disc. Locating the macula is facilitated by asking the patient, at the end of the retinal inspection, to look directly at the light. This maneuver brings the macula into the center of the examiner's vision. However, no patient can tolerate this light intensity exposure for more than a second or two.

On completion of the ophthalmoscopic examination, the examiner may replace the instrument head with that of the otoscope and turn the room lights back on.

Ears

INSPECTION OF EXTERNAL EARS (AURICLES OR PINNAE)

The two ears should be symmetrical in terms of their alignment on the head and their size and contour. Look at them as a pair and then examine each independently (see Fig. 4.10*A* for anatomic terminology and normal relationships). The external ear is largely composed of cartilage covered with skin and is semirigid. The earlobe is free of cartilage and made up of soft connective tissue and skin. Observe for swelling, redness, or skin lesions. Look carefully behind each auricle for cracks, erythema, or excoriation.

PALPATION OF EXTERNAL EARS (AURICLES OR PINNAE)

Palpate each auricle for tenderness, nodules, or discomfort on manipulation. Feel the area behind and below the auricles for subcutaneous nodules suggestive of lymph node enlargement.

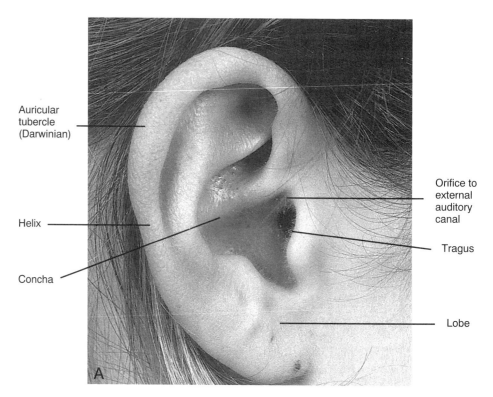

Auricular tubercle (Darwinian)

Helix

Concha

Orifice to external auditory canal

Tragus

Lobe

A

Figure 4.10   **A.** Anatomy of external ear. **B.** Schematic of coronal section of right ear. **C.** Schematic otoscopic view of right tympanic membrane.

CRANIAL NERVE VIII

Hearing Acuity

A second estimate of hearing acuity may now be made (a crude functional test has been performed previously in conducting the history). In the days of ticking watches, the symmetry of distance at which each ear perceived the watch sound was a good test for unilateral hearing loss. An alternative method is the use of the sound created by rubbing the thumb and middle finger together. The patient is asked to close his eyes and indicate the moment at which he first hears the sound as it moves closer to each ear in turn. The absolute distance at which sound is perceived by each ear is not critical in such a simple test. More significant is a difference in acuity between the two ears. Refinement of hearing acuity testing is indicated if the screening test is suspicious. If there is a difference in acuity between the two ears, the Rinne and Weber tests (see the Extended Examination section of this chapter) may be of help in differentiating conductive from sensorineural hearing loss.

Vestibular Function

Screening for dysfunction of the vestibular portion of CN VIII (and/or the labyrinthine apparatus) is accomplished by testing for **nystagmus.** The patient is asked to follow the examiner's finger with his eyes as it moves laterally in the visual field. The examiner observes for end-point vacillation (beating) of the globes, particularly if the duration of nystagmus movement is greater on one side.

OTOSCOPIC EXAMINATION

Auditory Canals

(For the anatomical markings of the canal and tympanic membranes, see Figure 4.10*B* and *C*).

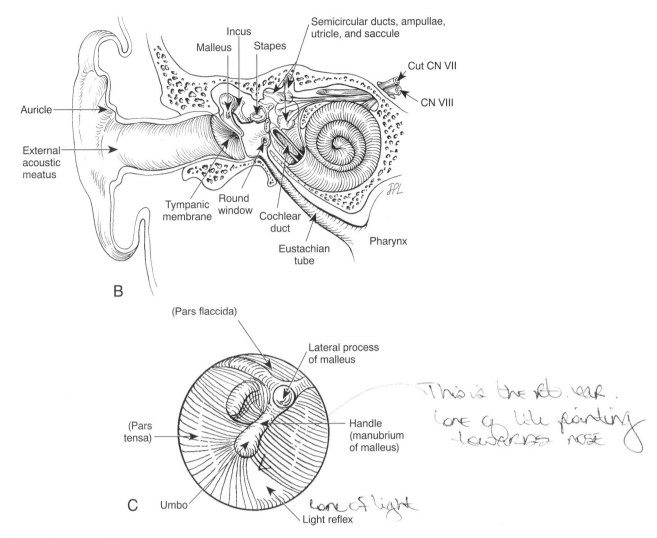

Figure 4.10   B and **C.**

An otic speculum is placed over the front of the otoscope. The patient is warned that this examination requires insertion of the speculum and is asked to indicate if he notes any discomfort. The examination of the auditory canals in adults begins by grasping the helix of the auricle and tugging it posterosuperiorly. This movement both reduces curvature of the external auditory canal to facilitate insertion of the otic speculum and provides a clue to tenderness indicating inflammation of the canal. With the auricle thus moderately stretched, the speculum is introduced, under direct and constant visualization, through its aperture into the ear canal (Fig. 4.11). To maneuver around the soft structures of the anterior canal, the speculum is initially directed 10° posterior to the coronal plane and shifted as indicated by the angulation of the canal until the tympanic membrane (eardrum) comes into view.

As the canal is traversed, it is inspected for scaling, erythema, bleeding points, or discharge. Cerumen may at any time partially or completely obstruct the view of the canal or of the tympanic membrane. (See the Extended Examination section of this chapter for procedures to deal with cerumen when direct visualization of the tympanic membrane is critical to diagnosis and/or treatment.)

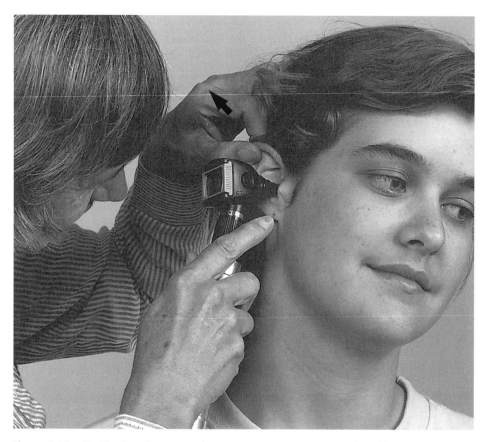

Figure 4.11   Positioning of otoscope for ear inspection; note upward and backward traction on the auricle to facilitate insertion of the speculum into the external auditory canal.

Tympanic Membranes

Inspection of the tympanic membrane requires full and painless insertion of the speculum to its comfortable maximum, as well as an awareness of the landmarks to be sought (Fig. 4.10C). The normally translucent eardrum is situated obliquely as a "dam" across the auditory canal and separates the external from the middle ear. It is gray-tan to pink-white, with the head of the bony malleus (umbo) showing up as a bright white central spot. Directed inferoanterior from the umbo is the conical **light reflex** of a normal membrane. This also shows up as a white and shining "pie slice" radiating from the "white cherry" made by the malleus at its apex. Anterosuperior to the handle of the malleus is the flaccid portion of the membrane, while posterior to the handle of the malleus lies the pars tensa. These terms describe mobility rather than truly anatomically separate structures. They are assessed dynamically with air insufflation, the technique for which is described in Chapter 15. The inspection of the canal and tympanic membrane should include observation of color, translucency versus opacity, visibility of normal anatomic landmarks, pain on manipulation, discharge, or a visible difference from one side to the other—asymmetry of appearance.

Nose and Paranasal Sinuses

See Figure 4.12 for nasal landmarks and the cross-sectional relationships of the nasal structures to the paranasal sinuses and other facial structures. The nose allows passage, humidification, and warming of inspired air into the nasophar-

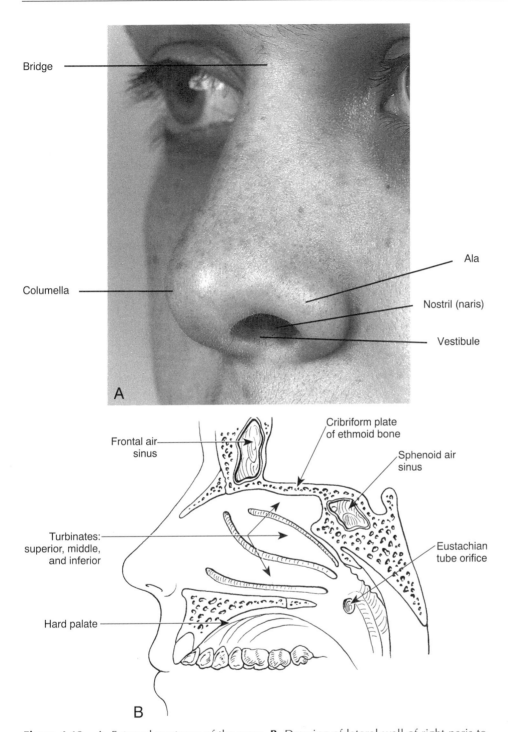

Figure 4.12   A. External anatomy of the nose. **B.** Drawing of lateral wall of right naris to illustrate nasal and related structures.

ynx; its sensors transmit data to the olfactory nerve regarding odors; it contains the exit of nasolacrimal and of paranasal sinus drainage. Indications and methods for assessment of olfactory function are described in the Extended Examination section of this chapter, as they are not considered a part of a screening examination.

INSPECTION

Look at the the nose for its centrality, its general configuration, and its skin surface. Noses are rarely symmetrical as facial structures. Most often they deviate slightly to one side or the other or have a bony or cartilaginous midline hump. The clinician is concerned with the septum and its relationship to free passage of air bilaterally. By compressing each nasal orifice (naris) in turn and asking the patient to sniff through the opposite opening, an estimate of patency is made. The nasal openings are noted for discharge or skin lesions.

The inspection of the nasal passages is facilitated by asking the patient to tilt his head backward while the examiner gently compresses the tip of the nose upward. This maneuver spreads the alae and flares the nares. A light shined into the openings should reveal color and consistency of nasal mucosa, major septal deviation, and mucosal discharge.

Further inspection of the nasal cavities can be carried out with the blunt-tipped nasal speculum—either the disposable plastic insert added over the otic light or a separate metal speculum with external light source. The nares are gently spread and the following observations are made:

- *Mucosa:* for color, discharge, bleeding sites.
- *Septum:* for centrality or deviation, for integrity, for mucosal characteristics.
- *Lateral walls:* for turbinates; the inferior two (inferior and middle) are usually visible. The meatus under each is studied to detect discharge. Again, note the mucosal characteristics.

(Note: Examination of the facial sinuses is not generally considered a part of the screening examination in the asymptomatic adult. See the Extended Examination section of this chapter for techniques of this assessment.)

Oral Cavity and Contents

The oral cavity is a complex set of structures that are all too often ignored by the medical clinician in the erroneous assumption that they are the province of the dental professional. Following is a systematic description of the approach to a basic screening examination of the oral cavity in the adult. See Figure 4.13 for a review of the anatomic relationships of the oral structures to be assessed in the screening examination.

Inspection and palpation of the oral structures require: (*a*) a good light source, either hand-held flashlight or floor lamp; (*b*) a tongue blade for retracting soft tissue; (*c*) gauze squares to assist in tongue inspection; and (*d*) gloves for palpation of oral structures.

The patient is seated at eye level with the examiner, and a good light source must be handy. The supplies should lie within ready reach.

The **steps of inspection** are as follows:

1. With the patient's mouth slightly open, his **lips** are inspected for color, lesions, and bleeding. Note the corners of the mouth for integrity of mucosal junctions.
2. With the patient's mouth opened wide, his oral cavity is assessed with a light shone back toward the throat. Note the dorsal surface of the **tongue**, the **soft and hard palates,** and the medial **gingival surfaces.**
3. Using the tongue blade, examine each quadrant of the **buccal mucosa** and **gingiva.** Note also the general condition of the **teeth.** Is there enamel decay or other evidence of poor dental care? Are there breaks in any mucosal surface? Are there exudates?
4. With the light cast centrally, ask the patient to elevate his tongue toward the roof of the mouth. Note the color and the vasculature of the undersurface. Observe for ulcers or patches of discoloration here and on the exposed floor of the mouth.

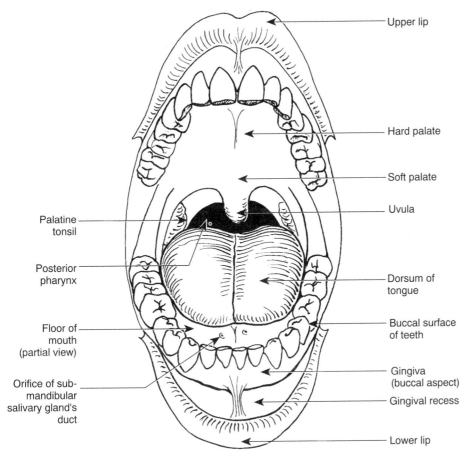

Figure 4.13 Anatomical structures of oral cavity as viewed on inspection.

5. With the light shone posteriorly, the patient is asked to pant or say "haaatt," in order to elevate the soft palate and contract the oropharyngeal muscles. The following observations are made:

    *   *Cranial nerve X—palatal elevation:* A branch of the vagus nerve is responsible for elevation of the soft palate. Ask the patient to say "hat" long and loud; observe the symmetry of palatal elevation (see Figure 4.14*A* and *B*).
    *   *Cranial nerve XII—tongue protrusion:* The paired hypoglossal nerves allow protrusion of the tongue anteriorly in the midline. Ask the patient to stick his tongue straight out. Inspect for lateral deviation, as well as for tremor or visible asymmetry (Fig. 4.14*D*).

6. Don gloves. With the nondominant hand, grasp the tongue in a gauze square and move it laterally in order to inspect its lateral surfaces.

    The **steps of palpation** are as follows:

1. With the examining fingers gloved, the tongue is palpated for lumps, irregularities, or tenderness

2. The patient is asked to elevate the tongue toward the roof of the mouth, and the floor of the mouth is systematically palpated for masses or tenderness

3. The index finger is passed along each gingival and palatal margin, seeking masses or tenderness previously undetected.

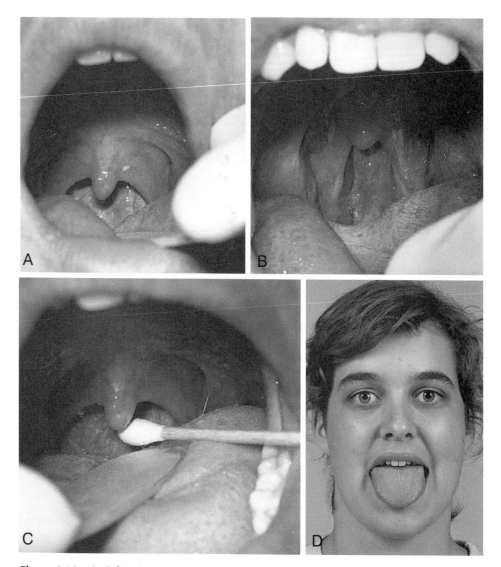

Figure 4.14 **A.** Palate in resting position. **B.** Palate elevated by vocalization. **C.** Approaching the posterior pharynx to elicit gag reflex. **D.** Normal midline tongue protrusion.

Oropharynx

The adult oropharynx is usually devoid of significant tonsillar or adenoidal tissue. The anterior tonsillar pillars define the foremost margin of the cavity in which the tonsils reside. Usually, there is little or no glandular tissue in the depression which at one time housed the tonsils. The posterior pharynx is usually smooth, glistening, and pink. Subepithelial elevations present on the posterior pharyngeal wall usually indicate lymphoid hyperplasia secondary to a recent local viral infection.

INSPECTION

Note the color of the posterior pharyngeal mucosa, the presence of hyperemic vasculature or exudate, and the smoothness of the mucosal surface.

CRANIAL NERVES IX AND X: THE GAG REFLEX

A sensory branch of CN X serves the posterior pharynx; motor branches of CNs IX and X are responsible for the muscular contraction of each side of the pharynx.

The combined integrity of these two branches may be tested by applying a stimulus (such as touching with a cotton swab) to each side of the posterior pharyngeal wall and observing for symmetrical muscle contraction—the gag that is so familiar to everyone ever so examined by a physician or dentist (Fig. 4.14C). It is important to learn the technique for eliciting the gag reflex, although the test should not be done unless specifically indicated (see the Extended Examination section of this chapter).

NORMAL AND COMMON VARIANTS

The discussion of the normal and variants of normal commonly encountered in the screening examination of the head and its organs (Table 4.4) follows the sequential pattern set out in Table 4.1.

Head and Scalp

The general shape and contour of the normal human head are functions of race, age, genetic specificity, and even sex, as well as of the effects of childhood trauma and nutrition on the ultimate fusion of skull sutures. Thus, the recognition of normal comes with extensive experience in observing variation before knowing when a particular shape lies outside the range of normal. A head that looks unusual in proportion to the rest of the body or is visibly asymmetrical from side to side may represent a pathologic abnormality. When the student's careful observation yields a "red flag," she should trust her intuition and ask for clarification by a more experienced clinician.

The scalp with its appendage, the hair, embodies skin, subcutis, and muscle. The "normal" scalp of an adult is smooth without skin lesions, and with hair evenly distributed in the pattern with which we are familiar. Most of us cannot boast perfection. Dandruff, the bane of "civilized" man, is the fine flaky matter on a scalp that may be shampooed too often with too many chemicals. The line between dandruff and seborrhea—the oily scales of a "pathologic" condition— can be murky. The beginning examiner should refrain from the temptation to make diagnoses; rather, she describes what she sees in the simplest language possible: the color, the palpable texture, the presence of areas of discoloration or flaking and their distribution—generalized or in localized patches—and the relationship of hair distribution to any visible skin variations noted.

Hair distribution and texture also have a wide range of normal. Male pattern baldness (thinning and recession at the temples and lateral forehead scalp line) is familial and can begin at any age after male pubescence. The same pattern in a woman suggests a pathologic (usually endocrine) entity. Generalized or patchy hair loss in any other pattern may represent local scalp disease or systemic abnormalities. A good history and a careful documentation of the change are the first steps in establishing abnormality. Hair texture, the coarseness or fineness of the individual shafts, is of importance clinically only if it represents a change from the baseline of the individual patient being examined. Hear what your patient says, and base your observations on his: If you notice something that doesn't look or feel right, ask the patient if he has noticed any changes. If the patient complains of a change, observe and record your findings and how they differ from the patient's description of his baseline.

Face

We speak extensively of "symmetry." Let's use the face as a case in point. Careful studies have shown that mild to moderate facial asymmetry is, in fact, the norm. This normal asymmetry is usually not prominent on visual scrutiny, however; it

Table 4.4
Common Variants[a]

Head and scalp
   Minor side-to-side asymmetry
   [Developmental anomalies]
   Dandruff
   Male pattern balding
Face
   Minor side-to-side asymmetry
     Static
     With movement
CN VII
   [Bell's peripheral facial palsy]
Eyes and periorbital structures
   Globe: range of normal protrusion
   Eyelids
     [Ectropion]
     [Hordeolum]
   Sclera, cornea, iris
     Arcus cornealis [under age 50]
     Defect due to cataract surgery, including iridodinesis
   Pupils
     Congenital anisocoria with preserved light reactions
Vision
   Myopia
   Presbyopia
   Hyperopia (farsightedness)
CNs II and III—pupillary responsiveness
   [Effect of blindness]
Ophthalmoscopic examination
   Wide range of normal color of retina
   [Effect of glaucoma]
   [Cataracts]
   Myelinated nerve fibers
External ear
   Asymmetry with variations in shape and size
Otoscopic examination
   [Cerumen in auditory canal]
   [Scarring of tympanic membrane]
Nose and nasal cavities
   Deviation of nose
     Congenital
     Posttraumatic
   Deviation of nasal septum
Lips, oral cavity and contents
   Lips
     Chapping
     [Angular cheilosis]
   Tongue
     "Geographic tongue" (atrophic migratory glossitis)
     Tight frenulum
   Palate
     Torus palatinus
   Teeth and gingiva
     [Dental defects]
     [Gingival inflammation]
Oropharynx
   Persistent tonsillar and adenoidal tissue in adults

[a]Note: structures without common variants are not included. **Boldface,** most common; and [. . .], common but considered abnormal.

is enhanced if photographic halves are studied in detail. The point is we expect the normal face to appear generally symmetric from side to side. A normal (or previously broken) nose may deviate to left or right, a smile may lift a little more at one corner of the mouth than at the other, one eyebrow may arch in reflection, but the "gestalt" examination of the facial structures should provide a sense of balance. The clinician looks for an asymmetry that exceeds the balance that we accept as usual.

If a disproportion strikes the examiner's eye, note whether it is truly asymmetry or merely a bilateral imbalance of the size or contour of the forehead relative to the jaw or of the eyes relative to the remainder of the facial structures. Does the face move symmetrically with conversation? Is there involuntary movement of one eyelid or a corner of one lip? No attempt will be made here to list all the possible variations of normal; the examiner needs to remember to look, see, and record anything outside the range of her perception of usual.

CRANIAL NERVE VII: MOTOR TO THE FACIAL MUSCLES

The movement of the facial muscles of each side is controlled by CN VII. If both tracts are intact from the cortex to the periphery, the muscles will move symmetrically. Temporary disability of one peripheral seventh nerve, the so-called idiopathic Bell's palsy, is sufficiently common as a transient phenomenon that its manifestations are discussed here. In this setting, the patient experiences a sudden loss of control of the muscles of the *entire* left or right half of the face, usually without other neurologic symptoms. When asked to smile, the patient's face sags and does not respond on one side. The lip corner lifts normally on the side of the unaffected nerve but does not move on the paralyzed side; the forehead remains smooth on the affected side, while the normal side wrinkles in response to a frown command; the eyelid on the affected side cannot be completely closed and will not resist an attempt to raise it with the examiner's finger. It is critical to differentiate this **peripheral nerve palsy** from a **central lesion** of CN VII, which will be manifest only in the lower divisions of the seventh nerve because of bilateral cortical representation. Thus, a central seventh nerve lesion involves only the lower face, while the usually benign and self-limited peripheral inflammation affects the entire half of the face on the affected side. The learner is not asked to determine the etiology of facial paralysis but should be prepared to indicate whether it is *central* (sparing forehead) or *peripheral* (impairing forehead wrinkling). Although the forced-smile/frown/resist-eyelid-elevation tests can be used for testing the motor branches of the seventh nerve, an astute observation of speech and facial response during ordinary conversation will usually provide the information necessary about function of the two nerves.

CRANIAL NERVE V

Sensory to the Skin

There is no variant in sensory perception to light touch or pain on the face that is considered normal. If the tests are administered accurately and the patient is alert and cooperative, sensory perception throughout the face is equal and nonextinguishing.

Motor to Muscles of Mastication

In the normal adult, the bulk and tension achievable in the masseter muscles of the face on a command of "bite down hard and keep at it" should be equal bilaterally. Any asymmetry is noted and considered abnormal until further assessed.

Eyes and Periorbital Structures

BROWS AND LASHES

The color, thickness, and length of the hair of the brows and lashes are determined by age, sex, race, and individual differences. Thus variants outside the realm of normal depend on other criteria that support a pathologic etiology. The normal eyebrow arches over the orbit and beyond the extremity of the eye on either side. Some normal brows meet in the midline over the bridge of the nose; others stop at the level of the medial canthus. The brows should be symmetrically placed. If there is thinning or absence laterally, note should be made of this variation. Some consider it related to hypothyroidism and call it Queen Anne's sign, while others dispute this association. If the brows are absent or very thin— including just laterally—inquire about plucking or shaving, or you may be tempted to a diagnostic wild goose chase!

LASHES

Lashes of the upper lid should curve gently upward; those of the lower lid, downward. If the lashes are absent, ask the patient if this is longstanding or represents a change. Again, a noted recent change in the appearance could indicate a problem.

EYELIDS

The eyelids should appear alike in any given patient. In the older person, they may have begun to evert (**ectropion**) such that a few millimeters of the tarsal conjunctival surface become visible to inspection. **Sties (hordeola),** or inflammatory nodules of eyelash (hair) follicles, are common but not normal. In this instance, there is a reddened mass at the lid margin, sometimes with a yellow dot of purulent inflammation at its center. Usually, the patient will report that it has appeared very recently and is slightly tender; also, sties tend to be recurrent and have a history of spontaneous regression.

If the lids do not close symmetrically or one lid seems "tighter" than the other, test for integrity of both seventh nerves. There should be no sclera visible on closure of the lids. A visible rim of sclera, especially if unilateral, is pathologic.

SCLERAE

The sclerae of the eyes are usually white. There is some normal variation dependent on general skin coloration, prior irritation, and age. A rim of red around the limbus of the iris is not normal, nor is a distinct yellow discoloration of the sclera. Some older persons will have bilateral yellowish deposits on the sclera medial or lateral to the limbus, **pinguecula.** If symmetrical and not impinging on the cornea, this may be considered a variation of normal.

In a significant number of older persons, there is a whitish ring at the rim of the cornea—**arcus cornealis** (once given the unfortunate adjective "senilis"). If queried, the patient will usually relate that this narrow circumferential band has gradually become apparent over time and has created no functional impairment. Its significance is nil in a person over 50 years of age, in whom it is considered a normal age-related change.

CONJUNCTIVA

The conjunctiva, the lining of the globe and lids (bulbar conjunctiva and tarsal conjunctiva, respectively), is transparent and glistening. In the setting of allergic response to environmental agents, the lower lid conjunctiva may appear pale, slightly edematous, and "pebbly." This is usually accompanied by a complaint of itching and is often associated with a runny, itchy nose and sneezing, as well as a slight to moderate increase in lacrimation. Although a few small vessels are visible in the normal conjunctiva, vascular prominence, especially if symptomatic, asymmetric, or associated with purulent discharge, is characteristic of infection or other local irritation.

CORNEA

The normal cornea is invisible, a transparent "window" to the iris, the pupil, the lens, and, for the examiner with an ophthalmoscope, the optic fundus. Unless the patient complains of anterior pain with the eye open or a sensation of "something in the eye," further inspection is unnecessary.

IRIS

The iris or colored central ring of the eye is normally perfectly round, fully responsive to light both directly and consensually, and completely regular at its peripheral margins. Any variation from this level of normal is to be considered pathologic. The only instance in which irregularity of the margins of the iris may be dismissed diagnostically is after cataract surgery has mechanically removed some iris. A keyhole-shaped iris defect may be present. On rare occasions, the two irides will differ in color; if this is noted, query the patient about the longevity of the difference. Normal asymmetry of iris color is congenital (heterochromia) and present since infancy.

PUPILS

In 80% of persons, the two pupils are equal in size. Congenital **anisocoria,** a discernible difference in the resting pupillary sizes, is noted as a normal variant in the remainder of the population. However, these variant pupils should be perfectly round and should react normally and equally promptly to both direct and consensual stimulation (see CNs II and III below). If the response to either stimulus is not normal, the asymmetry in size should be considered abnormal.

ORBIT

The bony rims of the orbit are smooth, nontender, and without irregularity in the normal person. Except in the instance of a history of orbital fracture, any asymmetrical deviation must be considered abnormal and evaluated as such.

Asymmetric protrusion of a globe or of bilateral protuberant globes needs to be evaluated for possible pathology, although there is some considerable variation between individuals and ethnic groups (see the Extended Examination section of this chapter).   **Oral Cavity**

CRANIAL NERVES III, IV, AND VI: EXTRAOCULAR MOVEMENTS

The movement of the two eyes should be uniformly symmetrical and should never result in a report of "double vision." If the examiner notes any variation from this normal pattern, it must be considered abnormal (see the Extended Examination section of this chapter).

CRANIAL NERVE II

Visual Acuity

Myopia, the inability to perceive distant objects clearly, is so common in the population that it is considered a normal variant. *Isolated* myopia is most unlikely to reflect any disorder beyond the optically imperfect shapes of lens or globe that underlie it. The extremes should be evaluated by an ophthalmologist, especially if they are new, markedly asymmetric, not correctable by lenses, or accompanied by other visual signs and symptoms. Aging of the normal globe leads to **presbyopia (difficulty with near vision)**—again considered to be a normal variant unless abrupt in onset, asymmetric, or associated with other signs and symptoms of ocular dysfunction.

Visual Fields by Confrontation

The estimate of optic nerve integrity and central connections by means of visual field testing by confrontation is crude at best. The test requires accuracy in distancing the test object equally between examiner and patient, as well as the full understanding and cooperation of the person being tested. Still, a loss in a peripheral (temporal) hemifield or a persistent quadrantic deficit must be taken seriously. There are no variants of normal in terms of visual field loss. Testing errors or preexisting disease states may alter the results of the test, however. If any patient's visual fields by confrontation do not conform to the expected range, more detailed mapping is indicated.

CRANIAL NERVES II AND III: PUPILLARY REFLEXES

Light Reflex

The patient with normal light sensitivity (transparent cornea, lens, and anterior chamber, normal retinal cells, and intact optic nerve) and with an intact third nerve branch to the pupil and pupilloconstrictor muscles will demonstrate the following responses to a light shown into the pupil:

- *Direct light response:* The pupil into which the light is shown will contract quickly to the stimulus.
- *Consensual light response:* The opposite pupil (unstimulated) will also simultaneously contract equally.

If one eye is blind to light for any reason, it will not respond directly but will respond consensually as long as its partner's vision and its own pupilloconstrictor innervation are intact. If both eyes are blind to light, no pupillary response will occur on direct stimulus or consensually, of course.

Asymmetry or absence of pupillary response, unless clearly accounted for on the basis of established blindness to light, should be considered indicative of local or central pathology.

Accommodation

As the focal distance shortens, i.e., the object on which the vision is concentrated moves closer to the eye, the pupils should symmetrically and progressively contract. A failure of both or of either to respond in this predictable manner is an indication for further evaluation. There are no normal variants to account for unilateral failure of accommodation, although blindness in either or both eyes will affect this response.

CRANIAL NERVES V AND VII: CORNEAL SENSITIVITY

It may be argued that testing for corneal response to noxious stimulation is not a part of the screening examination; however, the test has been described and is occasionally required. There are no variants of normal.

OPHTHALMOSCOPIC EXAMINATION

Anterior Chamber

The normally deep **anterior chamber** will be illuminated all the way to the nasal limbus by a light shined transversely from the temporal corner of the eye. Failure to illuminate the nasal margin by this method suggests an abnormally shallow chamber. This is almost always asymptomatic but is associated with enhanced risk of acute angle-closure glaucoma either spontaneously or with the use of mydriatics (chemical agents that paralyze the constrictor of the pupil and lead to temporary pupillodilation, thus enhancing funduscopic examination).

Lens

The **lens** in a normal eye is fully transparent and is not perceived as a visible structure on inspection; clouding of the lens indicates some disruption of its protein structure, i.e., **cataract.** A lenticular opacity sufficient to impair inspection of the deeper structures of the globe is abnormal and is discussed in the Extended Examination section of this chapter.

With the ophthalmoscope lens setting at +8 to +10 diopters and the light approximately 30 cm from the patient's cornea, the dull **red reflex** should become apparent to the examiner. Black shadows or dots anterior to the reddish background indicate opacities in the lens. If dark spots are seen, move the scope until they come into focus, then ask the patient to elevate the eye slightly. If the marks move upward with the eye, they are anterior and represent abrasions or scars on the cornea or an anterior cataract. If no motion of the dark reflections occurs with eye motion, a location in midlens is suggested; downward movement of the shadow with eye elevation may indicate a posterior lens lesion or one in the vitreous. Tiny vitreous floaters represented by tiny black dots or short strands are common, increase in number with age, and are seen most often in association with severe myopia.

Optic Fundus

A distinct view of the **optic fundus** requires relatively transparent anterior structures and an adjustment of lens diopters to correct for the refractive errors and degrees of accommodation of both the examiner and the patient. For example, if both persons are myopic, the additive diopter correction may be –2 to –4. If the patient or the examiner wears contact lenses, examine the eye with these lenses in place. Occasionally, it will be necessary to examine a markedly astigmatic patient with his glasses on.

Once the correct diopter setting has been located by moving the lenses through a plus (black) to minus (red) range until the retinal blood vessels are clear and sharply defined, the inspection of the fundus may begin. The fundus is studied systematically, usually beginning with the optic disc.

Optic disc. The optic disc is made up of the fibers of the optic nerve, and it is normally pale orange to yellow-pink ("butter-color") and distinctly lighter in color than the surrounding retina. The temporal margin should be sharp, and the nasal margin may be sharp or may seem very slightly blurred. More or less in the middle of the disc, a pale white area represents the **physiologic cup,** an area devoid of nerve fibers. Some normal persons and especially myopic persons have a crescent of dark pigmented dots at the temporal border of the disc. Note that you can focus on all retinal structures, including the optic disc, with a single diopter setting on the ophthalmoscope. If it is necessary to change the lens in order to obtain clear focus from one retinal structure to another, this indicates retinal or disc pathology.

An uncommon but dramatic normal variant of the optic disc is created by strands of **myelinated nerve fibers** that emerge from the disc as a white opaque "paintbrush" obscuring vessels and disc margins. The free ends of the "bristles" are actually the far ends of the myelinated segments lying in the retina. Why this should occupy only one eye and only part of the circumference of the optic disc is unknown. This variant, when first observed, may raise the question of pathology and should be confirmed by an experienced clinician.

Note the emergence of four pairs of vessels from near the center of the disc. Each pair is made up of a bright red artery (sometimes with a thin white stripe running along its center, a visual artifact created by light reflection) and a red-purple vein, which is without stripe and about one-fourth larger than its accompanying artery. Careful inspection will usually reveal faint pulsation in the portion of the vein overlying the disc. The artery is not visibly pulsatile. The vessels begin to branch and spread, like the limbs of a tree, at or near the disc margin, with each pair roughly serving a quarter of the retina. As the examiner traces each branching vascular pair toward the periphery, she observes their crossings. Normally, they are smooth without tapering or change in width. The details of the pattern of branching vary widely but should proceed progressively such that all areas of the retina (except the macula, see below) are uniformly vascularized.

Retina. The **retinal surface** varies in color intensity as a function of complexion and race but is normally uniform in pigment distribution and symmetrical bilaterally or shows faint variations called *tiger striping.* Patches of black, brilliant white, or deep red pigmentation must be considered abnormal.

Macula. The macula, the focus of central vision, is a darker red area lying on a horizontal plane with the optic disc, approximately 3 disc diameters temporal to the disc. It is devoid of vessels, is about one-fourth the size of the disc, and has a central dark spot, the **fovea centralis.** This tiny area is highly light-sensitive and thus difficult to examine for any length of time: The patient experiences the illumination as more noxious, the pupil constricts, and the patient involuntarily looks away—a move the examiner recognizes by the sudden disappearance of the retinal landscape!

Ears

EXTERNAL EARS (AURICLES OR PINNAE)

The appearance of the external ear (**auricle or pinna**) is widely variable. Minor asymmetry is not unusual. A number of congenital malformations have no functional significance. These include very small pinnae (microtia) or very large ones (macrotia), protrusion of both pinnae at right angles to the head, and variations in the shape of the individual portions of the external ear. Normally, manipulation of the pinna is painless.

Hearing is normally present equally in the two ears. By the completion of the medical history, the examiner should have a good sense of the patient's hearing acuity, both from direct discussion of the issue and from observations made during the history. If there is a question about hearing acuity, crude testing may substantiate a loss; the missions then become to determine whether the loss is bilateral or unilateral and whether it is related to nerve damage, dysfunction of the ossicles, or disease of the middle ear. The fine points of discrimination among these possibilities are discussed in the Extended Examination section of this chapter. Recall that some diminution of hearing is commonly found with aging; this becomes more than a variant of normal when it interferes with the patient's function. The most common hearing impairment in healthy adults is caused by **cerumen** (wax) accumulation in the auditory canal. This normal variant is easily discovered and remedied as the otoscopic examination is begun.

OTOSCOPIC EXAMINATION

Auditory Canals

The **auditory canals** are the deep extensions of the pinnae, about 2 ½ cm in length. They terminate as blind alleys blocked by the tympanic membranes. Initial inspection with stretching of the pinna upward and backward and the tip of the otoscope speculum just at the verge of the canal will reveal the normal pink, smooth lining of the canal. The acuteness of the canal angle varies individually, and thus the amount of "tug" on the pinna and manipulation of the speculum (**always under direct visualization**) will vary. No part of this examination should be painful. If it is, either the technique is incorrect, an oversized speculum has been employed, or a pathologic condition is present. If the view of the canal is obstructed by cerumen that is very soft and liquid, it may be removed by gentle swabbing with a cotton tip, under direct visualization. If wax resists such removal and still obstructs the view of the canal and/or tympanic membrane, the following procedures may be indicated: (*a*) removal of inspissated cerumen with an ear spatula; or (*b*) chemical softening of the wax with a product such as Debrox and subsequent warm water irrigation by syringe. Neither of these procedures should be carried out by the inexperienced examiner without the direct supervision of someone knowledgeable about the methods, potential contraindications to their use, and their complications.

Tympanic Membranes

The normal **tympanic membrane** is glistening, is gray-pink, and slants anteriorly and inferiorly. It is translucent, such that some of the middle ear ossicles are visible, notably the malleus as it presses on the eardrum from behind the membrane. Rarely are vessels visible on the surface of the eardrum, and if prominent, they usually indicate an inflammatory process. The eardrum should be totally imperforate. Its contour is minimally conical, with a slight concavity at the umbo. Occasionally, white scars are noted, usually the result of childhood perforation by spontaneous rupture or surgical incision during a bout of otitis media. The normal eardrum moves freely with gentle air insufflation via a bulb attachment. The indications for testing motion of the eardrum are limited in the adult and probably should be reserved for a specialist in the field to assess suspected middle ear disease or unexplained conductive hearing loss.

Nose and Paranasal Sinuses

The range of normal nasal contour is wide, with the nose being one of the facial characteristics that individualizes one's appearance. A "crooked" nose may be congenital or the result of an old fracture. The "sniff test" will help to determine whether and where nasal deviation has caused dysfunction (obstruction) of one passage and is indicated especially if the septum appears off center. Both nostrils should be approximately equal in terms of patency to air passage. A discrepancy directs the examiner to inspect carefully for extreme septal deviation, polyps, or enlarged turbinates as the basis for impairment of air movement.

Normal nasal **mucosa** is pink and glistening. The nasal vaults will have hairs visible, but there should be no discharge other than a thin layer of clear mucus on the mucosal surface. During an upper respiratory infection, the nasal mucosa may be swollen and irritated in appearance with some bilateral yellow mucus; allergic rhinitis presents as very pale and boggy mucosa with increased watery discharge. The **turbinates** are the same color as the surrounding mucosa and should not be large enough to obstruct air passage. Apparent asymmetric enlargement of a turbinate may, in fact, be a polyp when more carefully examined with the speculum. Pus in the nasal cavity suggests purulent sinusitis.

Oral Cavity and Its Contents

LIPS

Inspection of the normal **lips** should reveal unbroken skin without visible lesions. Occasionally, **chapping** or superficial cracking of the skin of the lips may be caused by wind exposure, especially if the patient has repeatedly licked his lips to moisturize them. The lips should be inspected (with all makeup removed) to note the normal pink to magenta color and the smooth margins and surface. Some persons with dental malocclusion will have intermittent **angular cheilosis** (cracks at the corners of the mouth) secondary to maceration from saliva accumulation. If such fissures are noted, it is not usually possible to differentiate those that are dentally related from those caused by riboflavin deficiency or candidal infection. If you are in doubt about the etiology of angular cheilosis, especially if the patient reports that it is longstanding and nonhealing, consultation and/or biopsy may be indicated.

TONGUE

The **dorsal surface** of the normal **tongue** varies widely. The **papillae** in some tongues are prominent; in others they give a velvety uniformity. The so-called **geographic tongue** is a variant that has the appearance of a map—with splotches of white atrophic surface scattered among areas of pink papillae. With experience, this normal variant can be differentiated by inspection from the tongue coated with fungal patches or displaying another glossitis. Deep, irregular **furrows** on the dorsum of the tongue are also seen as anatomic variants; the patient will be able to report that his tongue has "always looked like this."

The **underside** of the **tongue** is smooth and glistening, with salivary duct openings visible as pink carunculae at the base of the frenulum. The freedom of tongue protrusion and elevation is a function of the length and attachment of the frenulum, with its central membrane binding the tongue proximally to the floor of the mouth. Individuals born with a short frenulum may be "tongue tied," i.e., have limited protrusion. Only if the tight, short frenulum inhibits labial speech because of inability to place the tongue behind the upper teeth should this anomaly be considered for correction. In any event, tongue protrusion should be symmetrical and midline. On occasion, tiny, black-purple veins (sometimes called "caviar spots") may be prominent on the underside of the tongue; this is considered normal unless it is in the context of other indications of venous obstruction locally or of superior venal caval syndrome (see Chapter 8).

PALATE

The mucosa of the roof of the mouth is uniformly pale pink and glistening. There should be no lesion visible on the palate. An exception is the **torus palatinus,** a benign osseous overgrowth in the palatal midline, usually present since childhood. The uvula, the posterior extremity of the soft palate, hangs to varying lengths and is usually midline, sometimes partially bifid as a congenital anomaly (which is highly associated with submucous cleft palate of various degrees). The uvula displays the same color and surface smoothness as the remainder of the soft palate.

GINGIVAL AND BUCCAL SURFACES

The **gingival** and **buccal** surfaces of the interior of the mouth are covered with pale pink mucosae, free of lesions or significant color variation except a white "bite line" running horizontally. Bogginess, erythema, tenderness, local swelling, or purulence of the gingival mucosa may be a clue to periodontal disease and may indicate the need for a dental referral. The papillae through which the parotid glands empty their secretions into the mouth (via Stenson's ducts) are visible opposite the second upper molars on the buccal mucosal surfaces. They are normally pink, slightly raised, and without visible discharge. Ulcers, vesicles, white patches, petechiae, bleeding sites, or nodules on any mucosal surface must be considered abnormalities until proven otherwise.

TEETH

Inspection of the teeth should include an assessment of the fullness of dentition, general dental hygiene, malformation, and discoloration. A good dental history will assist the nondental examiner in determining the health of her patient's teeth and the need for intervention. Careful observation and documentation of unexplained variations in dentition are necessary during the screening examinations by medical personnel as well as in those conducted by dentists.

CRANIAL NERVE XII

Midline protrusion of the tongue is neurally controlled by the paired hypoglossal nerves. Deviation to one side or the other indicates a unilateral motor lesion. Occasionally, a fine tremor will be noted in the forcibly protruded tongue. This may represent a familial tremor of no functional consequence but must be considered in the context of other existing neurologic or systemic symptoms and signs.

Oropharynx

The designation, oropharynx, is an artificial division of the posterior portion of the oral cavity that is bounded anteriorly by the tonsillar pillars, inferiorly by the base of the tongue, posteriorly by the muscles of the pharynx, and superiorly by the soft palate and the nasopharynx. The entire visible mucosal surface should be pink, glistening, and free of lesions and exudate. Some normal adults retain visible tonsillar tissue protruding from behind the anterior pillars. These masses of lymphoid tissue may be pitted with visible crypts but should not be exudative (purulent) or reddened and should not have prominent surface vessels. During the course of a viral upper respiratory illness, there may be elevations of the posterior pharyngeal mucosa by a few patches of reactive lymphoid tissue (adenoids). These should disappear as the infection clears, although some adults retain small amounts of visible residual adenoidal tissue. Purulent discharge draining down the posterior pharyngeal wall suggests pathology in the sinuses or the nonvisible nasopharynx.

CRANIAL NERVES IX AND X

If the sensory branch of each glossopharyngeal nerve and the motor branch of each vagus nerve are functioning normally, the posterior pharynx will contract symmetrically ("gag") in response to touch stimulus of either side. Absence of this response would seem to be abnormal; however, gag reflexes are commonly absent without disease. Failure of one side of the palate to elevate, however, is indicative of a unilateral lesion of the motor branch of CN X.

RECORDING THE FINDINGS

Findings from the examination of the head and its structures are usually recorded immediately after those from examination of the SKIN. This part of the examination is typically labeled by the abbreviation used in this chapter, HEENT. It is permissible to further subdivide the heading, but space and time lead the experienced clinician to lump all observations. Note that some examiners choose to record all CN observations under the NEUROLOGIC heading. This example records II and III as part of the eye examination.

HEENT: Head symmetrical and free of palpable abnormalities. Scalp clear; hair distribution: normal male-pattern frontal balding; texture normal.

Facial structures symmetrical and move equally bilaterally. External eyes and periorbital structures normal. Pupils round, regular, equal and respond well to light and accommodation both directly and consensually (PERRL,D&C is a standard substitute for the preceding sentence concerning pupils). Visual acuity grossly normal bilaterally. Optic fundi clearly visualized; all structures present and normal.

External ears, canals, and tympanic membranes normal to inspection, although cerumen in left canal obscures full visualization.

Nasal septum deviated to right, but both nares patent. Mucosal surfaces normal without discharge.

Oral mucosa normal and without lesions. Tongue normally papillated. Several fillings in posterior teeth, otherwise dental status good. Posterior pharynx unremarkable; no tonsillar tissue seen.

Note the format for recording the remaining cranial nerve findings in Chapter 11. The pupillary responses are traditionally recorded with other pupil observations. Alternatively, all results of cranial nerve testing (with the exception of CN XI) could be entered in this part of the chart. In the instance of a normal examination, the cranial nerve testing could be appended: CNs II–X and XII, functionally intact.

EXTENDED EXAMINATION OF THE HEAD, EYES, EARS, NOSE, ORAL CAVITY, AND THROAT

INDICATIONS

Symptoms

A host of symptoms may lead to more detailed evaluation of these areas. Illustrative prototypes are listed here:

- *Hearing loss:* Evaluation of CN VIII (including vestibular as well as cochlear functions) and otoscopy are emphasized. Specific questions address etiology, e.g., sound pollution, physical trauma, prior otitis, presbycusis (age-associated high-frequency hearing loss), syphilis, hypothyroidism, Paget's disease with compression, acoustic neuroma, and Ménière's disease. Functional assessment includes severity of loss, *sound frequency range* that is most affected, and associated symptoms from adjacent cranial nerves or local structures.
- *Abuse of tobacco and alcohol:* Special attention is given to the face, oral cavity, and pharynx, because these habits promote cancers in these locations.
- *Ocular or visual symptoms:* These call for detailed assessment of the eyes and periorbital structures, all aspects of CNs II, III, IV, and VI, and ophthalmoscopy.

Abnormalities on Screening Examination

Because so many permutations exist, only a single illustrative example is provided: The patient who offers no symptoms but is found on screening examination to have Kaposi's sarcoma of the face requires detailed evaluation of the retinas and the mouth, since complications of HIV infection are particularly common and serious in those areas. Although parotid complications of AIDS have been reported, this gland does not require special attention, since enhanced diagnosis and improved management—the touchstones of performing an examination—would not justify this, barring symptoms. As the reader may already know, understanding when and what to focus on is much of the work of any clinician.

CONDUCTING THE EXTENDED EXAMINATION

More detailed inspection or palpation, using the techniques described earlier in this chapter, is vital. Beyond this, some special methods can help.

Head and Face

The face is studied in more detail with a good magnifying glass, as are the skin, external nose, scalp hair, external ears, eyelids, and globes.

Examination of the head in older persons calls for palpation of superficial temporal arteries (STAs). A pulse is palpable in the old as well as the young, a bit anterior to the tragus (the cartilage plate at the front of the auditory meatus (see Fig. 4.10)).

The various sensory modalities (except position) can be explored in relation to CN V, i.e., light touch, pain, temperature, and vibration. When precise localization is needed, test the three divisions of CN V separately. Otherwise, a single test in one territory per side, e.g., CN V1 on the left, CN V3 on the right, will suffice.

If sensory perception is intact but cortical disease is suspected, central connections can be evaluated by *bilateral simultaneous stimulation*, performed just as on limbs in the neurologic examination (see Fig. 11.18). If the patient can identify each separate stimulus correctly but does not recognize simultaneous stimulation and perceives it as unilateral, the ignored side shows *extinction*. A *consistent* pattern of extinction, e.g., always missing the left-sided stimulus, indicates a lesion of the cortical representation. Such a deficit is often particularly pronounced after a stroke affecting the nondominant parietal lobe. Similar defective integration and interpretation of sensory data apply to graphesthesia deficits (see Chapter 11, the Extended Examination section).

Eyes and Periorbital Structures

Both bulbar and tarsal conjunctivae can be inspected more widely by retracting the lower lid while having the patient look up. The maneuver elevates and rotates the globe, so that part of the membrane that lies deep in the recess (the conjunctival fornix) comes into view. For this purpose you press downward and slightly inward on the skin below the eye and do not grasp the lashes. Opposite techniques expose additional superior conjunctiva. To see still more, place a cotton swab such as a Q-tip (Fig. 4.15) firmly against the lid, then sharply grasp the lashes and, while having the patient look as far away as possible, *fold* the section of lid over the Q-tip as shown. Patients find this experience somewhat unpleasant and frightening, so one restricts its use to situations of genuine need.

The *"nipple test"* can demonstrate a shallow anterior chamber by revealing the associated anterior protrusion of the iris (Fig. 4.16). A light is shined medially across the globe, at the level of the limbus. If the medial iris is cast into shadow, the iris must be standing forward from the surface of the globe. This shadowing has been compared to a nipple above the breast or a volcano above the plain. In the normal eye no such shadowing is seen. For the non-ophthalmologist, the only use of this test is to consider the potential hazard of pupillodilation for ophthalmoscopy (see below).

For many years, generalists were urged to use the Schiötz tonometer to measure intraocular pressures in screening for chronic open-angle glaucoma. However, this instrument lacks the accuracy and safety of the gas-jet tonometer used

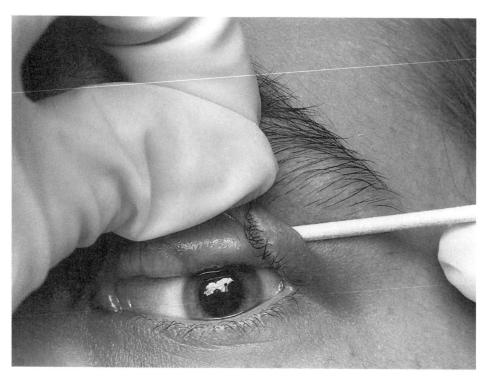

Figure 4.15   Elevating the upper eyelid to remove a foreign body.

by ophthalmologists. (Recognition of an enlarged optic cup on ophthalmoscopy is a preferable screening method for primary care physicians.)

If screening examination of the *extraocular movements* shows deficits in any cardinal direction of gaze, repeat the procedure with each eye separately while the other is closed or covered. If, on screening, the left eye fails to adduct (move medially, i.e., to the right) when the right eye abducts, you might infer that either the left medial rectus muscle or the third cranial nerve supplying it is dysfunctional. Yet if the *isolated* left eye adducts normally, you can exclude these hypotheses and can conclude that the problem lies in the integrative circuits that determine *conjugate binocular eye movements,* i.e., the median longitudinal fasciculus of the brainstem.

CRANIAL NERVE II: VISUAL ACUITY

Most visual impairment relates to **refractive errors** whereby the image produced by the lens is imperfectly focused on the retina. Refractive errors are overcome by examination with the patient's eyeglasses or contact lenses on. Alternatively, you can restrict the beam of light striking the retina to pinhole size by having the patient peer at the Snellen chart through a minute orifice. Plastic testing devices for this purpose are readily available. Testing with the pinhole will correct a refractive error but not rectify other difficulties in the visual axis.

CRANIAL NERVES II AND III: PUPILLARY REFLEXES

Multiple sclerosis often produces a *relative afferent pupillary defect,* which means that the affected structures transmit light-induced neural impulses poorly. Shine a flashlight first at one eye, then the other, as a means of comparing direct with consensual pupilloconstriction (see below).

When the iris is so dark that the pupil cannot be discerned, illuminate the pupil with an ophthalmoscope focused at the surface of the eye. Watch the pupil size, which is inferred from the size of the red reflex: It should shrink with the

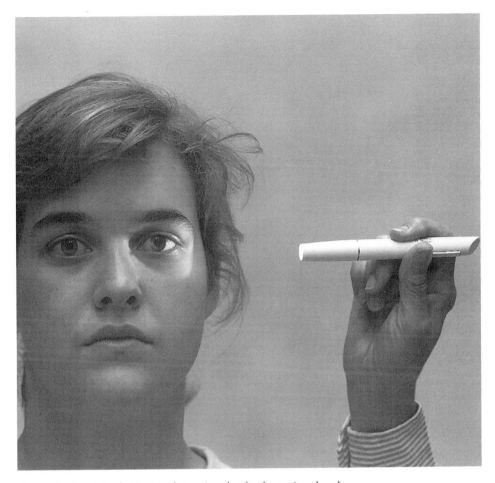

Figure 4.16   "Nipple" test to determine depth of anterior chamber.

application of light. This method permits assessment of direct pupillary light reactivity but cannot be used to show consensual pupillary reactions.

OPHTHALMOSCOPIC EXAMINATION

The chief method employed to ease and enhance this examination is administration of mydriatic (pupillodilating) drops. This should repeatedly be done under supervision before being performed alone. Be cognizant of contraindications and complications. If you're planning to perform pupillodilation, **ask the patient whether he has had cataract surgery and a lens implant.** If so, don't pupillodilate.

Most clinicians are intimidated by the prospect of precipitating glaucoma by this technique. A more frequent risk is *transmitting ocular infection* from patient to patient if the tip of the eyedropper is not kept sterile.

To perform **pupillodilation,** the clinician proceeds to

1. Pick a time at which she'll be available a half hour later.
2. Ask the patient about any history of acute angle-closure glaucoma. (Chronic open-angle glaucoma is not a contraindication to pupillodilation.) Eye pain that occurs only at night or in the dark is a rare but rather specific symptom of angle-closure glaucoma. If any response in this history is positive, the clinician consults an ophthalmologist before proceeding with pupillodilation. If the patient has had dilating drops as part of routine refraction (vision testing) previously and if they made everything blurry for an hour or two, they were

likely mydriatics. A successful dilation within the past 2 years strongly suggests that the patient will tolerate the procedure well.

3. Infer the anterior chamber depth by the nipple test. A positive nipple test means dilation is risky and should be done only by an ophthalmologist. A negative nipple test suggests that dilation is safe. Pupil size and the direct and consensual pupillary light reactions of each eye are recorded as baseline measurements.

4. Warn the patient that the drops sometimes sting for half a minute but this will abate and vision will be impaired, with some photophobia, for an hour or two after the examination. Inform the patient, family, and nurse that this test may rarely *unmask* acute angle-closure glaucoma. Failure of vision to improve, new headache, or eye pain should prompt a telephone call to consider this rare but important complication. The patient must not be heroic and "put up" with symptoms in this setting.

5. The patient lies down flat or at a 30° angle. He looks up and away from the side being instilled (Fig. 4.17*A*). The clinician can hold the inferior palpebral conjunctiva to make a receptacle sac. The solution bottle is held a few cm above the eye. A single drop is instilled. Tropicamide 1% ophthalmic solution is recommended. This nonabsorbable, short-acting topical anticholinergic is preferable to sympathomimetics such as phenylephrine because of efficacy and side effect profile. If the dropper touches the lash or any part of the patient, the bottle is bacterially contaminated and must be discarded.

6. After instilling the drops, the clinician notifies staff of the procedure and its consequences. Then no one is surprised to find the patient with dilated nonreactive pupils!

7. Excess dosage increases complications without raising diagnostic yield.

8. After 25 minutes, note pupil size. Direct and consensual light reactions should be nil. Ophthalmoscopy proceeds with remarkable ease and efficacy, revealing a spectacular panorama of the retina (Fig. 4.17*B*)

Ears

CRANIAL NERVE VIII

Hearing Acuity

By rubbing together your thumb and index finger successively at 2.5-cm intervals, beginning 10 cm from the external auditory canal, you can produce a reliable auditory stimulus to test hearing acuity. At about 21 cm, this test has a 90% sensitivity for detecting standard-definition hearing loss. The specificity compared with that of pure-tone audiometry is poor, yet this method is superior to tuning-fork tests and spoken or whispered voice tests.

An *audioscope* provides acoustic stimuli of different frequencies. It is conveniently built into an otoscope handle and shows good sensitivity and specificity for delineation of hearing loss. Diagnostic and predictive power is enhanced by combining this instrument with the Hearing Handicap Inventory for the Elderly—Screening Version, a set of self-administered written questions (Table 4.5). Each "no" answer represents 0 points, each "sometimes" answer represents 2 points, and each "yes" answer represents 4 points. A total score of 8 points establishes probable hearing loss, and a score of 24 or above shows almost certain hearing loss.

The Rinne and Weber tests help characterize hearing loss into its major subdivisions, sensorineural and conductive.

Rinne Test

The Rinne test is performed by setting a 512-Hz (cycles per second) tuning fork in motion. Hold the base of the fork against one mastoid process and ask the patient

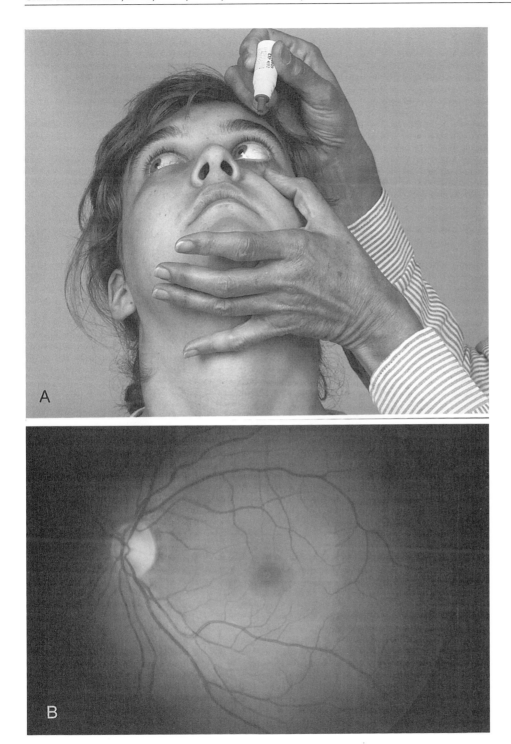

Figure 4.17 A. Instilling the drops for pupillodilation. **B.** Panoramic view of left retina. The optic disc is at left edge, and the macula is the darker area without vessels at dead center of the photograph.

to signal when he can no longer hear the hum. At this signal move the vibrating fork near the external auditory meatus of the ear on the same side and ask the patient to indicate whether or not he hears the sound. If the patient hears the hum conducted through the auditory canal (air) after it has disappeared from the mas-toid (bone) placement, he has a normal Rinne test—air conduction is better than

Table 4.5
Hearing Handicap Inventory for the Elderly—Screening Version

PLEASE CIRCLE THE BEST ANSWER FOR EACH QUESTION

1. Does a hearing problem cause you to feel embarrassed when you meet new people?
   NO　　　　　SOMETIMES　　　　　YES
2. Does a hearing problem cause you to feel frustrated when talking to members of your family?
   NO　　　　　SOMETIMES　　　　　YES
3. Do you have difficulty hearing when someone speaks in a whisper?
   NO　　　　　SOMETIMES　　　　　YES
4. Do you feel handicapped by a hearing problem?
   NO　　　　　SOMETIMES　　　　　YES
5. Does a hearing problem cause you difficulty when visiting friends, relatives, or neighbors?
   NO　　　　　SOMETIMES　　　　　YES
6. Does a hearing problem cause you to attend religious services less often than you would like?
   NO　　　　　SOMETIMES　　　　　YES
7. Does a hearing problem cause you to have arguments with family members?
   NO　　　　　SOMETIMES　　　　　YES
8. Does a hearing problem cause you difficulty when listening to television or radio?
   NO　　　　　SOMETIMES　　　　　YES
9. Do you feel that any difficulty with your hearing limits or hampers your personal or social life?
   NO　　　　　SOMETIMES　　　　　YES
10. Does a hearing problem cause you difficulty when in a restaurant with relatives or friends?
    NO　　　　　SOMETIMES　　　　　YES

bone conduction. On the other hand, if the patient cannot hear the air-transmitted sound after its disappearance from the bone placement, he has an abnormal Rinne test—air conduction is poorer than bone conduction. The test is then performed on the opposite ear and mastoid.

Weber Test

The Weber test is conducted by holding the base of the vibrating tuning fork on the midline of the skull (Fig. 4.18) and asking the patient to indicate where he perceives the sound. A normal response is "in the middle" or "all over my head." If the patient *clearly* hears the sound in only one ear or hears the sound substantially louder in one ear than the other, the Weber test is said to be lateralized and thereby abnormal. For use of these two tests to help distinguish between conductive and sensorineural hearing losses, see Table 4.6.

MASTOID TENDERNESS

Mastoid tenderness is elicited by pressing firmly on the mastoid eminence, an unmistakable bony knob behind the midportion of the external ear.

VESTIBULAR FUNCTION
Caloric Testing

Caloric testing causes nausea and profound discomfort to the conscious patient. Therefore it is reserved for assessing *brainstem function in the comatose patient.* **After otoscopy has shown an intact tympanic membrane,** the patient is kept supine, the trunk is flexed 30°, and the external auditory canal is irrigated via an ear syringe

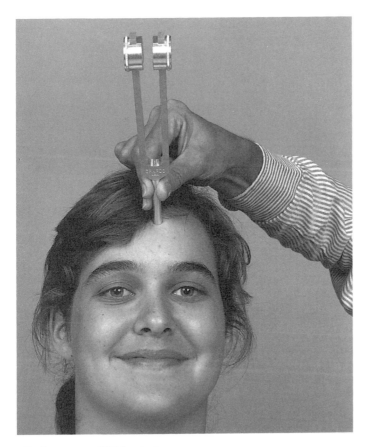

Figure 4.18   Performance of Weber test.

Table 4.6
Rinne and Weber Test Results Interpretation[a]

Description	Rinne	Weber
Left ear, pure sensorineural	AC greater than BC	Lateralizes to right
Right ear, normal	AC greater than BC	
Left ear, pure conductive loss	BC greater than AC	Lateralizes to left
Right ear, normal	AC greater than BC	
Left ear, mixed deafness	Cannot predict	Cannot predict
Right ear, normal	AC greater than BC	
Bilateral sensorineural deafness		
Left ear	AC greater than BC	Lateralizes to better
Right ear	AC greater than BC	(less diseased) ear
Bilateral conductive loss		
Left ear	BC greater than AC	Lateralizes to worse
Right ear	BC greater than AC	(more diseased) ear
Bilateral mixed deafness	Cannot predict any test results	

[a]AC, air conduction; and BC, bone conduction.

or bulb with 250 ml of water that is at least 7° *Centigrade cooler* than body tempera-ture (i.e., 30°C) or water run from the tap until it feels cold to the fingers. Look for nystagmus thereafter, and note whether it beats toward or away from the irrigated side of the body. The test can be repeated with warmed water, i.e., 44°C.

OTOSCOPIC EXAMINATION

Pneumatic otoscopy is a technique that is more widely employed in children than adults. See Chapter 15.

Cerumen Removal

Cerumen removal is necessary for visualization of the external canal and tym-panic membrane when they are obscured by wax. *Irrigation* is not safe unless the tympanic membrane is known (has been seen) to be intact. If there is a perfora-tion, irrigation may drench the middle ear, with the attendant hazards of physic-ochemical or bacterial otitis media. At best, in the patient with a wax-clogged ear you may have a record of a previous examination showing an intact tympanic membrane. More commonly, no data are available. Therefore, application of a *ceruminolytic agent* that will loosen wax physicochemically rather than mechani-cally is preferable. A *10% solution of sodium bicarbonate* in glycerol accomplishes this over the span of a day. Instill a few drops of this agent into the external canal. Leave the head tipped for a minute or two so as to allow maximal infiltration by gravity, and then, if necessary, place a cotton pledget at the external auditory meatus (Fig. 4.19) to prevent drainage when the opposite ear is turned upward. The pledget can be removed after the patient has had the second ear instilled. One day later, the wax should have softened and drained on its own, and oto-scopy can proceed without incident. If necessary, gentle irrigation with plain water can be added to this regimen. *Mechanical extraction* of wax with an instru-ment called a *cerumen spoon* is for the otologist, not the generalist.

Nose and Sinuses
INSPECTION AND TRANSILLUMINATION

Two methods are advocated for *transilluminating the maxillary sinus*. Both require a completely darkened room and the use of a penlight or a more narrow and directed *sinus transilluminator* (Fig. 4.20). Place the tip just under each inferior orbital rim (Fig. 4.21) in turn, and look for differential transillumination of each antrum. Alternatively, you can place the tip, covered by a disposable glove to stay sanitary, to each side of the palate in turn. Each time have the patient close his lips around the instrument so that transillumination can be compared from side to side.

The *ethmoid sinus* cannot be assessed by these methods, but you can draw an inference about it if crepitus is found in the infraorbital area.

The *frontal sinus* is studied with a variant of the first method, whereby the light source is placed under the *superior* orbital rim (Fig. 4.22).

PALPATION OF SINUSES

In general, palpation of the sinuses is less sensitive than percussion (below). The single exception is in the demonstration of *subcutaneous facial crepitus*, which is usually seen as well as felt. The sensation of this finding has been compared to moving air about in "bubble wrap."

PERCUSSION FOR TENDERNESS

Percussion in some areas is used not to create sound but to bring out *tenderness* that has not been elicited by simple palpation. Over the frontal sinuses, strike the

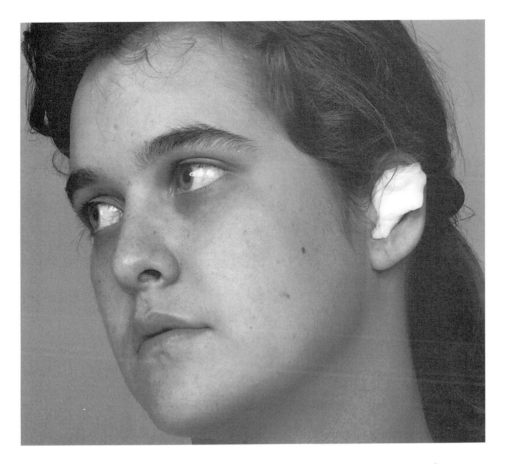

Figure 4.19   Pledget at external auditory meatus to keep ceruminolytic agent in place.

tip of the flexed middle finger against the midpoint of the cutaneous projection of the sinus (Fig. 4.23). The motion, just as for sonorous percussion of the thorax as described in Chapter 7, is entirely from the wrist: all joints below *and above* (proximal to) this one should remain immobile throughout the arc. The same technique is applied to the malar eminence or environs to delineate *maxillary sinus inflammation.* The difference from sonorous percussion is that no pleximeter is used; i.e., it is a one-handed procedure.

Strong lighting is essential for examining the oral cavity. A tiny or feeble penlight will not do. A flashlight or a large mobile light such as in a dental office is best. If the patient seems uncomfortable during routine examination from in front or if the tongue and floor of the mouth carry special import, ask him to hyperextend his neck over the back of the chair (Fig. 4.24), and then *reexamine the oral cavity from behind.* Since the floor of the mouth is a leading site for development of oral cancer, the technique is especially helpful for those at highest risk, i.e., abusers of alcohol and tobacco.

The tongue often gets in the way of seeing the floor of the mouth and sometimes even obscures the cheeks. When you need optimal visualization of the lateral and inferior aspects of the tongue itself, control its movement by using a *gloved* hand to *grip the tongue with a 2 x 2 gauze square.* Firmly pull or push the tongue so as to expose the tissues (Fig. 4.25). The tongue is very slippery: omit the gauze, and the tongue will slide out of your fingers.

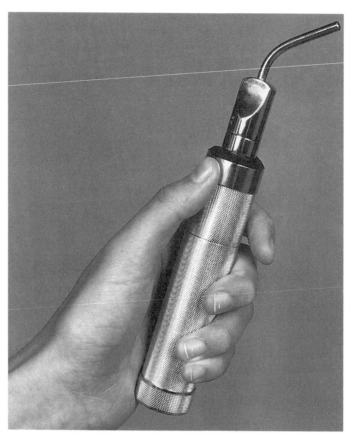

Figure 4.20   Sinus transilluminator.

If the posterior pharynx is not well visualized, passive anterior tongue protrusion may succeed in bringing it into view. However, many patients "buckle" the tongue upward. To see more of the throat, ask the patient to say the "aa" sound of the word *"hat."* You can increase and prolong exposure of the pharynx by asking him to give a *dragged out shout* of the sound he has just made. If he responds timidly, say "I want them to hear you in the next county, for 5 full seconds."

Dental mirrors are very helpful for observing the inner (lingual) aspects of the teeth. If the reflected structure is ill lighted, direct the light at the mirror such that it illuminates the tissue without coming back at you as glare.

CRANIAL NERVES IX AND X

If a patient's voice sounds strange or if he has a known problem with the larynx or its innervation, ask him to phonate various sounds. Record in your write-up whether all sounds are ill produced or whether there is hoarseness, a gritty or "throaty" quality, or difficulty only with high-frequency sounds such as "ai" as in the word "hail." The interpretation of phonation and laryngeal difficulty is best made during direct observation of the larynx with a mirror, a technique beyond the scope of this book.

Besides the gag reflex and voice quality, *deglutition* (swallowing) depends on the function of CNs IX and X. When you *have the patient swallow water* as part of the thyroid examination (see Chapter 5), observe the ease of swallowing (Fig. 4.26), and note whether any regurgitation or choking follows swallowing. If need be, use an additional water sip to study this separately. If the history points to dysphagia primarily for solids, ask the patient to chew and *swallow a suitable solid*

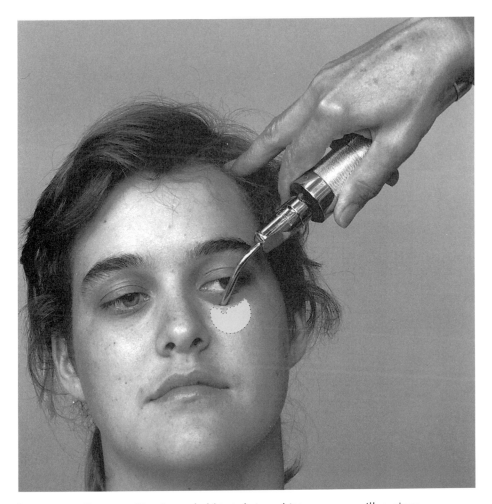

Figure 4.21   Sinus transilluminator held to inferior orbit to assess maxillary sinus.

in your presence, e.g., a slice of apple. A rough quantitation of efficiency of the entire swallowing apparatus (neural and muscular components, and esophageal patency) can be achieved as follows: The diaphragm of the stethoscope is placed on the skin overlying the stomach, i.e., in the epigastrium just to the left of the midline, with the patient seated comfortably. The patient is asked to hold a sip of water in the mouth and, at your signal, to swallow. Note with a stopwatch how many seconds elapse before you hear the unmistakable gastric rumbling that signifies the arrival of the liquid bolus in the stomach (Fig. 4.27). Try it on yourself to establish a normal. There is insufficient literature on the topic to provide a reference interval. A 10-second lag should indicate marked dysfunction, but the sensitivity and specificity of such a cutoff remain to be established.

CRANIAL NERVE XII

When the patient attempts to protrude his tongue forward, it should not deviate to either side. If it does, there may be unilateral *CN XII (hypoglossal)* disease *on the side toward which the tongue deviates*. Mechanical factors such as partial loss of dentition may displace a normal tongue without denervation. If hemiatrophy or fasciculation is seen on the presumably denervated half of the tongue, a neurologic cause is confirmed. However, these findings are often lacking even with established CN XII problems. To resolve the issue, ask the patient to *push the tongue*

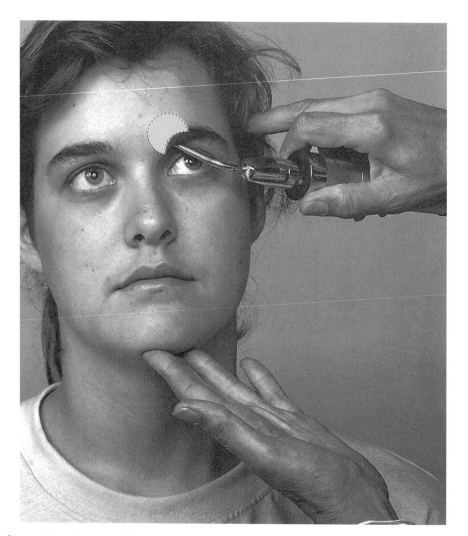

Figure 4.22   Sinus transilluminator under superior orbital rim to assess frontal sinus.

forcefully against your finger, through the cheek (Fig. 4.28), on each side in turn. Asymmetry of power will be evident.

If there is suspicion of *vascular insufficiency of the tongue*—a feature of *giant cell arteritis*—based on symptoms or setting, the tongue can be observed for blanching. To bring out this feature if it is not seen at baseline, you can employ exercise, analogous to the search for peripheral arterial insufficiency. Ask the patient to thrust the tongue forward repetitively or to talk at length, and then observe for blanching as dynamic blood demand exceeds the supply.

INTERPRETING THE FINDINGS

Head and Scalp

Frontal bossing, unusual prominence and curvature of the forehead, may be innocuous. It also occurs in patients with sickle cell anemia and as part of the HIV embryopathy complex. An upper part of the head that looks disproportionately large atop a normal jaw and lower face may reflect *hydrocephalus* or the platybasia of *Paget's disease of bone.* Distinction between these two conditions is made by history.

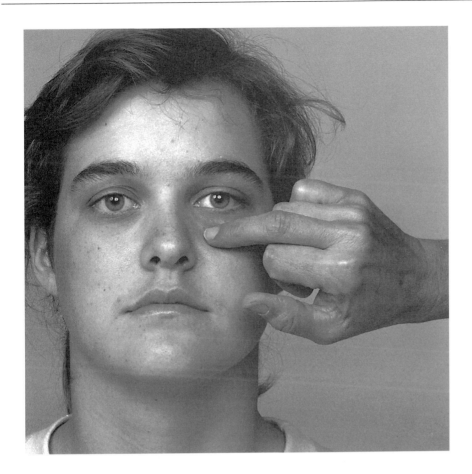

Figure 4.23   Percussing the maxillary sinus.

Palpable *subcutaneous masses* over the head are most commonly epidermal inclusion cysts, also called *sebaceous cysts* or *wens*. Lipomas and fibromas are also common. Multiplicity and chronicity together reinforce the likelihood of epidermal inclusion cysts or lipomas. Extraordinarily numerous epidermal inclusion cysts, particularly if accompanied by hard excrescences on bone (osteomas), can raise the question of *Gardner's syndrome,* a familial condition whose superficial component causes little trouble, while its internal component, colonic polyposis and premature colon cancer, can prove fatal if not recognized and treated promptly.

Face

The combination of swelling and crepitus without erythema implies communication between an air-containing space and the subcutis. Just below the eye, this suggests *ethmoid sinus fracture,* which is the etiology in Figure 4.31.

Visible or palpable *parotid enlargement* raises six differential diagnoses:

1. *Starvation,* including the self-starvation of *anorexia nervosa and bulimia.* These disorders may be present even in someone who does not appear cachectic.
2. *Sjögren's syndrome,* wherein autoimmune damage hinders production of saliva and tears. Often, lymphocytic infiltrate expands the parotids to a clinically detectable degree.

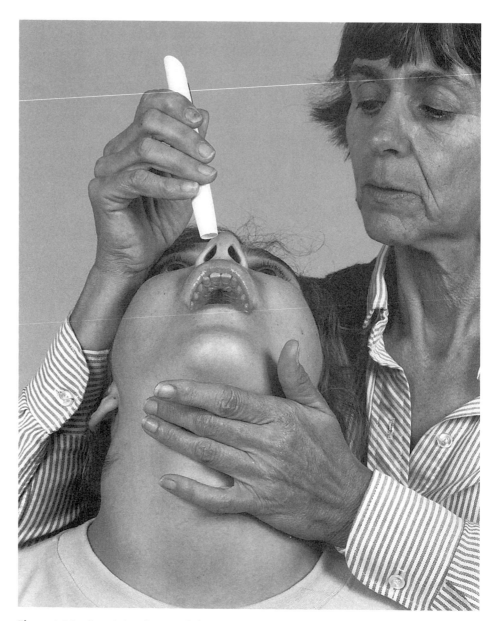

Figure 4.24   Examining the mouth from in back.

3. *Alcoholism*, in which fatty infiltration appears to be the histologic basis of the sign.
4. *Diabetes mellitus.*
5. *Acute parotitis*, classically from mumps.
6. *HIV infection*, in which the mechanism of parotid enlargement has been variously reported as associated with or independent of an excess of new Sjögren's symptoms.

The structural deviation or deformity caused by recent or remote *nasal fracture* is usually obvious.

In *fetal alcohol syndrome* there is often striking facial dysmorphism. Since the diagnosis is sometimes missed in infancy or childhood, observing for it in adulthood is more than a curiosity. Changes include **hypoplasia of the philtrum,** which is the little notch between nose and upper lip, so that it is invisible or incompletely

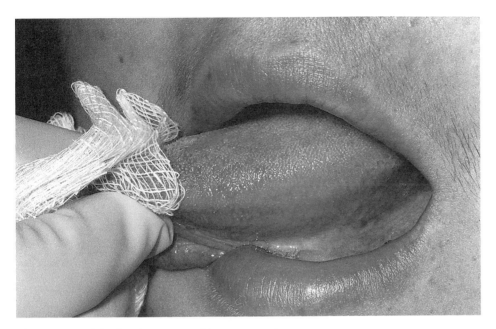

Figure 4.25   Gripping the tongue with a gauze pad.

"dug out" (Fig. 4.29 for normal philtrum), and **hypertelorism,** i.e., unduly wide-set eyes. Subtle cases may elude detection as the features blend with the normal range.

A spectrum from subtle to glaring applies in **acromegaly.** The full-blown case includes a *massive hypertrophic jaw,* an *overhanging forehead and eyebrows,* and *coarse features* (Fig. 4.30) with excess facial wrinkling in a pattern that has been called *leonine,* as well as extracephalic findings. There is overlap between persons who are constitutionally large-jawed and those with acromegaly. The diagnostic separation is more difficult because some normals also possess other large, prominent features. If in doubt, ask questions and perform examinations pertinent to the pituitary, e.g., visual fields by confrontation, measurement of blood growth hormone levels, and imaging of the pituitary.

Severe *hypothyroidism* can produce, besides the findings on trunk, limbs, and neck, a puffy, round, apathetic face with coarse features, dry coarse skin, and thick hair, along with a Queen Anne's sign. The latter, loss of the lateral third of the eyebrows, is seen, in addition to hypothyroidism, in (*a*) normal individuals, reflecting their particular distribution of hair follicles, (*b*) persons who pluck their eyebrows for cosmetic reasons or who have follicles ablated by electrolysis, and (*c*) some persons with leprosy.

The positive and negative predictive values of physical signs for hypothyroidism are reduced in middle age and beyond. Humility about the power of physical examination to rule in or rule out thyroid dysfunction is appropriate.

Severe *facial edema* can produce distortion of individual features or of the whole face and can even lead to a characteristic facies. *Allergy* is the commonest cause, including some cases of *angioedema.* The history may be of help in sorting this out. Facial edema is also seen in *anasarca* of any cause including end-stage heart failure or severe hypoalbuminemia from malnutrition, hepatic synthetic failure, or nephrotic syndrome. *Myxedema* in hypothyroidism can mimic facial edema. It can be surprisingly difficult to distinguish the facial disfigurement of *morbid obesity* from that of edema. Pitting—retention of indentation after a fingertip has been firmly applied for 15 seconds—supports fluid rather than adipose tissue as the cause. Edema limited to or maximal in the face raises the question of *superior vena caval syndrome.*

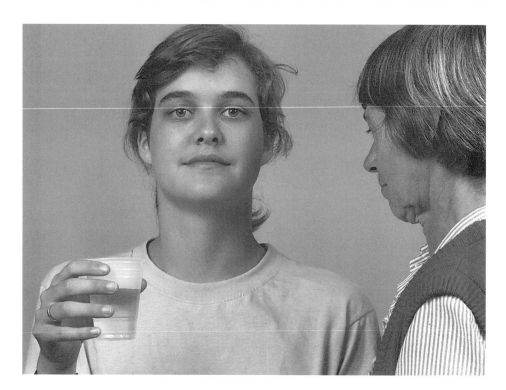

Figure 4.26   Observing the swallowing of water. Note that the chin is not elevated; the examiner has to tell the patient to keep the chin down.

Many *neurologic problems* can be identified from facial findings, even at rest. Asymmetry of mouth, nasolabial fold, and palpebral fissure suggest *facial nerve palsy,* although they do not distinguish central from peripheral (lower motor neuron) causes as delineated earlier in this chapter. It may be difficult or impossible to ascertain which is the normal side and which the abnormal side at rest. Neurologic examination and observation during speech for changing facial expression supply additional data.

CRANIAL NERVE V

The nuclei of CN V are set in the tight-packed pons, so that isolated fifth nerve problems without ocular palsies are likely to reflect disease of the peripheral (extracerebral, extra-axial) course of the nerve. The commonest problem is *dermatomal herpes zoster.* In this condition, one or more divisions—the ophthalmic (V1), maxillary (V2), and mandibular (V3)—are affected, usually unilaterally. The lesions may not appear for the first couple of days of pain. They begin as clustered vesicles on erythematous bases, then rupture with or without passing through a pustular phase, and eventually crust and dry. Ocular *(corneal) involvement* is a sight-threatening complication of herpes zoster in CN V1. For the generalist, the development of conjunctivitis or dulling of the corneal light reflex in the setting of facial shingles calls for prompt ophthalmologic consultation. The *otalgia* associated with facial zoster is serious but not as grave as ophthalmic involvement.

Eyes and Periorbital Structures

Periorbital edema, when not due to local causes such as blepharitis (see below), has been traditionally linked with glomerulonephritis and the nephrotic syndrome. Supporting data and a mechanism are lacking.

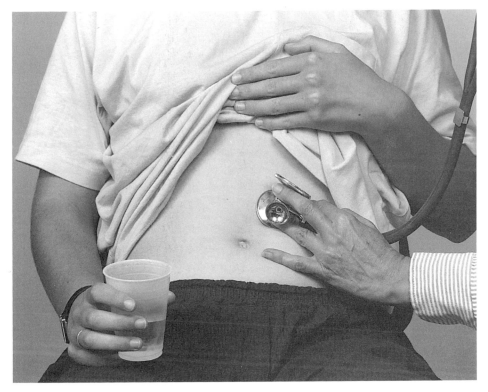

Figure 4.27 Auscultating a gastric air bubble with swallowing.

BLEPHARITIS

Blepharitis is an *infectious* or, more often, an *allergic* irritation of part or all of the lids and adjacent tissues. The physical findings are *swelling* and sometimes *purplish erythema* of the affected region, with or without an associated conjunctivitis (common) and with or without features of nasal allergy (less common). Excess tearing is common, an unduly dry eye less so. Edematous blepharitis is always mentioned in discussions of *trichinosis*, which is seen in the United States, especially in recent immigrants from Puerto Rico.

CONJUNCTIVAL IRRITATION

Conjunctivitis is among the commonest ocular disorders encountered by the primary care clinician. If yellow purulent exudate is found in the inferior conjunctival fornix, viral or bacterial infection is likely. If the conjunctiva is pink and the surface vessels visibly dilated but no pus is found, no conclusion can be drawn about etiology. *Physical irritation* produces conjunctivitis in persons exposed to excess particulate matter in the air and in those with inadequate tear formation, e.g., from Sjögren's syndrome.

The conjunctival vessels disappear at the margin of the cornea, which supplants the conjunctiva as the outermost covering over the iris, from the limbus forward. Therefore, prominent vessels in conjunctivitis should *not* be seen within the limbus, i.e., overlying the iris or within 0.5 mm of it: A hairline-thick preserved white zone should surround the iris. Reddening or ectatic vessels over the iris or in that zone implies inflammation of the uvea, which becomes inflamed with a variety of important systemic disorders. *Anterior uveitis* is synonymous with iritis and is seen in sarcoidosis, among other conditions. When you suspect uveitis, consult an ophthalmologist promptly.

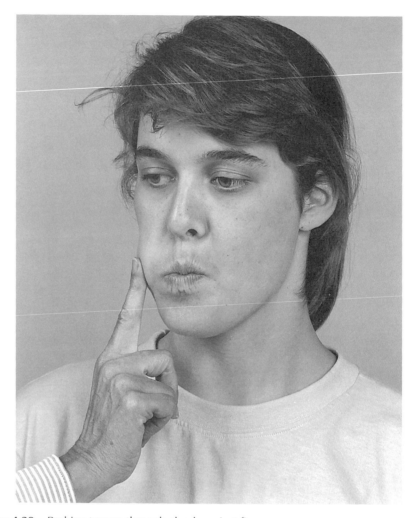

Figure 4.28   Pushing tongue through cheek against finger.

CHEMOSIS

Edema of the conjunctiva is *chemosis*. It is recognizable swelling, often with a buckling of the excess tissue and sometimes a degree of localized anterior protrusion at the inferior fornix. This finding may accompany several ocular disorders and also occurs in *superior vena cava syndrome*. For reasons that are not clear, it may be seen in *respiratory failure* (as can *papilledema* [see below]).

PTOSIS AND EXOPHTHALMOS

Ptosis means drooping. The *upper lid* can have ptosis in isolation (blepharoptosis), e.g., with a partial third nerve lesion, or with disease at or about the neuromuscular junctions of the levator palpebrae. Afflicted patients appear heavylidded. Eye carriage is so fraught with affective content in this society that such patients may mistakenly be considered drugged, sleepy, or disturbed. A first step in assessing patients with ptosis is to investigate for any local orbital problem displacing lid or globe. The second step is to assess extraocular motions and pupillary light reactions individually, directly and consensually, and aggregately, to seek deficits in other functions of the third nerve or its anatomic neighbors. Visual field testing also investigates the region.

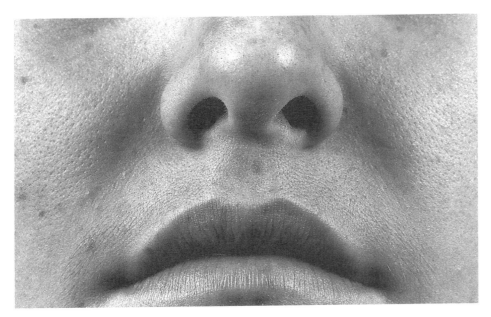

Figure 4.29   Facial view to show the philtrum.

Exophthalmos, also called **proptosis,** is a bulging of the eye. There is much racial and ethnic variation in normal protrusion of the globe. Healthy African-Americans *on average* show more anterior protrusion than healthy northern Europeans. Fruitless workups for exophthalmos can ensue if this is forgotten. The differential diagnosis of *symmetric exophthalmos* includes *Graves' hyperthyroidism* but not other forms of thyrotoxicosis. Exophthalmos and systolic anterior propulsion of the globes have been recorded in *congestive heart failure.* Unilateral exophthalmos may also reflect *Graves' disease,* as well as orbital or ocular *neoplasm* or *inflammatory lesions* including *infections* and idiopathic *orbital pseudotumor.* Audible systolic *ocular bruits* bolster the case for Graves' disease or neoplasm, but the finding is insensitive.

ARCUS CORNEALIS AND XANTHELASMA

Arcus cornealis is a lipid-rich corneal/pericorneal *whitening,* just inside the limbus, usually beginning at 12 and 6 o'clock. It can lighten the iris or render it an opaque white. The old name *arcus senilis* refers to its presence in many persons over age 50. In young-adulthood, it is a marker for hyperlipidemia and atherosclerotic vascular disease, but not in the aged.

Xanthelasma is a variant of *xanthoma* that correlates with premature coronary artery disease by reflecting substantial hypercholesterolemia. Xanthelasmas are yellowish to yellow-pink subepithelial excrescences, most commonly in the upper eyelids, especially medially, and occasionally in the lower lids. The predictive value is highest in children and young adults, but do seek this sign in every 40-year-old with chest pain. Some cholesterol-lowering drugs can cause visible regression of xanthelasmas.

CRANIAL NERVES III, IV, AND VI: EXTRAOCULAR MUSCLES

Cranial nerves III, IV, and VI share tight quarters in the brainstem. The first step in workup of an *apparent deficit* in a cardinal direction of gaze is to *repeat the test with the normal eye covered.* If the previously abnormal eye now shows full range of ocular movement, the problem lies in the median longitudinal fasciculus, the

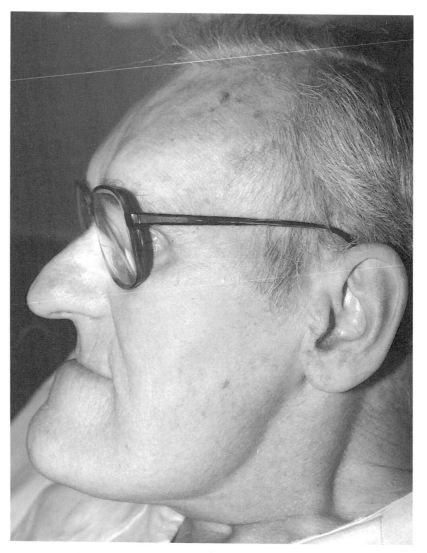

Figure 4.30   Facial appearance in acromegaly.

brainstem tract that "yokes" the two eyes, i.e., determines *conjugate* movement. A prime cause of dysconjugate movement is *multiple sclerosis*. A cause of *divergent (dysconjugate) gaze in rest position,* with normal bilateral extraocular movements, is **amblyopia,** the **"lazy eye"** that most affected patients will recount having had since childhood.

   If a deficit in gaze persists with monocular testing, think anatomically about its source:

1.   CN VI or the lateral rectus muscle if there is loss of lateral gaze,
2.   CN IV or the superior oblique muscle if there is loss of downward-inward gaze,
3.   CN III or any of the four extraocular muscles that it innervates (inferior oblique, medial rectus, superior rectus, and inferior rectus) for any other deviation.

   Hemorrhages and tumors in the brainstem can cause these deficits but seldom without associated abnormalities. Dysfunction within the orbit is another cause, both with local conditions such as *orbital cellulitis* and neoplasms and with relatively advanced *Graves' ophthalmopathy.* Extraocular movements are fre-

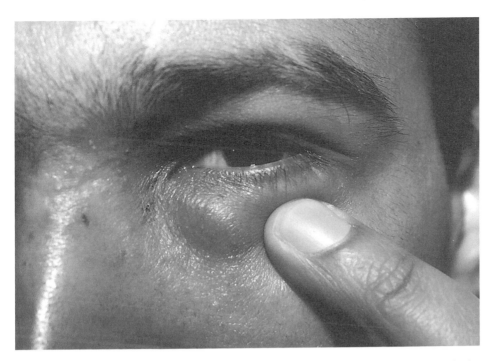

Figure 4.31   Infraorbital crepitus with minimal erythema after "blowout" fracture of ethmoid sinus.

quently studied in relation to *increased intracranial pressure*. Since the sixth cranial nerve has the longest extra-axial course, it may be impinged on first. The outermost fibers in the third nerve relate to pupilloconstriction, so that a *dilated, hyporeactive or unreactive pupil is expected to precede extraocular muscle palsies as intracranial pressure increases;* interpretation must be cautious rather than rigid.

Beware of what we call "conjugate paresis," whereby the eyes remain yoked but cannot move to the right, for example. *Factitious illness* offers one explanation of such a puzzling constellation, which would involve the right eye's abducent (sixth nerve–lateral rectus muscle) complex, and the left eye's third nerve–medial rectus muscle complex; if these were the only deficits, you would have to invoke two neurologic lesions rather than one. Although puzzling combinations of lesions can occur, especially in embolic disease and multiple sclerosis, the examiner must consider factitious physical signs when confronted with deficits that appear anatomically highly improbable.

CRANIAL NERVE II: VISUAL FIELDS

To make sense of large visual field cuts, remember that the temporal (lateral) half of the visual field projects onto the nasal (medial) half of the retina and retains that position in the optic nerve. Only the medial fibers of the nerve decussate at the optic chiasm. The temporal field is thus represented by calcarine radiation and occipital cortex contralateral to the eye on which the image fell. In successively more posterior order:

1. Transection of one optic nerve anterior to the chiasm produces unilateral blindness and no visual field cut contralaterally and in this sense is identical with disease of one globe.
2. Damage at the chiasm, classically from expansion of a pituitary mass, will damage fibers from both sides just as they cross. These fibers represent the *temporal* half of each eye's visual field. The result is a **bitemporal hemianopsia.**

3. Damage to the optic tract posterior to the chiasm destroys (*a*) fibers that have decussated from the temporal half of the contralateral eye's visual field and (*b*) fibers that have not decussated, from the nasal half of the ipsilateral eye's visual field. The result is a **homonymous hemianopsia.** A right calcarine lesion produces loss of the left (i.e., medial, nasal) half of the field of vision for the ipsilateral right eye and loss of the left (i.e., temporal, lateral, decussating) half of the visual field of the contralateral left eye. In contrast to the anatomic "impropriety" of "homonymous" paresis of extraocular muscles, this situation makes perfect pathophysiologic sense. By contrast, **binasal hemianopsia** should raise the specter of feigned dysfunction.

If only a portion of the craniocaudal dimension of an optic nerve is destroyed, there will be a corresponding (inverted) diminution of the lost portion of the visual field. By this mechanism there develop *quadrantanoptic* counterparts to the hemianopsias described above. In diseases of the retina, such as glaucomatous damage, more circumscribed visual cuts can occur.

CRANIAL NERVES II AND III: PUPILLARY REFLEXES

Sympathetic action dilates the pupils, while *parasympathetic (cholinergic)* impulses constrict them. Some drugs that mimic or block autonomic actions can produce effects. However, β-adrenergic blockade with antihypertensive drugs does not produce clinical pupilloconstriction, nor do systemic antimuscarinic drugs such as amitriptyline produce clinically useful pupillodilation. By contrast, endogenous discharge plays a role, so that excitement with epinephrine release enlarges the pupil. Heroin produces pinpoint pupils that dilate somewhat on administration of the opiate antagonist, naloxone. Cocaine can dilate the pupils.

Topical application of autonomic drugs to the eye affects pupil size. Ocular *pilocarpine* used for glaucoma constricts the pupil, as does ophthalmic timolol.

Many persons have *physiologic anisocoria,* wherein the "resting" size of the two pupils differs enough to be recognizable by an examiner. There are two approaches to confirming this innocuous state: the history and the examination.

History. Ask if the patient or any family member has noted the unequal pupils. If doubt exists, look at *unretouched* portrait photographs. If you discern the inequality dating from 2 or more years ago, no ominous cause is sought.

Examination. Check each pupil to see if it does the following:

1. Constricts normally in response to direct stimulation.
2. Constricts consensually on illuminating the opposite eye.
3. Dilates a bit after removal of the light source.
4. Constricts and converges with testing of accommodation.

If it does all this, the condition is almost certainly benign anisocoria.

A further step in evaluation of anisocoria is to determine whether it is the smaller or the larger pupil that is abnormal. A *very large pupil* (over 6 mm across), unless the result of topical medication, is likely to be the abnormal one. Also check extraocular motions, looking for evidence of dysfunction of the nearby cranial nerves or their effectors. Seek alterations in mental status, including change in level of consciousness, and focal neurologic deficits. Some possible underlying conditions are increased intracranial pressure, local compression by cerebral aneurysm, and neoplasia.

If accommodation (constriction on near gaze) is preserved in a large pupil whose light reaction is sluggish or absent, either *Argyll Robertson pupil* or *Adie's syndrome* is present. Neurosyphilis involving the midbrain is the best known cause of the Argyll Robertson pupil, although there are others, with *diabetic neuropathy* being commonest nowadays. Adie's syndrome is an innocent idiopathic polyneuropathy; its only other manifestations are reduced knee and ankle jerks.

Marcus Gunn Pupil

Marcus Gunn pupil is a *relative (i.e., incomplete) afferent pupillary defect.* The leading etiology today is multiple sclerosis. The ability of the optic nerve and visual apparatus to fire neural impulses in response to retinal illumination is reduced, often unilaterally, but the efferent limb for pupilloconstriction is not. Thus, illuminating the opposite eye, if the condition is unilateral, will cause prompt physiologic consensual pupilloconstriction of the diseased eye. However, shining the light on this eye will produce delayed or incomplete *direct* pupilloconstrictive reaction. If the light is moved from the unaffected eye to the abnormal eye, the pupil appears to dilate on illumination. What has really happened is that the consensual impulse to constriction from the intact pathway has been removed and nothing equally potent has replaced it.

CORNEAL REFLEXES

The afferent limb includes part of the trigeminal nerve (CN V), while the efferent is from the facial nerve (CN VII). Defective response is failure to contract orbicularis oculi and to blink. This can reflect problems with either limb. The distinction depends on comparing other functions of the two nerves. *Erroneous test results* are *avoided* by

1. Touching the cornea, not the conjunctiva, i.e., applying the stimulus over the iris rather than the white of the eye (a source of apparent loss of the reflex, i.e., false-positive tests).
2. Bringing the stimulus onto the cornea unseen. Tell the patient to stare straight ahead, then bring in the long wisp of cotton from the side (Fig. 4.8). Failure to heed this procedure may cause a *visual threat,* whereby the afferent limb is preempted by visual response to threat, resulting in a blink that could produce false-negative results.

OPHTHALMOSCOPY (FUNDUSCOPIC EXAMINATION)

Ophthalmoscopy (funduscopic examination) can only be touched on briefly because of space constraints. The reader who seeks more detail is referred to Sapira's monograph.

Lens Opacities (Cataracts)

Lens opacities (cataracts) produce black spots in the red reflex. For the generalist they raise two issues:

1. Do they interfere with vision and function sufficiently to warrant ophthalmologic consultation for possible surgical correction?
2. Do they interfere with funduscopy? If so, will *pharmacologic pupillodilation* allow you to look around them?

It is tempting to infer cataracts every time there is difficulty inspecting an old person's fundus, a difficulty that may also result from miosis, abnormal involuntary head movements, or noncooperation. The *specific* criteria for cataracts are black holes in the red reflex, best seen from a distance and with a high positive setting on the ophthalmoscope. If you are focused on the retina and suddenly everything disappears, it's not a cataract; rather, the light beam is falling outside the pupil, probably because somebody moved.

After Cataract Surgery

Today, it is standard practice to insert an intraocular lens prosthesis after cataract surgery. This improves vision for the patient, who will not need the thick spectacles that used to be the hallmark of the aphakic. For the examiner it means retinal landmarks look normal, not tiny and distant as in an aphakic eye. There is one major caveat, however: **Pharmacologic pupillodilation is contraindicated** in an eye with an intraocular lens implant.

You can no longer tell with certainty who has had cataract surgery by looking for a keyhole-shaped iridectomy defect. There may be only a minute defect hidden at the limbus or a minute scar running along the limbus.

Optic Cup and Glaucoma

The **optic cup** is the physiologic excavation or recess near the center of the optic disc. It ranges from inconspicuous to dominant in different individuals. An enlarged optic cup predicts, although imperfectly, chronic open-angle glaucoma. For practical purposes, a cup-to-disc ratio greater than 0.5, extension of the cup to meet the outer disc margin, or asymmetry in the cup-to-disc ratio greater than 0.2 requires ophthalmologic consultation about possible glaucoma.

Disc Margins and Papilledema

Papilledema results from increased intracranial pressure, an emergency that threatens both vision and brain function. The advanced state produces blurring of the disc margins, erythema of background disc and retina (often with hemorrhages), and eventually measurable elevation of the disc above the level of the adjacent retina. Among the mimics of this condition are (*a*) *pseudopapilledema* in marked hyperopia, and (*b*) *papillitis,* an inflammation of the optic nerve head that is part of the spectrum of optic neuritis.

Nasal Margins in Myopes

The nasal margin is often indistinct, especially in myopes. Therefore, it *cannot be relied on* as a sole sign of increased intracranial pressure (papilledema).

Crescents at the Temporal Margins

In myopes, crescents of dark pigment stipples frequently adjoin the temporal disc margin. These crescents consist of partly coalescent black granules. They are not hemorrhages, exudate, or the blackening that follows chorioretinitis.

Blood Vessels

Retinal venous pulsations. There is a major problem in using papilledema to infer increased intracranial pressure: Its appearance *and disappearance* may lag 24–48 hours behind alterations in intracranial pressure. By contrast, retinal venous pulsations respond within seconds or minutes to alterations in cerebrospinal fluid pressure. **In the retina it is the veins and not the arteries that pulsate.** Such pulsations reliably imply nonelevated intracranial pressure, barring special circumstances such as glaucoma. **In the absence of pulsations you can seldom make *any* inference,** since many normal persons lack these pulsations. However, if the patient has had demonstrated venous pulsations before and now lacks them, presume increased intracranial pressure.

Arteriovenous crossing changes ("nicking"). This widely misunderstood sign consists of disappearance of the venous blood column on both sides of an overlying artery. It is a useful optical illusion caused by thickening of the artery's adventitia and does *not* represent compression of the venous lumen. (If it did, the distal segment of the vein would be dilated, which it is not.) The sign has meaning only when it is peripheral, two disc diameters or more from the optic nerve head. Closer in, the density of glial tissue frequently produces the sign in the absence of disease. More peripherally, the sign is seen with *chronic moderate hypertension* and with normal aging. The sign persists even after sustained normalization of blood pressure.

Tortuosity. Prominent "squiggling" of retinal vessels, especially veins, is seen with hyperviscosity states. Examples include polycythemia vera, Waldenstrom's macroglobulinemia, and multiple myeloma with exceptionally large M-spikes. For reasons that are not understood, the same phenomenon is seen as a congenital variant in some normal persons and also in some persons with sickle diseases, especially S-C.

Background Retina

Color. The darkness of the retina tends to parallel that of the skin. Both relate to amount and distribution of melanin. Thus pale blonds have a very light background, and the darkest-skinned African-Americans can show a deep green-brown or umber.

Hemorrhages. Retinal hemorrhages occur in many settings, from severe hypertension—in which their appearance is a particularly useful marker to follow—to diabetes mellitus, leukemia, and severe anemia. *"Dot and blot" hemorrhages* are the smallest variety. They arise deep within the retina. Dot hemorrhages can result from any of the causes cited. Flame-shaped or *"splinter" hemorrhages* arise more superficially, in the nerve fiber layer. They do *not* usually reflect diabetes mellitus, and they are common in the syndrome of malignant hypertension.

Hemorrhages having a fibrinous (white) center, sometimes misdesignated *Roth spots,* occur not only in infective endocarditis and leukemia but also in extreme anemia of any cause, in various neurologic illnesses, in scurvy, and in other settings.

Soft "exudates" (cotton-wool spots). The key features of cotton-wool spots are *flatness, white color, indistinct edges,* and visual *obliteration of subjacent retina and vessels.* The lesion is localized infarction of the nerve fiber layer, which is seen in severe microvasculopathy (diabetes mellitus, hypertension, renal disease of any cause), almost any variety of vasculitis, or severe anemia. A common thread in all these situation is the potential for retinal hypoxia. Healing is followed by the restitution of normal-appearing retina. The mechanism of *cotton-wool spots in AIDS* is less clear, but the finding is common. They are usually transient and sometimes migratory. A major differential diagnosis for soft exudates in AIDS is cytomegalovirus retinitis (see below).

Soft "exudates" in diabetes mellitus mark the *preproliferative phase* of diabetic retinopathy and warrant ophthalmologic referral so that the patient can be considered for sight-preserving laser therapy. Since diabetic *nephropathy* should not occur in the absence of diabetic retinopathy, a normal retina in a diabetic with kidney failure prompts a search for nondiabetic renal disease.

Hard "exudates" (lipoprotein leakage). Sharpness of visible edge and a tendency to more yellowish color distinguish hard "exudates" from soft "exudates." They are sometimes shiny and vary quite a bit in both size and distinctness. They result from leaky microvessels. Many disorders cause both kinds of "exudates." Hypertension, diabetes, and intrinsic renal diseases head the list. Many infectious diseases, primary eye diseases, vasculitides, and other conditions may be added. Both hemorrhages and soft "exudates" can evolve into hard "exudates" on the way to resolution.

Macular degeneration. This is a common, frequently devastating cause of visual loss in the aged. It can produce diverse ophthalmoscopic findings, none specific enough to permit firm diagnosis by the generalist. Nor does a normal retinal examination by a nonophthalmologist exclude macular degeneration. Scattered exudates and scant hemorrhages from macular degeneration are sometimes overinterpreted as something else.

Chorioretinitis. True exudation of white cells occurs in this condition. Its most important causes are tuberculosis and toxoplasmosis. Distinction from soft and hard "exudates" can be impossible in the acute phase. After the passage of time, *black pigmentation* supervenes in chronic or healed chorioretinitis but not with the other entities named.

Cytomegalovirus retinitis. Cytomegalovirus retinitis occurs after organ transplantation, with various immune debilities, and most frequently with *HIV infection,* where it frequently progresses to blindness. Characteristic features are

1. A tendency to occur along blood vessels
2. A "brush fire" advance wherein the recognizably infected leading edge progresses peripherally, ultimately leaving normal-looking but damaged retina behind
3. A mixture of yellow exudate and small hemorrhages that has been described as "crumbled cheese and ketchup"

Ears

EXTERNAL EARS

Tophi are nodules of uric acid with associated inflammation and scarring in chronic gout. They may occur in skin and subcutis near joints or on fingertips but are also sought in the pinnae. Many "bumps in the ear" are benign fibromas. Nevertheless, discovery of tophi will raise the differential diagnosis of *gouty arthritis* in a patient whose joint complaints have previously been assumed to be rheumatoid.

Preauricular lymph node enlargement is a classic finding in *otitis externa* and in *adenoviral conjunctivitis.* Check that the apparent lymph node is mobile and not bony, or you may misdiagnose an exostosis of the skull. Preauricular nodes can also be found in any *generalized lymphadenopathy* but are seldom the group that announces the condition.

Just anterior to the external ears, the *superficial temporal artery pulsation* is palpable. To call a temporal artery normal, it must display three characteristics:

1. *It must be pulsatile.* This pulse is seldom if ever lost due to age alone. The vessel often has a faint pulse and almost never bounds as the carotid pulse can. The vessel is sometimes found anterior and superior to its traditional position 1 fingerbreadth anterior to the tragus. Occasionally, it is found more anteriorly and a bit inferiorly.
2. *It must not be tender.* This is usually straightforward. In the presence of diffuse scalp tenderness, an imperfect but important sign of giant cell arteritis, it may be difficult to decide, as it may be in persons who amplify bodily sensations.
3. *It must not be nodular or palpably thrombosed.*

If any of these features are lacking, giant cell arteritis is suspected.

CRANIAL NERVE VIII

Hearing Acuity

Beyond evaluating severity of loss, a major distinction lies in separating *sensorineural loss* from *conductive loss.* In *sensorineural loss,* bone conduction and air conduction are affected about equally on the diseased side. The Rinne test is expected to be normal; i.e., air conduction still exceeds bone conduction (Table 4.6). On a Weber test, sound lateralizes *away from* the affected ear, which has inferior capacities for both air and bone transmission compared with the normal ear. *Presbycusis* is a form of sensorineural deafness.

By contrast, in *conductive deafness*, the Rinne test becomes abnormal: Bone conduction is better than air conduction as vibrating bone "bypasses" some components of the abnormal vibration-conducting apparatus. In conductive deafness, the Weber test lateralizes to the deafer ear. Another way to think of this is that the ear with the conductive deficit is less distracted from the Weber stimulus by extraneous ambient sound.

In *mixed conductive and sensorineural deafness*, the Rinne test and Weber test may be misleading or mislocalizing, including falsely normal. The key to appreciating mixed deafness is to note *inappropriately little abnormality* of either test compared with a marked global auditory deficit.

Nystagmus

Nystagmus is a beating, abnormal involuntary eye movement named for the *fast component* that follows the initial deviation and produces a return toward rest position. It is observed most commonly in the course of testing extraocular movements and may also be seen while taking the history. To understand the significance of nystagmus, note the eye position in which the nystagmus occurs as well as its direction.

Horizontal nystagmus of three or fewer beats at the extremes of eye position is seen in normals and is disregarded. Sustained (for more than 5 beats) *horizontal nystagmus on lateral gaze* is a sign of *acute ethanol intoxication*, although the differential diagnosis also includes other *cerebellar and vestibular dysfunctions*. Nystagmus in any direction can occur with *phenytoin (Dilantin) toxicity* and may occur with therapeutic drug levels as well as with frank overdose and intoxication.

Vertical nystagmus shows beating up and down, *not necessarily abnormal movement elicited on vertical gaze*. It occurs in several *brainstem disorders*. *Rotary nystagmus* can occur with cerebellar disease, labyrinth dysfunction, or brainstem diseases and is also seen as a congenital disorder. Detailed assessment of nystagmus often calls for neurologic consultation, but the generalist clinician can optimize her own assessment by

1. Carefully instructing the patient in the extraocular muscle testing procedure
2. Not employing extremes of lateral gaze
3. Having the eyes kept (moderately) laterally deviated a full 10 seconds to give nystagmus time to appear

CALORIC RESPONSES

The assessment of the central connections of the eighth nerve can include caloric testing. The normal response will be nystagmus toward warm irrigation. With cold water (30° Centigrade), nystagmus is opposite, i.e., away from cold irrigation. Absence of response to both warm and cold is termed **canal paresis** and may lead to testing with much colder water to see if this restores a more recognizable pattern.

OTOSCOPIC EXAMINATION
Otitis Externa and Variants

Inflammation of the external auditory canal and adjacent skin produces reddening of the pinna and *tenderness to traction*. It may also lead to a *reddened external auditory canal* with or without purulent exudate. Tenderness may be especially prominent on compression of the tragus. Debris is often visible in the canal, and edema of the external auditory meatus can render it impassable by the otoscope.

Etiologies of external otitis include both *infective and allergic and/or toxic* causes. Many persons develop contact dermatitis to certain ceruminolytics, especially Ceruminex. The contact dermatitis can be followed by ear pain, discharge, and subsequent bacterial superinfection after toxic damage breaches the epithelial barrier.

A particularly virulent form of otitis externa is **malignant external otitis.** Otoscopically, there is profuse pus, a swollen canal lining, and often considerable granulation tissue. The condition is usually caused by invasive *Pseudomonas aeruginosa* infection and occurs predominantly in diabetics. Its characteristics include destruction of cartilage and eventually destruction of bone.

Otitis Media

A *reddened tympanic membrane* is the hallmark of acute otitis media, which is usually a bacterial infection. There are many variants; some cases of chronic otitis media lack distinct tympanic membrane erythema. Sensitivity to traction and an abnormal external canal should not be present in pure otitis media, and if they coexist with a red eardrum, the most probable explanation is combined otitis media and otitis externa.

Otologists mention a sequence of signs in the tympanic membrane affected by (untreated) **otitis media,** a sequence followed more commonly in children than in adults. These signs can coexist with a mucoid to purulent discharge, sometimes seen through the otoscope and sometimes also staining the area beneath the acoustic meatus. They are

1. The tympanic membrane loses its light reflex and its shininess.
2. The tympanic membrane becomes pink, and the vasculature becomes more prominent at its edges and on the handle of the malleus.
3. The eardrum becomes red and full.
4. The eardrum bulges and is plum colored, and landmarks cannot be seen.
5. Perforation occurs.

A *ciliary flush or red reflex* is a mimic of stage 2 otitis media changes. In this phenomenon, stimulation of the external auditory canal may result in reflex dilatation of precisely those blood vessels that stand out with inflammation. In adults, the distinction will depend on symptoms, but in children the distinction may not be apparent, since asymptomatic otitis media is well recognized in pediatrics.

Serous otitis media is a variant in which thin yellow (uninfected) serous fluid is visible within the middle ear, through the tympanic membrane, which is often *not* red.

Bullous myringitis is sometimes equated with mycoplasmal respiratory tract infection but is also seen in various viral infections. The *bullae* or blebs occur not only on the tympanic membrane but also on the skin of the nearby (bony) portion of the external auditory canal. The blebs contain clear to hemorrhagic fluid and are not to be confused with *air bubbles* entering via a patent Eustachian tube that are sometimes seen in the middle ear in both conventional and serous otitis media.

Nose and Sinuses

CRANIAL NERVE I

Loss of olfactory fibers occurs routinely with aging. In addition, many persons have *transient olfactory impairment* as a result of *viral or allergic rhinitis.* When should the function of CN I be tested? Testing is most useful when inspection of the nasal cavity is normal but the patient complains of loss of smell or when the olfactory brain (orbital surface of frontal lobes, cingulate gyrus) is being evaluated. Good stimuli are tobacco or *freshly ground* coffee in small pill bottles. Occlude one nostril while the patient's eyes are closed, let the patient inhale deeply, and then have him identify the substance. If he says he smells something but cannot identify it, olfaction is considered intact. Avoid irritant alcohol-based scents or pepper, with which a tactile *burning* may be misinterpreted as smell. *Bilateral anosmia* can be associated with nonnasal conditions such as Parkinson's disease and Kallmann's syndrome. The less common *unilateral anosmia* carries a restricted differential list once nasal normality has been established. Frontal lobe neoplasms and subdural hematomas are among the considerations.

NASAL POLYPS

Nasal polyps, which look like small intranasal "balloons," are usually associated with longstanding nasal allergy *(perennial allergic rhinitis)*. They are edematous, gray-blue to yellow-tan, soft, and not sensitive to touch. Sometimes they appear grape-like. Those arising from the ethmoid air cells may also occur in chronic ethmoid sinusitis. Others develop from the maxillary sinus and can protrude forward into the nose as an antronasal polyp or back through the posterior orifice of the nose, the *choana*, into the nasopharynx. Nasal polyps are sometimes found in a triad with *aspirin allergy* and *asthma*. The principal differential diagnosis of polyps is edematous turbinates, but turbinate mucosa is usually exquisitely sensitive when touched by any instrument.

NASAL MUCOSA

In **allergic rhinitis,** the nasal mucosa is pale, boggy (edematous) and often bluish in color. Yellowish, gray, and even slightly erythematous variants occur. In vasomotor rhinitis, one subtype of allergic rhinitis, the color is often more mauve. Swelling may be the most striking abnormality in this condition, but profuse clear discharge may dominate. In other cases, the mucosa makes nodules and folds that mimic polyps. One type of these, *moriform fringes,* arises from the lower borders of the posterior margins of inferior or less commonly middle turbinates. With *the common cold,* reddening is more prominent, and both watery and inspissated yellow-green nasal mucus may appear. Recognizably purulent secretions are uncommon and suggest acute sinusitis.

Erythema and tenderness of the skin of the nares are usual after frequent nose-blowing with colds and allergies. A red and swollen to dry and rubbery mucosa is seen with *prolonged nasal decongestant spray use,* which is toxic to the sensitive mucosa. This is called *rhinitis medicamentosa.*

Nasal septal perforation suggests two infectious diseases, tuberculosis and syphilis; two immune disorders, systemic lupus erythematosus and Wegener's granulomatosis; and two behavioral disturbances, cocaine abuse and intractable nose-picking. A subset of patients will have no apparent explanation.

SINUSITIS

Patterns of tenderness and reduced transillumination in sinusitis can be predicted from the cutaneous projections of each sinus: forehead, with frontal; malar, with maxillary; and periorbital, with ethmoid and sphenoid. In *ethmoid sinus fractures,* one clue is the presence of subcutaneous crepitus without erythema (Fig. 4.31).

Oral Cavity
LIPS

When a hospitalized woman who has worn no make-up during her stay is observed with lipstick on, this *"lipstick sign"* means she feels considerably better. Although the sign is not sensitive, it is specific for substantial functional, symptomatic, and physiologic improvement.

MECHANICAL AND BITE LESIONS

A number of oral lesions are due to injury from one's own teeth or from hard objects introduced into the mouth while eating, e.g., sharp bones, silverware. The history usually makes this obvious. The **bite line** is a horizontal white strip that appears quite distinct from the pink buccal mucosal background on which it is set. This variant represents a physiologic thickening of the epithelium and is not to be confused with any pathologic change including leukoplakia or the oral lesions of lichen planus.

CARIES AND ROOT CARIES

Cavities are familiar. They are defects in the structure of a tooth, usually on the bite surface but sometimes elsewhere on the tooth. They are typically irregular and may be accompanied by discoloration and plaque, as well as by gingivitis (see below). **Root caries** refers to similar lesions occurring below the gum line, usually in association with profuse gingivitis. These lesions reflect severe problems in oral hygiene practice, with or without defective wound healing.

GINGIVITIS AND GUM FINDINGS

The spectrum of lesions runs from mild erythema, edema, and hyperplasia to the rotting mouth of **pyorrhea,** with frank pus around exposed and carious roots of a few remaining teeth. Halitosis is foul breath caused by anaerobic oral bacteria, necrotic epithelium, and decaying food particles. It commonly accompanies moderate to severe gingivitis. Bony involvement is termed **periodontitis.** *Dark spots on the gingiva* are normal in dark-pigmented persons and can occur in light-skinned persons with Addison's disease.

CANDIDAL INFECTIONS

Candidal species flourish in the mouth whenever local or systemic factors permit. Precipitants include false teeth, antibiotic-induced alterations in flora, radiotherapy to the area, or abuse of tobacco, alcohol, or cocaine. Granulocytopenia and HIV infection also are major risk factors. Candidal stomatitis usually takes a *white pseudomembranous* form in which a white curdy membrane is found on the tongue, palate, buccal mucosa, or floor of the mouth. This material can be scraped off with a tongue blade, leaving raw, bleeding mucosa beneath. Similar scraping of *milk residues,* a major differential, reveals normal, intact underlying mucosa. The white patches of *leukoplakia, some early cancers, and hairy leukoplakia* do not scrape off.

Candida less commonly produces a flat red lesion without visible exudate. This variant, *atrophic oral candidiasis,* is common beneath ill-fitting dentures.

RECURRENT INTRAORAL HERPES INFECTION

Primary herpetic gingivostomatitis produces a painful mouth, fever, and debility. Subsequent attacks of recurrent oral herpes simplex virus infection produce *tiny vesicles,* often on erythematous bases. The vesicles quickly rupture and often coalesce to make ragged, *shallow ulcers* that are painful and retain their erythematous bases. They favor mucosa tightly bound to periosteum, such as hard palate and alveolar ridges. The lesions disappear without scarring over several days to 2 weeks. A major differential diagnosis is *aphthous stomatitis,* which begins as flat discoloration without vesicles, grows pale and necrotic centrally, and ultimately resolves. Aphthous stomatitis favors mobile mucosae such as the oral vestibule. Its lesions tend to be solitary or sparse. They are often larger than individual herpes lesions.

ATROPHIC GLOSSITIS

Atrophy of papillae and epithelium produces a shiny red **"beefy tongue"** that is not inflamed: The erythema comes from increased visibility of subepithelial vasculature. Many nutritional deficiencies can cause the lesion, and a specific etiology cannot be inferred from the appearance of the tongue. The best known cause is the vitamin B_{12} deficiency of *pernicious anemia.* Riboflavin deficiency and other nutritional problems can produce the same picture. **Migratory atrophic glossitis,** by contrast, is an idiopathic condition not associated with nutritional deficiency; it is better known as **geographic tongue** because of the island-like sharpness of the localized, transient patches of epithelial atrophy that it produces. These need not have regular outlines and are sometimes polycyclic. Often, there is an erythematous component that may mislead the examiner to consideration of an inflammatory lesion. A tongue stained green by Clorets suggests a cover-up, perhaps of alcohol odors.

EARLY ORAL CANCER

Historically, white discolorations of the oral mucosa were grouped as *leukoplakia,* a clinical term without a pathologic correlate. The color of frank *invasive squamous cell carcinoma* of the mouth is white. However, red lesions are much more significantly associated with early intraoral cancer. Other "classic" signs of cancer of the mouth—ulceration, induration, and an exophytic mass—occur late and carry ominous prognoses. In high-risk patients (alcohol and tobacco abusers and persons who have had prior upper aerodigestive tract cancer(s)), any red lesion that fails to clear within 2 weeks of conservative therapy is regarded as potentially malignant and is biopsied. The decision is also influenced by locale, with the floor of the mouth, retromolar trigone, lateral border of the tongue, and tonsillar pillars constituting high-risk areas.

One condition not to be confused with neoplasia is a sprinkling of yellow or yellow-white dots on the buccal mucosa. These **Fordyce spots** are merely aggregated "ectopic" intraoral sebaceous apparatuses of no significance.

On the lips, a premalignant dry roughening is called **solar cheilosis.**

INTRAORAL KAPOSI'S SARCOMA

Kaposi's sarcoma of the mouth, a nonepithelial cancer, has increased dramatically because of AIDS. This malignancy, which can be multicentric, also occurs on the skin. The neoplasm forms red to red-blue to purple intraoral nodules, macules, and patches. It commonly is seen on gingiva and palate but can occur anywhere in the mouth. Its color, the setting, and the normal overlying oral epithelium all help distinguish it from oral squamous cell carcinoma. With chemotherapy, the lesions can flatten and grow paler, but a residual "stain" may persist, relating to hemosiderin that is very slowly cleared by macrophages.

OTHER AIDS-ASSOCIATED ORAL LESIONS

Candidal infection, usually of the white pseudomembranous variety, is the commonest oral physical finding in persons with HIV. Another lesion found predominantly in AIDS is *hairy leukoplakia*. It is due, at least in part, to Epstein-Barr virus infection. This is a whitish-gray roughening and thickening of mucosa, most commonly on the lateral border of the tongue; the dorsum of the tongue is very infrequently involved. The lesion may include upward-extending points that contribute to its name. *It does not scrape off* with a tongue blade.

Gingivitis is more severe in many AIDS patients, and periodontitis and root caries can be seen even with careful oral hygiene. Many other intraoral findings have been reported in AIDS. Most relate to the plethora of conventional and opportunistic infections to which this populace is subject, while others are neoplastic or unclassifiable.

ORAL SIGNS OF SYSTEMIC DISORDERS

Several oral signs of systemic disorders are mentioned above. There are scores of others. Three prototypes are described.

In *Crohn's disease,* the oral mucosa occasionally takes on the same fissured, cobblestoned appearance as the diseased bowel, both clinically and histologically. In other instances, edema and inflammation of the lip *(cheilitis)* can accompany or even precede intestinal manifestations. So also can unusually numerous and persistent *oral aphthae.*

Angular cheilosis denotes cracking, atrophy, and irritation of the outer corners of the mouth. As mentioned earlier it is reported in nutritional deficiencies, immune deficits, with ill-fitting dentures, and in settings where saliva escapes and macerates the tissue repeatedly or constantly. Candidal infection is common to many cases but perhaps not all. Similar changes associated with syphilis are termed *rhagades.*

Persons with *bulimia and anorexia nervosa* can develop erosions of the posterior (lingual) surface of the teeth as a result of repeated acid exposure from self-induced vomiting. These erosions spare the fillings in the teeth, "etching" around them, and produce a highly distinctive appearance that may provide the first clue to the often-concealed underlying problem.

CRANIAL NERVE XII

Lesions of the hypoglossal nerve cause tongue deviation toward the affected side, since the lingual muscle normally pushes the tongue away. Coexistent fasciculation strongly supports a neural cause, but absence of fasciculation does not prove that the lesion is mechanical. Certain patients are at risk for both local causes in and about the tongue and damage to the hypoglossal nerve. For example, persons who have had oral resection, neck dissection, and local radiotherapy for cancer of the tongue or floor of the mouth may develop damage to the glossal muscle and its nerve.

Pharynx

NEOPLASMS

Much of the pharynx cannot be seen by examination. For what can be observed, the criteria for suspecting cancer are the same as for the mouth, above, and so are the risk factors.

PHARYNGITIS

The hallmark of all pharyngitides is *erythema,* which may occur exclusively in the posterior pharynx or may extend to uvula, soft palate, and tonsillar pillars. Some cases include *purulent exudate.* Bacteria such as streptococci are more apt to produce exudate than viruses, but exudate is neither sensitive nor specific enough to rely on for discrimination between the two classes of pathogens. If a *membrane* is seen on the palate and pharynx, consider *diphtheria* and obtain expert help at once. *Gonorrheal pharyngitis* can occur in any host who has had orogenital sexual contact with an infected person. The physical appearance of gonorrheal pharyngitis on inspection of the throat does not differ from that of other inflammatory disorders. Special culture media are required.

If multiple *telangiectases* are seen on palate and pharynx but not diffuse erythema, consider whether *cirrhosis* or *hereditary hemorrhagic telangiectasia (Osler-Weber-Rendu syndrome)* may be mimicking pharyngitis.

CRANIAL NERVES IX AND X

Gag Reflex

The gag reflex is difficult to interpret. Some normal people lack it on one side or both. It is absent in many acutely ill persons without neurologic syndromes. Finally, its predictive value for risk of pulmonary aspiration of gastric contents is poor. An intact gag reflex is no guarantee against aspiration, and a reduced or absent one does not guarantee that this complication will develop.

Voice Quality

Hoarseness can occur with any lesion of CN X, especially if bilateral. Most commonly, it is seen with any primary laryngeal pathology. In thoracic disease, especially lung cancer, it raises the question of recurrent laryngeal nerve paresis. It is also found in some cases of *hypothyroidism*. Hoarseness cannot be dismissed as psychogenic just because no anatomic basis is found in the larynx area.

RECORDING THE FINDINGS

An example of recording the findings of an extended examination of the HEENT follows.

Procedure note: Pupillodilation.
Indications: Miosis; rule out Roth spots.
PMH: Denies glaucoma, eye pain, use of drops. Dilated without incident last year. Thinks findings were normal then.
Baseline: Pupils 2.5 mm right, 3 mm left. Both react directly and consensually. Anterior chamber not shallow on nipple test.
Technique: One drop 1% tropicamide instilled sterilely in either eye at 2:40 p.m.
Findings: Pupils 7 mm OU, nonreactive to light both directly and consensually at 3:10 p.m.
Fundi: Normal background, no hemorrhage/exudate or Roth spots. Arteries and veins normal. Venous pulsations well seen. Disc margins sharp, and cupping is physiologic.
Impression: Normal extended ophthalmoscopic examination.
Follow-up: Patient, nurse, and intern on call warned to follow up any failure to improve vision in 2 hours, or any eye pain, or new headache with prompt evaluation by house officer and probable call to ophthalmology.

BEYOND THE PHYSICAL EXAMINATION
Laboratory Studies

Blood work depends on the condition. For example, a Bell's palsy may call for Lyme titers; a facial Kaposi's sarcoma, for HIV serology; and atrophic glossitis, for markers of malnutrition such as prealbumin. Thyroid function tests are done to investigate hoarseness and deafness. Serologic tests for syphilis are part of the study of deafness in some cases. Tests for antinuclear antibodies are part of the workup for systemic lupus erythematosus. The erythrocyte sedimentation rate usually, but not always, rises in giant cell arteritis. The antineutrophil cytoplasmic antibody (ANCA) may be positive in Wegener's granulomatosis.

Smears can be subjected to Gram's stain, modified Wright's stain, Papanicolaou stain for cancer cells, viral culture, or bacterial culture. Specialized culture variants include throat culture for group A β-hemolytic streptococci, diphtheria culture, or neisserial culture. The settings include lesions suspicious for diverse infections. Nasal secretion smears are typically stained to demonstrate eosinophils in establishing an allergic cause.

Imaging

The multiplicity of sites covered in this chapter precludes comprehensive listing of imaging procedures. Computed tomography (CT) and magnetic resonance imaging (MRI) are used in virtually all HEENT sites. Ultrasound is of help in the study of the eye and orbit and can establish information about the retina even when hemorrhage renders the vitreous impenetrable to the ophthalmoscope. Plain radiographs are used for sinus imaging and for study of dental disease and some other conditions of the mouth and jaws. Clinical photography is most useful for retinal lesions—employing pupillodilation and a special camera—and for oral lesions. Fluorescein angiography augments study of retinal pathology, especially retinal vascular disease. Applanation tonometry and formal computerized perimetry assist assessment of intraocular hypertension and glaucoma and their consequences.

Consultation

Depending on the site of the problem, one of the following colleagues is called: dentist, neurologist, otolaryngologist, ophthalmologist, plastic surgeon, head and neck surgeon, neurosurgeon, audiologist. The principal help from any of these consultants lies in their cognitive skills about this complex region and some of its parts. In addition, they may employ special techniques such as audiometry or various kinds of endoscopy.

RECOMMENDED READINGS

Ahola SJ. Unexplained parotid enlargement: a clue to occult bulimia. Conn Med 1982;46:185–186.

Anonymous. Orofacial manifestations of HIV infection. Lancet 1988;1:976–977.

Bloom JN, Palestine AG. The diagnosis of cytomegalovirus retinitis. Ann Intern Med 1988;109: 963–969.

Curran RE. Palpation of the superficial temporal artery in normal persons. Arch Ophthalmol 1986; 104:1756.

Landau WM. Clinical neuromythology. I. The Marcus Gunn phenomenon: loose canon of neuro-ophthalmology. Neurology 1988;38:1141–1142.

Levin BE. The clinical significance of spontaneous pulsations of the retinal vein. Arch Neurol 1978;35:37–40.

Mashberg A, Samit A. Early detection, diagnosis, and management of oral and oropharyngeal cancer. CA 1989;39:67–88.

Paton D, Hyman BN, Justice JJ. Introduction to ophthalmoscopy. Kalamazoo: Upjohn, 1983(1976):1–92.

Sapira JD. An internist looks at the fundus oculi. Disease-a-Month 1984;30(November):1–64.

Uhlmann RF, Rees TS, Psaty BM, Duckert LG. Validity and reliability of auditory screening in demented and non-demented older adults. J Gen Intern Med 1989;4:90–95.

Wood NK, Goaz PW. Differential diagnosis of oral lesions. 3rd ed. St Louis: C V Mosby, 1985:1–791.

5

Neck

APPROACH AND ANATOMICAL REVIEW

The neck contains multiple anatomical structures representing several organ systems. The entire neck examination, with the exception of assessment of the carotid arteries and the cervical veins, is routinely performed with the patient seated and immediately follows the examination of the head, eyes, ears, nose, oral cavity, and throat. Palpation of the lymph nodes of the lower head is conducted as a part of the neck examination for convenience. **Inspection** and **palpation** are the modes used in the screening examination of the neck. **Instruments** and **supplies** required include **warm hands,** a **strong light source** for cross-illumination of the anterior structures and inspection of skin lesions, and a **paper cup** containing **drinking water.**

The cervical structures to be examined include the skin, the cervical spine, the trachea and nearby cartilages, the thyroid gland, the chains of lymph nodes, and the sternomastoid and trapezius muscles with their innervations. An understanding of the anatomical relationships of these structures and the terminology used to describe them is requisite to successful performance of the evaluation and communication of findings.

The skull and its structures are supported in part by the **cervical spine** and its ligamentous attachments to the atlas (C1) and axis (C2) (Fig. 5.1*A*). Adding to this support system are the large paired muscles, the **sternomastoids,** which are attached superiorly to the mastoid processes of the skull and then pass anteriorly and inferiorly to their attachments to the clavicles and sternoclavicular joint. The **trapezius** muscles extend on the posterolateral neck from the occiput to the scapula and upper thoracic vertebrae (Fig. 5.1*B*). Nerve supply to these muscles is provided by **cranial nerve XI (CN XI), the spinal accessory nerve.**

Tracheal cartilages form the major midline anterior cervical landmarks. They are somewhat visible and readily palpable except with extreme obesity or anasarca. The **thyroid** gland, with its two lobes (right and left) and its flattened isthmus, clasps the anterolateral portion of the mid-lower trachea and extends upward for some distance along the larynx (Fig. 5.2).

For convenience of description, the neck is divided into regions: **occipital,** the portion contiguous with the occiput of the skull; the **posterior triangles,** each bounded at its superior apex by the occiput, medially by the paraspinal ligaments and muscles, anterolaterally by the posterior margins of the sternomastoids, and inferiorly by the superior border of trapezius muscle; the **anterior triangles,** bounded superiorly by the angle of the jaw and the ramus of the mandible, medially by the trachea and midline, posterolaterally by the anterior margin of sternomastoid, and having their apices meet at the sternal notch; the **supraclavicular fossae** are defined medially by the root of the neck, anteroinferiorly by the clavicle, and posteriorly by the anterior margin of trapezius. Each is a triangle whose lateral border is the point formed by the acromioclavicular joint. The apices of the lungs lie deep to the soft tissue structures of the supraclavicular fossae (Fig. 5.3).

The lymphatic drainage of the head is supplied by a series of nodal chains: the **mandibular and mental,** the **preauricular and postauricular,** the **occipital,**

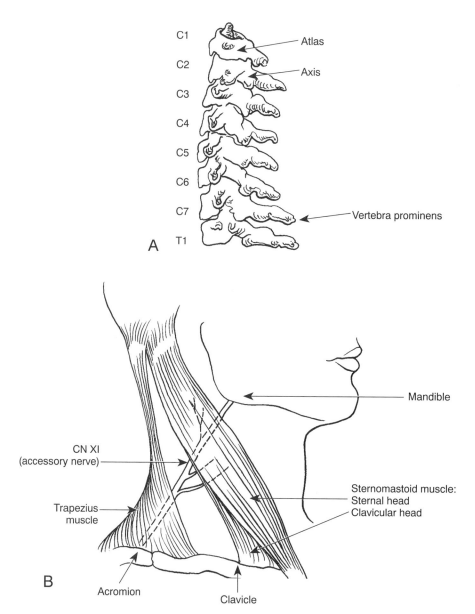

Figure 5.1 **A.** Anatomy of the bones of the cervical spine, lateral view. **B.** Placement of the major superficial cervical muscles.

posterior cervical, anterior cervical, and **supraclavicular.** The latter group also receives lymphatic drainage from thoracic and abdominal structures (see Fig. 5.4 for relationships of these nodal chains to the landmarks of the neck).

Other neck structures present, but not accessible for inspection or palpation, are

1. Esophagus, which lies immediately anterior to the bodies of the cervical spine
2. Larynx, which is just superior to the trachea (note that part of its outer surface is palpable, but the key aspect, its mucosa, cannot be assessed except with special instruments)
3. Cervical spinal nerves, which are discussed as a part of the neurologic examination (Chapter 11).

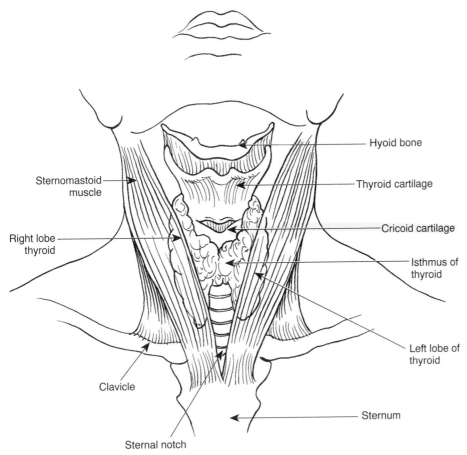

Figure 5.2   Relative positions of the bones near the trachea and of cartilages of the trachea and their relationships to the thyroid gland.

The visible and palpable vascular structures of the neck are assessed in concert with the cardiac examination (Chapter 8).

TECHNIQUE

The examiner works back and forth between inspection and palpation and will find it necessary to do some side-to-side shifting in order to make the necessary observations (see Table 5.1). The patient is seated at the end of the examining table. **Please note that the illustrations accompanying the neck examination picture the patient with gown open in front. This is done for clarity of demonstration. The gown, in ordinary clinical examination, is often worn open at the back.**

INSPECTION

General Inspection of the Neck

While standing directly in front of the patient with good cross-lighting available, the clinician assesses the contour and position of the neck. Is the head held straight and comfortably? Are the four major muscles symmetrical? Does the trachea seem to be in the midline? Are the superficial cervical veins distended?

Examination of the Skin of the Anterior Neck

The skin of the anterior and lateral neck is carefully inspected for lesions, discoloration, or scars. If anything abnormal is observed, it is palpated and measured as discussed in Chapter 3.

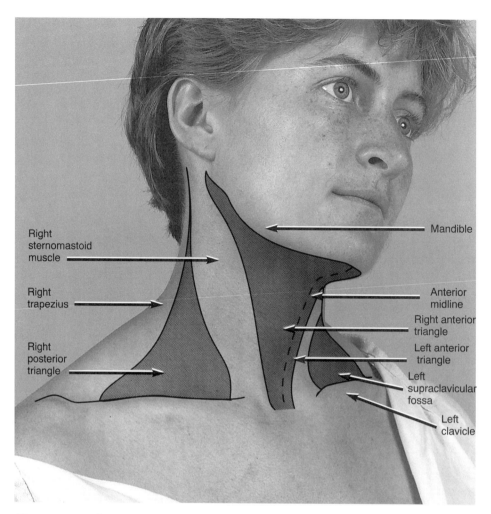

Figure 5.3 Surface projections of the major cervical triangles.

Assessment of Cervical Spine

The patient is asked to put the cervical spine through a range of motion encompassing six positions: hyperextension ("put your head all the way back"), lateral flexion to right and left ("try to put your ear on your shoulder"), flexion ("try to put your chin on your chest"), and rotation ("try to put your chin on your shoulder"). With the patient holding the flexed position, move to the patient's side and inspect the contour of the flexed neck, noting the normal protuberance of the spinous process of the seventh vertebra. While still standing at the patient's side, ask him to return his head to upright position. Note the curvature of the spine (Fig. 5.1*A*). Palpate the spinous processes for tenderness and alignment. This is a good time to **inspect the skin of the posterior neck.**

PALPATION

Head and Neck Lymph Nodes

Examination of head and neck lymph nodes is done with the examiner directly facing the patient and is conducted on both sides of the head and neck simultaneously. Use the pads and the tips of the three middle fingers for the examination. Hold them with the long axis of the respective fingers at 45° to the skin, which

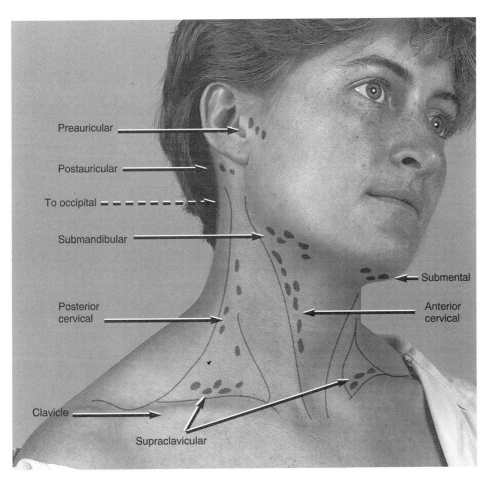

Figure 5.4   Surface projections of the chains of cervical lymph nodes.

avoids "digging in." Maintain constant skin contact while moving in small circles of palpation along each chain. Begin with the postauricular and preauricular nodal groups, then move the fingers to the angles of the jaw and palpate along the inferior ramus of the mandible until the fingers of the two hands meet under the chin. Start again at the occiput and palpate the posterior cervical triangle, feeling beneath the posterior margin of the sternomastoid as far as its clavicular attachment. It's also useful to "wander" a bit in the posterior triangle, since lymph node position is more variable in this chain than in the others. Now move laterally into the supraclavicular fossae, feeling for nodes along the clavicular margin, the center of the space, and the anterior borders of the trapezii. To examine the anterior cervical chains, start at the angles of the jaw and palpate downward along the anterior margins of the sternomastoids to their medial attachments at the clavicles (Fig. 5.5).

If at any point in the examination a subcutaneous nodule is felt, it should be carefully palpated for size (and measured), for mobility (freedom from attachment to underlying structures or overlying skin), for tenderness, for consistency (soft or fluctuant, normally firm, or rubbery, to even rock-hard), and for confluence with other nodes. Also look for any dimple or drainage onto the overlying skin. If a rounded anterior cervical lymph node that can be defined transversely but not craniocaudally is palpated, feel for pulsation; the carotid artery is easy to misperceive as a node.

Table 5.1
Steps in the Screening Neck Examination

Inspection
    Position of head and neck
    Symmetry of cervical musculature
    Position of trachea
    Skin of neck
    Cervical spine movement
        Flexion, anterior and lateral
        Extension
        Rotation

Palpation
    Cervical spinous processes
    Head and neck lymph nodes
        Preauricular and postauricular
        Mandibulomental
        Occipital
        Posterior cervical
        Anterior cervical
        Supraclavicular
        Infraclavicular

    Airway (trachea)
        Hyoid bone
        Thyroid cartilage
    Thyroid gland
    Cranial nerve XI
        Mass and strength of sternomastoids
        Mass and strength of trapezii

Trachea

With the fingertips, locate the hard, but retreating, **hyoid bone** inferior to the floor of the mouth. Move downward to the larger **thyroid cartilage.** At least two **tracheal rings** should be palpable below the thyroid cartilage. Are all structures midline or symmetric?

Thyroid Gland

Accurate, meaningful palpation of the thyroid gland is one of the most difficult skills to perfect. Each examiner has a favorite way of approaching this examination, and three variations are described. Begin the examination by inspecting the neck from in front with a strong cross-light. Sometimes, the gland will be visible, and palpation will be directed by inspection. Most commonly, the gland is too small and too deeply engaged with the trachea and behind the sternomastoids to be visualized. Many patients will try to help you with this inspection by extending the neck, raising the chin. This tightens the skin, however, and actually *impairs* inspection, so you should say, "Please just keep your head straight." You don't want the chin lowered unduly either, since that will close off visibility of part of the neck. Hand the patient a small cup of water to assist him in swallowing, and *watch* two swallows to see if anything in the zones of thyroid lobes or isthmus moves with deglutition. If so, you will approach palpation forewarned about a goiter or a thyroid nodule.

    Method A: posterior method (preferred by the authors). This method is conducted with the examiner standing behind the patient. It is facilitated by asking

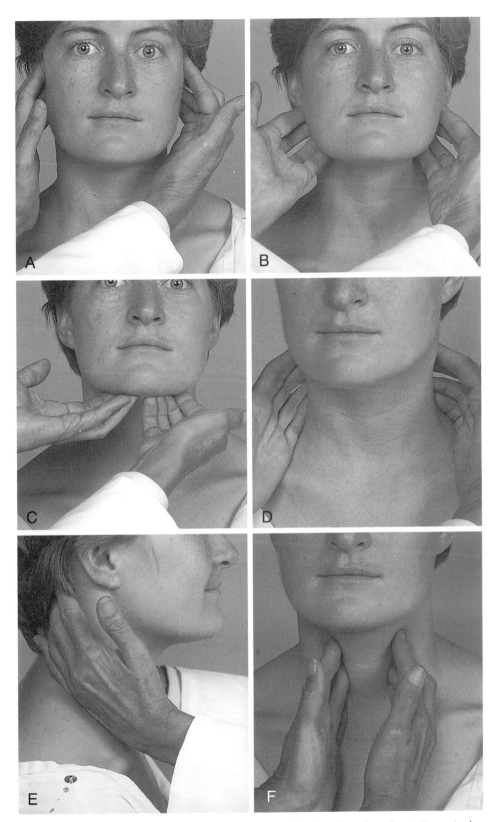

Figure 5.5 Technique of lymph node palpation of the head and neck. **A.** Preauricular nodes. **B.** Mandibular nodes. **C.** Submental nodes. **D.** Posterior cervical chains of nodes. **E.** Occipital nodes. **F.** Anterior cervical chains of nodes. **G.** Supraclavicular nodes.

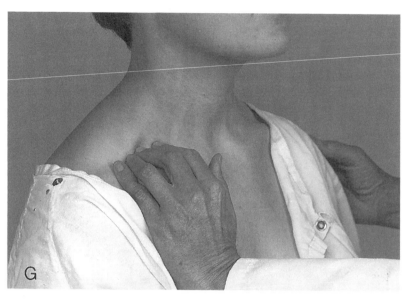

Figure 5.5   G.

the patient to sit sidewise on the table such that the examiner can reach the trachea from behind the patient's back. The fingers of the right hand are placed anterior to the right sternomastoid and pressed forward and medially against the right lateral trachea; the fingers of the left hand compress the left lobe of the gland from the front (Fig. 5.6*A*). When the gland is located, the patient is asked to swallow water from the cup. If your fingers are on the left thyroid lobe, you should feel the structure move upward with deglutition. Once the lobe is identified, palpate it for consistency, nodularity, or tenderness. If nodules or variations in consistency are found, an estimate of size is made, and they are characterized and localized (upper pole, lower pole, etc.). The procedure is repeated in reverse for the right lobe. The isthmus is felt by placing two fingers of each hand over the lower tracheal cartilage and palpating for the soft band of glandular tissue.

Method B: anterior method. Ask the patient to hold a small amount of water in his mouth. Place the three middle fingers of your left hand behind the patient's right sternomastoid, pressing anteriorly and toward the tracheal border (medially) to trap the thyroid and press it forward. Place the fingers of your right hand deep between the trachea and the anterior margin of the sternomastoid (Fig. 5.6*B*). You should feel a rim of soft tissue against the lateral margin of the trachea. With this tissue under your fingers, ask the patient to swallow the water in his mouth. Assessment then proceeds as in the previous method. Repeat the procedure for the left lobe, reversing hand positions. The isthmus of the gland is sought by palpating with three fingers superficial to the lower tracheal ring.

Method C: alternative anterior method. The three middle fingers of each hand are placed simultaneously, with pads to the trachea, under the anterior margins of sternomastoids, and the patient is asked to swallow. This method loses the advantage of "trapping" and is better for screening than for careful assessment of the individual lobes. The isthmus is examined as above.

Cranial Nerve XI: The Spinal Accessory Nerve

Cranial nerve XI, the spinal accessory nerve, innervates the sternomastoids and trapezii. The muscle mass and strength depend on intact innervation. The bulk of

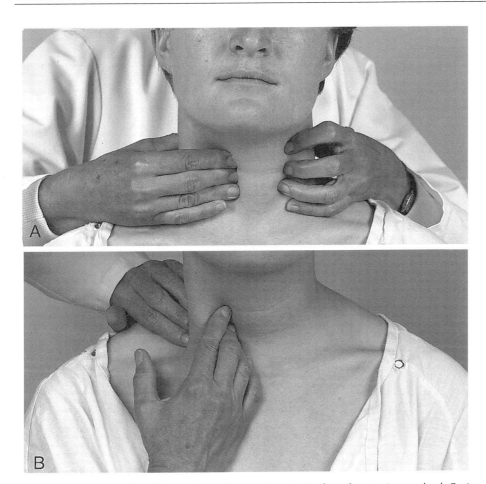

Figure 5.6 Two modes of thyroid gland palpation. **A.** Preferred posterior method. **B.** An anterior method.

the paired muscles should be symmetric, and they should carry out their normal function equally.

The nerve branch to the **sternomastoid** is assessed as follows: The patient is asked to rotate (not tilt) his head to the right. The examiner places her right palm against the patient's left cheek or mandibular ramus, and asks the patient to rotate toward midline against this resistance. This tests function of the **left** muscle and its nerve. Reverse the position of head and hand to test the **right** muscle and nerve.

Trapezius strength is tested bilaterally at once by placing the examiner's hands on top of the muscle mass and asking the patient to shrug his shoulders upward. The shoulders should rise symmetrically against this downward hand pressure, and both muscle bodies should be felt in equal contraction (Fig. 5.7).

NORMAL AND COMMON VARIANTS

Examination of the neck will reveal some, but relatively few, variants from normal that do not require further investigation. Some of the variants described are congenital and will occasionally require correction because of complications or for cosmetic reasons; others are self-limited and need only observation; still others relate to aging and, although sometimes symptomatic, are not problems and need no workup treatment. The following variants occur commonly enough or are sufficiently striking as physical findings that every clinician needs to become familiar with them (Table 5.2).

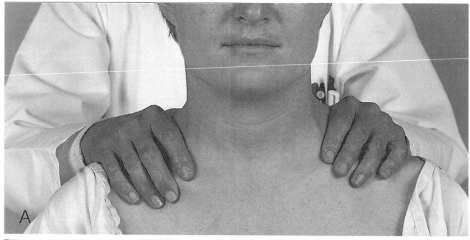

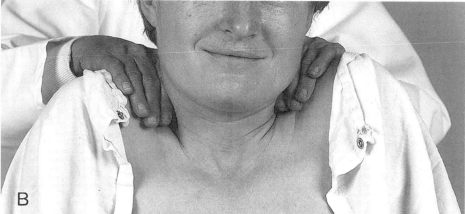

Figure 5.7 Testing cranial nerve XI—shoulder shrug component. **A.** Resting position of shoulders and examiner's downward pressure. **B.** Shrug against examiner's downward pressure.

Soft Tissue Masses

There are several masses that may be noted by the patient or discovered on routine examination of the neck that represent developmental abnormalities, although they may not become apparent until adulthood.

PYRAMIDAL LOBE OF THE THYROID

Pyramidal lobe of the thyroid must be distinguished from a thyroglossal duct cyst, lymphadenopathy, or thyroid nodule. This projection of normal thyroid tissue arises from the isthmus and extends upward, sometimes as high as the hyoid bone. It is triangular, with its base contiguous with the isthmus of the gland. It has the consistency of thyroid tissue and moves accordingly, i.e., rises with deglutition.

THYROGLOSSAL DUCT CYST

Thyroglossal duct cyst is a projection that arises from remnants of the primitive thyroglossal duct and may appear at any time in life, although it occurs most commonly in childhood or adolescence. It is a painless, soft mass that may present above or below the hyoid bone in the midline. If the cyst presents at the level of the thyroid cartilage, it may protrude laterally. It is distinguishable from an

Table 5.2
Common Variants^a

Masses in the neck
    Pyramidal lobe of thyroid
    [Thyroglossal duct cyst]
    [Branchial cleft cyst]
    [Diverticulum of pharynx or larynx]
    [Diverticulum of esophagus]

Cervical spine
    Klippel-Feil anomaly
    [Torticollis]
    [Spinal limitation of motion or pain upon motion]
      [Osteoarthrosis]
      [Posttraumatic]

Lymph node enlargement
    [Local infection]

^a[. . .], common but abnormal; and **boldface,** most common.

enlarged lymph node by its *upward movement on protrusion of the tongue,* to which it is connected.

BRANCHIAL CLEFT CYST

Branchial cleft cyst is a mass appearing in childhood or adulthood, usually just anterior to the upper third of sternomastoid muscle. Unless secondarily infected, it is painless and soft and contains cloudy, cholesterol–crystal-laden fluid on aspiration. The branchial cleft cyst forms in an area of incomplete closure of branchial arches of the developing fetus.

DIVERTICULA OF THE PHARYNX OR LARYNX

Diverticula of the pharynx or larynx are uncommon, intermittent, pressure-dependent masses of the neck. They are described by the patient as "coming and going," fading with swallowing and reappearing with blowing the nose, executing a Valsalva maneuver (bearing down with the glottis closed), or playing a brass or wind instrument.

DIVERTICULUM OF THE ESOPHAGUS (ZENKER'S DIVERTICULUM)

Diverticulum of the esophagus (Zenker's diverticulum) is an unusual, typically symptomatic lateral cervical mass that is also a pressure anomaly created in a congenitally defective segment of esophageal muscularis. It is mentioned here because of its potential confusion with branchial cleft cyst or diverticula of the pharynx or larynx. The esophageal diverticulum may become quite large and may store swallowed food that is periodically regurgitated (undigested) back into the patient's mouth. The history is usually very helpful in differentiating this cystic pouch from those that are less troublesome to the patient. (See Figure 5.8 for surface projections of the cervical masses described.)

Klippel-Feil Anomaly

Klippel-Feil anomaly refers to a congenital fusion of cervical vertebrae that results in a very short neck with resultant limitation of head movement. It is rare and seen more commonly in women than in men. The trapezii appear shortened, thus giving the neck a "webbed" appearance. History will indicate that the anom-

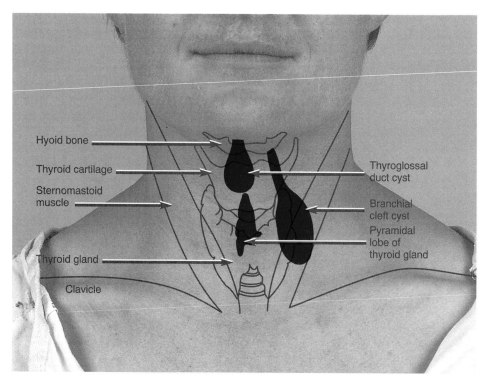

Figure 5.8   Surface projections of several cervical masses.

aly has been present since birth. The condition should present no differential diagnostic problems.

Cervical Musculature

Torticollis is a term that refers to a twisting of the neck secondary to spasm or disease of one or more of the muscles controlling cervical motion. Most commonly, the patient will complain of having awakened from sleep with an acute fixation of the neck muscles in an abnormal position, correction of which is very painful. This is considered to be the result of muscle inflammation with spasm, either viral or traumatic (such as sleeping with the head unusually placed) in etiology. Despite its dramatic inconvenience and discomfort, "wryneck" usually remits spontaneously. The other form of acute spastic torticollis occasionally encountered is caused by a dystonic reaction to phenothiazines or related compounds. The history of medication intake and the frequent accompaniment of dystonic movements of the jaw and mouth should differentiate this torticollis from the other form of "wryneck," which is not accompanied by any involuntary movements.

Cervical Spine

With the patient sitting erect, there is normally a gentle extension curve to the cervical spine when viewed from the side (physiologic cervical lordosis). Palpation or percussion with the middle finger should not elicit tenderness.

In the aged person having some osteoporotic compression of the anterior portion of the thoracic vertebral bodies, the head and neck may be thrust somewhat forward by the change in spinal alignment. Old cervical trauma or spinal surgery may account for some variation in the curvature of the cervical spine; this should be confirmed by a history of the deviation dating from the event and/or by surgical scars.

The normal movement of the cervical spine allows for 45° of anterior flexion from the rest position, 40° of extension, and 45° of lateral flexion to each side. Most of this movement occurs at the C3-C4 and C4-C5 articulations. Rotation should be about 70° to either side (Fig. 5.9). If **limitation** of motion occurs during any of these routine maneuvers, the patient is queried about the duration of the limitation and its possible relationship to trauma or surgery. **Pain** on cervical motion is **not normal** and requires investigation.

Osteoarthrosis (spondylosis or degenerative arthritis) of some degree is common in the aged. It is painless unless nerve root irritation occurs (see the Extended Examination section), although it may lead to moderate generalized limitation of neck motion. In this case, the patient may report a crunching sound with hyperextension of the neck, and the examiner may feel a grating sensation (**crepitus**) while palpating the cervical spine during flexion and extension.

Lymph Nodes of the Head and Neck

A clear understanding of the drainage pattern of the lymphatic system is important to assessment of any nodal enlargement (Fig. 5.10). When a lymph node or group of nodes proves palpable, examine the area drained by these nodes for evidence of mass or, more commonly, of infection. For example, scalp infections or a wound may lead to tender enlargement of the occipital or postauricular nodes. An abscess of a lower molar can cause submandibular nodal enlargement. Anterior cervical chain nodes are frequently enlarged during the course of, and after, acute tonsillitis or a pharyngeal infection. Palpable posterior cervical lymph nodes are seen in rubella and quite often in infectious mononucleosis. Preauricular lymphadenitis commonly accompanies otitis and adenoviral conjunctivitis.

A few palpable, small, mobile, nontender nodes may be discovered in a perfectly healthy adult. One study of well persons showed a high prevalence of this finding. If a palpable cervical node **feels normal**, i.e., is less than 2 cm in its greatest dimension, is soft, freely movable, and unattached to other structures, but cannot be accounted for on the basis of local infection, it should be carefully described in the patient's record and reexamined for change in 2–3 weeks. Because of their drainage of deep and nonaccessible structures, palpable supraclavicular nodes must be investigated promptly.

Trachea

The normal trachea is midline and somewhat movable from side to side. Any deviation, fixation, or pain on gentle movement by the examiner's fingers is outside the range of normal.

Thyroid Gland

In the adult, the normal thyroid gland weighs 25–30 g. However, norms vary inversely with dietary iodine content. Each lateral lobe is elongated, 4–5 cm in height and about 2 cm in width. Because of its configuration and placement beneath the sternomastoids, it is commonly not palpable in adults—especially if the neck muscles are well developed or if the neck is fat. The right lobe is often somewhat larger than the left; therefore, it is not unusual to feel only the right lobe in a normal person. The entire gland may enlarge slightly during adolescence and pregnancy but should retain its normal shape and consistency and be free of nodules or tenderness.

Cranial Nerve XI: The Spinal Accessory Nerve

The sternomastoids and trapezii are normally symmetrical in position, size, and strength. Any appreciable deviation from this symmetry implies either disease of

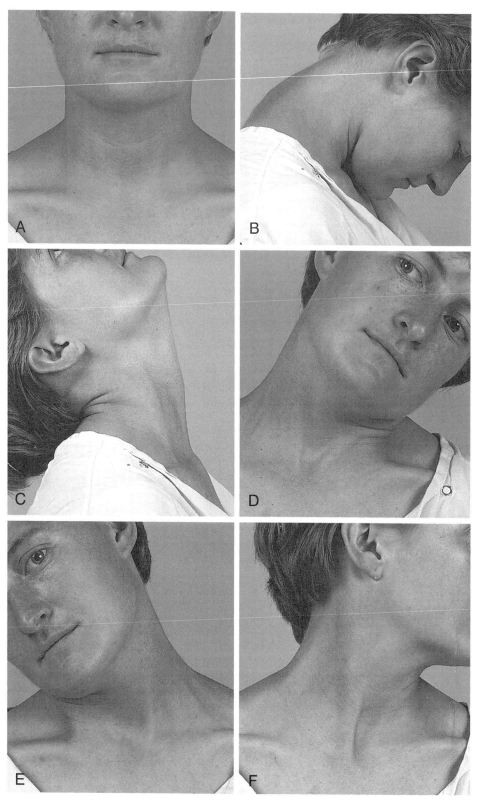

Figure 5.9 Normal cervical spine range of motion. **A.** Resting position. **B.** Anterior flexion. **C.** Extension. **D.** Lateral flexion ("tipping") to left. **E.** Lateral flexion ("tipping") to right. **F.** Lateral rotation to left. **G.** Lateral rotation to right.

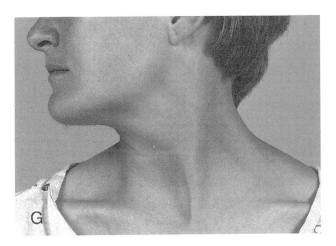

Figure 5.9   G.

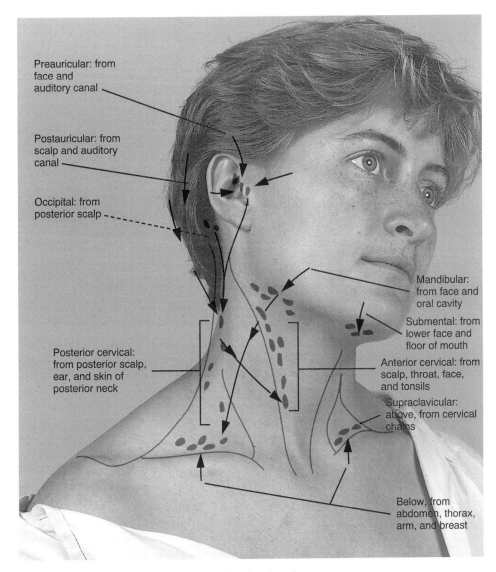

Preauricular: from
face and
auditory canal

Postauricular: from
scalp and auditory
canal

Occipital: from
posterior scalp

Posterior cervical:
from posterior scalp,
ear, and skin of
posterior neck

Mandibular:
from face and
oral cavity

Submental: from
lower face and
floor of mouth

Anterior cervical: from
scalp, throat, face,
and tonsils

Supraclavicular:
above, from cervical
chains

Below, from
abdomen, thorax,
arm, and breast

Figure 5.10   Lymphatic drainage of the head and neck.

the muscle body itself or loss of normal motor function of the **spinal accessory nerve** on the affected side or its nucleus. Keep in mind that pain in a shoulder, cervical spine disease, or "wryneck" may cause the patient to resist attempts to test the strength of an otherwise normally innervated muscle. In these instances, testing of the motor integrity of the cranial nerve may be rendered invalid.

RECORDING THE FINDINGS

The description of the neck examination is regionally partitioned in the patient's record. Position, active range of motion (AROM), and the thyroid examination appear under the heading NECK. Skin of the neck joins its organ system, SKIN, and the lymph nodes may be recorded with all others under a separate heading, LYMPH NODES. Description of the trachea is most logically recorded with the THORAX AND LUNGS (RESPIRATORY).

EXTENDED EXAMINATION OF THE NECK

The neck is a complex crossroads of respiratory, digestive, vascular, lymphatic, vertebral, and neural structures, with most of them conveying matter or information between thorax and head but with some branching out to the arms. For this reason, regional examination of the neck is intimately tied to a functional approach. So many organ systems converge here that a single disorder may affect several, and the discussion that follows will frequently point to other regions.

INDICATIONS
Symptoms
PAIN IN THE NECK

The most common question requiring a more probing study of the neck is why a person has acute or chronic pain in some part of the neck. Sometimes the history is obvious, e.g., musculoskeletal strain. At other times it is obscure.

CEREBROVASCULAR OR NERVE ROOT SYMPTOMS

The carotid and vertebral arteries traverse the neck. Symptoms of stroke or transient ischemic attack (TIA)—lateralized motor or sensory loss, amaurosis fugax, or transient aphasia—lead to consideration of extracranial arterial obstruction. The delineation has particular importance, since carotid endarterectomy can dramatically decrease the risk of permanent and disabling neurologic deficits in highly selected subgroups. Symptoms associated with vertebrobasilar disease such as dizziness and vertigo carry no such surgical implications. Sensory or motor dysfunction in the distribution of cervical spinal roots, in the arm or hand, will also lead to extended assessment, but of the cervical spine and neural structures rather than of the carotid arteries.

Physical Findings
LYMPHADENOPATHY

The patient in whom abnormal lymph nodes are detected elsewhere in the body or in whom a disorder associated with diffuse lymphadenopathy is suspected will have assessment of all chains in the head and neck, for diagnosis and staging.

In any patient with an established **primary cancer of the head and neck** (mouth, larynx, cervical esophagus, etc.), the lymph nodes are inspected and palpated with great care in the search for metastases, inasmuch as *confirmed* metastases alter goals and details of management.

Mixed Symptoms and Signs
FEVER AND HEADACHE

Fever and headache lead to careful assessment of the neck for signs of acute meningeal irritation. Unfortunately, such signs are sometimes seen without inflammation and are frequently lacking in the presence of irritation. Thus the decision for or against the key diagnostic procedure, lumbar puncture, does not always correspond to findings in the neck examination. Meningeal signs are discussed in detail in the Extended Examination section of Chapter 11.

WEIGHT CHANGE

Unexplained weight change can result from many causes including neoplasm, chronic infection, or thyroid dysfunction. The search for these problems will include detailed study of several cervical structures.

RESPIRATORY ABNORMALITIES

Respiratory symptoms, especially if positional or confusing, may lead to investigation of the trachea. So will **stridor,** the noisy and distressed inspiration that arises from the larynx or trachea in several physical disorders and, rarely, in psychogenic distress. **Hoarseness** is seen with local disorders of the larynx, most often transient inflammation. When the symptom persists, the larynx is evaluated by using methods outside the scope of this book. The generalist has a contribution to make in evaluation of the thyroid: Hypothyroidism is a "non-anatomical" cause of hoarseness that cannot be detected by visualization of the larynx.

In the **cigarette smoker,** cancer of the larynx is a special concern. The extended examination of the neck will include careful palpation of cervical lymph nodes for metastatic laryngeal cancer.

A RARE ENTITY

Finally, a personal or family history of a **multiple endocrine neoplasia syndrome** calls for careful study of the thyroid and the cervical lymph nodes. Various proliferations in thyroid and parathyroid can occur in these conditions. The malignant neoplasms among them can produce lymph node metastases.

Abnormalities Noted on the Screening Physical Examination

A patient in whom an **oral or head and neck cancer** is suspected from screening physical examination will require the same extended cervical lymph node examination as one in whom there is an established history.

The patient with a **neck mass** always needs workup. This is addressed in detail below.

Any patient with an **abdominal, pelvic, or pulmonary cancer** needs extended examination of supraclavicular lymph nodes. Enlarged nodes will alter staging, management, and prognosis.

Abnormalities on Routine Laboratory Studies

The most common and pertinent scenario is an **abnormal thyroid function test.** Goiter will be sought in cases of hypothyroidism, and both diffuse toxic hyperplasia (Graves' disease) and nodular lesions are considered when the bloodwork shows hyperthyroidism. The extended physical examination of the thyroid is most often, however, inconclusive in assigning a cause to thyroid dysfunction.

CONDUCTING THE EXTENDED EXAMINATION

As with the basic examination, the patient is seated, with his legs dangling, except as noted.

Skin

The **"neck sign"** is elicited by having the patient drop the relaxed arms to his sides. Then he extends the head so that the chin points forward and a bit up. He looks up. The examiner looks for tightness and ridging of the longitudinal skin folds that run up the sides of the neck, anteriorly over the throat, and down to the sternal notch. If such ridges are found, they are palpated to determine whether they are lax or tight and taut.

Cervical Spine

There are 35 joints in the cervical spine, so except for the subspecialist, precise localization is seldom feasible. The examiner should know that C2-3 is the "headache joint" and C5-6 is commonly an "osteoarthrosis joint" that typically produces arm as well as neck symptoms. In general, extended examination of the cervical spine is directed toward reproducing symptoms and seeking the anatomic level of a problem, either for definitive management or to direct intelligent selection of tests and consultants.

INSPECTION

Inspection is accomplished by observing motion both supine and seated. First, the examiner checks active range of cervical motion in the six cardinal directions, as described in the Screening Examination section. Note especially how **comfortable** or **willing** the patient appears about **moving the head and neck.** Focus on **neck flexion,** since this is often the most uncomfortable movement with neck arthritis. Is the rest position of the head normal or deviated? If it is deviated, the first question is whether this is simple torticollis or something else. Excess sagging of the shoulders and a hunched appearance suggest different problems.

On attempting lateral flexion of the neck, some patients with pain or limited range of motion will compensate (sometimes unconsciously) by elevating the ipsilateral shoulder toward the head. If this is observed, the examiner asks the patient to lower the shoulder. If she is unsure, when attempting to assess **rotation,** that rotation has been isolated from lateral flexion, the examiner can specify, "Look backward over your shoulder." If the active range of motion seems disproportionately slight, so that **voluntary** limitation of motion is suspected, the six directions are retested while distracting the patient with engaging questions, e.g., "Can you name all the members of the Cabinet?", or activity, e.g., "Tap your toes rapidly, then roll your eyeballs."

PALPATION

Spinous processes are palpable in the midline posteriorly. C2 (the axis) is the first large projection you can feel inferior to the occiput. C3–C5 are impalpable. C6 can be felt but disappears with extension of the neck. C7 is the **vertebra prominens** that forms a familiar bump at the base of the neck. The **facet joints** lie 2 cm lateral to the midline. The **transverse process of C1** (the atlas) can be felt as a deep indistinct firmness between the angle of the jaw and the mastoid.

For the examiner to study **joint pain** contributing to neck pain, the patient holds the head immobile while the examiner presses down on the head in flexion, extension, and rotation to either side. Since the joints should produce little discomfort while held still in this way, pain with these maneuvers points toward a nonarticular origin unless there is *severe* inflammation or malalignment.

The **compression test** is performed as follows. The head is laterally flexed by the patient toward the painful side. The neck is actively extended slightly. The examiner places steady pressure downward on the head, compressing the ipsilateral articular pillar. The **quadrant test** consists of the same but, in addition, with the neck **actively rotated** toward the painful side. This maneuver achieves narrowing of the intervertebral foramina.

Upper Airway and Digestive Tract

The **hyoid** is palpated by pressing superoposteriorly, well above the thyroid cartilage and below the mandible.

Mirror or endoscopic examination of the **larynx,** while vital to diagnosis of laryngeal disease, lies outside the realm of this textbook.

TRACHEA

On inspection, the normal trachea lies in the midline or within 4 mm to the right of this line with the patient seated upright. Detection of asymmetry is improved by observing the trachea at end-inspiration with a deep breath, when deviation may be accentuated or may first become visible.

Palpation of the trachea can corroborate displacement and disclose tenderness. A special assessment is for **tracheal tug.** The patient is seated, mouth closed and chin fully elevated. To elicit a tug, the examiner holds the cricoid cartilage between thumb and index finger and presses upward.

Auscultation of the trachea (Fig. 5.11) may reveal wheezes of pulmonary as well as laryngotracheal origin, for example, in an asthmatic attack without wheezes on **pulmonary auscultation.** For the patient with stridor, tracheal auscultation may show intense wheezing that is not well heard elsewhere. Tracheal auscultation can confirm a functional or structural critical narrowing of the upper airway.

Various writings have described changes in wheeze pattern with head position and other variables when a partial obstruction of the trachea acts as a ball valve. However, wheezes are routinely sought with the head in rest position. If they are heard, they should be characterized with regard to phase of the respiratory cycle. Wheezes are expected in expiration but may be heard throughout the cycle. When present, they should be compared to auscultatory phenomena over the chest, i.e., both extent and severity of thoracic wheezing, if any, and should be compared to thoracic breath sound intensity as a first approximation of global air exchange.

The **esophagus** lies so deep that inspection and palpation of the neck are likely to offer no insights regarding this organ even when it is severely disordered. Observed swallowing may transiently enlarge a Zenker's diverticulum. There is also indirect assessment of obstruction and dysfunction via timing esophageal transit (see the Extended Examination section of Chapter 4). Discovery of metastatic supraclavicular lymphadenopathy from a primary esophageal cancer carries no helpful therapeutic implication in 1994.

Thyroid

Extended examination of the thyroid entails additional attention and repetition, rather than more maneuvers. The import of inspection requires reemphasis. Many goiters and nodules are *visible as well as palpable.* Strong cross-lighting is indispensable. A well-directed flashlight can bring out landmarks and lumps with surprising frequency (Fig. 5.12). You must look low enough in the neck: A search at midneck will be fruitless, since the isthmus lies only a few centimeters

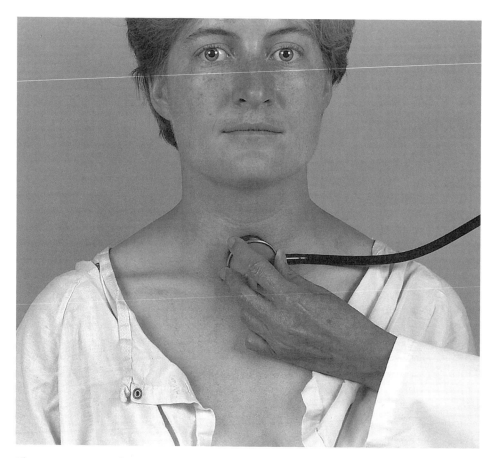

Figure 5.11 *Auscultation of the trachea* may reveal wheezes even when conventional pulmonary auscultation does not. Furthermore, by changing the patient's neck position, the examiner may hear different airflow in the presence of partial obstruction.

above the suprasternal notch. The lobes extend upward 4 or 5 cm. For any swellings visible at rest, the **absence of visible elevation on swallowing** usually excludes a thyroidal origin. This liberates the examiner from having to dig in with palpating fingers in an attempt to delineate gland, goiter, or nodules. If the neck is thick or short, the patient can extend the neck moderately and clasp his hands behind him, and the examiner can reinspect both the contour at rest and the effect of swallowing a sip of water.

The fingers can be run up and down the anterior midtrachea to seek the thyroid isthmus and laterally to try to delineate the lobes. If the sternomastoids feel tight, the examiner can have the patient laterally flex his neck *slightly* toward the side being assessed. This will relax, soften, and to some degree mobilize the ipsilateral sternomastoid. This way, a previously impalpable thyroid lobe or nodule will sometimes pop out at the examiner's fingertips or become distinct from background cervical tissues. Some patients have a central *pyramidal lobe of the thyroid* extending well up from the isthmus. This may be discovered with a *broadly pinching palpation* (Fig. 5.13) that spans the midline. The touchstone is whether the tissue rises with swallowing.

Auscultation of palpable thyroid lobes with the bell of the stethoscope (Fig. 5.14) can reveal systolic arterial murmurs, i.e., bruits. These occur in diffuse toxic hyperplasia of the thyroid (Graves' disease). High bloodflow to endocrine glands explains how such a small organ can engender an arterial sound. If a low-pitched

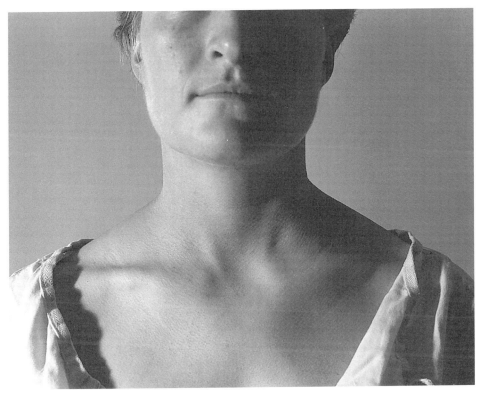

Figure 5.12 *Cross-lighting of the neck* is essential in any detailed assessment. The thyroid gland is often *visible* as well as palpable, particularly if goitrous (enlarged). So are many other anatomical landmarks, such as the clavicular heads of the sternomastoid, the trachea, and the supraclavicular fossae. Many masses also become visible in this setting; the rarity of employing this method of investigation contrasts starkly with its ease, simplicity, lack of cost, and utility.

sound is heard, check whether it persists when pressure is applied to the bell. Pressure converts the skin to a diaphragm, filtering out low frequencies and leaving only high ones. If such is the case, inch up the carotids and down to the base of the heart. If need be, also, reauscultate the lobes after occluding external jugular outflow with light finger pressure just above the clavicle.

Humility about the power of physical examination is an essential component of extended examination of the thyroid and environs.

The **parathyroids** are almost never palpable even when massively enlarged. The absence of physical signs does not exclude thyroid or parathyroid disease.

Cervical Lymph Nodes

In searching for lymph nodes, feel widely in the posterior triangle for **posterior cervical lymph nodes.** They do not cluster within a centimeter or two of the posterior border of sternomastoid the way anterior cervical lymph nodes do anteriorly. **Wandering fingers** often detect them 4 or even 8 cm posteriorly and at any craniocaudad level in the neck. Let the wandering fingers ascend the anterolateral margins of trapezius, and finish by repalpating for occipital nodes.

LEFT SUPRACLAVICULAR LYMPH NODE (VIRCHOW'S SENTINEL NODE)

To bring out a left supraclavicular lymph (Virchow's sentinel) node(s), three techniques are advocated:

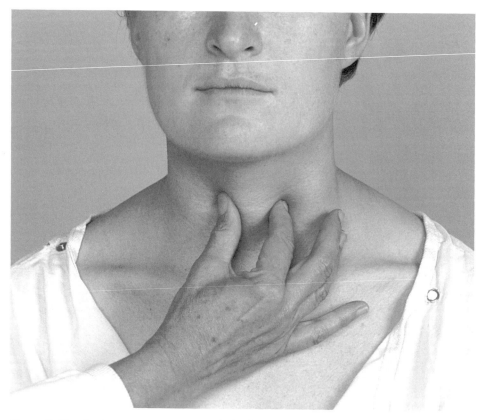

Figure 5.13   A pincers movement may help the examiner feel the *pyramidal lobe of the thyroid gland,* especially on scouting 2 cm below the level illustrated. Have the patient swallow, preferably from a cup of water, to ascertain that the putative thyroidal tissue rises with deglutition. If it does not, it isn't thyroid.

1. **Palpate from behind**. For this, the key feature is *adaptation of the examiner's anatomy to that of the patient.* Her flexed fingers curl over the shoulder and slip deeply into the supraclavicular fossa (Fig. 5.15).
2. Have the patient perform a **Valsalva maneuver.** The increased intrathoracic pressure should push the supraclavicular nodes superiorly, bringing them within reach of probing fingers.
3. If need be, repeat the examination with the patient *supine.* In this case, gravity redistributes the tissues favorably. The examiner positions herself at the head of the bed for best results with this maneuver, i.e., to enhance retroclavicular reach.

What feels like a rock-hard supraclavicular lymph node may actually be the tip of a *cervical rib.* To distinguish the two, the examiner's thumb "pops" or "twangs" the ipsilateral posterior area where such a rib would articulate with the spine, at a point just anterior to the trapezius and due posterior to the lymph node. If the "node" reliably moves with each push of the thumb, it is actually a rib tip transmitting movement initiated at the end of a rigid bone.

INFRACLAVICULAR LYMPH NODES

The chain of infraclavicular lymph nodes is traditionally checked with the lymph nodes of the neck and axilla. It is easy to explore. The fingertips are swept along the anteroinferior aspect of the clavicle, from shoulder to sternal notch. Regionally metastatic breast cancer is the commonest source of enlargement.

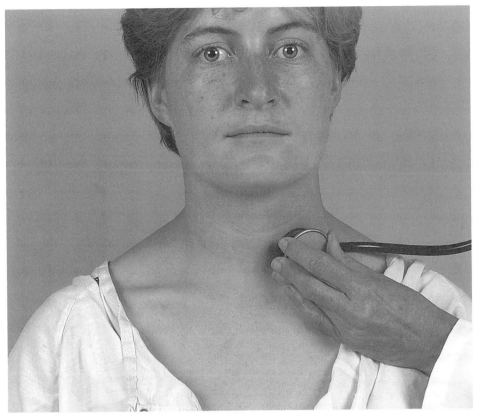

Figure 5.14 *Auscultation of the thyroid* may reveal a bruit in some goiters. The bell is placed lightly over palpable thyroid lobes. The sign is not sensitive; however, its specificity is greatest when alternative sound sources such as carotid bruits are unlikely. The patient at greatest risk, a young woman, fits this profile.

CHARACTERISTICS

When enlarged nodes are detected in the neck or elsewhere, the examiner automatically performs an extended examination by feeling the area carefully for

1. *Tenderness.* Extremely tender lymph nodes are usually inflamed, but some malignant nodes are tender too. Tuberculosis is variable. Large nontender lymph nodes are often but not always cancerous.
2. *Size.* What is the largest dimension? Under 1 cm is usually innocuous; over 5 cm, almost always cancer–often a hematologic malignancy. However, other conditions can rarely produce nodes as large or larger.
3. *Consistency.* Rock-hard nodes are often malignant. Fluctuant nodes raise the question of suppuration, which is commonest in bacterial lymphadenitis but not confined to that condition.
4. *Fixation.* Three separate components must be elucidated.
    a. Is the node *stuck to the overlying skin?*
    b. Is it immobile with respect to the *subjacent fascia* or body wall?
    c. Is it *matted* to one or more other nodes? In this last case, the examiner may feel a multilobar or dumbbell-shaped mass rather than two clear-cut masses.
5. Is there a *pore or sinus* overlying the mass, and if so, what sort of *drainage* has come from it?

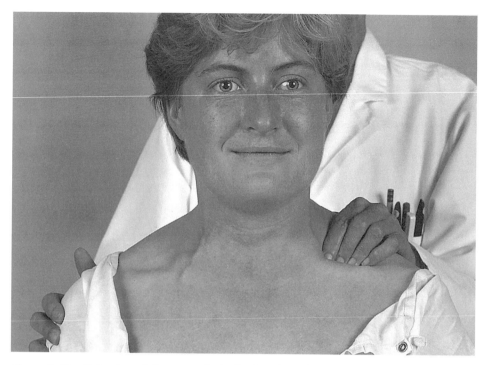

Figure 5.15   *Palpation of the supraclavicular lymph nodes* may reveal metastatic cancer from abdomen, esophagus, lung, or rarely breast. The nodes are best appreciated from behind, with the fingers curled over the shoulder; both sides can be assessed simultaneously, or for anatomic reasons the examiner may focus on the left side. See text for further means of enhancing this examination.

Muscles and Nerves

Detailed assessment of the muscles and nerves is found in Chapters 10 and 11, but a few issues arise so commonly in relation to neck disorders that they need review here.

The **trapezii and sternomastoids,** the largest muscles of the neck, are both innervated by cranial nerve XI, the spinal accessory nerve. Dysfunction of either may reflect local neuromuscular injury in the neck or damage to the lower brainstem.

The principal nerve roots that exit the spinal cord in the neck innervate muscles and skin in the upper limb. Thus the search for abnormalities in or about cervical vertebrae encompasses the following:

1. *C5:* Check sensation of upper arm and upper outer forearm, forceful abduction of arms held at 45° to the vertical against resistance (deltoid muscle), and biceps reflex.
2. *C6:* Check sensation over palmar surface of thumb and index finger, flexion of supinated forearm against resistance (biceps muscle), and brachioradialis reflex (C5-**C6**).
3. *C7:* Check sensation over middle finger, extension of partially flexed elbow against resistance (triceps muscle), and triceps reflex (C6-C7-C8).
4. *C8:* Check sensation over fifth finger and extension of wrist against resistance.

Since innervation of muscles and reflexes often encompasses multiple nerve roots and since dermatomes overlap, sometimes no deficit is present despite a lesion. Conversely, any deficit is highly significant.

Handgrip encompasses muscles innervated from spinal segments C7–T1. Hence, in the absence of cerebral or brainstem pathology, grip also serves as an indicator of lower cervical spinal cord and root function.

Vascular System

The principal blood vessels of the neck, the carotid arteries and jugular veins, are considered along with the heart and other great vessels in Chapter 8. In the extended examination, however, three other arteries in or about the neck are sometimes assessed: the vertebral artery, the subclavian artery, and the innominate artery–aorta complex.

VERTEBRAL ARTERY

Bruits arising from the vertebral artery are best heard with the *bell* held to the *lower posterior border of sternomastoid.* This location makes sense in relation to the ascent of the vessel through the foramina at the lateral edges of cervical vertebrae. A bruit heard here is assessed further as described with thyroid bruits. At present, a vertebral bruit lacks surgical implications but might be adduced in support of antiplatelet therapy.

SUBCLAVIAN ARTERY

Although the subclavian artery lies just below the neck, it is examined from the neck. It may seem counterintuitive that a *sub*clavian artery is best appreciated from superiorly, but the direction of sound propagation and the anatomic barriers from beneath so dictate. A subclavian arterial pulsation can be felt in many normal persons by pressing down and back from the posterior margin of the junction of the medial and middle thirds of the clavicle. Auscultation with the bell "snuggled" in at this point—something that cannot always achieve an acoustic seal—may also disclose an innocent subclavian bruit. When there is a need to listen at this site and the patient is too thin and bony, an acoustic seal can be achieved if

1. A smaller pediatric stethoscope bell is employed, or
2. The diaphragm is removed from the stethoscope.
3. Failing these, obtain a 150-mL flexible bag of fluid for intravenous infusion and with needle and syringe withdraw enough fluid to render the bag moderately floppy, without introduction of air. The bag is placed so as to fill in the contours of the supraclavicular triangle. Auscultation proceeds through the bag by placement of the stethoscope bell on the outer surface.

INNOMINATE ARTERY–AORTA COMPLEX

The root of the neck serves as a "window" to intrathoracic arteries otherwise protected by the thoracic cage. The examiner observes the jugular notch for pulsations and introduces a fingertip from above a bit inferiorly into the notch. Pulsations are often felt even when not seen.

Neck Masses

Several features and maneuvers assist the evaluation of cervical lumps. This is fortunate, since the differential diagnosis is long.

LOCATION

Precise delineation and description are essential. A high posterior mass cannot be thyroid, and a soft tissue mass arising beneath the midmandible will almost certainly be lymph node or salivary gland. A lump that "peeks" forward from the superior third of the sternomastoid suggests a branchial cleft cyst.

SOLITARY OR MULTIPLE?

Single lumps may mean anything. Multiple masses are likely to be lymph nodes, much less likely to be multiple thyroid masses or multiple diseased salivary glands.

TEXTURE

The texture of lymph nodes has been addressed above. A cystic-feeling neck mass can be a cyst, any of various swellings (–celes), or a degenerated thyroid colloid nodule. The sensation of a half-full hot water bottle has been proffered to describe branchial cleft cysts.

MANEUVERS

The following maneuvers are used to evaluate cervical masses:

1. See if the lesion can be **transilluminated** with a bright narrow beam directed to minimize intervening normal tissue. Do the test in a thoroughly darkened room.
2. Have the patient stick out his tongue, and both watch and feel for elevation of the mass.
3. Observe and, if necessary, feel for the effect of swallowing. Does the lump rise or enlarge?
4. Assess the impact of having the patient blow hard through the nose or pursed lips for 10 seconds. Does the mass enlarge?
5. Watch what happens with the Valsalva maneuver.
6. Finally, assess for attachment to the sternomastoid. This is accomplished as follows. The patient reclines comfortably supine, with a small pillow beneath the head producing slight passive flexion of the neck to relax the sternomastoids. Then he lifts his head a few (2–5) centimeters from the pillow and rotates his neck *away from the lump.* These maneuvers maximally contract both heads of the sternomastoid ipsilateral to the mass and cause them to stand out sharply. The examiner can assess the relation of the mass to the muscles and, in particular, whether the mass is visibly attached to or continuous with the tightly contracted and prominent muscle.

INTERPRETING THE FINDINGS

Skin

A positive "neck sign" consists of the formation of *tight, hard cords* on the skin surface with the neck extended. In small series, to date, this sign is found in persons with progressive systemic sclerosis (scleroderma) but not in normal persons or in those with uncomplicated Raynaud's disease. Normal aged persons may have **soft cords** from skin laxity, readily distinguished by texture. Further studies are needed to establish positive and negative predictive values in larger populations.

Cervical Spine

Painless restriction of neck motion suggests cervical spine osteoarthrosis or voluntary restriction of neck movement as a result of anticipation of pain or a psychologic issue. Voluntary restriction is confirmed if range of motion increases with distraction. *Pain* with decreased range of motion can also signify osteoarthrosis, cervical disc disease, or other conditions. Local tenderness over a particular **spin-**

ous process or facet joint suggests pathology there but does not distinguish between common problems such as **cervical spondylosis** and ominous rarities such as **osteomyelitis.**

It is essential to keep in mind the limitations of examination. In particular, *atlantoaxial instability* (a special concern with patients who have *trisomy 21*), which predisposes to calamitous spinal cord injury, cannot be detected or excluded on physical examination.

Positive compression and quadrant tests may localize the pathologic process, particularly if pain is reproduced in a small, sharply circumscribed area. A positive quadrant test with a negative compression test localizes the difficulty to the intervertebral foramina. However, the etiology will remain obscure.

A **short webbed neck** suggests Turner's syndrome (XO karyotype), but the suggestion often proves false, especially in adults. Klippel-Feil, as mentioned above, is also rare.

An **anteriorly thrust neck** may be due to spondylolisthesis. The more common association is far-advanced osteoarthrosis.

Upper Airway and Digestive Tract

TRACHEA

Visible **deviation of the trachea** can occur toward an atelectatic lung but away from large pleural effusions and pneumothoraces. Consolidation can push the trachea away or, if there is associated bronchial obstruction and atelectasis, draw it in. However, tracheal displacement is not a sensitive marker, and much pleuropulmonary disease may coexist with a negative sign.

Tracheal tenderness is characteristic of nonpyogenic ("atypical") pneumonias.

As to **tracheal tug,** a palpable outward pulsation or a pulsation palpable only in inspiration is not important. However, a **systolic downward-inward pull on the fingers** that persists in expiration means the aorta is tethered to the carina or left main-stem bronchus, so that the attached airway transmits aortic pulsations. Local inflammation at the site of a leaking aortic aneurysm is possible.

Tracheal **wheezes** can reflect turbulent airflow isolated to the upper respiratory tract or the propagation of turbulent noise from the lower airways. Because of the physics of sound transmission, the limitation of audible expiratory or panrespiratory wheezes to the trachea does **not** prove that the origin of the adventitious noises is there and does not rule out asthma. Purely **inspiratory wheezes** are stridorous and indicate a laryngotracheal origin.

Thyroid

INSPECTION

The full-looking lower neck that fails to rise with swallowing usually means a nonthyroidal cause of neck enlargement, most commonly simply prominent or excess fat and muscle. A rare exception is **Riedel's thyroiditis,** a fibrosing condition that can anchor the gland to surrounding tissues in addition to the normal firm attachment to the airway. Such anchoring could abrogate the expected "yoking" of thyroid to airway that underlies normal elevation on swallowing. Another exception is **locally advanced thyroid cancer** if it has followed an atypical biologic behavior and infiltrated widely beyond the capsule, plastering the gland to all nearby tissues.

PALPATION

Tenderness of an enlarged, firm thyroid suggests thyroiditis. It usually accompanies a history of neck pain with recent symptoms and signs of hyperthyroidism.

An apparent **pyramidal lobe** may occasionally turn out to be a Delphian lymph node, a midline cervical lymph node found in some cases of thyroid disease. Another differential diagnosis is a thyroid nodule arising from the thyroid isthmus or from a pyramidal lobe. In the presence of diffuse thyroid enlargement, especially if there is clear evidence of hyperthyroidism—exophthalmos being the most specific *in this setting*—lymphadenopathy should raise two prospects. One is metastatic thyroid cancer, which can produce cervical lymphadenopathy. The other, involving nodes throughout the body and producing splenomegaly, is the *lymphoid hyperplasia of Graves' hyperthyroidism.*

AUSCULTATION

Thyroid bruits are usually low-pitched, whereas their differential diagnoses—cervical venous hum, carotid bruit, and transmitted basal cardiac murmurs—are higher pitched. Thus, pressure exerted on the bell should reduce a thyroid bruit or cause it to disappear, whereas the other conditions should change little if at all. Localization plays a major role too. A systolic sound that is louder high in the neck should be a carotid bruit. A sound of thyroidal origin should be maximal over the palpable gland. A transmitted cardiac murmur usually, although not always, progressively attenuates as the stethoscope is inched up the neck from the root toward the angle of the jaw. A subclavian artery bruit should be louder in the supraclavicular fossa than over the thyroid. A cervical venous hum is often continuous rather than systolic and abates when the patient reclines. Furthermore, digital pressure over the superior aspect of the midclavicle should compress the external jugular vein, interrupt flow through it, and abrogate the sound. A Valsalva maneuver may cause a venous hum to disappear. Active rotation of the neck away from the side being auscultated may increase the pitch or intensity of a cervical venous hum.

A restatement of *limitations* is in order. Besides the lack of sensitivity of all *local signs* for thyroid disease mentioned earlier, there are no *extrathyroidal* clinical features that allow confident exclusion of thyroid dysfunction, particularly in older patients. A pulse of 80 beats/minute, normal eyes, and an apathetic demeanor does not exclude hyperthyroidism. Nor do normal skin and hair, facies, and habitus reassure that hypothyroidism is absent.

Lymph Nodes
LOCATION

Submandibular lumps usually represent submandibular salivary glands or submental lymph nodes. In the aged, salivary glands can descend and become *ptotic.* Hence, a lump that can be nearly completely encircled with the fingers or that lies a couple of centimeters below the jaw may be this. It may feel more *pebbly-surfaced* than a node.

Occipital lymph nodes, at the junction of head and neck, are common in childhood infection but much less so in adults. Their discovery in an adult, if there is no local source of antigenic stimulation such as a scalp infection, prompts consideration of causes of generalized lymphadenopathy including HIV infection. Occipital nodes were found with considerable frequency in early reports of progressive generalized lymphadenopathy resulting from HIV.

When *hard* lymph nodes are found or other features suggest metastatic cancer (multiplicity, fixation, matting, risk factors), sublocalization of the most probable *primary tumor site* can be suggested by the particular cervical lymph node chain involved. Thus, high posterior cervical lymph nodes, especially bilateral, suggest a nasopharyngeal primary. Submental and submandibular nodes occur with cancers of the nose, lip, anterior tongue, and—the most frequent—anterior floor of the mouth. Midjugular lymph node metastases suggest a primary at the base of the tongue or in the larynx. Lower jugular nodes point to the thyroid or cervical esophagus.

Left supraclavicular lymph nodes are known by the eponym "Virchow's," for a great pathologist who recognized their frequent involvement with metastatic cancer of the stomach. Based on lymphatic drainage patterns and perhaps on reflux from the termination of the thoracic duct in the subclavian vein on the left, they can harbor metastases from any abdominal or pelvic cancer, including pancreatic and endometrial, as well as cancer of the left lung or cancer of the esophagus. Hence, they can be "sentinel nodes," signaling deep internal carcinoma.

Right supraclavicular lymph nodes have a parallel significance but are less common. They are sometimes associated with an *accessory right thoracic duct,* but the nodes do not serve as sentinels so often. Right supraclavicular nodes can be involved with metastases from cancer of the right lung and, because of bilateral crossed drainage, from cancer of the base of the *left* lung.

GENERALIZED LYMPHADENOPATHY

Generalized lymphadenopathy with involvement of the neck nodes suggests a host of causes including

1. Hematologic malignancies, especially Hodgkin's disease, non-Hodgkin's lymphomas, and chronic lymphocytic leukemia
2. HIV infection with progressive generalized lymphadenopathy; or other viral illnesses, notably Epstein-Barr virus disease (infectious mononucleosis) and cytomegalovirus infection
3. Mycobacterioses and other granulomatous infections
4. Syphilis or toxoplasmosis
5. Immune-stimulated lymphoid hyperplasia, as in Graves' disease
6. Phenytoin (Dilantin) therapy, which causes generalized lymphoid hyperplasia as an adverse effect
7. Sarcoidosis

CHARACTERISTICS

Tenderness has been described previously. **Massive cervical lymph nodes**, over 5 cm across, can be seen in the hematologic malignancies most prone to generalized lymphadenopathy. Much less commonly they harbor reactive hyperplasia, often from unknown stimuli; or untreated diphtherial pharyngitis in which a "bull neck" or "yoke collar" is illustrated, in textbooks from the pre-antibiotic era; or solid neoplasms with unusually large nodal metastases; or extraordinarily proliferative HIV lymphadenopathy.

Consistency is discussed earlier. The lymph nodes of Hodgkin's disease are often described as *rubbery,* whereas those of non-Hodgkin's lymphoma may be compared with the texture of *fish flesh.* The major lesson is to *avoid equating hardness with malignancy.* Hardness is based on the stromal response to many breast cancers, not on intrinsic characteristics of cancer. In the pathology laboratory, *soft cancers* can often be felt among both surgical and autopsy specimens. Hardness is not sensitive or specific for neoplasia. One of the authors has had a stable, small, hard posterior cervical lymph node for 19 years, which arose with chickenpox (varicella) and must have undergone calcification.

Soft, fluctuant lymph nodes suggest necrosis with suppuration (purulence). Bacterial infection is the usual etiology. Sometimes the term bubo is employed, but usually this is specific for inguinal nodal suppuration. *Fistulization* is suggestive of mycobacteriosis. The combined involvement of cervical lymph node and skin by mycobacterial infection is designated **scrofula** and is a major differential in children. Suppuration with or without skin involvement can also occur in cat-scratch disease and occasionally with spontaneous necrosis in the center of a cancerous metastasis.

Fixation to skin, subjacent tissue, or other lymph nodes bespeaks a process extending beyond the lymph node capsule. In addition to malignant neoplasia, the cause can be any aggressive form of infective inflammation. In general, fixed or matted nodes call for rapid evaluation by special investigation rather than for observation over time.

Muscles and Nerves

Most inferences about disordered spinal segments or roots are made in the discussion under Conducting the Extended Examination. In attempting assessment of the neck, think about neural representation not only in the spinal cord but also in the pyramids, the internal capsule, and the cerebral cortical homunculi. Thus a weak grip accompanied by spasticity and arm weakness means upper motor neuron damage, probably at the frontal lobe cortex or the internal capsule. A chronically flaccid hand with reduced muscle stretch reflexes could reflect damage anywhere in the lower motor neuron course, from the anterior horn cell to anterior roots, brachial plexus, peripheral nerves, and even the neuromuscular junction, or the muscle. An *acutely* flaccid areflexic forearm could represent, besides all these, the first phase after upper motor neuron injury, so-called **spinal shock.** The principles of seeking a **unitary hypothesis** and a **solitary lesion** of whatever size apply as in other neurologic reasoning. In the neck, perhaps the commonest striking neuromuscular sign is **torticollis.**

Vascular System

Palpable aortic pulsations in the jugular notch often reflect *uncoiling* of an aged, atherosclerotic aorta, without aneurysm. Unfortunately, the paucity of reliable signs and symptoms made authors refer to thoracic aneurysm as the most humbling of diseases at the turn of the century, and that statement still applies.

The distinctions between one noise and another in the neck are discussed with the interpretation of thyroidal bruits above. Cervical venous hums are common in children and less so in young adults. However, they can also occur in adults with high cardiac output resulting from anemia, cirrhosis, pregnancy, or hyperthyroidism. A **continuous cervical murmur** is usually a venous hum.

Neck Masses

HISTORY

A mass that appears, rises, or enlarges with swallowing—as determined by history and examination—is likely to be a Zenker's diverticulum. The history of regurgitation of undigested food well after eating supports a pharyngeal or esophageal diverticulum as the cause of a mass. A woodwind or brass instrument player has increased risk for laryngocele.

Age is a pertinent part of the history, as an increasing percentage of neck masses prove malignant with advancing age.

LOCATION AND CHARACTERISTICS

Both midline and low lateral masses require inclusion of *goiter* in the differential diagnosis. An overlying *dimple* in a lateral mass raises the question of branchial cleft cyst. A sinus suggests scrofula. The triad of fixation, skin breakdown, and drainage raises the additional specter of a primary cancer or a nodal metastasis with extranodal extension.

TENDERNESS

Tenderness, a characteristic of inflammation, no more reliably separates it from neoplasia with neck masses than with lymph nodes, as discussed above.

TEXTURE

A *fluctuant* mass, i.e., one that retreats and to some slight degree springs back or moves aside when one presses on it, is likely to be suppurative, as described under Lymph Nodes in the Extended Examination section above. Branchial cleft cysts and any palpable laryngocele or achalasic mass may share this characteristic.

MANEUVERS

The following characteristics of responses to maneuvers help evaluate cervical masses:

1. A mass that can be **transilluminated** can be a cystic hygroma (lymphangioma) or, if accessible, a diverticulum or swelling (–cele) arising from any cervical part of the upper aerodigestive tract.
2. A mass that **rises with sticking out of the tongue** is likely to be a **thyroglossal duct cyst,** since this is firmly attached to the tongue.
3. The interpretation of the impact of *swallowing* is addressed in the discussion of the Thyroid under Conducting the Extended Examination.
4. **Blowing the nose or pursed lips** can enlarge a laryngocele. This maneuver is especially worthwhile if the history reveals enlargement with crying, coughing, or laughing.
5. The **Valsalva maneuver** can also enlarge a laryngocele. **Jugular venous ectasia,** a rare condition of the internal jugular vein in children, can be highlighted this way when the history so directs. The mass will be soft, diffuse, and deep to the inferior margin of one sternomastoid. Venous ectasia and laryngocele may subside completely at rest.
6. **Attachment to sternomastoid** suggests (*a*) fixation from inflammation, (*b*) neoplasm that has not respected fascial planes, or (*c*) origin from the muscle proper, e.g., fibroma of sternomastoid.

RECORDING THE FINDINGS

Sample Write-up

22-year-old nonsmoking printer with a lump in the neck of 3-months duration. No prior history of same, no known occupational risks, and has not noticed that it changes with any activity of daily living.

Examination: 2×2-cm midline mass at midanterior neck. Not hard or fluctuant and cannot be transilluminated. Overlying skin normal, no pore. Lump rises with tongue protrusion, but not with swallowing; no change with deep inspiration, nose-blowing, or Valsalva maneuver. No associated lymphadenopathy or thyromegaly.

Impression: Thyroglossal duct cyst.

BEYOND THE PHYSICAL EXAMINATION

Laboratory Studies

The most frequently useful bloodwork consists of **thyroid function tests,** particularly the thyroid-stimulating hormone (TSH) and the free thyroxine (free T_4) tests.

Specialized thyroid tests are useful in subsets of patients. **Calcium, phosphate, and parathormone** measurements are routine when parathyroid disease is under consideration. There are no consistently helpful tests of blood, urine, or body fluids in regard to salivary gland pathology or head and neck neoplasms. **Biopsy and aspiration cytology,** often under ultrasonic guidance, play critical roles in some selected cases.

Imaging

Plain *cervical spine radiographs* are sometimes useful in the assessment of neck pain, particularly of suspected osseous, disc, or ligamentous origin. *Chest radiographs* may disclose a source of cervical pathology, e.g., a lung cancer presenting with metastases.

Ultrasound delineates a large variety of conditions of the neck noninvasively, at relatively low cost, and with minimal discomfort. Ultrasound can be enhanced with the same maneuvers used to alter visible or palpable neck masses, for example, by repeating the study while the patient performs a Valsalva maneuver. Ultrasound is a principal tool used in distinguishing solid from cystic masses, since this differentiation can sometimes be impossible on examination. *In general,* a cystic lesion reassures one that cancer is not the cause—although there are exceptions. There are also preliminary reports that ultrasound may detect small cervical lymph nodes containing metastatic cancer in patients with head and neck primary carcinomas who have had a negative physical examination for this complication.

More expensive, complex, and invasive imaging includes **computed tomography (CT)** and **magnetic resonance imaging (MRI).** Either of these techniques can be combined with the introduction of radiopaque contrast agents into the subarachnoid space to produce **CT myelography,** for example. Plain myelography is less used now than formerly.

Vascular imaging of the principal arteries and veins in the neck includes duplex ultrasound studies, digital subtraction angiography, and conventional contrast angiography.

The **usual contrast study** in this region is the **barium swallow** to delineate the esophagus.

Functional Studies

Electromyography (EMG) and nerve conduction velocity studies (NCV) can be used for further assessment of neurologic and root problems.

Flow-volume loops play a role in delineation of obstructive respiratory disorders including those of the trachea.

Thyroid scans and **radioactive iodine uptake (RAIU)** scans assist in evaluation of thyroid function, thyroid nodules, and the extent of proven thyroid cancers.

Consultation

As with the head, eyes, ears, nose, oral cavity, and throat, many potential helpers exist. The *otorhinolaryngologist* brings expertise to conventional examination, to endoscopic evaluation of all aerodigestive mucosae, to biopsy, and to surgical exploration when necessary. Many *head and neck surgeons,* some *general surgeons,* and all *endocrine surgeons* have special interest and expertise in the neck. So do some *plastic surgeons.* Laryngoscopy may be performed by these or by properly credentialed internists.

Thyroid aspiration is often performed by an *endocrinologist,* although at some institutions a *surgeon,* a *general internist,* a *cytopathologist,* or an *interventional radiologist* performs this function.

Both *rheumatologists* and *orthopedic surgeons* offer much knowledge about the musculoskeletal components in the neck. *Neurosurgeons* know these well and know the spinal cord, roots, and peripheral nerves that exit the central nervous system in the neck better than anyone. *Gastroenterologists* can perform esophageal function studies and endoscopy that includes the cervical part of the alimentary canal, i.e., esophagoscopy.

Anesthesiologists know the neck well and the airway best of all.

Conclusions

The plethora of experts on the neck underscores the theme stated earlier, namely, that this structure is a *crossroads* with which every clinician needs familiarity. In addition to all the tests mentioned, it is often appropriate to evaluate an abnormality of the neck by simple *observation over time,* which may provide diagnosis and lead to optimal management with less physical, psychic, and financial stress on the patient.

RECOMMENDED READINGS

Barnett AJ. The "neck sign" in scleroderma. Arthritis Rheum 1989;32:209–211.

Bruneton JN, Normand F, Balu-Maestro C, et al. Lymphomatous superficial lymph nodes: ultrasound detection. Radiology 1987;165:233–235.

Drumm AJ, Chow JM. Congenital neck masses. Am Fam Physician 1989;39(1):159–163.

Hurst JW, Hopkins LC, Smith RB. Noises in the neck. N Engl J Med 1980;302:862–863.

Kenna C, Murtagh J. Examination of the neck. Aust Fam Physician 1986;15(1):1015–1020.

Linet OI, Metzler C. Practical ENT: incidence of palpable cervical nodes in adults. Postgrad Med 1977;62:210–211, 213.

Morris MR, Woody EA. A closer look at the thyroglossal cyst. Ear Nose Throat J 1987;66(9):364–368.

Pyman B. Practical procedures: examination of the nose, pharynx, larynx and neck. Aust Fam Physician 1981;10:90–92.

Rood SR, Johnson JT. Examination for cervical masses. Postgrad Med 1982;71:189–194.

Shepherd JJ. Attached to sternomastoid? Aust N Z J Surg 1979;49:704.

6

Breasts and Axillae

APPROACH AND ANATOMICAL REVIEW

Approach

The screening examination of the breasts and axillae is next in the sequence of a routine complete examination. It begins after the pulmonary assessment is completed while the patient remains seated. Full inspection of the breasts is done first, followed by palpation of the axillae. The patient then reclines, in which position palpation of the breast is completed, and the bulk of the remaining general examination is conducted.

Before beginning inspection of the breasts, explain this portion of the examination to the patient, especially the need to have the chest bared to the waist. History of breast symptoms and cancer risk factors (Table 6.1), which should have been acquired before beginning the examination, will help direct the examiner's attention to areas of special concern. Also, to avoid creating undue worry on the part of the patient, even the experienced clinician who has become sufficiently adept to incorporate the review of systems into the physical examination should *ask routine breast-related questions before initiating inspection* (see Chapter 1).

Anatomical Review

The glands, ducts, fibrous tissue, and fat making up the substance of the female breast are supported by the fascia and the underlying pectoralis major muscle. Fibrous bands known as Cooper's ligaments pass between the glandular lobules from their deep fascial attachment. These ligaments provide additional support for the mass of glandular and fatty tissue. Each glandular lobule consists of clusters of potentially milk-producing cells that empty into collecting ducts. The ducts track centripetally to the nipple, where they open onto the surface through several principal lactiferous sinuses just visible to the naked eye as tiny pores. Relative proportions of glandular tissue, fibrous tissue, and fat vary widely depending on age, hormonal status, body weight and habitus, and the presence or absence of pregnancy or lactation (Fig. 6.1).

The lymphatic drainage of the breast area is complex; the critical chains are: The upper outer quadrant drains to the scapular, subhumeral (brachial), and anterior pectoral nodes, all of which are part of the axillary group. The two medial quadrants empty lymph into the internal mammary chain, which is nonpalpable unless greatly enlarged and even then may not be appreciable. The lower outer quadrants drain into the axillary chains as well as into the abdominal lymphatic system. Drainage of the areola and nipple is via the infraclavicular, supraclavicular, and midaxillary nodes (Fig. 6.2).

For anatomical location and description, the surface of the breast is divided into four quadrants as illustrated in Figures 6.1 and 6.3. The elongated segment of the upper outer quadrant, which extends in some women high along the border of the pectoralis muscle, is called the tail of the breast, sometimes referred to by the eponym "tail of Spence." The inferior border of the breast may contain a cres-

Table 6.1
Breast Cancer Risk Factors

Family history of breast cancer in sister, mother, grandmother, daughter, granddaughter
History of nulliparity or late childbearing (after age 30)
Personal history of previous **breast** cancer
Alcohol use
Obesity

cent of dense fibrous tissue known as the inframammary ridge. This structure is palpable in some breasts and is not appreciable in others. The quadrantic designations are used by the examiner as a mental map to help guarantee comprehensiveness and as a framework for describing and recording the findings of the examination.

TECHNIQUE

Inspection

Inspection of the breast includes observation of the integument, the nipple and areola as specific structures, the contour of the breasts themselves, and the effect

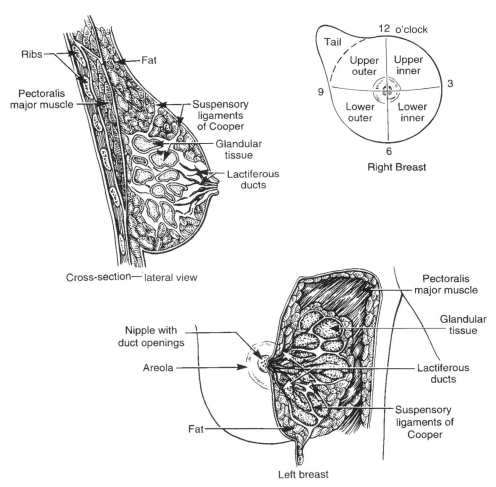

Figure 6.1 Schematic representations of major structures of female breast and nomenclature for describing breast findings.

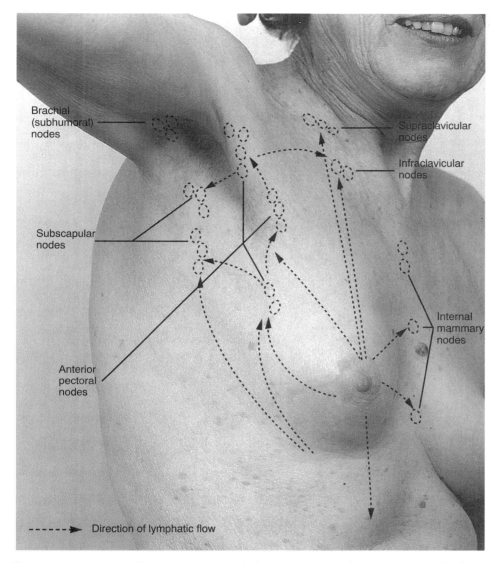

Brachial
(subhumoral)
nodes

Supraclavicular
nodes

Infraclavicular
nodes

Subscapular
nodes

Internal
mammary
nodes

Anterior
pectoral
nodes

- - - - - ▶ Direction of lymphatic flow

Figure 6.2 Major lymphatic drainage of right breast. *Interrupted arrows* indicate the direction of lymphatic flow from breast tissue to node clusters.

of movement on the organs and their overlying skin (see Table 6.2 for the sequence).

The examiner faces the seated patient, both of whose breasts should be fully and simultaneously exposed, since side-to-side comparison is critical. A systematic visual inspection is made, with the presence of any skin lesions noted (refer to Chapter 3 for methods of describing and recording skin findings). The symmetry and general contour of the two breasts are observed. The nipples are inspected for symmetry and particularly for the presence of inversion.

Next, the examiner asks the patient to perform a series of maneuvers. As the patient raises her arms above her head, the clinician observes the symmetry of breast and nipple motion and end-position. The breasts should lift evenly, as should the nipples. **Watch for dimpling of the skin, deviation of a nipple, or change in skin contour that could indicate an underlying abnormality.** The patient is asked to place her hands on her waist and to press inward, thus tensing

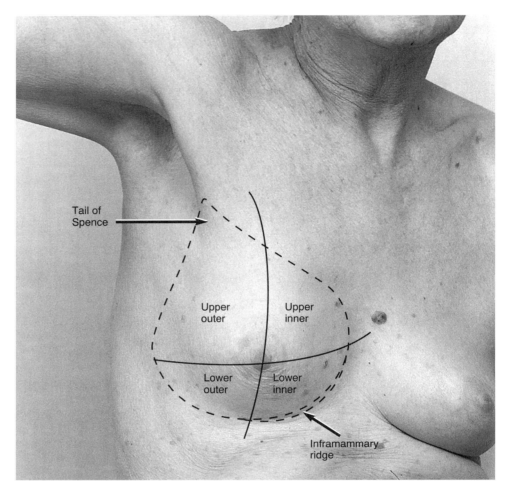

Figure 6.3 Designated quadrants of right breast, useful for describing local findings.

the pectoralis muscles. The examiner observes for skin dimpling, nipple deviation, or asymmetric movement. On occasion, especially with very large or pendulous breasts, it is useful to ask the patient to lean forward from the waist. This
motion puts tension on the suspensory ligaments. Again, the breasts are observed
for symmetry of movement and alteration in surface structure (Fig. 6.4).

Palpation

Before asking the patient to change to the supine position for breast palpation,
the examiner should inspect and palpate the axillae (see below). Some clinicians
prefer to palpate the tail of Spence and its adjacent pectoral nodes at this time
(Fig. 6.5) by compressing the tissue between the thumb and finger pads. If the
breasts are large or pendulous, it is helpful to palpate the dependent breast
between two hands as illustrated in Figure 6.6. Little is gained by palpating a
small or nonpendulous normal-appearing breast with the patient seated.

  With the patient supine and draped and with the examiner standing on the
patient's right, each breast is exposed and palpated individually. The patient is
asked to raise and place under her head the arm corresponding to the breast to be
examined. If the breast is large, a small towel is folded under the same shoulder to
allow further spreading of breast tissue on and across the chest wall. The success
and thoroughness of breast palpation depends on a systematic sequence and the

Table 6.2
Sequence for the Routine Breast Examination

Inspection, patient seated
   Observation of skin, nipple, and areola
   Observation for symmetry
     At rest
     With tension of the pectoralis
     With dependency and movement
   Inspection of the axillary area

Palpation, patient seated
   Axillae, right and left
     Pectoral (anterior axillary) nodes
     Subscapular (posterior axillary) nodes
     Brachial nodal chain

Palpation, patient supine
   Breasts, right and left
     Four quadrants
     Tail of Spence (tail of breast)
     Subareolar area
     Nipple

effective use of the sensitive palmar surface of the examiner's fingers, as well as on letting gravity spread the tissue so that the depth to be assessed between palpating fingers and subjacent ribs is minimized (Fig. 6.7).

SEQUENCE OF PALPATION

Any one of several systems for comprehensive palpation is acceptable.

- The "spiral" (or concentric circle) is begun with the tail and moves inward to terminate with the nipple and areola.
- The "spokes of a wheel" is a centripetal pattern moving from the periphery of the breast toward the nipple in a series of adjacent radial lines.
- The "back-and-forth" technique is an approach to the breast as if it were transected vertically and involves palpation from superior to inferior.
- The "quadrantic" method is particularly useful for small breasts with little pendulous tissue (Fig. 6.8).

METHOD OF PALPATION

A few general principles are essential to effective palpation:

- The pads of the fingers should be utilized, not the tips. "Digging" with the fingertips is not only uncomfortable for the patient but can result in skipping over mobile glandular abnormalities.
- An attempt should be made to maintain continuous skin contact as the fingers move over the surface, in order to avoid missing areas.
- The breast tissue is gently compressed between the examining fingers and the underlying chest wall structures. Keep in mind that the ribs and cartilage of a very thin woman must be discriminated from breast mass.
- The motion of the fingers is that of "rolling" the mobile underlying tissue.
- Do not neglect the confluence of ducts beneath the nipple. The nipple and areola should be palpated as discrete structures by pressing them against the chest wall.

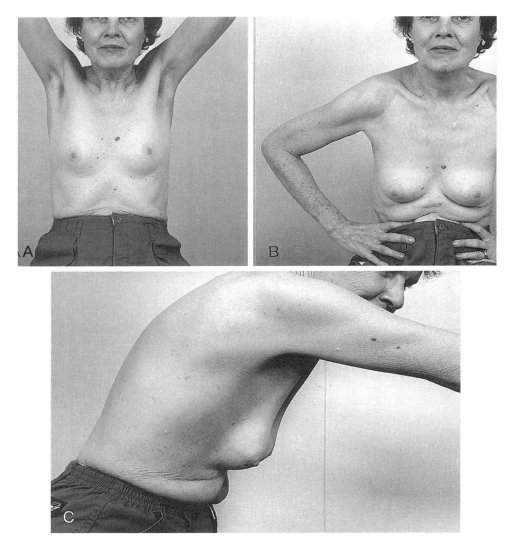

Figure 6.4   Three positions to observe the breasts for asymmetry on movement, skin dimpling or retraction, or nipple deviation. **A.** Arms elevated over head (the slight asymmetry of nipple position raises suspicion; in the case of this patient, however, no pathology was evident on further examination). **B.** Hand pressing on hips with pectoralis muscles tensed. **C.** Leaning forward with breast tissue dependent.

To effect adequate spread of the large breast for thorough palpation, it is sometimes necessary to support or move the breast during the examination. The assistance of the patient may be required to aid in distributing the tissue evenly while the examiner palpates. If, for example, a heavy breast falls over the pectoral border, ask the patient to cup her hand under the dependent tissue and hold it medially so that the outer quadrants may be more effectively palpated.

Finally, each nipple should be examined for secretion. The patient should be informed that some pressing of the nipple is required for this portion of the examination. This may be accomplished with minimal patient discomfort by gentle compression of the areola at the base of the nipple between the examiner's thumb and forefinger or first and second fingers. The tissue is "milked" toward the surface of the nipple in order to express any fluid present within the ducts (Fig. 6.9).

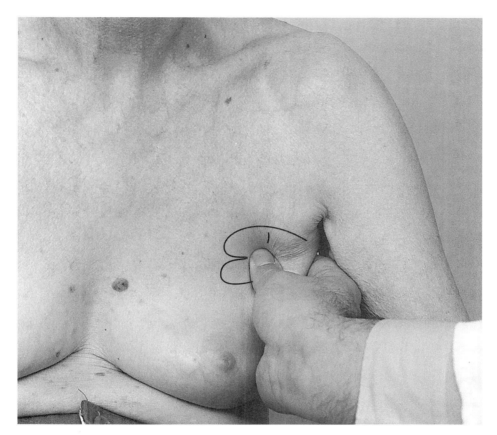

Figure 6.5 Palpation of tail of Spence. The examiner compresses the tail of the breast between thumb and forefinger to seek masses or tenderness in this high pectoral extension of breast tissue. Posterior digit position, behind fold of pectoralis, is shown by sketched lines.

Axillary and Periclavicular Lymph Node Examination

If the supraclavicular and infraclavicular lymph nodes have not been sought during the cervical and supraclavicular examination, they should be assessed at this time via the technique for nodal palpation described in Chapter 5. The axillary examination is conducted with the patient seated and the examiner standing on the side to be examined. Inspection of the axilla is best accomplished by having the patient raise the arm over the head. Note the axillary hair, and carefully inspect the skin for lesions or inflammation.

Many textbooks on physical examination recommend that palpation of the axilla be conducted with the patient's flexed arm supported by the examiner. Maximal pectoralis and shoulder muscle relaxation is obtained, however, by having the patient let the arm hang limp at the side. For the patient with hypersensitive or "ticklish" skin, this examination can be unpleasant, and the examiner should inform the patient that this is a normal response. The maintenance of firm, continuous skin contact will help to minimize discomfort. The examiner slides the appropriate hand (right for the left axilla, left for the right axilla) upward along the midaxillary chest wall until the bone resistance of the shoulder joint is met. The examiner should palpate three chains of nodes: the pectoral (anterior axillary), the subscapular (posterior axillary), and the subhumeral (brachial) (see Fig. 6.2). From high in the axilla, the examiner palpates, with the palmar surface of the fingers, downward along the border of the pectoralis muscle, compressing

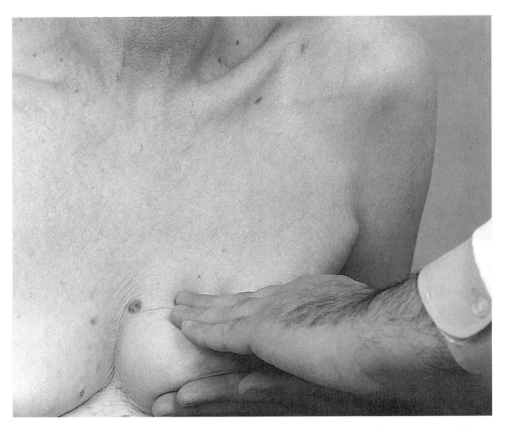

Figure 6.6   Palpation of dependent breast with patient seated. This technique, especially for the large or pendulous breast, is an adjunct to the more common supine palpation.

the tissue against the chest wall to about the level of the nipple (anterior axillary chain). Returning to the apex of the axilla, the examiner repeats the procedure at the posterior extremity of the axillary hollow, i.e., along the anterior border of the latissimus dorsi muscle (subscapular chain). Reversing the hand such that the palmar surface lies against the humerus, search for the subhumeral nodes. Any palpable node or nonnodal mass located is characterized as to size and other features as described in Chapter 5. The examiner then moves to the opposite side of the patient, changes hands, and repeats the procedure for the other axilla.

NORMAL AND COMMON VARIANTS

Inspection

The shape, size, and symmetry of the female breast is widely variable. Visible difference in size between the two breasts is the rule rather than the exception, with the left breast slightly larger in most instances of normal asymmetry. The skin over the surface of the breast should be smooth with unbroken contour. A venous pattern over the surface of the breast is visible in many women. If the pattern is present and generally symmetrical bilaterally, it may be considered normal.

The pigmentation of the areola varies with general skin pigmentation from fawn to very dark brown and tends to darken during pregnancy and retain the darker coloration permanently. The areola is normally dotted with tiny papular structures, the sebaceous glands of Montgomery, which are of variable prominence. The adult nipples are usually everted symmetrically. On occasion, one or both nipples may never have everted. A lifetime inversion is considered a normal variant,

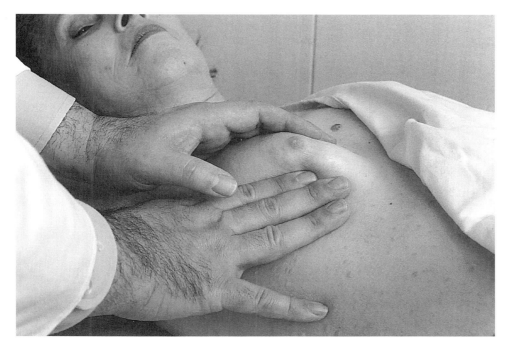

Figure 6.7 Hand placement for supine palpation of breast. Note that the examiner's right fingers are compressing tissue of the right lower quadrant against the chest wall, while the examiner's left fingers stabilize the medial breast.

but if inversion is noted, the examiner should ask about its duration. An acquired inversion demands further investigation. Note that rudimentary nipples or even palpable supernumerary breasts may normally be discovered along the embryonic "milk line" that extends on each side of the anterior trunk from the axilla to the proximal medial thigh. These minor congenital anomalies, when discovered, are occasionally difficult to differentiate from nevi. Except during pregnancy and lactation, nipple secretion is considered abnormal until proven otherwise.

Palpation

The consistency of the normal female breast varies widely. The normal breast in an adult woman of reproductive age who is neither pregnant nor lactating is coarsely granular and uniform in consistency. The so-called fibrocystic breast occurs commonly enough to be considered a normal variant, but it may present recurrent diagnostic problems. The intermittent and often asymmetric dilatation of lacteal ducts, which make up the "cystic" dimension of fibrocystic breasts, may occasionally require confirmation via mammography, aspiration, or biopsy. The appearance of any new mass, even in the setting of underlying fibrocystic tissue, must be approached as suspicious. Any mass should be carefully measured, recorded, and reassessed as described in Extended Examination of the Breasts and Axillae.

In addition to individual variations, the breast, as a hormonally sensitive organ, is subject to changes dictated by age and cyclic events. In the female, full breast development is usually reached by age 14–15, although there is a wide range of normal (see Fig. 6.10 for stages of breast development). Once menstrual cycling is established, there are alterations in the normal breast related to estrogen and progesterone levels. The breasts may become tense, slightly swollen, and tender during the postovulatory phase of the cycle. Examination of the breast during

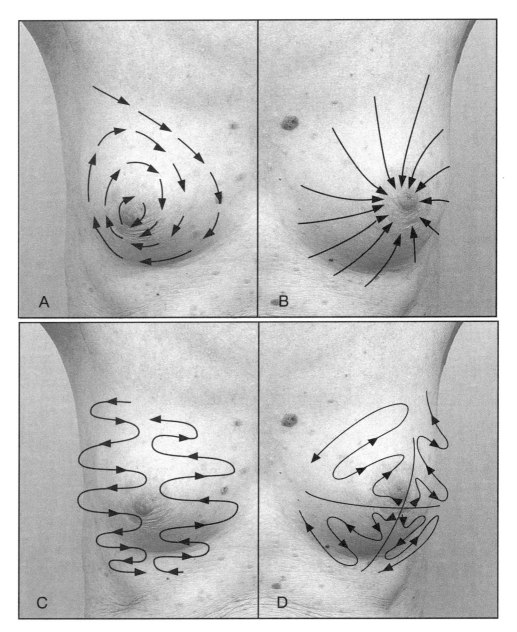

Figure 6.8   Four alternative methods for systematic palpation of breast. **A.** Spiral, beginning with the tail. **B.** Spokes, periphery to center. **C.** Back-and-forth method. **D.** Quadrantic, i.e., palpation of each quadrant from areola to periphery.

the week preceding menstruation may reveal an increase in palpable dilated ducts, particularly in the woman with fibrocystic breasts. For this reason it is suggested that, *when possible, breast examination be conducted soon after the end of menses.*

The Breast in Pregnancy

During pregnancy, the breasts enlarge and may secrete colostrum on minimal stimulation. As pregnancy advances, the clear discharge becomes more viscous and slightly yellowish, the nipples and areolae darken, and the glands of Montgomery often become strikingly prominent. On palpation, the breast is found to be

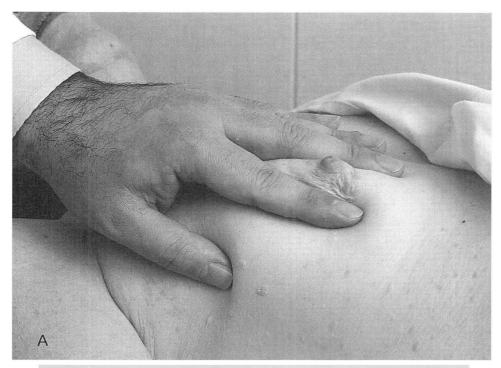

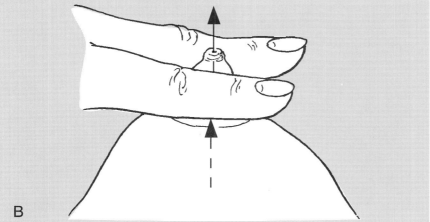

Figure 6.9 Assessing for nipple secretion. **A.** Placement of fingers beside areola, to begin upward compression of lactiferous ducts. **B.** Continuous upward compression of nipple, to bring any secretion into view at duct orifices.

lobular, even nodular, as the glandular tissue hypertrophies. The venous pattern is accentuated because of vascular dilatation, and sometimes an audible sound of blood flow, referred to as a mammary souffle, develops. If lactation is sustained during the puerperal period, the breasts remain firm and enlarged. When lactation ceases, the breasts slowly return to their prepregnancy state, but with sustained darkening of the areolae and sometimes a lessening of their prior firmness.

The Postmenopausal Breast

After menopause, with the reduction in estrogen stimulation, the glandular tissue of the breast atrophies and is gradually replaced by fibrous tissue and fat. The suspensory ligaments "relax" and the breast may appear elongated and flattened.

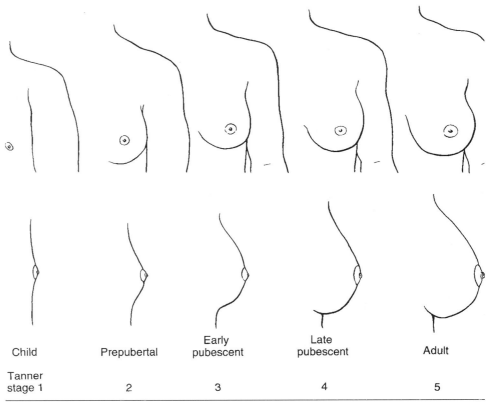

Child	Prepubertal	Early pubescent	Late pubescent	Adult
Tanner stage 1	2	3	4	5

Figure 6.10 Normal sequence of female breast development. Note Tanner stage terminology as the standard description.

With the reduction of glandular tissue, the breast feels more uniform and more finely granular.

The Male Breast

The male nipple and areola are assessed visually as a part of the inspection of the anterior chest wall. They may be palpated with the patient in the sitting position. A small disc of fatty and fibrous tissue may be appreciated directly under the areola in adolescent boys and some adult males. If distinct glandular enlargement is noted on inspection or initial palpation, more careful palpation using the techniques described for the examination of the female breast is indicated.

During early adolescence, the male breast may go through a period of hypertrophy, either bilateral or unilateral. There is sometimes a small amount of palpable glandular tissue immediately under the areola in the normal adult male; more commonly, the nipple and areola lie flat against the subcutaneous tissue of the chest wall. In the obese male, there may be an accumulation of fat beneath the areola, giving the visual impression of gynecomastia. Careful palpation will usually enable the examiner to determine whether the enlargement of the male breast is a result of development of glandular tissue (true gynecomastia), fatty deposition (pseudogynecomastia), or tumor.

RECORDING THE FINDINGS

The results of a breast examination are, by convention, **recorded** immediately before the results of the pulmonary examination. The description should include:

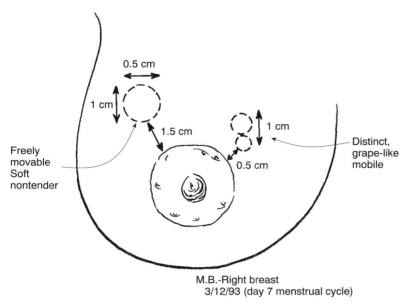

Figure 6.11   Sample chart entry of breast examination.

size, symmetry, and surface contour; symmetry of nipple movement and state of eversion; palpation findings such as nodularity, tenderness, and general consistency; and the finding of any discrete cysts (with the fibrocystic breast), which should be measured and recorded by quadrant location and distance from the rim of the areola. A sketch is very useful for "mapping" cystic dilatations and should be entered into the record (see Fig. 6.11 for an example). Any nipple secretion should be noted and characterized.

Skin lesions on the breast may be recorded with the breast examination or may be included with the skin examination. The results of axillary inspection and palpation are usually recorded with all other lymph nodes; some clinicians prefer to include the axillary examination with the breast examination in the record, but this makes the reader's work more difficult.

Because of the very wide range of normal in the adult female breast, considerable experience is required to become fully comfortable with these variations. While learning this range, the beginning examiner should call freely on supervisors for confirmation of the significance of any variant.

EXTENDED EXAMINATION OF THE BREASTS AND AXILLAE

INDICATIONS

Indications for additional breast or axillary physical examination maneuvers are detailed in Tables 6.1 and 6.3.

Breast Cancer Risk Factors

Immediate and long-term evaluation of the patient with one or more risk factors for breast cancer includes

- **Immediate:** A careful complete examination of the breasts and axillae as described earlier

- **Long-term:** A three-part management plan consisting of:
  - **Annual** physician examination
  - Instruction of patient in a method for **monthly** self-examination
  - Tailoring an individual schedule for **regular** mammography reevaluation

Breast Symptoms

A history of any of the breast symptoms listed in Table 6.3 and elicited by the interviewer or offered by the patient demands special attention during the breast examination.

Breast or Axillary Findings Noted on the Screening Examination

When during inspection or palpation in the screening physical examination any one of the abnormal signs in Table 6.3 is noted, a more detailed appraisal is indicated. This, like symptoms, applies to patients of either gender.

CONDUCTING THE EXTENDED EXAMINATION

Should any of the signs or symptoms listed in Table 6.3 apply to the patient being interviewed and examined, the examination is focused and expanded to maximize discrimination among regional features. If the patient has raised the concern during the history, obtain the details of the complaint—such as its duration, precise location, course since first noted, and any associated symptoms—*before* initiating the examination itself. If the examiner has discovered an unexpected abnormality during the screening examination, additional history may be necessary before proceeding with the more detailed maneuvers described below. It is critical, when assessing a suspected or observed breast abnormality, to remain sensitive to the fact that *most women equate breast problems with cancer.* When this specter is raised by the examiner's questions or by the examination itself, the physician must be prepared to discuss the implications of the findings.

Table 6.3
Indications for Extended Examination

Increased risk factors by history
Breast symptoms *in either sex*
    Swelling, discoloration, localized pain, or change in contour
    Lump in breast or axillae
    Nipple discharge in nonlactating *patient*

Breast or axillary findings on screening examination
    On inspection
        Asymmetry of contour or dimpling of skin
        Localized redness of skin
        Asymmetry of venous pattern
        Lymphedema of skin
        Skin abnormalities of nipple or areola
        Unilateral nipple inversion or deviation
    On palpation
        Mass in the breast or axilla
        Localized tenderness
        Localized warmth
        Palpable lymph nodes in breast drainage
        Nipple discharge

Skin or Contour Abnormalities

Evaluation of skin or contour abnormalities begins with detailed inspection. The patient is seated, with both breasts exposed. Observe the suspicious area as the patient raises her arms over her head. Does it move freely with the rest of the breast, remain stationary, or retract? When the patient tenses the pectoralis muscles by pressing her hands on her hips or clasping them behind her back, does the abnormal area move differently from the remainder of the breast? Retraction or asymmetrical movement suggests fixation of the skin to underlying tissue.

Observe for nipple deviation of the involved breast while the patient raises her arms and contracts the pectoralis muscles. A nipple that does not move symmetrically with the opposite nipple or that is deviated in the relaxed position also implies fixation to the suspensory ligaments or to an underlying mass. Is the nipple unilaterally inverted or flattened?

Next, palpate the skin area for tenderness, induration, or increased temperature. Compress it between thumb and forefinger. Does it feel edematous? Does it resist tenting away from the underlying tissue? Does it appear to be fixed to structures beneath it?

Palpate the tissue deep to the skin abnormality. Is there induration beneath the skin? Is there a mass?

With the patient supine, repeat inspection and palpation of the skin abnormality. If nipple deviation, retraction, or flattening has been noted, the areolar area is palpated against the chest wall for mass or thickening, and the nipple is compressed and milked for secretion.

Breast Masses

Physical evaluation of a breast mass reported by the patient is preceded by a complete history including the circumstances of its discovery, the length of time the patient has known it to be present, any past history of mass or other breast problems, and the date of the last menstrual period. Inquiry should be made as to attendant symptoms, such as pain, nipple changes or discharge, and trauma to the area.

Inspection of the breasts is conducted in the usual manner with particular attention given to the area of patient concern and observations of overlying skin, symmetry of movement, nipple abnormalities, and venous patterns. If the mass is visible when the patient is seated, it may be palpated first in this position. After careful axillary palpation, the patient is asked to lie down. The noninvolved breast is thoroughly palpated first in order to ascertain its normal consistency and density. The examination of the involved breast should begin with the uninvolved quadrants and progress to the area indicated by the patient. When the suspicious area is located by the examiner, and if a mass is palpated, the following features are noted and subsequently recorded as indicated in Figure 6.1:

- **Size** of the mass in its vertical and horizontal dimensions, measured with a ruler or tape measure
- **Location** of the mass by quadrant and by distance from the areolar rim
- **Consistency** of the mass, such as compressible or cystic, firm or rock-hard
- **Shape and character of the edges** of the mass, i.e., round, elliptical, or diffuse and ill-defined
- **Character of the overlying skin** as to the presence or absence of increased temperature, erythema, edema, or retraction
- **Attachment** of the mass to overlying skin or deep structures or absence of attachment

If a mass unreported by the patient is discovered in the course of the screening breast examination, the same procedure for its extended examination and full assessment and recording is followed.

Nipple Secretion

The evaluation of nipple secretion is dictated by the circumstances under which it appears. If the patient reports new or unilateral nipple secretion, historical data should include duration, characteristics such as color, ease of expression, associated pain, or other changes observed in the breast. If the secretion is reported to be bilateral, additional information concerning medications, possibility of pregnancy, unusual stimulation, or systemic symptoms such as increased facial hair or change in menstrual pattern is sought.

If in the course of a screening examination any secretion is expressed from the nipple, except colostrum in the pregnant patient or milk in the lactating woman, it should be evaluated further. The secretion is characterized by its color, viscosity, and laterality. Both breasts are fully examined for other evidence of local abnormality as indicated above. A clean glass slide can be pressed directly against the secretion on the nipple and sprayed immediately with fixative for a Papanicolaou smear. An interpretation of "acellular specimen" by this test usually indicates simple galactorrhea. On the other hand, a Papanicolaou smear report of "cellularity without evidence of malignant cells" does not definitively rule out cancer. If there is heat, tenderness, purulent discharge, or other indication of infection, prepare a smear for Gram stain, and obtain a specimen for culture.

Axillary Masses

A patient-reported or examiner-discovered axillary mass should include the detailed breast examination described above as well as an assessment of the limb drained by the axillary nodes and a full lymphatic system examination (see Chapter 10).

INTERPRETING THE FINDINGS

Once the full history and extended physical examination of the breast are completed, decisions regarding technical studies or referral are made, based on the potential health significance of the constellation of findings. Guidelines for interpreting the more common abnormalities are summarized below (see also Table 6.4).

Nipple Abnormalities
INVERSION, FLATTENING, FIXATION, OR DEVIATION

Longstanding inversion of the nipple may be normal; in this instance, the nipple can usually (but not always) be pulled out by gentle manual traction. If the patient is uncertain about the duration of the inversion, the prudent clinician will consider it as new and therefore a potentially dangerous finding. The recently inverted, fixed, flattened, or deviated nipple is a signal for further workup, even when the remainder of the breast examination is normal. It may indicate scarring from inflammation or, much more commonly, cancer.

SECRETION IN THE NONPREGNANT, NONLACTATING PATIENT

The most common cause of serous or serosanguineous discharge from the nipple is not cancer but is intraductal papilloma. However, papillary carcinoma or other carcinoma cannot be excluded without further study. Galactorrhea—discharge of a milky substance from the breasts of a nonpregnant person—is seen as a result

Table 6.4
Abnormalities of the Breast and Axilla

Nipple abnormalities
  Inversion, flattening, fixation, or deviation
  Secretion in the nonpregnant, nonlactating patient
  Lesions of the skin
Breast masses
  Discrete, nontender masses
    Cyst
    Fibroadenoma
    Cancer
    Fat necrosis
    Chronic abscess
    Idiopathic granulomatous mastitis
    Tuberculosis
    Galactocele
  Discrete tender masses
    Acute abscess
    Cancer
    Cyst
    Tuberculosis
  Diffuse tender masses
    Acute mastitis
    Inflammatory carcinoma
Axillary lymphadenopathy
  Secondary to distant or local infection
  Secondary to systemic disease
  Secondary to mammary neoplasm

Male breast abnormalities
  Gynecomastia
  Mass in breast or axilla

of drugs (estrogens, tricyclic antidepressants, phenothiazines, and some antihypertensives) or secondary to endocrine problems such as hyperthyroidism, hypothalamic or pituitary tumors, or Cushing's syndrome. A common denominator in many of these conditions is hyperprolactinemia.

Nipple secretion of purulent material with other manifestations of infection, such as a hot, tender mass or acute pain and diffuse redness and swelling in the lactating woman, is usually clear-cut and diagnosed by physical examination, Gram stain, and culture of the secretions. If the history and physical examination do not clearly indicate infection or suggest endocrine dysfunction, however, a newly manifest or a bloody discharge calls for exclusion of causative malignancy. The role of Papanicolaou preparations in diagnosis is unclear. Today, the best next step in the face of nipple secretion is mammography in the case of absence of a mass on palpation and referral for evaluation and probable biopsy in the instance of palpable breast mass.

ABNORMALITIES OF SKIN OF THE NIPPLE OR AREOLA

The nipple and areola, as part of the integument, are subject to most of the common skin lesions, such as nevi, psoriasis, and eczema. Because of its protuberance, the nipple may be subject to irritation by clothing fabrics, atopic reactions to local contactants (contact dermatitis), or fissure. The latter is especially frequent with breast-feeding. The three most common causes of scaling and excoriation of the nipple are trauma from nursing, simple eczema, and Paget's disease of the breast. This form of Paget's disease is a growth of cancer cells from lactiferous ducts into the epidermis, which then becomes irritated. The carcinoma is called to the patient's attention by itching, crusting, and erosion of the nipple with or without a palpable subjacent mass. Most experts in the field of breast disease would recommend that redness and thickening of the nipple epidermis with erosion be biopsied as suspicious of Paget's carcinoma. If microscopy confirms simple dermatitis, no harm has been done; if the pathology indicates carcinoma, the appropriate interventions may then be accomplished promptly and with a better prognosis than if delayed until a mass becomes palpable.

Breast Masses
DISCRETE, NONTENDER MASSES

The most common breast lump is a **benign cyst,** usually in the setting of the fibrocystic process. These cysts are associated with cyclic hormonal stimulation and tend to regress after menopause. The cyst is typically round to slightly elliptical, soft and elastic, and freely mobile. There is no attachment to surrounding structures, and thus no dimpling or nipple retraction is associated. Although usually nontender to palpation, cysts may become tender prior to menses. Cysts are often multiple and bilateral and are commonly symmetric both within a breast and between breasts. They usually vary in size with the menstrual cycle, being smallest just after menses—hence the desirability of scheduling routine examination of reproductive-age women to this phase, in order to minimize cyclical "positives."

Fibroadenoma is a benign solid mass that may appear any time after puberty but presents less commonly after menopause. It is usually a single lesion. The fibroadenoma, like the cyst, is well demarcated, freely mobile, and usually nontender. It tends to be round, but its shape is variable. There should be no retraction or other sign of fixation.

Cancer of the breast may present at any age after puberty; its frequency increases progressively with age and does not decline, as previously thought, with extreme old age. Carcinoma can exist as a single lesion in an otherwise completely normal breast, or it may coexist with benign lesions. Characteristically, the malignant breast lesion is irregular in contour, very firm to hard in consistency, and not clearly delineated from surrounding tissue. *These features are not uniformly present, however, and their absence does not exclude cancer.* Fixation to skin, ligaments, and/or chest wall will eventually occur, but early tumors will seldom have retraction signs. Intraductal carcinomas occasionally produce a serous or serosanguineous nipple discharge. Cancer of the breast is usually painless; however, the examiner cannot rely on tenderness of a breast lesion to exclude the possibility of malignancy, since some cancers are tender to palpation whether or not they are reported as painful.

Other, less common nontender solitary masses include **fat necrosis, chronic abscess, idiopathic granulomatous mastitis,** and **tuberculosis.** Because each of these lesions may be irregular and nondiscrete, they often require biopsy to differentiate them from carcinoma. **Galactocele,** the cystic dilatation caused by duct blockage in the lactating breast, is a noninflammatory soft mass that can usually be made to disappear by use of a breast pump to enhance drainage.

DISCRETE TENDER MASSES

Acute abscess of the breast presents as a well-localized, hot, tender, and often fluctuant mass. It is frequently accompanied by systemic signs and symptoms such as fever, chills, and leukocytosis. Abscess usually arises as a sequel to acute mastitis, and therefore most frequently during lactation, but it may also develop de novo.

DIFFUSE TENDER MASSES

Acute mastitis is a diffuse infection of the breast, most commonly occurring during lactation. The involved portion of the breast, usually a single quadrant, is red, indurated, and exquisitely tender. There are often systemic physical and laboratory signs such as fever and leukocytosis.

One neoplasm, **inflammatory carcinoma** of the breast, may present as an acute process resembling mastitis. It tends to involve an entire breast rather than a single quadrant and is accompanied by axillary lymphadenopathy. Biopsy is often indicated, especially outside the lactational period, to differentiate between acute mastitis and inflammatory carcinoma, particularly if a suspected mastitis does not promptly and completely respond to antibiotic therapy.

Axillary Lymphadenopathy

In the thin patient, small, mobile, soft nodes are occasionally palpable in the axillary chains. The axillary nodes will enlarge and become tender in response to small wounds or infection located distally in the arm. If such nodes are found unilaterally, the examiner should ask about possible cat scratches, look carefully at the ipsilateral hand and forearm for inflammation, and inspect the axilla for infected hair follicles. Very hard, fixed, or matted nodes in the axilla mandate careful assessment of the breast that they drain. If nothing is found there on examination, the search for breast problems should proceed while a search for causes of primary nodal processes such as lymphoma takes place. The infectious or neoplastic implications of bilateral axillary and/or diffuse lymphadenopathy are discussed in Chapters 5 and 10.

Abnormalities of the Male Breast

Gynecomastia, i.e., enlargement of the male breast, occurs in adult males as a result of hormonal stimulation. The use of exogenous estrogen, such as in the treatment of prostatic carcinoma, regularly produces bilateral breast enlargement. Endogenous secretion of feminizing hormones from the adrenal gland (Cushing's syndrome or adenoma) or from germ cell tumors (choriocarcinoma) may also result in gynecomastia. The male breast may hypertrophy in the setting of hepatic cirrhosis in relation to impaired estrogen metabolism. A number of drugs have been observed to induce gynecomastia.

Approximately 1.5% of breast cancers arise in males. A visible or palpable subareolar mass, nipple retraction, or secretion may herald neoplasia and such signs are indications for referral for tissue biopsy. Unfortunately, male breast cancer is often diagnosed only at an advanced stage because of patient and examiner prejudice that breast cancer is an exclusively female disease.

RECORDING THE FINDINGS

An example of recording the findings of an extended breast and axillary examination follows.

Breasts: On inspection, slight retraction of skin in upper outer quadrant of left breast. Left nipple flattened and deviated to left. Right breast appears normal. With elevation of arm, dimpling of skin visible in left upper outer quadrant with restriction of elevation of left nipple. Right breast tissue moves normally. On palpation, right breast is granular and free of mass or tenderness. In left breast, there is a hard, irregular mass in upper outer quadrant, measuring 2×1 cm and surrounded by a ring of edema. Mass is fixed to overlying skin but appears free of underlying tissue. No secretion expressed from either nipple.

S.W.--43-year-old -white female 4/2/91

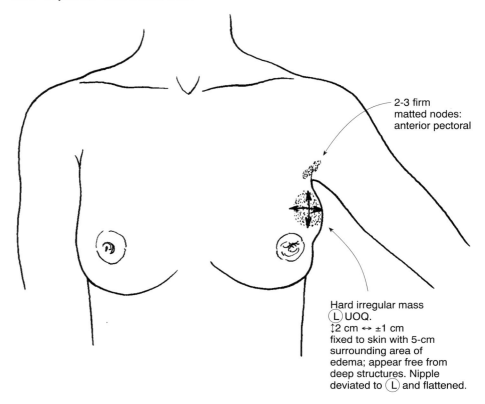

2-3 firm matted nodes: anterior pectoral

Hard irregular mass
(L) UOQ.
↕2 cm ↔ ±1 cm
fixed to skin with 5-cm surrounding area of edema; appear free from deep structures. Nipple deviated to (L) and flattened.

Axillae: Right axilla normal to palpation. In left axilla, a small cluster of firm, matted nodes is felt in anterior chain. No middle, posterior, or high nodes felt.

Impression: Left breast mass, upper outer quadrant, with skin fixation and palpable anterior axillary nodes, probable carcinoma with nodal metastases.

BEYOND THE PHYSICAL EXAMINATION

Mammography as a screening and follow-up procedure continues to evolve in terms of recommendations for frequency and indications. Current recommendations of the American Cancer Society and the American College of Radiology are for every woman to have a baseline study between ages 35 and 40, a repeat mammogram every other year from ages 40–50, and annually thereafter. These recommendations may change as new information is collected.

For the generalist who discovers a suspicious mass, access to the **consultation** of a general surgeon with expertise in breast disease is necessary. Aspiration cytology is an effective, easy way to get fluid for a Papanicolaou smear. **Biopsy** under the guidance of mammography is performed by interventional radiologists in some institutions or by surgeons in concert with radiologists in others. Since the definitive diagnosis of any suspicious breast lesion resides in the histopathologic specimen, biopsy is often the best route to resolving the questions of causality and appropriate management. If there is any doubt—after a careful history and physical examination—about the cause of a breast abnormality, surgical referral should be the next step.

RECOMMENDED READINGS

Carlson HE. Gynecomastia. N Engl J Med 1980;303:795–799.

Fariselli G, Lepera P, Viganotti G, Martelli G, Bandieramonte G, DiPietro S. Localized mastalgia as presenting symptom in breast cancer. Eur J Surg Oncol 1988;14:213–215.

Goodson WH III, Mallman R, Jacobson M, Hunt T. What do breast symptoms mean? Am J Surg 1985;1 50:271–274.

Haagensen CD. Diseases of the breast. 3rd ed. Philadelphia: WB Saunders, 1986.

Hall FM. Screening mammography—potential problems on the horizon. N Engl J Med 1986;314: 53–55.

Health and Public Policy Committee, American College of Physicians. The use of diagnostic tests for screening and evaluating breast lesions. Ann Intern Med 1985;103:143–146.

Lynch HT, Watson P, Conway T, Fitzsimmons ML, Lynch J. Breast cancer family history as a risk factor for early onset breast cancer. Breast Cancer Res Treat 1988;11:263–267.

Nattinger AB, Panzer RJ, Janus J. Improving the utilization of screening mammography in primary care practice. Arch Intern Med 1989;149:2087–2092.

Tabar L, Faberberg G, Day NE, Holmberg L. What is the optimum interval between mammographic screening examinations?—An analysis based on the latest results of the Swedish two-county breast cancer screening trial. Br J Cancer 1987;66(2):251–256.

Winchester DP, Sener S, Immerman S, Blum M. A systematic approach to the evaluation and management of breast masses. Cancer 1983;51:2535–2539.

7

Thorax and Lungs

APPROACH AND ANATOMICAL REVIEW

The regional approach demands that the chest, including its skin, skeletal structure, and the lungs, be examined as a unit. The review of anatomy moves from the surface inward, with particular attention given to surface projections of deep structures and the language necessary to understand and describe the locations of the examination findings.

Surface Landmarks

Three views of the chest are presented. For ease of visualizing the deep structures as they relate to the surface divisions, each of the three chest wall surface views is accompanied by a sketch of skeletal and pulmonary structures. Please note that the position of the nipples is so variable that they must not be used as landmarks for inferring visceral or skeletal locales; skin lesions, however, may be described in terms of their position relative to a nipple rather than to conventional anatomical lines.

ANTERIOR

The clavicles and supraclavicular fossae define the superior limit of the chest. The inferior tip of the sternum and approximately the seventh ribs define the lower margin. For clinical description, two conventional lines are projected onto the chest wall. The **midsternal line,** running from the sternal notch to the xiphoid process, indicates the (anterior) midline of the thorax, and the right and left **midclavicular lines** pass from the midpoint of each clavicle downward, parallel to the midsternal line (Fig. 7.1).

LATERAL

The upper portions of the lateral borders of the chest are covered by the attachment of the arms to the chest wall. With the arm raised over the head, imaginary lines delineate relationships between axillae and deeper structures. The **anterior axillary lines (right and left)** begin at the upper limit of the anterior axillary fold, which is created by the border of the **pectoralis major muscle,** and drop inferiorly parallel to the midsternal line. The **midaxillary lines** (right and left) are drawn from the midapices of the axillae downward, parallel to the anterior ancillary line. The **posterior axillary lines** (right and left) commence at the upper extremity of the posterior axillary fold, which is formed by the latissimus dorsi muscle, and drop downward parallel to the midaxillary line (Fig. 7.2).

POSTERIOR

Two lines are imagined on the posterior chest wall. The **midvertebral or midspinal line** descends from the C7 spinous process downward and marks the midposterior chest. The **scapular lines** parallel the midspinal line and cross the palpable inferior angle of the scapula (Fig. 7.3).

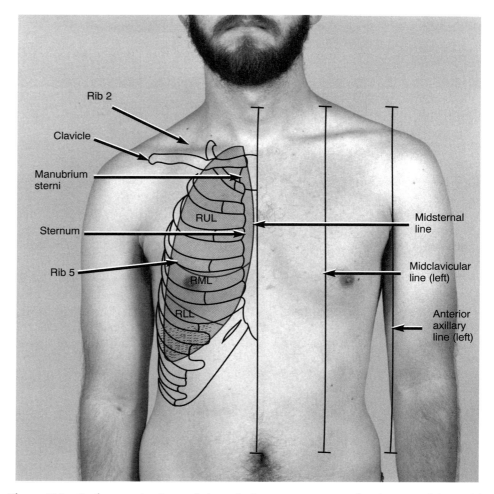

Figure 7.1   Surface projections of thoracic bone structures and pulmonary lobes with placement of anterior thoracic lines.

Thoracic Skeleton and Muscles

The anterior bony thorax consists of the **clavicles, the ribs** and their **cartilaginous attachments** to the **sternum,** the **xiphoid process,** and the remainder of the **sternum.** The **suprasternal notch** is palpable between the medial ends of the clavicles. Also palpable is the **sternal angle (angle of Louis)** at the junction of the **manubrium** and the **body (corpus)** of the sternum. The second costal cartilage is at the level of the sternal angle. These landmarks remain palpable even in morbid obesity or massive pectoral development and in patients with very large breasts.

The posterior skeletal structures of the chest include the **ribs, thoracic spine, and scapulae (shoulder blades)** (Fig. 7.4*A* and *B*).

The large, superficial, and usually palpable muscles of the chest wall are the bilateral (right and left) **pectoralis major and latissimi dorsi** muscles. Each pectoralis major muscle traverses the chest wall diagonally from the proximal humerus down and toward the xiphoid. Each latissimus dorsi muscle lies along the lateral posterior thorax, from the upper humerus to the lumbar and lower thoracic spine.

The primary chest wall muscles of respiration are the **intercostals,** which connect one rib with the next and provide the bellows action for the lungs. The other-

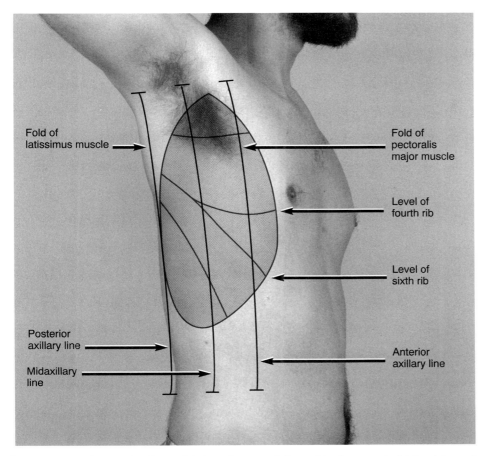

Figure 7.2 Surface projections of right pulmonary lobes with placement of lateral thoracic lines.

major muscle involved in ventilation is the **diaphragm**, which contracts and moves downward during inspiration. Accessory muscles of respiration include the **serrati, scaleni, sternomastoids, and the two rectus abdominis** muscles (Fig. 7.5A and B).

Contents of the Thoracic Cavity
PLEURA

The pleura are thin layers of mesothelium and connective tissue that line and adhere to the inner thoracic wall (**parietal pleura**) and the lungs (**visceral pleura**), respectively. Between these two layers of pleura in each hemithorax is a potential space, the **pleural cavity**, which contains a small amount of fluid to lubricate the surfaces as they slide over one another during inflation and deflation of the lungs. The normal pleural cavity contains no air. The parietal pleura is sharply reflected at the **costophrenic angle** to extend over the thoracic surface of the diaphragm.

MEDIASTINUM

The mediastinum is the space between the two lungs, in which are contained the **aorta**, the lower **trachea** and its division into the **right and left main-stem bronchi, lymph nodes, the vagus nerves (cranial nerve X), the esophagus**, and,

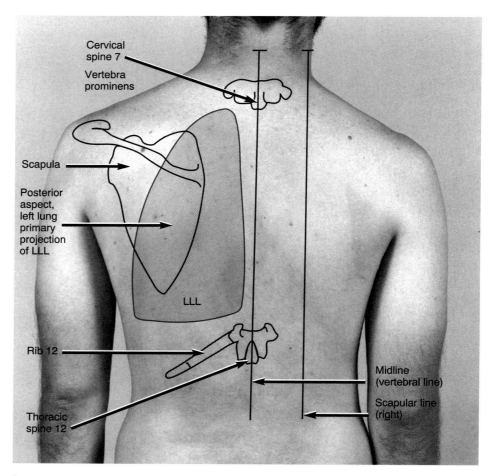

Figure 7.3   Surface projections of posterior pulmonary viscera with placement of posterior thoracic lines.

anteriorly, **the heart and pericardial sac.** This chapter is concerned with the airways (the tracheobronchial tree) and the lungs.

TRACHEOBRONCHIAL TREE

The trachea bifurcates at or just below the level of the sternal angle into the right and left **main-stem bronchi,** with each providing the airway into the respective lung. The site of division is called the **carina.** The **right main-stem bronchus** sends a trunk to each of three lung lobes; the **left main-stem bronchus** divides into two **lobar bronchi.** Each lobar trunk arborizes into branches of decreasing diameter, which eventually become **bronchioles** (twiglets) that ultimately serve the alveolar sacs of the pulmonary parenchyma. Each bronchus is accompanied by a **pulmonary artery** and its branches. The **pulmonary vein** divisions follow intersegmental septa instead.

LUNGS

The lungs are clusters of air sacs (**alveoli**) grouped around terminal bronchioles. The right lung is divided into three distinct **lobes,** each of which is separated from the others by a visceral pleural reflection that forms the **fissures.** They are the **upper, middle, and lower lobes.** The left lung has two major divisions, the

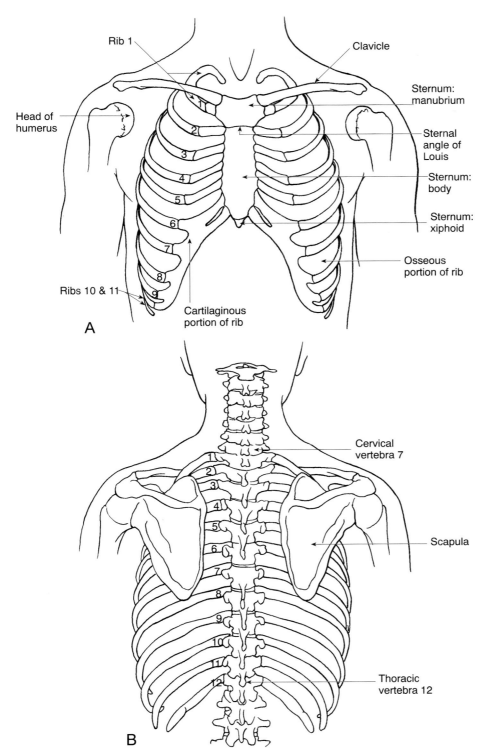

Figure 7.4   Schematic representation of structures of the bony thorax. **A.** Anterior view.
B. Posterior view.

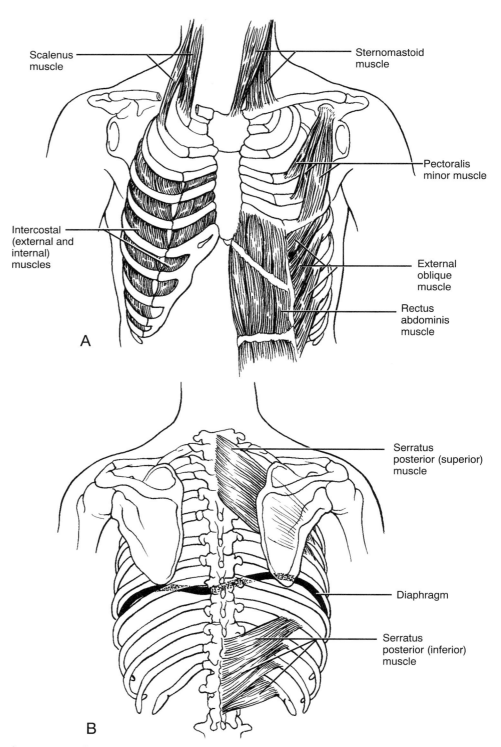

Figure 7.5 Schematic representation of major muscles of respiration. **A.** Anterior view. The pectoralis major has been removed to demonstrate relationships of deeper musculature. **B.** Posterior view.

upper and lower lobes. Although there is no middle lobe in the left lung, the segment of the left upper lobe positionally analogous to the right middle lobe is referred to as the **lingula** (Fig. 7.6). It is much smaller than the right middle lobe because it is indented by the heart. Each lung is roughly conical in shape. The apices extend in the circle above the first rib and the clavicle, to lie beneath the subcutaneous structures of the supraclavicular fossae. The broad base of each lung is concave and fits over the convex surface of the respective hemidiaphragm. With quiet respiration, the most posteroinferior part of the lung extends to approximately the level of the eleventh thoracic vertebra.

The **mechanics of respiration,** which play a major role in interpretation of pulmonary physical findings, are reviewed briefly. At the initiation of **inspiration (inhalation),** the diaphragm descends and the ribs flare. The intrapleural pressure drops from –5 to about –15 cm of water relative to atmospheric pressure. This differential assists the inflation of the alveolar sacs by oxygen-laden air entering the tracheobronchial tree from the atmosphere via the oropharynx and nasopharynx. During **expiration (exhalation),** the process is reversed but is much more passive in normal persons. The rib cage contracts, the diaphragms rise, the negative pressure in the pleural space diminishes, the alveoli lose some content, and the bronchial tubular structures narrow—all of which expels the oxygen-depleted air from the airways along with its burden of carbon dioxide.

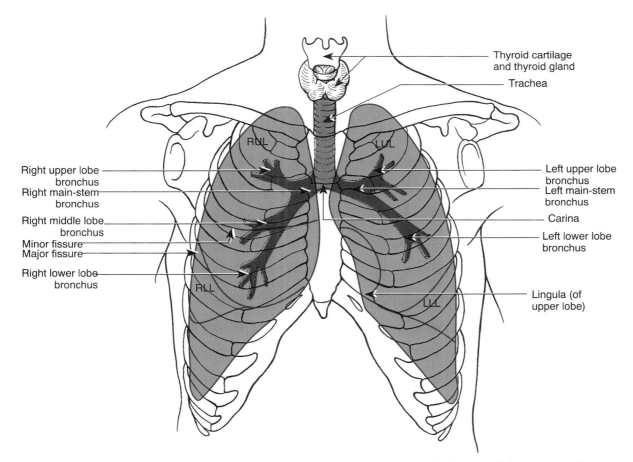

Figure 7.6 Drawing of major respiratory structures: tracheobronchial tree and pulmonary lobes. *RUL,* right upper lobe; *RLL,* right lower lobe; *LUL,* left upper lobe; and *LLL,* left lower lobe. Lung volume represented in mid-respiration.

TECHNIQUE

Although all four modes—inspection, palpation, percussion, and auscultation—are utilized in the chest examination, they are mixed to facilitate an efficient *regional* examination. Thus, the examination is begun with the examiner facing the seated patient for inspection (only) of the anterior chest, followed by complete examination of the posterior and lateral thorax and lungs and ending with auscultation and percussion of the lungs anteriorly.

The patient remains seated throughout this examination, and the examiner moves from front to back to sides, returning lastly to the front of the patient. See Table 7.1 for the sequence of the chest and lung examination.

Equipment for this portion of the examination includes good lighting, warm hands, the stethoscope, and a skin pencil.

As the examiner moves from front to side to back, she conducts a (regional) portion of the examination of the skin, looking for, measuring, and describing any skin lesions that are noted on the chest wall (see Chapter 3).

Respiratory assessment at first contact and during the interview includes noting the effort, general rate, and depth of breathing and whether it is noisy. Decades ago, noisy breathing (apart from snoring) was identified as a valid sign of disordered respiratory-pulmonary function. It retains this significance now. Although the etiology may not be apparent, if the breathing is loud—in the ambient atmosphere—to the unaided ear, it is abnormal.

Anterior Chest Wall Inspection

With the patient seated at the end of the examining table, the examiner faces him directly and observes the chest wall for its shape and symmetry. The respiratory movement of the chest is noted for rate, rhythm, evidence of labored breathing, symmetry of movement from side to side, and visible retraction of the intercostal muscles. The examiner then inspects and palpates the trachea to determine if it is in the midline and, if relevant, whether it is tender.

Table 7.1
Sequence of the Chest Examination[a]

Examiner Position	Maneuver
Facing patient	Inspect anterior chest wall
	Inspect and palpate tracheal position
Facing patient's back	Inspect respiratory motion
	Count respirations
	Inspect and palpate thoracic spine
	Percuss costovertebral angles
	Palpate respiratory motion
	Percuss diaphragmatic excursions
	Percuss lungs (posterior)
	Auscultate lungs (posterior)
At patient's left and right sides, respectively	Inspect lateral chest walls
	Percuss lungs (lateral)
	Auscultate lungs (lateral)
Facing patient	Auscultate lungs (anterior)[b]
	Percuss lungs (anterior)[b]

[a]Patient is seated for entire examination.
[b]Including Krönig's isthmus.

Lateral Chest Wall Inspection

The examiner asks the patient to raise his arms over his head and then moves to the patient's right, then to his left side, noting the overall shape and the **anteroposterior diameter** of the thorax as well as the lateral configuration of the **thoracic spine**.

Full Posterior Thorax Examination

With the patient holding both arms at his sides and the examiner facing his back, **inspection** of the posterior thorax is begun.

RESPIRATORY MOVEMENT INSPECTION

From this position, it is possible to note the resting respirations. If movement of the chest wall is visible, count the **respiratory rate** in cycles (breaths) per minute. As emphasized in Chapter 2 under the discussion of technique for taking vital signs (Respiratory Rate and Rhythm), this must be done with the patient unaware. Note the **rhythm, the amplitude,** and the side-to-side **symmetry** of movement.

THORACIC SPINE INSPECTION, PALPATION, AND PERCUSSION

Note the contour of the thoracic (dorsal) spine by studying the alignment of the dorsal processes. With fingertips, locate the prominence of C7, and run the fingers inferiorly along the processes to determine the contour of the column. With your dominant hand curled into a fist, percuss gently with the ulnar surface of the fist over each dorsal vertebral process from the level of T1 to the level of L1, asking the patient to indicate any area of tenderness. Note that as with sinus percussion (Chapter 4 Extended Examination section) this percussion is designed to elicit tenderness, *not* to create audible or palpable vibration of diagnostic significance.

COSTOVERTEBRAL ANGLE PALPATION

Just beneath the twelfth rib and lateral to the last thoracic vertebra (T12) is the surface landmark known as the costovertebral angle (CVA). The kidney lies deep to the long paraspinal muscles in this angle (Fig. 7.7). Using a single finger, press firmly against each CVA, asking the patient to indicate any discomfort created by this pressure. Although many authors have advocated fist percussion at this site, the specificity is so poor (with many false-positives occurring in tense or apprehensive persons) that any putative gain in sensitivity is offset.

RESPIRATORY MOVEMENT PALPATION

Place both hands on the lower rib cage, with the palms flat against the patient's back and the fingers spread. Watch the movement of the hands. Do they move symmetrically with the patient's respiratory cycle? Does one hemithorax move more or less widely than the other? If the respirations could not be counted visually, count them now as they are palpated.

POSTERIOR AND LATERAL LUNG PERCUSSION

The **indirect** technique of percussion is carried out as follows: The palmar surfaces of the fingers of one hand are spread over the area to be percussed. Using the middle finger of the other hand, the dorsum of the spread middle finger is struck quickly and sharply, with the wrist of the percussing hand used as the fulcrum of motion (Fig. 7.8A).

The finger held to the chest wall is the *pleximeter,* while the one striking it is the *plexor.* The middle finger of the nondominant hand is a fine pleximeter, and the best place to strike it is directly on the midpoint of the distal interphalangeal joint (DIP). The pleximeter is held firmly but not rigidly to the surface to be

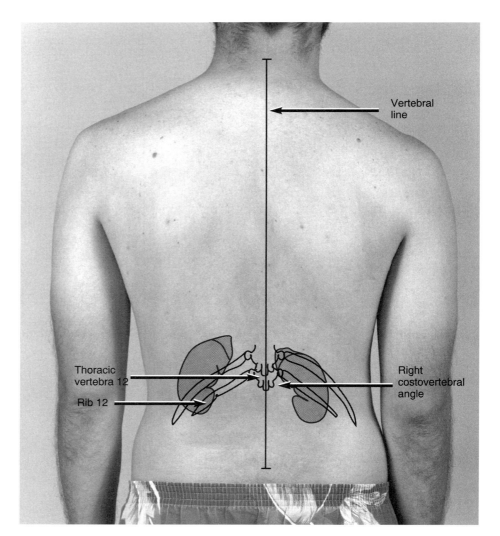

Figure 7.7   Surface projections of costovertebral angle and underlying kidneys.

assessed, with the parts of this digit just above and below the DIP apposed lightly and with the remaining digits and palm apposed more lightly still, if at all. The plexor is the pulp tip of the middle finger of the dominant hand (Fig. 7.8). It is touched to the pleximeter at the joint to be struck. Ignoring the thumb, all finger joints of the plexor hand are flexed. The wrist is extended about 45°, so that the plexor finger describes an arc of a few centimeters above the point to be struck on the pleximeter. The wrist is then flexed to a little below rest position, using very little force. In this maneuver sound vibration is produced. The pleximeter perceives tissue vibration as a second, parallel information source. THROUGHOUT PERCUSSION, the only joint to be moved is the wrist. The remainder of the plexor hand is held as a static but not rigid unit.

    Practice the correct movement by gently squeezing your dominant wrist to mark its use (Fig. 7.8B) and then bringing down your dominant middle finger tip against any surface (for this exercise, forget the pleximeter). Your puffed-out cheek makes a good hyperresonant to tympanic note. A deflated cheek is dull. Your thigh is flat. Once you've done this until you are confident that your hand works as a unit, moving only at the wrist, take away your nondominant hand

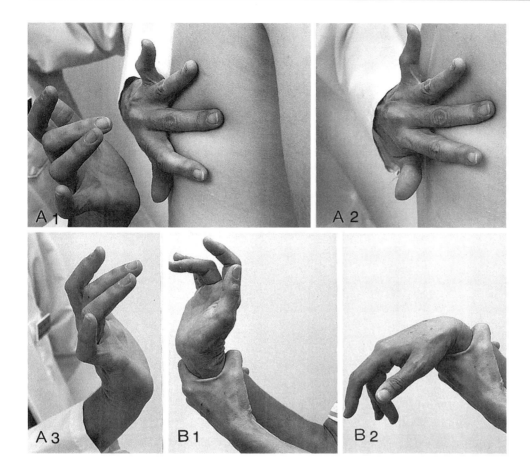

Figure 7.8 A. Chest wall percussion techniques. **A1.** Relative position of plexor and pleximeter at beginning of percussion stroke. **A2.** Pleximeter placement. **A3.** Plexor in position to begin percussion stroke. **B.** Practicing percussion, with fixation of wrist by opposite hand. **B1.** Full extension at beginning of stroke. **B2.** Full flexion at time of contact of plexor with pleximeter.

from the plexor wrist and use it as the pleximeter. Go over the same sites again, and note how you now *feel* as well as *hear* something with each percussion blow you strike. It is conventional to retain the pleximeter at the site percussed for a moment after the percussion blow is struck, to permit the palpatory component to be maximized; however, the plexor is usually removed immediately after striking, by reextension of the wrist.

There are four distinct notes that may be elicited by percussion: (1) **flat** as over the muscle of the thigh, (2) **dull** as over the liver in the right upper quadrant of the abdomen, (3) **resonant** as through the chest wall over normally inflated lung, and (4) **tympanitic** as over the gas bubble of the stomach. (For the anticipated percussion notes over the adult thorax, see Figure 7.12.) These are gradations, but with practice the student will learn to discern them quite distinctly from one another.

The purpose of percussion of the chest is to define the anatomic limits of the normal pulmonary resonance and to locate areas of abnormal percussion note within the lung parenchyma.

Percussion of the posterior and lateral chest proceeds as follows:

1. Determine the range of diaphragmatic excursion.
   a. Ask the patient to take in a deep breath, exhale fully, and maintain this full expiration. Then begin percussion in the scapular line downward from about the T8 level until the percussion note changes from resonance to the dullness below the diaphragm. With a skin pencil, mark the point of transition on each posterior hemithorax.
   b. Ask the patient to take a deep breath and hold it in full inspiration. Then begin percussion downward in the scapular line, starting at each previously marked skin line, marking the new transition with another line. The distance between the two marks indicates the extent of downward hemidiaphragmatic movement with inspiration cycle. This distance is measured and recorded (Fig. 7.9).
2. Percuss the lungs posteriorly (Fig. 7.10A).
   a. The patient may be asked to cross his arms in front of his body in order to spread the scapulae laterally, or he may be asked to sit and breathe normally.

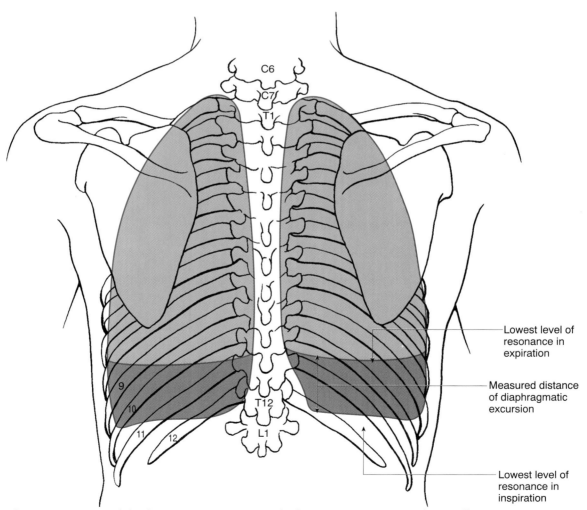

Figure 7.9   Range of diaphragmatic excursion, marked on patient's posterior chest wall at maximum expiration (*upper mark*) and maximum inspiration (*lower mark*).

b. Beginning high on the chest wall, between the vertebral column and the scapula of each hemithorax (scapular line), the examiner percusses downward toward the marked base of each lung, moving from side to side in order to compare the percussion note of symmetrical lung segments.
3. Percuss the lungs laterally (Fig. 7.10C and D).
   a. The examiner moves to the right side of the patient and asks the patient to raise his right arm over his head to reveal the lateral chest wall.
   b. The chest is percussed from high in the axilla to the level of the diaphragm.
   c. The examiner then moves to the left side of the patient, and the procedure is repeated over the left lateral chest. **Note that the right middle lobe and the lingula of the left upper lobe are assessed laterally, not anteriorly or posteriorly.** The percussion note and, in particular, the projections of breath sounds from them project to the axillae.

POSTERIOR AND LATERAL LUNG AUSCULTATION

The purpose of auscultation of the lungs is to assess air movement in the large to medium-sized airways and to make inferences about airways, parenchyma, and pleural space. The **diaphragm of the stethoscope** (warmed by holding or rubbing it vigorously in the palm of the hand) is used for routine pulmonary auscultation.

Three kinds of breath sounds are heard in normal adult lungs: **vesicular, bronchovesicular, and bronchial.** See Figure 7.12 for the characteristics of these sounds and their usual locations.

The technique of chest auscultation is as follows:

1. Ask the patient to breathe through the mouth *with the mouth well open.* The positioning of the stethoscope on the chest wall follows the pattern defined for percussion. The breath sounds are compared from side to side, and each area is assessed through one complete respiratory cycle.
2. The procedure is continued into each lateral hemithorax, positioning the instrument as described for percussion.

ANTERIOR CHEST PERCUSSION AND AUSCULTATION

The examiner now comes around front again and faces the patient to complete the screening chest examination. This begins with percussion and is followed by auscultation. Percussion and auscultation should include the **apices** of each lung, located in the supraclavicular fossae (Krönig's isthmuses). If this space is too narrow to allow full apposition of the diaphragm of the stethoscope to the skin, the examiner can press the smaller **bell** firmly against the skin and achieve similar sound transmission. The **anterior lung fields** are further auscultated and percussed from immediately below the clavicles to the level of the anterior diaphragmatic limits (at approximately the fifth intercostal spaces). Routinely, the "supradiaphragmatic" portion of the dome of the liver renders the lower right anterior thorax dull. Depending on body habitus, the breasts may interfere, the examiner may encounter the dullness of the heart on the left anterior hemithorax before reaching the level of the diaphragm, or both may occur. For the appropriate positions for percussion and auscultation during the anterior chest examination, please refer to Figure 7.10B.

NORMAL AND COMMON VARIANTS

The range of normal in the examination of the thorax and lungs is relatively narrow. Body habitus, sex, and age will account for most of the variants ac-

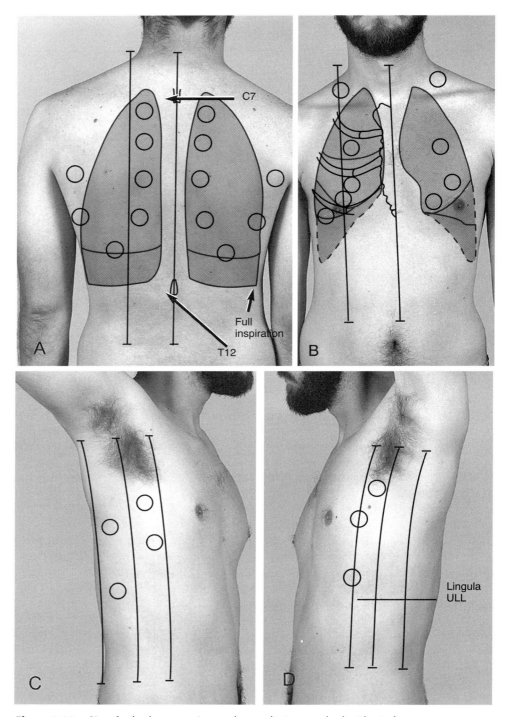

Figure 7.10   Sites for both percussion and auscultation marked with circles.

cepted as either normal or not requiring further diagnostic workup or consideration for therapeutic intervention. A few structural abnormalities not amenable to treatment are discussed; when discovered they should be described in the patient's record even if there is no intent to pursue them further at the time.

Chest Wall Inspection

Respirations are evaluated for rate, rhythm, and evidence of increased work of breathing (see also Chapter 2 for details on respiratory rate variables). **Respiratory rate** in the normal adult ranges from 12 to 18 cycles/minute. **Tachypnea** is defined as a respiratory rate greater than 20/minute. Occasionally, an anxious patient may exhibit tachypnea, but calming should reduce the rate to normal. Also, the tachypnea of anxiety can usually be consciously controlled by the patient's will, whereas tachypnea of pathologic origin is subject to only short-lived voluntary slowing. Tachypnea of pathologic origin has a long differential diagnosis. **Bradypnea,** or a respiratory rate of 10 or less, in a conscious adult is very unusual as a normal variant and is generally volitional. When distracted, such a person's respiratory rate may return to the normal range. If the examiner observes either mild tachypnea or bradypnea in a patient who seems to be otherwise comfortable and breathing without effort, she should repeat the observation at another point in the examination. For example, take the respiratory count during the posterior thoracic examination when the patient is not conscious of having his respirations watched. Any *obstructive airway disease* such as emphysema or asthma can reduce efficiency and thereby slow respiration. *Narcotic drugs* can produce bradypnea even when they do not impair consciousness.

Respiratory rhythm is normally very regular, with the duration of expiration slightly longer. It is common for the rhythm to be occasionally punctuated by a single deep and slow cycle, a **sigh,** a physiologic adjustment of the O_2-CO_2 balance. Frequent sighing may be seen in an emotionally depressed or very anxious patient who has no cardiopulmonary or central nervous system pathology. **Hyperpnea** and **hyperventilation syndrome** are covered in the Extended Examination section of this chapter under Interpreting the Findings.

The **work or effort of respiration** should not appear laborious. Normal breathing at rest is an effortless, quiet, automatic action. The muscles involved in normal respiration do not appear to be working hard, and expiration is passive. The accessory muscles of respiration, such as the sternomastoids and the abdominal muscles, do not visibly participate in normal breathing. An exception to this general rule may occasionally be found in the very elderly patient in whom calcification of the rib cartilages limits rib cage motion, so that the accessory muscles are required for chest wall movement to accommodate the function of normal lungs.

The shape of the thorax is symmetrical from side to side and is wider in its frontal dimensions than in its anteroposterior (AP) dimensions, although questions have been raised about the significance of an increase in AP diameter. There are skeletal variants that alter the normal chest contour. Two of these anomalies are present since birth or childhood (a congenital form and one that is acquired as a result of vitamin D deficiency during skeletal growth) and are permanent and stable in adulthood. **Pectus carinatum (pigeon breast)** is a result of anterior projection of the sternum and costal cartilages into a form resembling the keel of a boat. **Pectus excavatum** is created by a depression or sinking inward of the lower sternum. A second set of deformities occurs with thoracic spine variants that are developmental or may be acquired by way of anterior collapse of osteopenic thoracic vertebral bodies. Pathologic **kyphosis** of the thoracic spine leads to an increase in the AP diameter of the chest and a reduction in stature (height). The most striking form of kyphosis is the **gibbus** deformity in which an acute angulation at the midthoracic spine accentuates the kyphosis (Fig. 7.11). **Scoliosis,** or lateral curvature of the thoracic spine, is discussed in Chapter 12.

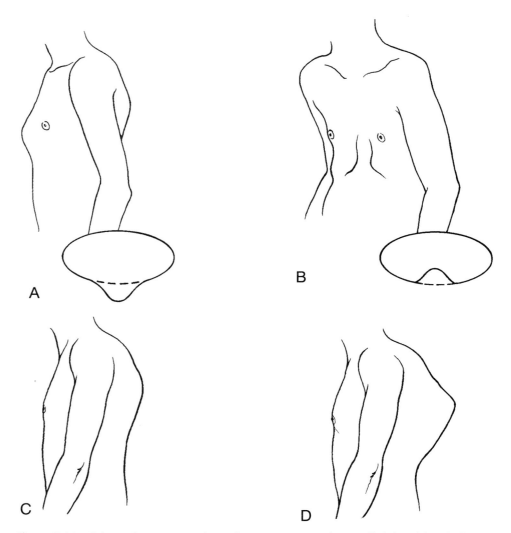

Figure 7.11   Schematic representations of some common chest wall deformities. **A.** Pectus carinatum. **B.** Pectus excavatum. **C.** Mildly exaggerated (pathologic) dorsal kyphosis. **D.** Severe dorsal kyphosis (gibbus deformity).

Costovertebral Angle Percussion

Percussion over the CVAs should elicit no tenderness. Discomfort (especially unilateral) with this maneuver is suggestive of inflammation of the deep muscles of the back or of the kidney in the retroperitoneum (see the Extended Examination section of this chapter and Chapter 12), although minor discomfort may be elicited in the anxious but otherwise normal patient.

Percussion of Diaphragmatic Excursion

The right hemidiaphragm is normally slightly higher than the left, perhaps because of its position over the larger right lobe of the liver. Thus, there is often a slight difference in the two sides in terms of end-inspiratory and end-expiratory position, particularly anteriorly. The excursion of each leaf of the diaphragm should be 3 cm or more posteriorly. The inability to detect a change in diaphragmatic position with respiration indicates pathology, as does failure of either muscle to move the predicted distance.

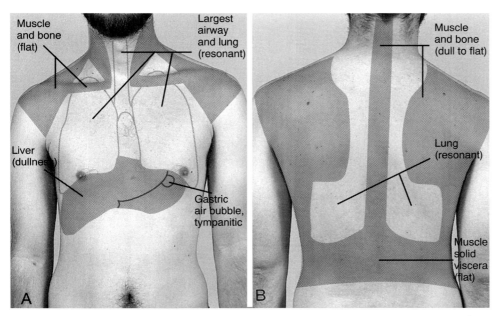

Figure 7.12   Normal percussion notes. **A.** Over anterior chest wall. **B.** Over posterior chest wall. *White areas* represent resonance of pulmonary parenchyma; *red crosshatched areas,* the dullness of non-air-filled tissue; and *solid red areas,* the tympany of hollow viscera.

Lung Palpation, Percussion, and Auscultation

The normal range of findings resulting from palpation, percussion, and ausculta-tion of the lungs is a function of chest size, muscle development, fat distribution, and breast contour. For example, bodybuilders, with their massive pectoralis and latissimus muscles, may have distant breath sounds simply because of the vol-ume of acoustically impedant tissue between the airway and the examiner's hand or stethoscope. However, these findings should be continuous and symmetrical. The same premise holds true for morbidly obese persons. By contrast, very thin persons without lung abnormality may manifest more intense sounds from air movement. Symmetry from side to side, normal duration of the inspiratory and expiratory phases of the cycle, and a normal distribution of the quality of the vibrations should be present.

   The usual distribution of normal variations in the percussion note over the chest wall is depicted in Figure 7.12. Expected auscultatory findings in the nor-mal person are represented in Table 7.2. **Any variations from normal in percus-sion note or breath sounds on auscultation, other than those accounted for by organ position and body habitus, indicate pathology and are discussed in the Extended Examination section.**

RECORDING THE FINDINGS

The chest examination is usually recorded after the breast examination in the patient's record. Any skin abnormalities may be recorded with the SKIN exami-nation or regionally as illustrated below.

Respiratory system: Trachea midline and mobile. Thorax normal to inspection, except for mild pectus excavatum. Several small, bright red, slightly palpable lesions over anterior chest wall; one dark, palpable lesion with a single hair growing from its center, inferior to the left nipple. Well-healed midsternal sur-gical scar from suprasternal notch to tip of xiphoid.

Respiratory movements easy, without use of accessory muscles. Diaphragmatic excursion 3 cm bilaterally. Percussion note normal over all lobes. Breath sounds vesicular posteriorly and over upper lobes. Normal bronchovesicular sounds to right and left of sternum. No adventitious sounds present.

Musculoskeletal system: No spinal tenderness nor CVA tenderness.

Impression:
1. Normal respiratory examination with mild pectus excavatum
2. S/P sternotomy, remote
3. Skin lesions: cherry angiomata, nevus

Table 7.2
Normal Breath Sounds Heard on Auscultation

Sound	Quality	Location
Bronchial	Loud, pitch high, dominant in expiration	Trachea, anterior
Bronchovesicular	Medium volume and pitch, heard equally in inspiration and expiration	Main bronchi, anterior and some interscapular
Vesicular	Soft to medium, pitch lower, dominant in inspiration	Over remainder of lung fields

EXTENDED EXAMINATION OF THE THORAX AND LUNGS

INDICATIONS

Indications are best subdivided into history and symptoms, physical findings, and laboratory abnormalities, most commonly those seen on the chest radiograph.

Symptoms and History

The most prominent symptoms of lung disease are *cough* and *dyspnea.* Barring a clear answer from another organ system or from a screening thoracic evaluation, these symptoms call for extended examination and a search for assessment of both etiology and functional consequences (severity). *Chest pain* commonly leads to cardiac evaluation as well as extended examination of the thorax, but the results are often disappointing. The same is true of a search by thoracic examination for the cause of *weight loss, failure to thrive, or hoarseness.* Although a cause often lies within the chest, lung cancer being the feared prototype, it is seldom discovered by physical examination. The same limitation applies to screening *heavy cigarette smokers* for cancer. Extended thoracic examination of smokers is warranted, however, because it provides information about chronic bronchitis, emphysema, and function.

The search for evidence of *occupational lung disease* by extended thoracic examination is undertaken for some persons at risk, such as fire fighters, smelters, silica workers, and miners.

Persons with an *established lung disease,* such as asthma, or *heart disease,* such as cardiomyopathy, also need regular and probing thoracic examinations.

A report by patient or spouse of *audible nocturnal wheezing* will also prompt further examination.

Physical Findings

The patient with the greatest probability of pneumonia is the febrile immunode-bilitated patient in hospital, whether with iatrogenic neutropenia or HIV disease. In such instances, the search for a source of fever includes careful thoracic examination.

Patients with unexpected pulmonary crackles, wheezes, or rubs also require thorough thoracic evaluation.

As to noncardiorespiratory disease, signs of *osteoporosis* such as localized spinous process tenderness will prompt extended thoracic examination, as will persistent unexplained *back pain*, particularly in a host with major risk factors, e.g., a thin woman of northern European ethnicity who is not a regular exerciser and has had early menopause. Anybody who has suffered *major trauma* to the chest, as from a motor vehicle crash, needs extended thoracic examination in search of musculoskeletal as well as cardiorespiratory injuries.

Laboratory Imaging Findings

The commonest investigation of the chest is the plain posteroanterior chest radiograph. Although evidence supporting the use of the test in *screening* is lacking, the practice is widespread. As a result, patients frequently have abnormalities identified—including trivial ones. Then they receive a careful thoracic examination! This technology-driven scattershot approach is condemned but prevalent.

CONDUCTING THE EXTENDED EXAMINATION
Respiratory Examination
BODY POSITION

Although the screening respiratory examination is conducted with the patient seated, reauscultation with the patient standing (Fig. 7.13) can increase diagnostic yield. In the obese or ascitic patient, the diaphragm may be displaced upward by abdominal contents in the seated position, with some gravitational descent on standing. Thus the standing examination might eliminate false-positive abnormal findings resulting from extrinsic compression of basal portions of the lung. It is not clear that standing adds diagnostic help in a patient who does not have abdominal distension. The weak patient can lean against a support without hampering upright lung examination. There are scant data on improving other examination modalities by specific body position, but visualization of abnormal diaphragmatic motion may be enhanced with the patient *upright.* In the patient lying on either side, some lung zones are compressed by body weight and become artifactually dull to percussion (Fig. 7.14).

Several features of general appearance are so characteristic of chest and respiratory problems that they are recounted here. Respiratory airflow mechanics are worst in the supine position. Thus the patient with obstructive airway disease will choose to sit up rather than lie flat. The patient with *advanced* obstructive disease tends to assume either of two positions that minimize discomfort and work of breathing. The first is the *seated position, with elbows on knees* and head in hands; skin calluses on the anterior thighs imply extreme chronicity and severity. The second, characteristic and grave, is the *professorial position* that resembles a speaker at a lectern. Whether seated or standing, the patient leans forward, bracing the trunk with arms and hands so that arms and trunk form a tripod.

Sometimes the neck is slightly hyperextended, and the lips may be pursed in expiration. The patient with extraordinary emphysema can end life on all fours,

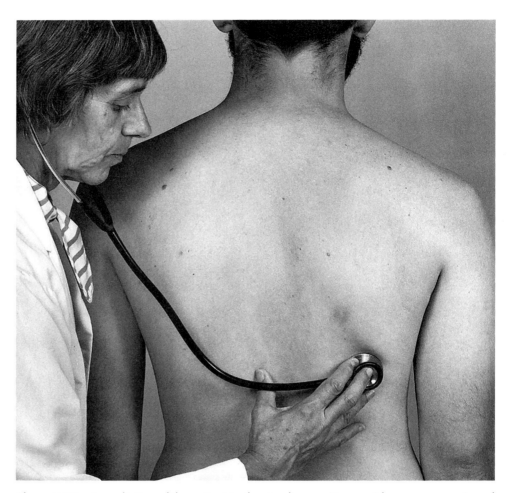

Figure 7.13 Auscultation of the patient in the standing position avoids any compression of diaphragm and thorax by abdominal contents. This is a major consideration in the obese. Patient's arms need not be crossed anteriorly.

seeking relief from dyspnea. Looking for such features constitutes part of the extended thoracic examination and helps distinguish obstructive from restrictive lung disease (see Interpreting the Findings, below).

ACCESSORY MUSCLES

The accessory muscles do not contribute visibly to either inspiration or expiration in the normal host. With labored breathing, they may be called into use for either phase or both phases. In adults, the commonest recognizable extra effort is by tight strap muscles (sternomastoids) in inspiration, with global thoracoabdominal expulsive expiration. Exaggerated inspiratory intercostal muscle retraction is only occasionally prominent in adults, and the diagnosis of respiratory distress does not depend on observing accessory muscle use. More often this is an ancillary sign.

COORDINATION, DEPTH, AND SYNCHRONIZATION OF BREATHING

Look to see if chest movements are symmetric. This is best done by looking up from the foot of the bed or with a tangential look down onto the upper anterior chest from behind, while the patient takes a deep breath. Clearly, the chest should not rise on one side (nor in one zone) in inspiration while falling in another.

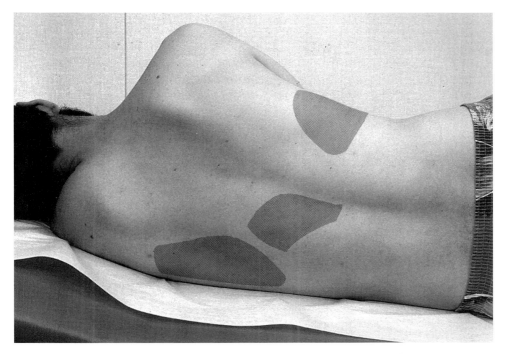

Figure 7.14 Special zones of percussive dullness appear as a gravitational and/or compressive artifact in the lateral decubitus position and are indicated by *hatched zones* overlying the photograph.

Note whether abdomen and thorax work together appropriately. Expect the abdomen to protrude when the diaphragm descends and the chest expands during inspiration. Likewise, the abdomen should retract as expiration proceeds. When in doubt, multiple respiratory cycles are observed. Dyssynergy that occurs only intermittently is ignored. Unduly deep breathing is discussed in Chapter 2.

Look also for the points in lung inflation from which inspiration and expiration begin. Two vivid patterns are: *"off-the-top" breathing,* in which inspiration begins without much preceding chest deflation, and *shallow panting breaths* taken from a midposition that is neither full chest inflation nor full deflation.

Use a tape measure to check chest circumferences at full inspiration and full expiration, then subtract the latter to quantify chest expansion.

PALPATION FOR SUBCUTANEOUS EMPHYSEMA

Air escaping from airways or lungs can dissect through the chest wall, root of the neck, and subcutis and then produce mobile soft bumps that "squish" distinctively. Subcutaneous emphysema under the hand feels like popping plastic "bubble wrap" but is more delicate. The sign is sought about the jugular notch, manubrium, clavicles, and supraclavicular fossae, because they are close to airways and pulmonary parenchyma, or in the vicinity of a possible air leak, e.g., about a site of recent chest tube insertion or removal. Subcutaneous emphysema tends to migrate up into the loose skin and subcutis of the face, head, and neck.

PALPATION FOR TACTILE VOCAL FREMITUS

Fremitus is the palpable vibration of the chest wall transmitted from the phonating larynx. Intensity of fremitus tends to parallel breath sound intensity. Yet the method is not redundant with respect to auscultation, since the vibratory frequencies best appreciated by palpation are lower than those best appreciated with the stethoscope and since the vibratory source in one case is respiration and in the other is phonation. Thus findings with the two modalities may differ. Tactile vocal fremitus is sometimes the more sensitive test.

Detection of vibration is greatest when the joints are used as sensors. The side of the hand (Fig. 7.15A) or the DIPs or metacarpophalangeal joints (Fig. 7.15B) are used. These joints are apposed to a portion of chest wall, and the patient repeatedly vocalizes a stock phrase, "ninety-nine." Normally, moderate vibration is palpable unless the chest wall is very thick. Symmetric points on the two hemithoraces are compared (Fig. 7.15A). Sequential assessment is preferred over simultaneous bimanual assessment (Fig. 7.15C) by some examiners. The intensity of tactile vocal fremitus varies considerably from front (stronger) to back and from apex (stronger) to lung base in normal persons. Thus the key comparison is between symmetric points. Abnormalities can lead to an increase *or* a decrease in intensity, so the examiner cannot assume, for example, that the more intensely vibrating side is the abnormal one.

PERCUSSION: REPETITION FOR GRAVITATIONAL REDISTRIBUTION

If pleural effusion is suspected, the examiner can further assess the subjacent lung by repeating conventional percussion and auscultation after having the patient lie with the apparently fluid-filled zone uppermost for a period of 20 minutes. In this position, *free-flowing (nonloculated)* pleural effusion settles gravitationally away from the zone in question. If the patient remains in this position during reexamination, the lungs are more amenable to assessment by percussion, tactile vocal fremitus, and auscultation. If the fluid has caused *compressive atelectasis* nearby, however, the findings there may not be normalized. If local *pleuropulmonary* disease is the cause of the fluid accumulation, the findings may remain highly abnormal.

PERCUSSION OF THE APEX

It is sometimes not feasible to place a conventional pleximeter in the supraclavicular fossa. Therefore, to percuss the pulmonary apex (Krönig's isthmus) the examiner faces the patient, rests the left hand at the root of the neck in the posture of touching a friend while speaking, and drops the left thumb into the patient's right supraclavicular fossa to serve as pleximeter. The usual plexor strikes the ulnar side of the thumb's interphalangeal joint from above. For the left fossa, the examiner's hand curls around the back and left side of the patient's neck, in intimate-conversation style, so that the tip of the left middle finger falls into the supraclavicular fossa and becomes the pleximeter, with the radial side of its DIP joint being struck by the conventional plexor.

PERCUSSION LATERAL TO SCAPULAE

Scapulae can dull the percussion note. Therefore, thorough chest examination requires percussion lateral to them, particularly lateral to their lower portions. Since the scapulae are mobile, they can be brought out of the field by having the patient elevate and protract the arms (reach forward). Both percussion and auscultation can be redirected to the newly uncovered zones.

AUSCULTATORY PERCUSSION

The sound-impedance characteristics of normal and diseased lung, pleura, and chest wall affect sound vibrations generated at one point and received at

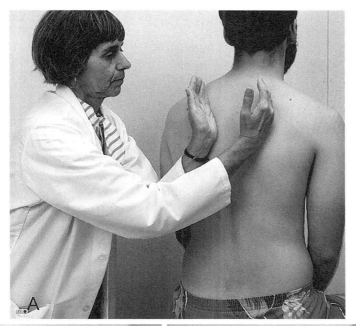

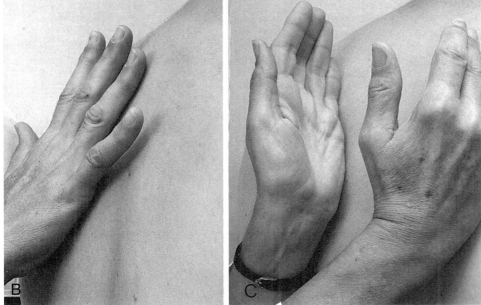

Figure 7.15   Fremitus is best assessed by comparing side-to-side at a given level. **A.** This examiner uses the sides of both hands. **B.** This technique, better still, employs the metacarpophalangeal joints and sequential testing. **C.** Here the sides are checked simultaneously. Any combination of sensor and timing can be productive *except* use of fingertips, which are poor vibratory sensors.

another. Repetitively tap lightly on the manubrium sterni with the plexor alone, without a pleximeter. Each time assess the sound transmitted through the chest and lung to the diaphragm of the stethoscope, which is held at symmetric points along each hemithorax posteriorly. As with tactile vocal fremitus, significance is attached to *asymmetry* of sound transmission rather than to change from one craniocaudad level to another. Each blow struck on the manubrium *must* have equal force, or false-positive results may be produced. Because the whole depth of the lung lies between sound source and receiver, this modality might be superior to conventional percussion in detection of deep lung lesions, inasmuch as conventional percussion only assesses the most superficial 5 cm of lung and chest wall combined. Most work on this modality has arisen from a single investigator. Supporting controlled scientific experiments and clinical data show impressive sensitivity of this modality, but further correlation is urgently needed.

VARIATIONS OF UNIFORM SOUND GENERATION

Pectoriloquy refers to clear audition of spoken or whispered speech through the stethoscope applied to the chest. The normal lung filters speech sounds made by the larynx so that they are muffled when auscultated through the stethoscope. Consolidated lung, however, loses its filter function. If the patient whispers, "sixty-six whiskies, please," the stethoscope applied to the chest transmits comprehensible speech over an area of pathology associated with loss of air in the alveoli. Normal muffling is demonstrated by auscultating the chest of a healthy colleague. Well-transmitted whispered sounds, by contrast, are heard with the stethoscope over the trachea, as the sound is unattenuated by lung.

   Egophony is a variant in which, through the stethoscope, a spoken "ee" sounds more like "ay." To elicit this sign, ask the patient to "say 'ee' each time I touch you with the stethoscope," and then survey areas in question, using the diaphragm pressed firmly to the chest.

AUSCULTATION WITH MEASUREMENT OF FORCED EXPIRATORY TIME

Auscultation with measurement of forced expiratory time is a technique that assesses adequacy of expiratory airflow. It is the only test for chronic obstructive lung disease that does not depend on lung overinflation. The patient is told, "When I say so, please take a big slow breath in and hold it a second. When my finger drops, push every bit of air out of your open mouth, as fast and as hard and as completely as you can." A demonstration is useful. The examiner auscultates over the trachea anteriorly or over the posterior projection of the trachea (observing chest motion is not accurate enough) and drops the finger, timing with the watch until the last expiratory noise ceases (Fig. 7.16).

AUSCULTATION OF FORCED EXPIRATION TO PRODUCE WHEEZING

With any extra-deep breath, the examiner may provoke wheezes that were not heard during auscultation during ordinary tidal breathing. To accomplish this, say to the patient, "Please breathe in and out through your mouth, extra deeply and extra fast." This quickly tires patients, so it should be performed for a few breaths only.

REMINDING AND REINFORCING THE PATIENT DURING AUSCULTATION

Many persons seem to have difficulty following directions for lung auscultation. Most commonly, they stop breathing through the mouth, or exaggerate depth of breathing, or stop after inspiration and await a signal to exhale. Sometimes, failure to follow directions is recognized when breath sounds grow faint or inaudible despite normal chest movement; at other times it is missed, and diagnostic sound is not discovered. The remedy is to repeat the instructions and to demonstrate steady open-mouth breathing. For the patient who still can't get it right, say, "I need to hear many breaths. Each time my stethoscope touches a new place, please begin a new breath in. It's important to take each of these breaths through

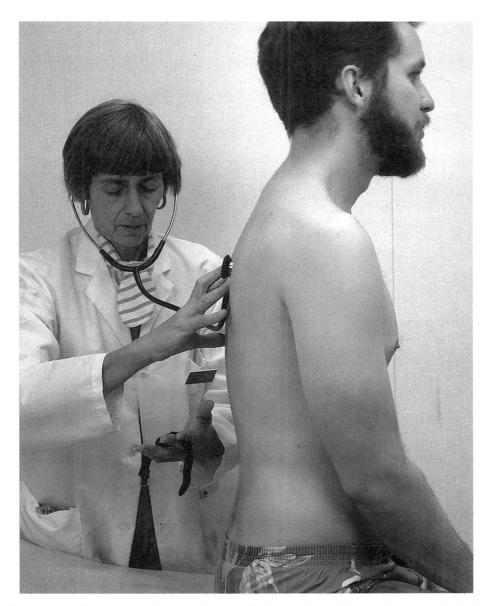

Figure 7.16 The patient is instructed to breathe in deeply and slowly, then to push all air out quickly. Timing of full exhalation is measured with a stopwatch. This sign has predictive value, while production of wheezes with forced expiration does not.

your mouth, with your mouth wide open. Don't breathe deeper than normal unless I tell you to, and don't hold your breath—let each breath out as usual, but through your mouth."

POST-TUSSIVE AUSCULTATION AND POST-DEEP-BREATHING REAUSCULTATION AND REPOSITIONING

Many abnormal lung sounds relate to transient medium-sized airway closure from atelectasis or secretions. These findings can be distinguished, in part, by reauscultating an abnormal area after having the patient take two deep breaths or coughs. Difficulty with directions comes into play, so say, "Now stop coughing—

just take a regular breath when the stethoscope touches your chest ... and please breathe with your mouth wide open." Auscultation can also be repeated after a period with the patient in a body position designed to move a free-flowing pleural effusion out of the field.

Nonrespiratory Components

PALPATION

Firm pressure over a bone or cartilage can demonstrate tenderness or fracture. Pressure is not applied abruptly, lest false-positives be increased. **Springing a rib** consists of pressing hard against it, some 6 cm from a suspected fracture. The temporary deformation of the flexible bone reproduces pain *not* at the site of pressure but at the discontinuity in osseous cortex. As a screening test for rib fracture in the patient with trauma or chest pain, a tight fist is pressed, using the dorsa of all proximal phalanges jointly, against the lateral chest wall. This broad flat surface avoids the point pressure of knuckles or proximal interphalangeal joints. In seeking *costochondritis,* a single fingertip is pressed firmly against each costochondral junction, 2 cm lateral to each sternal border.

HOOKING RIB MANEUVER

In **slipping rib syndrome,** chest pain is reproduced by the hooking rib maneuver. With the patient supine, the lower anterior rib cage is grasped firmly with one or both hands and drawn upward, i.e., anteriorly. A mild ache is not a positive test. Rather, the patient must exclaim that the maneuver has precisely replicated the character of his pain if not its severity.

INTERPRETING THE FINDINGS

Respiratory Examination

OBSTRUCTIVE VERSUS RESTRICTIVE PATTERNS

Two principal sources of disordered respiratory physiology are *restrictive* and *obstructive* disease. **Restrictive lung disease** encompasses parenchymal loss and disordered gas exchange at the alveolar level. **Obstructive airway disease** involves inappropriately slow airflow, especially in expiration, between terminal bronchioles and atmosphere. Often the two processes coexist. Although much obstructive disease is fixed, *asthma* is a prototype of **reversible** obstruction.

GENERAL INSPECTION

Some general appearance pertinent to respiratory function is described above. The *use of accessory muscles* in an adult bespeaks trouble. Obstructive disease produces this finding earlier than restrictive disease, but the common denominator of air hunger can bring it about with either. In general, use of accessory muscles in both inspiration and expiration portends worse than does one-phase use.

Barrel chest as an indicator of lung hyperinflation has been discredited. The same finding occurs, independent of respiratory status, with osteopenic anterior thoracic vertebral compression fractures and in some normal aged persons.

Cyanosis—blue discoloration of lips and skin—can be a feature of severe lung disease. It is discussed fully in the Extended Examination section of Chapter 10. *Clubbing,* another important but nonspecific sign of respiratory disease, is described in the Extended Examination section of Chapter 3.

When *hyperpnea* is observed and the context suggests hyperventilation, ask the patient to breathe into a paper bag held over his mouth and nose. Rebreathing will interrupt the hyperventilation cycle. However, if in doubt about pulmonary status, check oxygenation by laboratory methods or obtain consultation, since rebreathing is contraindicated with hypoxemia.

BODY POSITION AND SKIN SIGNS

The *professorial position* is a sign of advanced obstructive airway disease, typically end-stage emphysema. Other positions maintained to ease the breathing include *seated sleep* rather than reclining sleep; sitting with the trunk leaned forward, elbows on knees and head in hands; and, in the extreme, on hands and knees. The *head-on-hands-on-knees position* produces erythema of the apposed surfaces and sometimes calluses (hyperkeratotic skin from chronic minor trauma). Symmetric *calluses* or hyperpigmented patches (Dahl's sign) on the anterior thigh just above the knee underscore severity. *Pursed lips* also suggest expiratory difficulty.

BREATHING PATTERNS AND MOVEMENTS

The off-the-top breathing pattern is seen in obstructive small-airway disease including asthma and emphysema. Panting from midposition is described in pulmonary edema.

With *asymmetric movement* of the two hemithoraces, the side with decreased movement is the abnormal one. If *both* sides are diseased, the one with less movement is more abnormal. Women have more thoracic breathing movement than men, in whom abdominal motion sometimes predominates. Symmetric, clear-cut decrease in chest expansion compared with the normal range of chest expansion for gender suggests disease of the chest wall, pleura, or lung. Ankylosing spondylitis is cited as a cause of chest expansion of less than 5 cm, especially in a young man with longstanding back pain and the absence of other lung signs. However, the specificity of the sign is unknown.

In assessing extent of movement, recall that *absence of abdominal movement* occurs with any marked abdominal distension or peritoneal pain. *Completely abdominal respiratory movement,* without visible thoracic movement, is seen in lung or chest wall disease and particularly with severe pleuritic pain, e.g., from multiple rib fractures.

Even if the relative proportions of respiratory movement of abdomen and chest seem normal, *poor coordination* of the two is both a sign of disease and an exacerbating factor. *Abdominothoracic dyssynchrony (or dyssynergy)* consists of *abdominal wall retraction during inspiration.* The pathophysiology begins with a weak or paralyzed hemidiaphragm, whether from unilateral phrenic nerve palsy, from muscle disease, or from overwork in severe respiratory disease. This muscle fails to contract properly on inspiration, so that the diaphragm is drawn upward by the intercostal muscle contraction that is doing the work of inspiration, namely, reducing intrapleural pressure. The upward movement of the diaphragm causes the abdominal wall to sink with inspiration, a striking deviation from normal. This pattern has been called *respiratory paradox* by strained analogy with pulsus paradoxus. The sign is a grave (but seldom isolated) harbinger of impending respiratory failure.

Respiratory alternans consists of a few normal breaths followed by a few with the paradoxical dyssynergy described above, reflecting *temporary* exhaustion of the diaphragm. It is considered less grave than sustained respiratory paradox. On occasion, these two signs are best seen with the patient upright rather than supine.

INSPECTION IN THE DRUG ADDICT

As intravenous drug abuse destroys veins, addicts become progressively more desperate for vascular access. Some hire an accomplice to inject the junction of the subclavian vein and the jugular, via a supraclavicular approach. Predictably, pneumothorax, hemothorax, and infection commonly result. Thus if needle punctures are observed in the supraclavicular fossa of a patient with thoracic problems, this disease mechanism should be considered.

SUBCUTANEOUS EMPHYSEMA

Subcutaneous emphysema is distinguished from edema by its softness and failure to "pit," i.e., to retain a relatively crisp-edged indentation made with the examining finger. Unlike inflammatory edema, subcutaneous emphysema does not redden the skin. The usual cause in the chest is air leakage, e.g., pneumothorax with dissection of air out of the pleural space and into the subcutis. Auscultation of the occasional "mediastinal crunch" heard with pneumomediastinum, evaluation for pneumothorax, and inspection of the mechanical ventilator if the patient is on one—as is quite often the case—are productive follow-up examinations.

In the face, fracture of any air sinus provides another mechanism.

Rarely, subcutaneous emphysema *and* inflammatory signs coexist when the cause is infection with a gas-forming bacterium. Such patients are acutely ill and usually toxic. Retained air in the superficial layers of a chest wound is a separate differential that is obvious from context.

TACTILE VOCAL FREMITUS

The wide range of normal for fremitus depends largely on habitus and muscular development. In the very obese, vibrations cannot be felt simply because the chest wall dampens their transmission. In the cachectic, every nuance of spoken sound seems to reach the palpating fingers.

Generally, decreased fremitus is found with barriers to transmission of sound waves. Intrapleural fluid or air provides a particularly strong barrier. Pleural scarring has the same general effect. By contrast, consolidation of the lung *augments* transmission, so that the classical feature of a well-developed pneumonia is increased tactile vocal fremitus along with its acoustic counterpart, bronchial breath sounds. If bronchial obstruction or pleural effusion supervenes, fremitus and breath sound intensity decrease and may be obliterated.

LOUD SOUNDS ON PERCUSSION

Hyperresonance on percussion is common in pulmonary hyperinflation, both in asthmatics and in patients with chronic obstructive pulmonary disease with or without bullae. *Tympany* is not encountered in the chest unless a significant air pocket, i.e., a large bulla or a large pneumothorax, is separated from the pleximeter by only a thin chest wall.

REDUCED SOUNDS ON PERCUSSION

Dullness on percussion is produced by pulmonary disease or a thick chest wall. Sometimes the entire (normal) posterior chest is dull in weight lifters and obese persons. The axillae and anterior chest usually remain evaluable in such cases. *Localized dullness* is a hallmark of *consolidation* of the lung, as from pneumonia or pulmonary edema. *Flatness,* the sound made by percussing the thigh, implies absence of contained air within the zone, usually from *pleural effusion* or thick *pleural scarring;* consolidated lung tends not to become flat, because some air remains in it, unless its airway becomes obstructed.

PERCUSSION WITH NO DIAPHRAGMATIC MOVEMENT

Dullness and then flatness are normally encountered at the inferior borders of the lungs. The transition from resonance to dullness is expected to descend with the diaphragm on deep inspiration. When no such descent occurs, the examiner should suspect hemidiaphragmatic paralysis from *phrenic nerve palsy.* This sign is sought with mediastinal masses and in lung cancer, where it represents a major complication having therapeutic and prognostic implications. In the patient whose whole posterior chest is dull, the sign is impossible to elicit. The examiner must then rely on observed hemithoracic asymmetry of inspiratory movement. Large pleural effusions can also hamper this assessment.

AUSCOPERCUSSION

Asymmetry of sound transmission determined by auscopercussion does not permit etiologic diagnosis. Solid matter, such as tumor or granuloma, or alveolar fluid infiltrate with or without cellularity alters auscopercussive transmission.

AUSCULTATION WITHOUT THE STETHOSCOPE

When wheezes are heard before the stethoscope is put in the ears, they must be loud. If they are not then encountered by stethoscopy and the patient is not holding his breath, the following explanations apply in descending likelihood:

1. The stethoscope is not working properly, usually because its "silent" head has been applied to the patient's chest.
2. The listener is distracted.
3. Airflow is so reduced that no air exchange or wheezing is audible.
4. A sudden marked improvement has terminated the wheezes, e.g., expulsion of a large mucus plug.

PROLONGED EXPIRATION ON AUSCULTATION

Prolonged expiration noted on auscultation demonstrates diminished expiratory function. The responsible airway obstruction may include any combination of mucus plugging, bronchial smooth-muscle spasm, and inflammatory alteration of physical properties of the airways. In addition, in emphysema (and to a lesser degree in old age) the elastic recoil of the lung is reduced. Prolongation of the expiratory phase may be noted during ordinary auscultation or may be quantified by measurement of forced expiratory time. The latter is a convenient serial measurement to assess disease progression or benefit from bronchodilators. Forced expiratory time exceeding 6 seconds indicates considerable obstructive airway disease.

The usual causes of airway obstruction—asthma and chronic obstructive pulmonary disease—produce multifocal abnormalities. However, *localized* wheezing or prolongation of expiration suggests (*a*) a mucus plug, (*b*) an inhaled foreign body (uncommon in adults), or (*c*) bronchial neoplasm.

REDUCED BREATH SOUNDS

A thick chest wall can attenuate breath sounds. When airflow is reduced, breath sounds are correspondingly faint or even inaudible. This can occur globally with severe emphysema or locally over consolidated lung with an obstructed bronchus. Interposition of air or fluid in the pleural space provides a potent vibratory muffler, so that in pleural effusion and pneumothorax both fremitus and breath-sound intensity are sharply reduced.

INCREASED AND BRONCHIAL BREATH SOUNDS

On auscultation, bronchial breath sounds are normally heard over the largest airways. Elsewhere, they indicate enhancement of the sound-transmitting properties of the lung between the airway of origin and the auscultatory site on the chest wall.

That is, alveolar air spaces contain less air and are *consolidated.* Alveoli may be collapsed (atelectatic), but they more commonly contain fluid (pulmonary edema) or inflammation (pneumonia). Any process that replaces sufficient air in the alveoli can produce this finding, including scarring, granulomata, and neoplasia.

CRACKLES

Crackles are the most commonly recognized pulmonary auscultatory abnormality. They are short discontinuous explosive sounds heard in inspiration. Crackles reflect the sudden popping-open of small airways that were previously closed. Sparse basilar crackles are present in a few normal persons, particularly among the aged. However, crackles in a patient who did not have them before, or who has them in new locations, are abnormal. You may be able to produce a few crackles in a normal colleague on the first inspiration after a very deep, slow, complete expiration. Very deep exhalation probably produces crackles by creating some temporary regional airway closure. Atelectasis, fibrosis, inflammation, pulmonary edema, granuloma, bronchospasm, emphysema, and tumor can all do the same.

One erroneous teaching deserves mention only because the reader will encounter it, namely, that crackles arise from air bubbling through fluid. This is wrong. Crackles arising from airways shut by pulmonary edema ("wet rales") cannot be distinguished from those reflecting other causes ("dry rales"): The putative distinction is based on presumptions about etiology, not on acoustic characteristics. Nor are there any differences between crackles, rales, and crepitations.

There are two subcategorizations of crackles. The first addresses abundance and intensity, i.e., fine, medium, or coarse. However, no specific diagnosis can be made from crackle type.

The second distinguishes between **early inspiratory crackles** and so-called **late inspiratory crackles.** The latter are far more common. They begin at any point in inspiration and *extend into the second half of inspiration.* They are seen in various kinds of lung disease. By contrast, **early inspiratory crackles do not extend into the second half of inspiration** or barely do so. Early inspiratory crackles are associated with severe obstructive airway disease. Because of these counterintuitive definitions, the patient with paninspiratory crackles may have only so-called "late" crackles from restrictive disease or a mixture of both late ones and the early crackles of concomitant obstructive disease!

Profuse crackles are generally accorded more weight than scant ones, but there is no cutoff. Crackles that disappear post-tussively, or after a deep breath or two, are usually considered insignificant and perhaps as arising from gravitational or dependent nonpathologic small-airway closure. Thus a first step in the workup of crackles must be to check if they can be abated with a few breaths (i.e., a few cycles of listening) or a cough or two.

WHEEZES

Wheezes noted on auscultation indicate markedly reduced airflow. They are high-pitched, continuous vibrations of the air column and/or airway wall, usually detected at multiple sites simultaneously. They have a musical quality and are continuous, in contradistinction to crackles. Wheezing inevitably is expiratory. Sometimes, inspiratory wheezes are also heard, but never inspiratory wheezes alone. When continuous expiratory sounds are heard that are low pitched and not musical, they are labeled rhonchi. In older terminology, wheezes were called sibilant rhonchi, and rhonchi were called sonorous rhonchi. Rhonchi are believed to be more common with transient mucus plugging and poor movement of airway secretions, whereas the classical setting for wheezes is bronchospasm.

Some wheezes are audible to the patient or any nearby person without a stethoscope. Sometimes, the patient will be confused when the doctor tells him he has wheezes, although he can no longer hear them with his unaided ear.

When wheezing disappears on serial auscultation, one of two scenarios may apply. Therapy may have relieved airway obstruction. In this case, dyspnea will be less, respiratory rate will fall, wheezing will be gone, and breath sounds will be easier to hear both over the lungs and over the large airways, reflecting improved air exchange. In the opposite setting, air movement has become so impaired that wheezing is lost because of reduced flow. Such a patient will have more dyspnea, usually stays quite still, and may have poor skin color. The examiner will hear neither wheezes nor much in the way of breath sounds. Loss of wheezes in this setting is *not* reassuring! This patient is desperately ill.

Most wheezing is widespread, although intensity and pitch may vary from site to site. Sharply localized wheezing has the significance of localized airway obstruction delineated above. In adults, localized wheezing has long been considered a sign of lung cancer, although neither a sensitive nor specific sign.

Interpretation of localized wheezing is different when *wheezing is audible only over the trachea.* This can occur in ordinary asthma, perhaps related to propagation of sound in the direction of airflow. The practical considerations are

1. Don't look for tracheal obstruction based solely on this finding.
2. In the asthmatic without wheezes on chest auscultation, auscultate at the trachea also. It may be the first site at which wheezes appear or the last to lose them.

PLEURAL RUBS

Pleural rubs are noises that occur in both inspiration and expiration. They sound like two leather surfaces creaking over one another. They are heard with inflammation of the pleura and usually disappear if substantial pleural effusion accumulates. Pleural rubs are sought in relation to pleuritis and pulmonary infarction. Four caveats apply:

1. At and just below the scapular tip, a sound is heard in some normal persons that closely mimics a pleural rub. If a rub is heard here and at the symmetric point opposite, be wary.
2. Pulmonary embolism per se does not produce a rub. Rather, this sign indicates inflammation at the site of pulmonary *infarction,* a complication that afflicts only a minority of patients with pulmonary emboli. Thus the rub is not a sensitive indicator, and its absence does not exclude embolization.
3. Rubs are not specific for pulmonary infarction. They are also found with viral and immune pleuritides, with pneumonias that reach the pleural surface, with pleural metastases of carcinoma, and occasionally with chest tubes.
4. Sometimes, it is difficult to know if a rub near the precordium is pleural or pericardial. Have the patient hold his breath for a few seconds. A rub that persists without respiratory movement must be pericardial. Sound that disappears during apnea and reappears on rebreathing must be pleural.

FORCED WHEEZING

Some literature states that wheezes produced by forced expiration (forced expiratory wheezing) indicate airway obstruction. There is, however, poor correlation between this phenomenon and a standard measure of pharmacologically provokable bronchoconstriction in the laboratory.

MEANING OF EGOPHONY AND WHISPERED PECTORILOQUY

Egophony is common at the top of pleural effusion, perhaps relating to compression of adjacent pulmonary parenchyma. Thin persons may have egophony over the entire area of an effusion. The finding is also present over consolidated lung when the bronchus to the segment is patent. Egophony may be among the most sensitive signs for consolidation. Some but not all pulmonary fibrosis produces egophony.

Whispered pectoriloquy indicates pulmonary consolidation. It is recognized if whispered words form comprehensible phonemes through the stethoscope placed on the chest wall.

Nonrespiratory Examination
SCOLIOSIS

Scoliosis implies inequality in vertebral height or strength of paraspinal musculature. When scoliosis is marked, there may be compression of lung and the production of restrictive respiratory disease despite intrinsically normal lungs. The convex side of the spine is likely to produce pulmonary compression, especially basally and medially, and so crackles are frequently present in this zone as a result of regional atelectasis from external pressure.

BONY TENDERNESS IN THE THORAX

If the examiner *pounds on the spine,* excess false-positives are produced. Consistent gentle punches with the hypothenar eminence of the fist or *taps* with the reflex hammer are preferable. For the jumpy patient who gives a positive tenderness response that the examiner suspects is false, a second pass is made after asking, "Are there one or two spots that hurt *much* more when tapped?" Tenderness from paravertebral structures can produce false-positives, e.g., a trigger point in fibrositis that overlies paraspinal muscle. False-negative tests with metabolic bone disease are common except when complicated by fracture. Spinal tenderness can arise from any inflammatory disorder, from cancer, from fractures, and from other processes.

Tender ribs carry a similar differential diagnosis, with costochondritis added to the possibilities. Although anterior chest wall tenderness is sometimes adduced as evidence against coronary disease in a case of chest pain, such tenderness does *not* reduce the likelihood of myocardial ischemia.

A *positive springing test* of the rib consists of localized, usually severe pain at a distance from the sites compressed by the examiner's knuckles. It is diagnostic of rib fracture.

CVA tenderness is most familiar in pyelonephritis. Positive tests may occur, however, in tense persons, with perinephric inflammation, in some musculoskeletal strains and inflammations of the midback, or when a pounding fist rather than a single probing finger is used as a stimulus.

Patterns of Physical Findings

Several patterns of respiratory physical findings are highly characteristic and very useful diagnostically (Table 7.3).

PNEUMONIA

The classic pneumonias of the past century consolidated whole lobes. Similar cases are seen only occasionally today. A *consolidated lobe* with a patent bronchus typically produces an increased respiratory rate, diminished visible and palpable movement of the affected hemithorax, increased tactile vocal fremitus, dullness to percussion, egophony and perhaps whispered pectoriloquy, bronchial breath sounds, and profuse late inspiratory crackles over the auscultatory areas corresponding to the involved lobe. Stasis of secretions may lead to rhonchi; if an asso-

Table 7.3
Patterns of Abnormal Lung Findings

Disorder	Tracheal Deviation	Percussion Note	Breath Sounds	Crackles	Wheezes	Rhonchi	Egophony	Other
Pneumonia, lobar	Usually away, often none	Dull	Increased, tubular	Prominent	Rare	Variable	Variable	Fever common
Pneumonia, other	None (usually)	Often normal	Normal	Scant to absent	Absent	Usually absent	Rare	Fever common
Pneumonia with bronchial obstruction	Toward lesion	Flat to dull	Decreased to absent	Scant or none	Rare	Usually none	None	Fever common
Atelectasis	Toward, if any	Normal to dull	Normal or reduced	Scant or none	None	None	None	Fever sometimes
Pleural effusion	Away, if any	Flat to dull	Reduced or absent	Scant but variable	None	None	Usual	Chest wall may bulge
Pneumothorax	Away, if any	Hyperresonant or normal, rarely tympanic	Reduced or absent	None or few	None	None	Variable	Can be difficult diagnosis
Pulmonary embolism	None	Normal to dull	Normal	Usually none	Rarely prominent	None	None	Fever sometimes, difficult to diagnose
Pulmonary edema	None	Normal to dull	Normal	Prominent	Variable (cardiac asthma)	Variable	None usually	Features of heart failure
Asthma	None	Tympanic to normal	Reduced or absent	Rare	Prominent	Variable	None	Paradoxus
COPD[a]	None	Hyperresonant to normal	Reduced	Variable, often early inspiratory if present	Common	Usual	None	Paradoxus

[a]COPD, chronic obstructive pulmonary disease.

ciated acute bronchitis provokes local airway spasm, there will be localized wheezes. If the pleura is affected, a rub may develop and, later, signs of pleural effusion. Tracheal deviation is away from the side of consolidation.

If the bronchus leading to a pneumonic lobe or segment is obstructed, either by a neoplasm with a *postobstructive pneumonia* or by inspissated inflammation and mucus, the following signs change from those of the previous paragraph: Respiratory movement of the zone decreases further, tactile vocal fremitus is markedly decreased, dullness may become flatness, egophony and whispered pectoriloquy are lost, breath sounds become faint, and crackles diminish or disappear. Tracheal deviation may be lost as an atelectatic component draws the airway back toward the midline.

When pneumonia produces lesser pulmonary infiltration, physical signs are fewer and subtler. Tachypnea is almost always present, and crackles are common although not inevitable. Tracheal tenderness may be present especially in so-called atypical pneumonias. However, other signs mentioned above may be lacking.

ATELECTASIS

Atelectasis commonly produces fever, tachypnea, perhaps decreased respiratory motion, tracheal deviation toward the affected side, sometimes *decreased* fremitus, sometimes dullness, decreased or absent breath sounds, and a few crackles. The physical findings can be subtle, and *an apparently normal respiratory examination does not exclude atelectasis.*

PLEURAL EFFUSION

Small pleural effusions are notoriously difficult to detect by physical examination. Larger effusions produce decreased movement of the hemithorax, absent tactile vocal fremitus, percussive flatness, egophony at the upper edge of the effusion, absent or attenuated breath sounds, and, occasionally, bulging of the chest wall. Sometimes there are crackles just above the effusion, from secondary compressive atelectasis. When tracheal deviation occurs, it is away from the side of the effusion.

PNEUMOTHORAX

A small pneumothorax is as elusive as a small pleural effusion. Larger pneumothoraces can shift the trachea away and can produce localized hyperresonance or even tympany. Parallels between the effects of intrapleural air and pleural effusion include marked attenuation of palpable and audible respiratory and vocal vibrations. However, air rises in the pleural cavity, whereas fluid sinks, so the findings in lung above a pleural effusion have no parallels in pneumothorax. Depending on the source of the pneumothorax and whether there is a ball-valve effect or a tension pneumothorax, some patients are suddenly desperately dyspneic and hypotensive. Sometimes, subcutaneous emphysema may supervene.

PULMONARY EMBOLISM

Physical findings in pulmonary embolism are inconsistent, scant, and nonspecific. *A normal chest examination does not exclude even a large pulmonary embolism,* although severe cases usually show hypotension, tachycardia, and tachypnea.

Compensatory airspace deflation sometimes decreases ventilation-perfusion mismatching; when this happens, local findings of atelectasis can appear, i.e., crackles and dullness. Pulmonary embolism can precipitate bronchospasm, so that new wheezing in someone at risk for pulmonary embolism raises this differential. Pulmonary embolism *with infarction* can produce pleural rubs, dullness, and sometimes crackles. Occasionally, hemorrhagic pleural effusion supervenes, and in such cases the findings shift to flatness, absence of breath sounds, and loss of the rub.

A **phantom infarct** is hemorrhage without necrosis distal to the pulmonary artery branch obstructed by a pulmonary embolism. This may produce pneumonia-like rather than infarct-like pulmonary signs.

PULMONARY EDEMA

Pulmonary edema due to left-heart dysfunction produces a lesser degree of consolidation than does pneumonia, probably because the edema fluid is thinner. The first findings are bibasilar pulmonary crackles, which can progress up the chest. The topmost height of crackles may be asymmetric. Crackles may even be lacking on one side if emphysema has obliterated the potentially leaky pulmonary capillary bed on that side. Dullness is less prominent than in pneumonia and is variable.

Since right-sided pleural effusions or bilateral pleural effusions commonly complicate biventricular heart failure, findings related to these may coexist or supervene.

In the extreme case, the patient is hypotensive, cyanotic, gasping for breath, and foaming or spitting yellow, white, or pink-tinged frothy pulmonary edema fluid at the mouth.

The more proteinaceous noncardiogenic pulmonary edema fluid of adult respiratory distress syndrome (ARDS) tends to produce about as many crackles as, and perhaps more dullness than, cardiogenic pulmonary edema.

ASTHMA

In the patient with asthma, the findings relate to both air trapping and poor flow. Respiratory rate is often elevated, and the patient is apprehensive or even panicky as well as dyspneic. Deep breathing on command, for examination, is often difficult or impossible; attempts may lead to paroxysms of coughing or wheezing. Wheezing is frequently audible on entering the room, even before the examiner employs the stethoscope. Noisy breathing may be prominent. The patient may be in the professorial position and is almost certain to be seated rather than supine. If fatigued, the patient may compromise by lying with head and trunk raised 45° from the horizontal or even with the trunk bolt upright at 90°. Accessory muscles of respiration are often in use, and cyanosis may be recognized peripherally and centrally. Fremitus may be decreased but may be unassessable, since speech is whispery and exhausting in the midst of an attack. The percussion note is resonant to diffusely hyperresonant. Auscultation reveals faint breath sounds, widespread expiratory wheezes, and sometimes also inspiratory wheezes (see below). The wheezes are often polyphonic, and there are sometimes rhonchi also. Local wheezes that persist beyond end-expiration into the start of the next inspiration represent persistent outflow across stenoses, despite traction exerted by inspiration, and indicate severe obstruction.

Diffuse inspiratory as well as expiratory wheezes correspond to disordered inward airflow across very tight airways. Since airway caliber enlarges with inspiration, the addition of inspiratory wheezes to expiratory ones implies more severe narrowing than purely expiratory wheezing.

Crackles are less common. Attempts to observe the effect of deep breaths or coughs on the physical signs usually result in a paroxysm of coughing or wheezing and cannot be successfully completed. Forced expiratory time usually cannot be measured, since the maneuver precipitates bronchospasm. If measurable, it is prolonged, and a wheeze usually constitutes the final sound that this test reveals, long after the last conventional breath sound has disappeared.

Pulsus paradoxus, a key element in assessing these patients, is described in the Extended Examination section of Chapter 2.

CHRONIC OBSTRUCTIVE PULMONARY DISEASE (EMPHYSEMA AND CHRONIC BRONCHITIS)

In chronic obstructive pulmonary disease (emphysema and chronic bronchitis), many signs of asthma can be found, with variable severity and chronicity. In addition, early inspiratory crackles are sometimes present. Forced expiratory time is more easily measured and is always prolonged. In patients with large *bullae* from emphysema, areas with absent breath sounds and hyperresonance and even tympany are common. Chronic air trapping in emphysema attenuates transmitted respiratory, vocal, and cardiovascular vibration. In severe cases, the examiner hears no breath sounds or heart sounds at all. Abnormal right-heart findings are common in this setting and are described in the Extended Examination section of Chapter 8.

LUNG CANCER

Unfortunately, physical examination does not yield early diagnosis of lung cancer. Preliminary reports about auscopercussion are encouraging. Depending on the size and location of a lung cancer and complications such as malignant pleural effusion, almost every possible chest finding can be produced during the course of the disease.

RECORDING THE FINDINGS

Sample Write-up

29-year-old man with AIDS who has had a week of malaise, high fevers, dry cough, and progressive dyspnea. No prior respiratory symptoms. His only AIDS complications in the past have been oral Kaposi sarcoma and thrush, both treated successfully, and a depressed T-helper (CD4) lymphocyte count of 150/cu mm. He receives zidovudine and inhaled pentamidine prophylaxis against *Pneumocystis carinii* pneumonia and oral antimycotic agent, ?which.

Examination: Temperature 39.2°C, pulse 124 and regular, respirations 32/minute, slightly toxic look.

Chest symmetric in contour and movement. Fremitus symmetric, universally prominent (thin habitus). Percussion resonant except for a 4 × 4-cm area in left midaxilla, dull. Air exchange good, breath sounds vesicular where expected. A few late inspiratory crackles in same area. These diminish but do not disappear post-tussively or after three voluntary deep breaths. No crackles elsewhere. No wheezes or rhonchi. Krönig's isthmus normal by percussion and auscultation bilaterally.

Impression: Left upper lobe pneumonia involving the lingula.

BEYOND THE PHYSICAL EXAMINATION

In the chest more than in any other region, technology is called on frequently to aid in diagnosis. The advantages of **chest radiographs** are *high sensitivity* and *localizing value.* One disadvantage is encroachment on bedside clinical skills and clinical thinking, so that eventually these atrophy and the care of patients suffers. Humility about limitations of chest examination is essential for clinicians, but nihilism is counterproductive.

Radiography and Imaging

POSITIVE FILM, NEGATIVE EXAMINATION

When cough, fever, tachypnea, or other indicators point to the chest, but physical examination is negative, the answer lies sometimes in a chest radiograph. Among pneumonias notorious for this combination are *Mycoplasma, Legionella, Chlamydia,* and *Pneumocystis carinii.* The last can also produce hypoxemia with a normal chest radiograph, underscoring its elusiveness.

In screening for lung cancer, radiographs do not meet criteria of efficacy or cost-effectiveness. Nor have they been shown to be worthwhile in seeking the cause of fever in the granulocytopenic patient in hospital who has had a negative physical examination of the chest. Pneumothorax and pleural effusion sometimes are found radiographically even after an expert physical examination has been negative.

NEGATIVE FILM, POSITIVE EXAMINATION

Patients with a negative film but a positive examination for chest pathology would go undiagnosed if clinical examination of the chest were cursory or deleted. The commonest setting is *asthma,* where pulmonary hyperinflation is radiographically inconspicuous or unchanged during an acute attack. In early *bronchopneumonia,* radiographic evolution commonly lags 24–48 hours behind both symptoms and physical signs. The novice must not disbelieve the physical findings because "the x-ray was negative!" In *acute bronchitis,* wheezes and a few crackles are heard, and the patient is sick, but there is no radiographic abnormality. *Atelectasis* and early *bronchial stenosis*—classically from cancer—may also be missed on the chest film. *Foreign bodies* can lead to positive examination with a negative radiograph. *Chronic obstructive pulmonary disease* of mild degree is more clearly shown by percussion and auscultation than by chest radiograph. Acute complications in the patient whose chest x-ray is chronically abnormal are particularly likely to be unrecognized radiographically and to depend on new physical findings.

OTHER IMAGING

Lateral decubitus chest radiographs can "uncover" pulmonary parenchyma obscured by a (free-flowing) pleural effusion. *Apical lordotic* radiographs are especially good in evaluation of possible apical tuberculosis. *Computed tomography* and *magnetic resonance imaging* are applied frequently to the chest, as are *gallium scans.* *Ultrasound examinations* of lung are usually confined to real-time imaging of possible loculated pleural effusion during thoracentesis.

Functional Testing: Blood-Gas Analysis

Arterial blood-gas samples provide unique information about acid-base status. Since marked hypoxia does not always cause symptoms or tachypnea, measurement of blood oxygen can be valuable. Assessment of pCO_2 delineates whether compensatory hyperventilation is adequate. *Pulse oximetry* provides frequent, cheap, and noninvasive data that are reliable but do not provide information on CO_2 status or hydrogen ion balance. Bedside *spirometry* involves measurement of flow rates and is a splendid adjunct to the management of asthma.

In the patient with airflow limitation, spirometric measurements are repeated after administration of a bronchodilating agent to explore pharmacologic reversibility. Other *pulmonary function tests* assess volumes and carbon monoxide diffusion. The latter can be deranged without physical signs. *Bronchoprovocative tests* are performed when asthma is suspected but unconfirmed. They include administration of methacholine, followed by repeat spirometry and pulmonary function tests to seek a decrement in airflow.

Pulmonary Vascular Testing

Pulmonary embolism is often difficult to diagnose or exclude technologically as well as clinically. Pulmonary ventilation-perfusion scans use minute quantities of radioisotopes that are inhaled and injected intravenously. Mismatches of ventilation and perfusion are characteristic of emboli but fraught with interpretative problems. *Pulmonary angiography* is more expensive, invasive, and dangerous but is more accurate; there are perhaps 1% false-positive and false-negative results. The primitive state of pulmonary embolism diagnosis has led to use of *Doppler examination of leg veins* to establish the diagnosis backhandedly.

For determinations of pulmonary vascular pressures and for inference of left-heart pressures, *flow-directed pulmonary artery catheters* with manometers are used (*Swan-Ganz catheters*). These also measure right-heart pressures and serve diverse diagnostic and management needs, primarily in patients with heart disease or multiorgan failure but also in patients with respiratory disease and, especially, pulmonary hypertension. This extraordinary tool has not yet been demonstrated to improve outcome.

Infections

The most direct investigation is *study of the sputum. Gram's stain* and *culture* are usual. Smear and culture for mycobacteria (*acid-fast bacilli*) are also important, as are studies of sputum for *Pneumocystis carinii* by silver staining or by direct fluorescent antibody assay. In the patient at special risk, other studies are undertaken for fungi, cytomegalovirus, or other pathogens in sputum.

Skin testing for evidence of past exposure to mycobacteria (purified protein derivative or *PPD testing*) is important in workup for mycobacterioses but not specific for *Mycobacterium tuberculosis.*

Neoplasia

Histologic diagnosis is ideal, and cytologic diagnosis is acceptable. For histology, endobronchial biopsy, mediastinoscopic biopsy of lymph nodes, and open-lung biopsy are the chief methods. Major cytologic methods involve expectorated deep sputum, bronchoalveolar lavage, and bronchial brushings.

Other Tests

Progressively more invasive methods can secure diagnoses in obscure instances of infectious, immune, and neoplastic diseases of the chest. These include: bronchoscopy, with or without brushing and biopsy; bronchoalveolar lavage, in which fluid is injected down a bronchus from the bronchoscope and then reaspirated and spun to concentrate the recovered cells, which are then stained; transbronchial biopsy of peribronchial lung parenchyma; and thoracotomy with open-lung biopsy. Each method has advocates. The gentlest test having reasonable diagnostic success is chosen.

Pleural Fluid

Principal methods are decubitus radiographs as described above and thoracentesis with aspiration of intrapleural fluid for analysis and sometimes as therapy. The analysis typically includes studies for infection and neoplasia, as well as chemical studies. Cell counts and differential cell counts help distinguish transudate from exudate and may provide a specific etiologic diagnosis. Repeat chest radiography after pleural drainage is useful.

Nonrespiratory Thoracic Problems

Radiographs of the spine can show some kinds of lesions. *Plain films of the ribs* can help delineate fractures. *Radionuclide bone scans* have better sensitivity and specificity. Osteoporosis investigations such as *bone densitometry* are sometimes indicated, although the thoracic spine is not frequently studied.

Regarding renal disorders that may produce CVA tenderness, the key investigations are *urinalysis and culture* and imaging techniques ranging from *renal ultrasound,* to *nuclide blood flow scans,* to *abdominal computed tomography and magnetic resonance imaging,* to *excretory urography* (intravenous pyelography, or IVP), to *cystoscopy with retrograde cannulation of the ureters and retrograde pyelography.*

Consultants

A *chest physician* has special training and certification in *pulmonary medicine* and substantial secondary expertise in *cardiology.* Some cardiologists also develop a special interest in the lungs. The interdependence of the two systems is both anatomic and functional: Problems of the left heart tax the lungs, and many lung problems eventually damage the right side of the heart.

Thoracic surgeons frequently contribute. In selected cases, the medical oncologist or infectious diseases physician is brought in on a chest problem. The latter is sometimes needed to help untangle complex pulmonary issues in persons with AIDS.

For the thoracic skeleton, the orthopedic surgeon and osteoporosis expert can be helpful. When neural structures are involved or pain is intractable, the neurologist, neurosurgeon, or pain consultant, who is often an anesthesiologist, occupies center stage.

For renal disorders, the nephrologist and urologist can be vitally important.

RECOMMENDED READINGS

Baughman RP, Shipley RT, Loudon RG, Lower EE. Crackles in interstitial lung disease. Chest 1991;100:96–101.

Campbell EJM. Physical signs of diffuse airways obstruction and lung distension. Thorax 1969;24:1–3.

Carroll JL, Clayton JE, Lemen RG. The physiology and clinical usefulness of common pulmonary physical findings. Arizona Med 1983;40:408–414.

Forgacs P. Noisy breathing. Chest 1973;63(suppl):38S–41S.

Guarino JR. Auscultatory percussion of the chest. Lancet 1980;1:1332–1334.

Loudon R, Murphy RLH Jr. Lung sounds. Am Rev Respir Dis 1984;130:663–673.

Mulrow CD, Dolmatch BL, Delong ER, et al. Observer variability in the pulmonary examination. J Gen Intern Med 1986;1:364–367.

Murphy RLH Jr, Holford SK, Knowler WC. Visual lung-sound characterization by time-expanded wave-form analysis. N Engl J Med 1977;296:968–971.

Nath AR, Capel LH. Inspiratory crackles—early and late. Thorax 1974;29:223–227.

Parrino TA. The art and science of percussion. Hosp Pract 1987;22(9A):25–36.

8

Heart and Great Vessels

SCREENING EXAMINATION OF THE HEART AND GREAT VESSELS

APPROACH AND ANATOMICAL REVIEW

The heart and its great vessels, the inferior and superior venae cavae, aorta, and pulmonary veins and arteries, lie about the thoracic midline surrounded laterally and posteriorly by the two lungs and bounded anteriorly by the sternum and central rib cage. The esophagus, traversing the thorax from the neck to the abdominal cavity, lies between the midline vascular structures and the anterior surfaces of the vertebral bodies (Fig. 8.1). The vascular structures discussed in this chapter are the pericardium, the three anatomical layers of the heart, the chambers and valves of the heart, the great vessels (aorta and its major thoracic branches, venae cavae, pulmonary arteries and their proximal divisions), the carotid arteries, and the jugular veins.

Vascular Structures

PERICARDIUM

The fibrous pericardial sac, which encases the heart, is separated from the surface of the heart by a space that contains a few milliliters of pericardial fluid—just enough to prevent friction as the contracting and relaxing heart moves with the cardiac cycle with respect to the outer protective covering.

THREE LAYERS OF HEART WALL

The **epicardium** is a thin mesothelial and fat layer that covers all chambers of the heart. Mesothelium extends a short way out onto the great vessels. Deep to the epicardium is the thick **myocardium** that makes up the contractile muscle mass of the heart. The thickness of the myocardium varies from chamber to chamber, being greater in the ventricles than the atria and greater in the left ventricle than the right ventricle. The chambers, valves, and valve infrastructures (chordae tendineae, papillary muscles) of the heart are lined by thin **endocardium.**

CHAMBERS OF THE HEART

The heart has four chambers. The relatively thin walled **atria** (auricles) receive venous blood from the systemic venous circuit (**right atrium**) and from the lungs (**left atrium**). From each atrium, the blood passes into the **respective ventricle.** The **right ventricle** handles desaturated blood to be moved into the pulmonary circulation; the **left ventricle** accepts oxygenated blood for subsequent systemic distribution.

VALVES OF THE HEART

Two **atrioventricular (AV) valves** separate atria from ventricles: the triple-leaflet **tricuspid valve** that admits blood from the right atrium to the right ventricle, and the double-leaflet **mitral valve** between the left atrium and left ventricle. Two valves control outflow from the heart; both normally have three cusps and are collectively referred to as the **semilunar valves:** the **pulmonic valve,** which

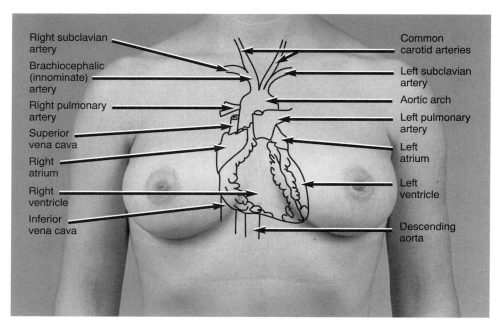

Figure 8.1   Heart and great vessels: anatomical placement in chest.

admits desaturated blood to the pulmonary arteries, then to the lungs to pick up oxygen for ultimate transport to the tissues of the body and to release carbon dioxide for excretion as the other component of respiration; and the **aortic valve,** past which oxygenated blood leaves the left ventricle, enters the aorta, and is thus distributed systemically.

GREAT VESSELS

The great veins bring systemic or pulmonic blood into the atria. From the head, neck, upper limbs, and part of the upper trunk, desaturated blood enters the right atrium via the **superior vena cava;** and from the abdomen, lower chest, and lower limbs, deoxygenated blood enters the right atrium via the **inferior vena cava.** Oxygen-saturated blood enters the left atrium via the two **right** and two **left (superior and inferior) pulmonary veins.**

The **pulmonary artery** exits the right ventricle and soon divides into a **left** and a **right** pulmonary artery, each of which carries desaturated blood into the respective pulmonary circulatory system (Fig. 8.2).

The **aorta** courses cephalad, then arches into its descent after sending branches to the head and upper limbs **(innominate,** thence right subclavian and right **carotid arteries,** left **common carotid** and left **subclavian arteries).** The more distal aorta conducts oxygenated blood from the posterior thorax into the abdomen.

Cardiac Cycle

The mechanical activity of the cardiac cycle is stimulated and, in part, controlled by an **electrical** conduction system. The electrical impulse is normally generated in the **sinoatrial (SA) node** that lies high in the wall of the right atrium; the impulse passes to the **AV node** that lies in the fibrous skeleton of the heart, just above the tricuspid valve. From the AV node the impulse, after a brief delay, passes through the **bundle of His,** the two **bundle branches, right (RBB) and left (LBB),** and subsequent ramifications to terminate in the **Purkinje fibers** of the

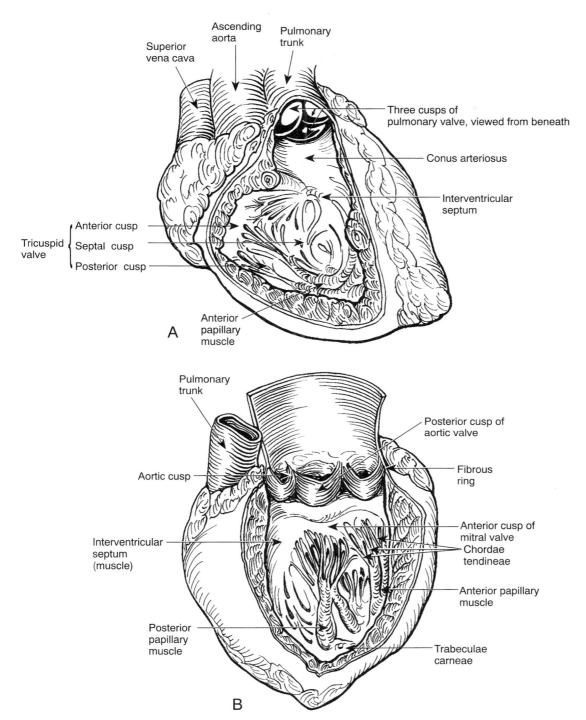

Figure 8.2   Cross-sectional views of interior of heart. **A.** Anterior dissection of right ventricle. **B.** Dissection of left ventricle.

ventricular myocardium. In response to these electrical stimuli, the chambers contract. A refractory period to permit repolarization occurs before the cycle is repeated. Left ventricular myocardial depolarization and the linked event of mechanical contraction occur slightly earlier than the analogous right heart events.

The **mechanical** cycle set in action by the electrical cycle results in rhythmic contraction and relaxation of the heart as pump for the circulatory system. The contractile phase is termed **systole;** the resting phase, **diastole.** When not further specified, these terms refer to *left ventricular* systole and diastole, respectively. During early diastole and later, in **atrial systole,** blood is pumped through each open AV valve into the respective ventricle; during ventricular systole, it is expelled through the open pulmonic or aortic valve into the pulmonary artery or aorta, respectively. Early in systole, when ventricular pressure exceeds atrial pressure, the AV valves close (corresponding to the sound known as S_1). The semilunar valves close (S_2) at the end of **ventricular systole,** and the ventricles receive atrial blood through the open AV valves during **ventricular diastole.** At heart rates less than approximately 120, diastole is longer than systole; the duration of systole and the duration of diastole are equal at greater rates.

TECHNIQUE

The physical examination of the heart and great vessels, in regional sequence, is begun after inspection of the breasts and palpation of the axillae have been completed. The precordium can be inspected and initially palpated with the patient in the sitting position. Usually, auscultatory maneuvers are conducted and the apical impulse is reassessed with the patient supine. In special circumstances, standing or squatting examination is also performed. See Table 8.1 for sequencing of the cardiac examination.

Table 8.1
Steps in the Screening Examination of the Heart and Great Vessels[a]

Patient seated
  Inspection
    Anterior chest wall motion
    Apical impulse
  Palpation
    Apical impulse (PMI)
    Base and sternal borders

Patient supine
  Inspection
    Height of jugular venous column
    Anterior chest wall motion, base, and sternal borders
    Apical impulse
    Jugular venous waves a, c, and v
  Palpation
    Carotid artery pulse
    Apical impulse
    Apical impulse and carotid artery synchrony
    Base and sternal borders
  Auscultation
    Carotid arteries
    All components of cycle with diaphragm and bell of stethoscope
      Apex
      Fourth intercostal space, left of sternum
      Third intercostal space, left of sternum
      Second intercostal space, left of sternum
      Second intercostal space, right of sternum
    All components of cycle with bell of stethoscope at apex, left lateral decubitus position

[a]**Boldface,** universally performed; lightface, elective.

Equipment required for the examination includes a quiet room to maximize auscultatory accuracy, good cross-lighting and fully bared patient chest for precordial inspection, warm room and warm examiner hands for comfortable palpation, and a stethoscope with both bell and diaphragm.

Supine Inspection

After initial inspection and palpation of the precordium, the patient is moved to the supine position. The examiner faces the patient, who is supine with the trunk—not just the head—raised 30° from the horizontal. There must be good lighting across the anterior chest wall for adequate inspection of the precordium. The examiner looks for visible pulsations, retractions, or any chest wall motion related to cyclic cardiac events and makes a systematic evaluation of the apex, left lower sternal area, and pulmonic and aortic valve areas.

Supine Palpation

With distal interphalangeal joints of the index and middle fingers (not fingertips), the examiner seeks the **apical impulse** usually found in the fourth or fifth intercostal space (ICS) at or about the midclavicular line. Location of the apical beat can be facilitated by asking the patient to roll slightly leftward, thus bringing the apex closer to the chest wall. However, the patient is then restored to supine before any conclusions about the locale, force, and character of the impulse can be drawn. The sometimes visible, and often palpable, apical thrust at this "point of maximal impulse" (PMI) is created by anterior cardiac motion coincident with ventricular systole. Its **location, size, force, and duration** are noted. When the apical impulse has been located, the examiner places two fingers of her other hand on the right carotid pulse (see below) and feels through a few cardiac cycles for the relative timing of the **carotid pulse.** It should follow, after a slight delay, each apical impulse (Fig. 8.3A) corresponding to later systole.

The examiner next places the palmar surface of one hand along the left lower sternal border to feel for **heaves** (diffuse cardiac movement) or **thrills,** which are vibrations caused by turbulence of blood flow (Fig. 8.3B). Similarly, the right and left second intercostal spaces at the **base of the heart** are palpated (Fig. 8.3C).

Supine Auscultation

Meaningful auscultation of the events of the cardiac cycle requires a consistent system and careful concentration on the part of the examiner. For definitions of the terms used to describe these events, see Table 8.2.

Where to listen. There are five primary sites at which the stethoscope is placed for auscultation. The order of placement is less important than is the understanding of the expected findings at each site and the use of a systematic approach in listening. The sites (Fig. 8.4) are

1. **Apex or mitral apical:** best located by palpation of the apical beat; if no impulse can be felt, listen at the left fifth intercostal space in the midclavicular line
2. **Lower left sternal border (LLSB) or tricuspid** focus: fourth intercostal space just at left side of the sternal border
3. **Third left intercostal:** just left of the sternal border ("accessory pulmonic focus")
4. **Second left intercostal,** also called left upper sternal border (LUSB) or **pulmonic valve** focus: second intercostal space, just left of the sternal border
5. **Second right intercostal or aortic valve** focus: second intercostal space, just right of the sternal border

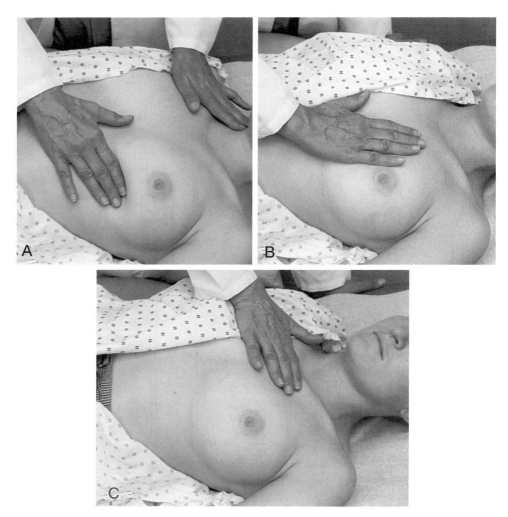

Figure 8.3   Precordial palpation. **A.** Synchrony of apical impulse and carotid pulse. **B.** Left sternal border. **C.** Base.

Each of these areas is auscultated first with the diaphragm, listening through enough cardiac and respiratory cycles at each site to determine the effect of respiration and to describe all the events discussed below. The procedure is repeated with the bell of the stethoscope *held lightly to the skin* to listen for lower-frequency sounds.

How to listen.   Create and maintain a regular **system** for listening. Each event in the cardiac cycle is auscultated individually at each chest wall site. One suggested system follows. At each site, isolate and concentrate on each event in the cycle and listen through enough cycles to be able to characterize

1. S_1, the sound corresponding to closure of the AV valves
2. S_2, the sound corresponding to closure of the semilunar valves
3.   Systole, the time after S_1 and before S_2
4.   Diastole, the time following S_2 and preceding S_1

When all four components of the cycle have been appreciated, move to the next site and repeat the system.

What to listen for.   While listening to each component of the cardiac cycle at each site, the examiner makes a series of observations and answers a set of questions:

Table 8.2
Terms for Describing Common Auscultatory Findings

Sites: equivalent terminology
    Mitral focus, apex, point of maximum impulse (PMI), fifth left intercostal space (5LICS) at midclavicular line (MCL)
    Tricuspid focus, lower left sternal border (LLSB), fourth left intercostal space (4LICS)
    Secondary pulmonic focus, third left intercostal space (3LICS)
    Pulmonic focus, second left intercostal space (2LICS), left base, left upper sternal border (LUSB)
    Aortic focus, second right intercostal space (2RICS), right base, right upper sternal border (RUSB)

Heart rate and rhythm
    Rate = number of cycles per minute
        Bradycardia = less than 60/minute
        Tachycardia = greater than 100/minute
    Rhythm = regularity of heart beat
        Normal sinus rhythm (NSR) = perfectly regular rhythm at rate between 60 and 100/minute
        Sinus arrhythmia = variation in heart rate with the respiratory cycle

Sounds of the cardiac cycle
    First heart sound
        S_1 = atrioventricular valve closure-associated sound
        M_1 = mitral component (= S_1M)
        T_1 = tricuspid component (= S_1T)
        Split S_1 = M_1 and T_1 heard as separate sounds
    Second heart sound
        S_2 = semilunar valve closure-associated sound
        A_2 = aortic component (= S_2A)
        P_2 = pulmonic component (= S_2P)
        Split S_2 = A_2 and P_2 heard as separate sounds
    Systole = period of ventricular ejection occurring after S_1 and before S_2
    Diastole = period of ventricular filling occurring after S_2 and before S_1
    Third heart sound
        S_3 = occurs in early diastole, after S_2
    Fourth heart sound
        S_4 = occurs in late diastole, before S_1
    Murmur = prolonged vibrations in systole or diastole, created within the heart (analogous term in artery is *bruit*)
    Venous hum = prolonged vibrations in systole and diastole, created within the venous system

1. **Rate and rhythm.** With the diaphragm placed at the apex:
   a. Count the apical cardiac rate. (This may exceed the radial pulse rate, especially if there are some unconducted weak cardiac cycles, e.g., in atrial fibrillation.)
   b. Is the rhythm perfectly regular?
   c. If not, is the **arrhythmia** regular or irregular in its pattern of recurrence?
   d. If an irregularity is noted, does it vary with the respiratory cycle or appear independent of respiration?
2. **S_1.**
   a. What is the relative intensity of S_1 at each site? Is it louder at apex than base, as expected? Is it louder than S_2 at the apex, and softer than S_2 at the base, as expected?

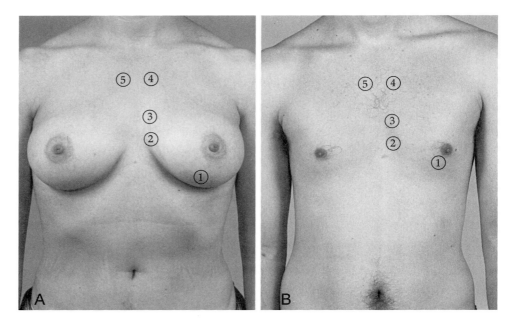

Figure 8.4   Auscultatory sites in women (**A**) and men (**B**): *1,* apex; *2,* 4LICS (LLSB); *3,* 3LICS; *4,* 2LICS; and *5,* 2RICS.

    b.   Is S_1 a single sound or is it split? If split, is the split heard at every site, only at LLSB, or only at the apex? Does the split vary in width with the respiratory cycle, or is it constant throughout respiration? If it is split, is the first component of S_1 louder than the second, as expected, or not?

3.   **S_2.** Repeat observations as for **S_1.**

4.   **Systole.**

    a.   Is systole silent, or does it contain sound(s)?

    b.   If sounds are heard in systole, they fall into one of the following categories:

         Murmurs are relatively prolonged vibrations, which are characterized in terms of their **loudness (intensity), shape (configuration), pitch (frequency), duration** and **timing within this phase of the cycle, site of greatest intensity,** direction of **radiation** (Table 8.3), and response to maneuvers (see the Extended Examination section).

         Venous hums are usually continuous (systolic and diastolic) soft, low-pitched vibrations of passive flow in large veins. *Mammary souffles* are continuous arterial murmurs arising in the mammary vasculature during pregnancy and lactation.

         Systolic clicks, prosthetic valve sounds, and extracardiac sounds such as friction rubs and mediastinal crunch are discussed in the Extended Examination section.

5.   **Diastole.**

    a.   Repeat observations as for *systole* above.

    b.   If sounds are heard in diastole, consider:

         Murmurs, which should be characterized by the parameters outlined above.

         S_3 (third heart sound), which is a low-pitched extra sound coinciding with early diastolic ventricular filling and heard 0.12–0.18 seconds *after S_2.*

Table 8.3
Murmurs: Definition of Descriptive Terms[a]

Loudness (intensity) of systolic murmurs
  Grade I: barely audible with careful concentration
  Grade II: faint but readily detected
  Grade III: prominent, easily detectable
  Grade IV: louder still; palpable thrill associated
  Grade V: audible with only rim of stethoscope touching chest wall
  Grade VI: loud enough to be heard without stethoscope

Shape (configuration)
  Crescendo: rising in intensity

  Decrescendo: falling in intensity

  Crescendo-decrescendo (diamond-shaped): rising,
    then falling in intensity

  Plateau: even in intensity

  Uneven: varying irregularly in intensity

Pitch: a description of the frequency characteristics of the sound, e.g., low-pitched, high-pitched (other terms such as harsh, grating, whistling, rumbling, scratchy, blowing, and musical relate to pitch and to additional characteristics that are more difficult to describe and define scientifically)

Timing and duration in cycle
  Systolic or diastolic
  Duration or relationship to S_1 and S_2, including obliteration of either or both of them

Site of greatest intensity: the auscultatory site at which the murmur sounds loudest

Direction of radiation: sites away from that of greatest intensity at which the murmur remains audible although reduced

[a]Sample description of a murmur: There is a grade II midsystolic, medium-pitched harsh murmur heard best in the 4LICS, (LLSB) radiating to the apex but not to the axilla, base, or carotids. It decreases with the Valsalva maneuver and is augmented during deep inspiration.

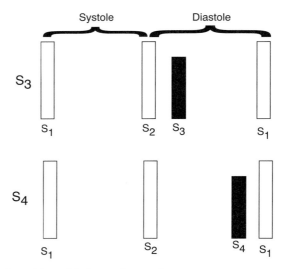

Figure 8.5   Timing of S₃ and S₄ in cardiac cycle.

S_4 *(fourth heart sound),* a low-pitched atrial contraction sound that occurs in late diastole, *preceding* S_1 (Fig. 8.5). **If you are uncertain whether a double sound represents an S_4 or a split S_1, take advantage of the differential pitch (S_1 high, S_4 low) and differential filtering properties of stethoscope heads cited above:** S_1 is well heard with the diaphragm; S_4 is far better (and often exclusively) heard with the bell held *lightly* to the skin. When the bell is pressed firmly, the skin is stretched and functions as a diaphragm, so that transmission of high-pitched sounds suddenly predominates. **Apply firm pressure with the bell. A fourth heart sound is damped or completely obliterated by this maneuver, whereas S_1 is unchanged or intensified.** Location also assists this common problem in distinction. Split S_1 sounds are usually best appreciated at LLSB, whereas S_4 sounds of left heart origin are clearest at the apex.

Bell auscultation at the apex is repeated with the patient in a modified lateral decubitus position, since several low-pitched diastolic sounds may become audible only in this way, namely S_4 sounds, S_3 sounds, and rumbling murmurs of mitral stenosis. Higher-pitched mitral opening snaps may also emerge with this maneuver.

Supine Inspection of Vessels

Observe the lateral neck for visibility of the jugular venous blood column and its height. With a light beam directed tangential to the right side of the neck, observe for pulsations (Fig. 8.6). Inspect the *right* external jugular vein for its three positive (outward) wave components while palpating the *left* carotid artery:

1. The **a wave,** produced by atrial contraction, occurs just before the carotid pulse.
2. The **c wave** (mechanism disputed) is essentially the transmission of the carotid pulse wave, i.e., ventricular ejection.
3. The **v wave** comes after the c wave and relates to later ventricular contraction.

Transmitted carotid artery pulsations are sometimes difficult to distinguish from venous a and v waves. The following observations assist in differentiating the two:

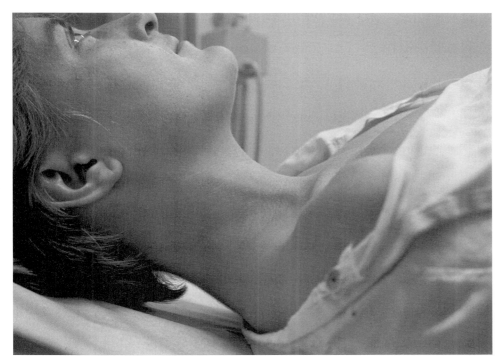

Figure 8.6   Patient positioned for observation of cervical veins.

1. The jugular venous pulse can have up to three positive components, whereas the carotid artery pulse has only one.
2. On inspiration, the level of the venous column normally descends, whereas the carotid pulsation remains visible above this point.
3. *Light* pressure over the vein just above the medial clavicle will eliminate any visible venous pulse but will not affect carotid pulsation.

Supine Palpation of Vessels

Palpate each side of the neck separately, inferior to the mandibular ramus and lateral to the trachea, for the **carotid artery pulse.** Its upstroke coincides with the midpoint of ventricular systole. If you auscultate the heart while feeling the carotid, the carotid pulse will accompany S_1 or follow shortly after it. The value of the simultaneous study of the two areas is, in part, to help figure out which auscultatory phenomena are systolic, which are diastolic, or even which is S_1 and which is S_2—not always an achievable goal, especially at high heart rates. The right and left carotid pulsations should be equal in amplitude and should have a single positive wave (Fig. 8.7*A*).

Supine Auscultation of Vessels

With the patient's face turned *very slightly* toward the opposite side, gently press the stethoscope (diaphragm, if full skin contact can be made, or the bell, if it cannot) over the palpable pulse of each **carotid artery** (Fig. 8.7*B*). One or two systolic sounds are usually audible, corresponding to transmission of S_2 and sometimes of S_1. The intensity of these transmitted sounds should be more or less equal bilaterally. Listen for bruits or transmitted aortic valve murmurs (see the Extended Examination section).

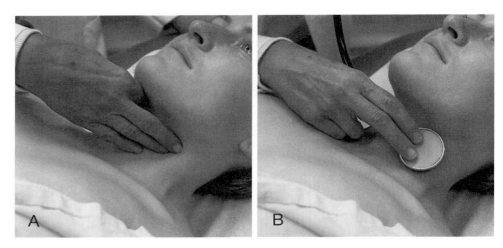

Figure 8.7   Examination of carotid artery pulse. **A.** Palpation of left carotid artery. **B.** Auscultation of left carotid artery.

NORMAL AND COMMON VARIANTS

The expected ranges of normal and the common variants are described as they pertain to the young or middle-aged adult at rest (Table 8.4). Physiologic changes common to pregnancy and anticipated in the aged are noted under separate headings.

Inspection

Chest wall thickness and body habitus affect visibility of cardiac motion on the anterior chest wall. In a minority of adults, the apical impulse is visible in the fourth or fifth intercostal space 5–6 cm to the left of the midsternal line (usually at, just inside, or just outside the midclavicular line). In tall, thin individuals, the impulse may lie lower and/or more medially. Obesity, highly developed pectoral muscles, and large pendulous breasts can all obscure the apical cardiac impulse. Note that in the rare developmental anomaly **dextrocardia,** in which the position of the heart is rotated, the left ventricular apex presents to the right of the sternal border. In **situs inversus,** most organs, including the heart, occupy mirror positions to those of normals. The effect on locale of cardiac impulse is evident.

Other than the apical impulse of early systole, the chest wall on inspection does not usually reveal events of the cardiac cycle. In very thin young adults, the lower parasternal region may retract slightly during systole, with outward pulsation of the lower sternum. This movement is accentuated in response to noncardiac systemic events demanding increased cardiac output and/or rate, e.g., anemia, anxiety, or fever. With the head and thorax elevated at 30°, venous pulses should not ascend more than 4 cm above the level of the jugular notch (top of the sternum). If distension of the veins exceeds this height, measurements are made as described in the Extended Examination section.

Palpation

The apical impulse, when palpable, occupies an area less than 2.5 cm in diameter and is felt in early systole. Its amplitude and duration may be increased in the patient with a thin chest wall or during periods of increased cardiac output. Under the same circumstances, a brief tiny pulsation of the pulmonary artery may be appreciated in the second or third left intercostal space. Other vibrations or palpable movements of the chest wall with the cardiac cycle must be considered abnormal.

Table 8.4
Variant Findings Encountered on Screening Examination of the Heart and Great Vessels[a]

Inspection
   No visible apical pulsation
   Apical impulse to right of sternum (dextrocardia)
   Lower left parasternal retraction
   In the elderly, supraclavicular arterial pulsation, unilateral distension of left jugular vein
       [unilateral or bilateral visibility of jugular vein(s)]

Palpation
   Nonpalpable apical impulse
   [Pulmonary artery pulsation, 3LICS]
   [Late pregnancy, left displacement of apical impulse]
   In the elderly, increased frequency of nonpalpable apical impulse

Auscultation
   Regular heart rate at 50–60/minute or 100–110/minute
   Sinus arrhythmia
   [Occasional (sometimes frequent) premature contractions]
   [Atrial fibrillation (irregularly irregular rhythm)]
   S_1 split at the apex or LLSB
   S_2 split at LUSB, with respiratory variation
   Systolic sounds
       [Pulmonic systolic murmur]
       Still's murmur and other unclassified innocent systolic murmurs
       Brachiocephalic bruits
       [Aortic sclerotic murmur]
   Cervical venous hums
   [S_3 in children and young adults]
   [S_4]
   In pregnancy
       [Midsystolic murmur]
       Mammary souffle

[a]**Boldface,** common; lightface, uncommon; [. . .], potentially abnormal.

Auscultation

CARDIAC RATE

The range of normal heart rates is conventionally 60–100 cycles/minute. The well-conditioned athlete's heart may have a resting rate in the 40s, however. Anemia, hyperthyroidism, fever, or anxiety may push the rate well over 100 in adults with intrinsically normal cardiovascular systems.

CARDIAC RHYTHM

Two basic rhythm patterns are considered normal:

1. **Normal sinus rhythm** (NSR) consists of perfectly regular beats within the range assigned above; **sinus bradycardia** refers to slow regular beating including that of the athlete; **sinus tachycardia** refers to rapid regular heart action over 100 beats/minute.
2. **Sinus arrhythmia** is a physiologic irregularity associated with the respiratory cycle in which the heart rate momentarily increases detectably with inspiration and correspondingly decreases with expiration.

Premature contractions (ventricular or atrial) commonly occur in normal hearts. These irregular irregularities are usually asymptomatic. They may be noted on physical examination as "extra" or "skipped" beats, without a break in the underlying rhythm pattern. For further definition of these irregularities, see Chapter 2 and the Extended Examination section of this chapter.

S_1

The **intensity** of the first heart sound is always greater at the apex than at the base, barring disease (Fig. 8.8*A*). Hyperkinetic states that shorten the interval between atrial and ventricular contraction (P-R interval), such as anemia or fever, may increase S_1 intensity. Because of minor asynchrony between left and right ventricular contraction, S_1 may be **split** at the LLSB (Fig. 8.8*B*), the loud mitral closure (S_1M) occurring slightly before the softer tricuspid closure (S_1T).

S_2

As the examiner inches the stethoscope toward the base of the heart, the second heart sound becomes louder than the first heart sound at the upper sternal borders. Normal **splitting** of S_2 occurs because right ventricular ejection time is slightly longer than left ventricular ejection, resulting in a delay of pulmonic valve closure. This asynchrony is exaggerated during inspiration such that the split widens as the patient breathes in and narrows or disappears as he breathes out (Fig. 8.8*C*). This split is best appreciated in the second (or third, or occasionally fourth) left intercostal space and is not normally audible at the apex. When both components of S_2 can be heard, note that the first (aortic valve closure) should be of greater **intensity** than the second (pulmonic valve closure) in normal adults over age 25. The relative intensities cannot be predicted in normal children, teenagers, or younger adults.

SYSTOLE

Systole is usually silent, although sounds of turbulent flow without cardiac pathology are heard during systole in some patients. The following systolic sounds fall into the category of normal variants:

- **Innocent murmurs** are defined as those flow sounds that do not appear to be associated with anatomic or functional abnormality. All are midsystolic in timing and include the following:
    —**Pulmonic systolic murmurs,** heard in some older children and young adults, represent exaggerated ejection vibrations in the pulmonary trunk. They are relatively brief and soft and are heard best along the left upper sternal border (pulmonic focus). They begin well after S_1 and end before S_2.
    —**Still's murmur** is a short, medium-frequency buzz, probably created by vibration of the attachments of the pulmonic valve leaflets.
    —**Brachiocephalic murmurs** are heard best in the supraclavicular fossae, although they may be heard faintly below the clavicles. They represent vibrations in brachiocephalic and/or subclavian arteries and are typically diminished by hyperextension of the shoulders.
    —**Benign aortic sclerosis** gives rise to a midsystolic murmur appearing at the second right intercostal space (aortic focus) in aging adults.
- **Cervical venous hum** is a continuous murmur caused by flow in normal veins. It may be discovered incidentally during auscultation of the neck or of the base of the heart, or picked up when listening with the bell in the supraclavicular fossae. Obliteration of the sound by application of light pressure to the jugular vein, with a transient intensification of the sound as pressure is released, assists in proving the venous origin of this innocent systolic-diastolic murmur.

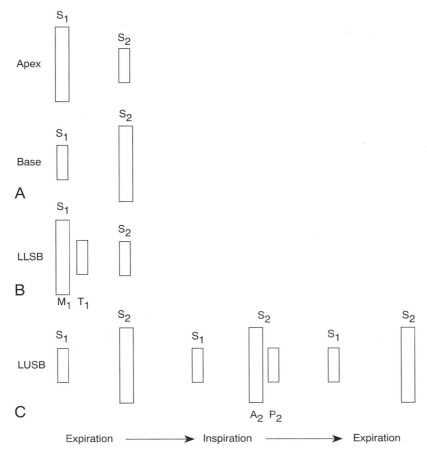

Figure 8.8   Normal variants of S_1 and S_2. **A.** Intensity variations by auscultatory site. **B.** LLSB split of S_1. **C.** Physiologic splitting of S_2.

DIASTOLE

There are few normal variants that result in diastolic sounds. One is the continuous cervical venous hum noted above, which is typically louder in diastole than in systole. In addition, the examiner may hear:

- *Third heart sound (S_3)*. This low-pitched sound, best heard at the apex with the bell of the stethoscope and with the patient in the modified left decubitus position, occurs in many normal children and healthy young adults. It rarely presents as a normal variant in individuals over age 30, and is a prototype of a physical finding that must be interpreted in a total-patient context.
- *Fourth heart sound (S_4)*. This later diastolic sound is often heard in persons over age 50 and is sometimes heard in younger persons without evidence of cardiac disease.

Variants Related to Pregnancy

Pregnancy produces a physiologic circulatory hyperdynamic state related to the increased blood volume necessary to support the growing fetus and placenta. Altered cardiovascular physiology may produce the following physical examination variants.

On *inspection and palpation*, the elevation of the diaphragms by the enlarging uterus may tip the left heart border up and out, often moving the apical impulse lateral to the midclavicular line and superior to the fourth intercostal space. The impulse may be increased in intensity and diameter.

On *auscultation,* two phenomena may appear during pregnancy:

1. **Midsystolic murmur** generated by rapid ejection into a normal aortic root or pulmonary trunk is best heard along the left upper sternal border.
2. **Mammary souffle** is created by increased flow in the internal mammary arteries. The (sometimes) continuous souffle tends to be loudest in the second or third right or left intercostal space, although it may be audible anywhere over either breast. It is best heard with the patient supine and may disappear when she sits. The systolic component is loudest, with a perceptible silence after S_1. Firm pressure with the stethoscope diminishes the sound, whereas light pressure augments it. The souffle may persist throughout the lactation period and reflects the increased flow associated with the physiologic functional hypertrophy of lactation.

Variants Related to Aging

Aging brings about cardiac alterations that may be reflected in the physical examination.

On *inspection,* a visible and palpable **arterial pulsation** resulting from tortuosity of the aortic arch is often detected in the supraclavicular area or in the suprasternal (jugular) notch. The elongated, tortuous, and uncoiled thoracic aorta may, in turn, compress the left innominate artery, giving rise to apparent **distension of the left jugular venous system.** Under this circumstance, the right jugular venous column remains at normal height with the patient's head and chest raised to 30°.

On *palpation,* because of muscular wasting and/or thoracic spine kyphosis, as well as in the setting of chronic obstructive pulmonary disease, **position of the heart relative to the chest wall** may be distorted, making meaningful precordial palpation difficult or impossible. A subxiphoid approach may permit better assessment of the ventricular impulse in this group of patients.

On *auscultation,* **fourth heart sounds** are heard frequently enough in the elderly to be considered a normal phenomenon when not accompanied by evidence of valvular disease, myocardial hypertrophy, or compromised cardiac function. The **midsystolic murmur** of aortic sclerosis has been mentioned earlier. It has been placed at the benign end of the spectrum of aortic valve calcification because of the absence of left ventricular compromise (see the Extended Examination section) as well as because of some characteristics of the murmur itself.

RECORDING THE FINDINGS

In the patient's record, the findings from the screening examination of the heart and great vessels are entered after the RESPIRATORY SYSTEM. The findings on palpation of the peripheral vasculature, *although performed* while examining the neck, abdomen, and limbs, can also be recorded here as a part of the CARDIO-VASCULAR SYSTEM.

Sample Write-up

Cardiovascular system:

Heart: No visible pulsations. Apical impulse normal size, in 5th ICS, 4 cm to left of LSB. No other precordial movement. On auscultation, S_1 narrowly split at LLSB, normal intensity throughout. S_2 physiologically split along LUSB, $A_2 > P_2$. No gallops, murmurs, or rubs.

Arteries: Carotid pulses equal bilaterally, without bruit.

Veins: Cervical veins just visible above clavicle at 30°. No aberrant waves. Soft, low-pitched midsystolic murmur or bruit just inferior to both clavicles; disappears completely with hyperextension of shoulders.

Impressions:

1. Normal cardiovascular system.
2. Brachiocephalic bruit, innocuous.
3. Split S_1, probably normal variant.

EXTENDED EXAMINATION OF THE HEART AND GREAT VESSELS

INDICATIONS

Symptoms and History

The most common symptom prompting extended cardiovascular examination is *chest pain,* which raises such cardiac differential diagnoses as coronary artery disease and pericarditis. *Dyspnea,* like chest pain, may reflect either cardiac or pulmonary problems. Underscoring the functional link between the systems mentioned at the end of Chapter 7, this symptom will usually lead to extended evaluation of both.

A history of a known *cardiac murmur,* established heart disease, or open-heart surgery also calls for extended examination, as does the presence of a cardiac *pacemaker. Palpitations* or the report of severe irregularity of the heartbeat or a very slow or fast heart rate may also lead to further cardiac evaluation.

Physical Examination

The patient with highly abnormal heart rate or rhythm, tachypnea, hypotension, or hypertension is likely to receive thorough cardiac examination, particularly if no clear extracardiac explanation has been achieved. Likewise, new or etiologically obscure physical signs of congestion in the systemic veins (edema) or the pulmonary veins (unexplained late inspiratory crackles) will lead to extended cardiac evaluation. A cardiac murmur discovered by screening cardiovascular examination suggests the need for extended examination. Stroke, especially a new one, stimulates extended examination of the great arteries, while superior vena cava syndrome will lead to limited extended examination of the great veins.

Laboratory and Imaging

A newly or severely abnormal electrocardiogram (ECG) may lead back to the bedside for further assessment, as can a chest radiograph showing any abnormal cardiac chamber silhouette or any suggestion of pulmonary edema. A positive blood culture, especially with "endocarditis genera"—staphylococci or streptococci—will direct an extended search for infective endocarditis.

CONDUCTING THE EXTENDED EXAMINATION

Heart

INSPECTION

The principal maneuver is *repeated inspection* of the entire precordium, with good cross-lighting, in an unhurried manner and in several positions if necessary. The supine position is standard, but the examiner may also carry out reinspection with the patient seated, lying in left lateral decubitus position, and lying halfway between the supine and left lateral decubitus positions.

PALPATION
Position and Characteristics

Some impalpable apical impulses can be rendered palpable in the left lateral decubitus or semi-left lateral decubitus position (Fig. 8.9). Once the impulse has been discovered, it may remain perceptible even after return to the supine position. Although in the left lateral decubitus position the location of the apex impulse is not a reliable indicator of heart size, some characteristics can be assessed in either position: **diameter** (2.5 cm or smaller is normal); **duration,** since the impulse is not expected to last beyond the first third of systole; **force,** compared with a large personal series of normals; and any associated vibratory sensation (**thrill**) or palpable heart sounds.

Comparison to Audibility

Any **cardiac sound**—a generic term embracing both discrete heart sounds and murmurs—including a gallop (S_3 or S_4), may be palpable. Audibility is more common, and palpation tends to be overlooked; some low-frequency heart sounds or gallops are *palpable but not audible,* however, and thus are missed if only a cursory precordial palpation is done. If S_1 is palpable, it is perceived just before the apical impulse, perhaps producing a double apical impulse. A palpable S_4 would occur just a bit earlier. S_2 is produced at the base and should not be palpable at the apex. A palpable S_3 will follow systole and might also suggest a double impulse at the apex. The thrill most frequently felt at the cardiac apex is that of mitral regurgitation, which will feel like the purring of a tiny kitten.

Right Heart Events

Palpation may permit appreciation of a prominent S_2P (pulmonary component of the second heart sound) at the left upper sternal border. A left parasternal lift

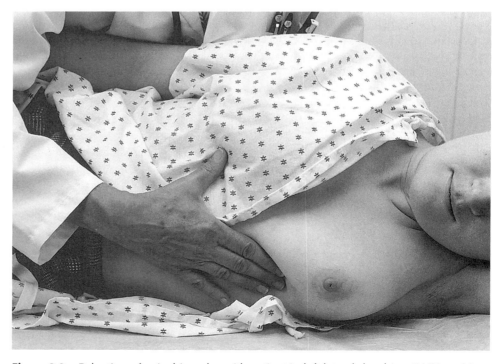

Figure 8.9   Palpation of apical impulse with patient in left lateral decubitus (LLD) position: valuable for discovery but not for localization.

indicates *right* ventricular hypertrophy and forceful contraction in any setting that taxes the right side of the heart. At the aortic valve focus (right upper sternal border), a systolic thrill is sought to diagnose the cause and severity of a systolic ejection murmur.

Technique Revisited

For all cardiac palpation, the use of vibratory receptors is essential: The interphalangeal or metacarpophalangeal joints—as many as can comfortably be employed—are used to study maximal area. Pushing down *harder* to locate an obscure finding guarantees failure. The hand must settle on the chest under its own weight, without exertion or additional downward force or pressure. The examiner needs to hold still for 20 seconds to "tune in" on precordial impulses. Finally, contouring the examiner's anatomy to that of the patient is essential. The examiner's right hand, with thumb pointed more or less toward the patient's chin, falls naturally onto the patient's anterior left precordium, without hyperextension or twisting that impairs perception. This positioning is the reason for preferentially examining from the *right rather than the left* side of the patient.

AUSCULTATION
Environment and Instrument

When trainees are dismayed at their inability to hear findings described by other examiners, the answer often lies in the room or in the stethoscope rather than in the acoustic or cognitive skills of the examiner.

It is hard enough to hear everything, without stacking the deck against oneself. Specific steps include those mentioned in Table 8.5.

The cheapest stethoscopes often have inferior sound transmission capability. When subtle distinctions are to be drawn or soft sounds are to be appreciated, a fine stethoscope repays its cost a hundredfold. Examiners become quite attached to their instrument. Obtaining a good stethoscope at a planned step-up in auscultatory skill makes sense. To those who rejoin that the most important component is "what is between the ears," we respond: "Good equipment stimulates thinking. Poor equipment stifles its growth and development."

Maximal Intensity

A simple method of probing cardiac sound is ascertaining where it is *loudest*. The examiner may reauscultate the four principal auscultatory sites, concentrating exclusively on the particular sound or murmur's relative intensity from site to site. Heart sounds and murmurs usually follow true. Forward flow from the aortic valve and environs is maximal in the right upper sternal border or aortic focus (Fig. 8.10) (aortic insufficiency may be loudest over the sternum or at either sternal edge, halfway down). Sound best heard at the left upper sternal border should arise from forward flow across the pulmonic valve (Fig. 8.11), as should that in the third left intercostal space—unless it comes from the interventricular septum.

Table 8.5
Steps to Improve Auscultation

Make the room quiet.
Don't be shy. Proper diagnosis and the welfare of the patient are at stake.
If the room cannot be made quiet, remove the patient to a place that is quiet.

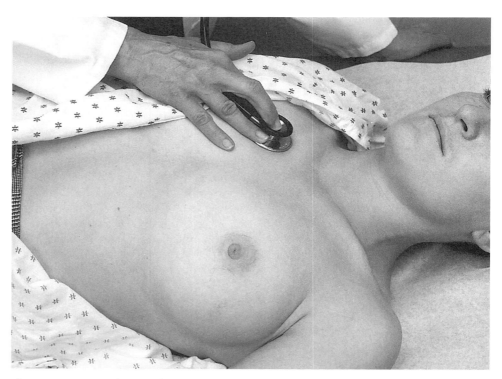

Figure 8.10   Auscultation of aortic valve focus (right upper sternal border or RUSB). Localization of the area where a sound or murmur is loudest is among the easiest, most important evaluations of the heart and great vessels.

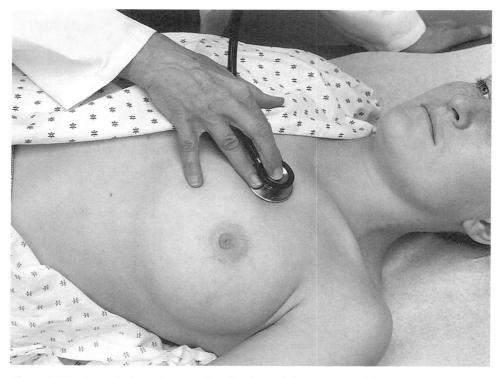

Figure 8.11   Auscultation of pulmonic valve focus (left upper sternal border or LUSB).

The left lower sternal border reflects right ventricular and tricuspid valvular events (Fig. 8.12). The apex—best located as the apical impulse rather than the arbitrary fifth intercostal space at the midclavicular line—is the prime auscultatory window for left ventricular and mitral valvular events.

Distortions of anatomy can change the acoustic projections, for example, in a patient whose mediastinum has shifted after pneumonectomy. Barring such distortions, maximal intensity points to the source of any cardiac vibration. The information is no more reliable or precise than the report; e.g., describing a systolic murmur as maximal "at the left sternal border" introduces needless ambiguity, suggesting both the pulmonic valve and the tricuspid valve.

Sound Radiation

Many murmurs propagate in an attenuated form for some distance from the point of origin. Very loud sound may be audible all over the precordium and epigastrium and even over the back. Several patterns of radiation are characteristic (Table 8.6).

To find axillary radiation, the examiner slides the stethoscope laterally from the apex, stopping in the midaxillary line (Fig. 8.13). Some experts move the stethoscope high in the axilla, reasoning that the gain in specificity for mitral origin outweighs the loss in sensitivity (Fig. 8.14). Sound radiation is delineated on a pass focused on one acoustic event *only*. If a cardiac sound is maximal over the pulmonic focus, for example, there is little point in checking for axillary radiation but higher yield in going through the principal cardiac sites and then the interscapular area.

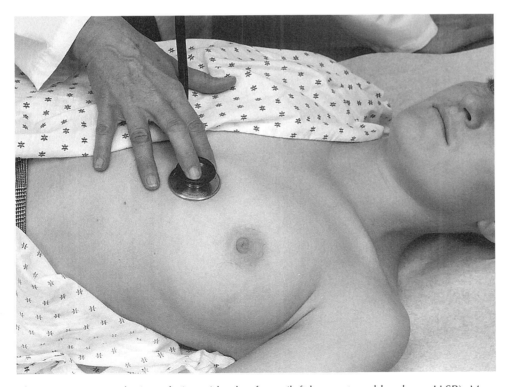

Figure 8.12   Auscultation of tricuspid valve focus (left lower sternal border or LLSB). Murmurs are often described as best heard "at the left sternal border," i.e., half-characterized.

Table 8.6
Sound radiation

Site	Principal Radiation	Secondary Radiation	Not Heard
Aortic valve systolic (forward flow) murmurs	Up the carotids	Cardiac apex	Axilla, posterior chest
Loud pulmonic valve systolic (forward flow) murmurs	Audible posteriorly	Aortic focus	Inconsistent
Subvalvular stenoses of aortic and pulmonic valves	Inconsistent	Inconsistent	Inconsistent
Aortic and pulmonic insufficiency (backflow diastolic murmurs)	Down sternal borders	Inconsistent	Inconsistent
Tricuspid regurgitation murmurs	Rightward, epigastrium	Apex	Axilla
Mitral regurgitation murmurs (Fig. 8.13)	Axilla (with left ventricular dilation)	Base	Inconsistent
Gallops of right-heart origin	Supraclavicular fossae, especially the right	Not known	Base
Left-heart gallops	None	None	Base

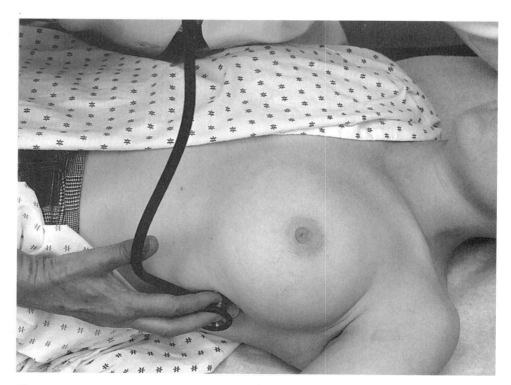

Figure 8.13 Determination of radiation of sound is vital also. Mitral murmurs tend to radiate to the axilla if there is left ventricular enlargement.

Changing Frequency Spectrum

The bell of the stethoscope provides a variable-frequency filter to characterize cardiac sound. Anything well-heard with the lightly apposed bell must include low-frequency components. As the examiner presses the bell firmly, low-

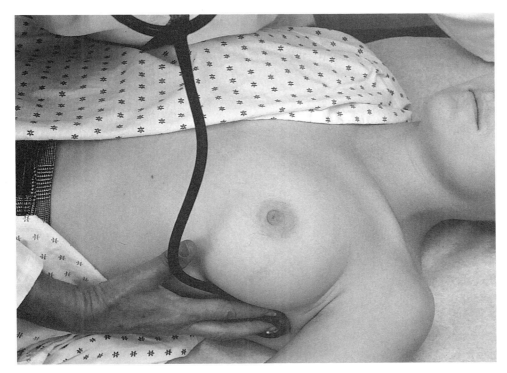

Figure 8.14   The examiner can increase the specificity of the sign—i.e., make a surer inference that axillary audibility implies a mitral origin—by listening in the upper axilla; however, the sensitivity of the sign will drop accordingly.

frequency components are attenuated. If the sound softens or disappears, it is of low frequency, but if it gets louder, high frequencies must predominate. This method helps discriminate S_4 from a split S_1 and, occasionally, abnormal S_2P from S_3. It helps characterize the frequency of *any* cardiac sound. If in doubt, again reduce the pressure: If it is still unclear whether the change augments or diminishes the sound, both high- and low-frequency components must be present.

Respiratory Variation

The effect of respiration is most helpful. Cardiac sound that neither increases nor diminishes with inspiration is indeterminate. However, that which *softens on inspiration* and loudens on expiration usually comes from the *left heart*, and that which *increases with inspiration* usually comes from the *right side of the heart*. The only common exceptions are patients with marked air trapping in whom *all* cardiac sound diminishes *in concert* on inspiration and those with pulmonic stenosis murmurs that soften on inspiration.

Left Lateral Decubitus Position

The rollover from supine to left lateral decubitus position increases the audibility of S_3 and S_4 gallops and the murmur of mitral stenosis, among other phenomena. The increased cardiovascular work of the mild exercise or perhaps "flopping" of the heart toward the chest wall may do this. Key points of technique are

1.   The sounds you seek to amplify or detect in this position are most often *apical.* The bell of the stethoscope is usually placed on the apex with the patient supine, and the examiner listens here as the patient turns.

2. Stay in place. With the stethoscope in the ears and the stethoscope head held lightly on the apex, say, "Now *while I listen,* when I say so, roll halfway over onto your left side, away from me."

3. Give the signal, and listen during the transfer—and for a few seconds afterward.

4. If the patient feels unsteady, allow him to lean his upper back against your trunk, since, although standing, you will be curled around him somewhat. If his right hand is in the way, have him rest it on his right hip.

Supraclavicular, Epigastric, Clavicular Sites

Listening in the supraclavicular fossa and epigastrium can help detect cardiac sound when the chest is noisy. The sites are subject to sounds of their own—subclavian and celiac bruits—that complicate interpretation. They are rementioned here because they are easily forgotten, being nonprecordial. They can assist investigation in the following instances:

1. A right versus a left heart origin cannot be established otherwise, e.g., an S_4 that is equally loud in both tricuspid and mitral foci and in both phases of respiration.

2. Abundant wheezes or crackles obscure precordial sounds.

3. Severe pulmonary hyperinflation attenuates precordial sound.

4. Multiple cardiac sounds and murmurs produce a cacophony that is difficult to analyze one piece at a time without "division and conquest."

In follow-up of a murmur that appears to be maximal at the right upper sternal border or of one that has characteristics of aortic insufficiency, the examiner can listen with the stethoscope directly applied to the midpoint of the right clavi-

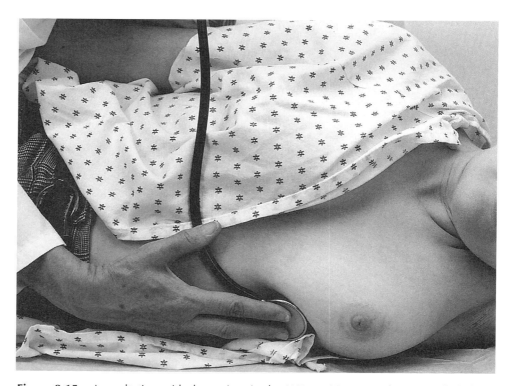

Figure 8.15   Auscultation with the patient in the LLD position provides particularly high yield, using the bell in search for gallops (S_3 and S_4 sounds).

cle. Some aortic valve murmurs are actually louder here than at the right upper sternal border, rather than attenuated by distance.

Simultaneous Palpation and Auscultation

The eye-hand-ear coordination required is considerable. The examiner palpates the right carotid pulse while auscultating the heart. This can help with timing of events, since the carotid pulse occurs during systole, shortly after S_1 or *apparently* coinciding with it (Fig. 8.16). If, alternatively, the examiner is confident of which heart sound is S_1 and which is S_2, this method can help demonstrate a delayed carotid upstroke, an important if insensitive sign of aortic valvular stenosis *or* significant aortic, innominate, or common carotid arterial obstruction.

Rarely, the examiner may time the apical impulse with regard to other events, and for this, the right hand palpates the apex while the left holds the stethoscope at the base or palpates a right carotid pulse previously timed with respect to S_1, using the prior maneuver. Simultaneous carotid and apical palpation has been employed in assessment of the severity of aortic stenosis.

Common Auscultatory Errors

Some auscultatory errors are so detrimental and so commonly repeated even by seasoned clinicians that they require further emphasis here.

Futility of listening in a noisy room. The futility of listening in a noisy room cannot be repeated too often. Regrettably, in the acute hospital setting, somebody walks in during *every* examination and inevitably leaves the hall door open. The open door lets in noise and destroys privacy.

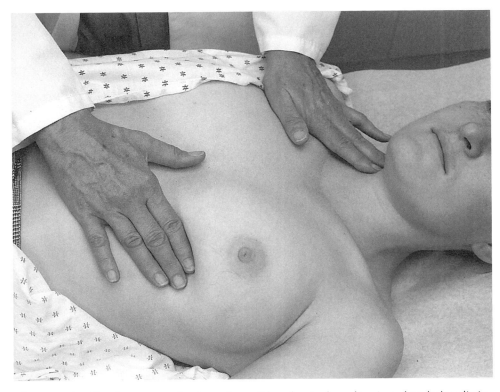

Figure 8.16 Simultaneous palpation of carotid and apical cardiac impulses helps distinguish abnormal cardiac pulsations; delineation of delayed carotid upstroke is better accomplished by timing the arterial pulse to the first heart sound while *auscultating* the latter.

Disrobing issues. *Privacy and modesty* do need to be respected. The former is obtained by pulling the bed curtain all the way around *and* closing the door. *Modesty* is served with a respectful and serious demeanor and the absence of non-professional comments about the patient's body. Failure to disrobe has many consequences (Table 8.7).

Upper body garments must be removed completely so that the entire pre-cordium is visible at once. Examination through clothing (Fig. 8.17) attenuates all cardiovascular and respiratory vibrations both for palpation and for auscultation and renders both inspection and percussion meaningless. Motion of the stetho-scope against clothing—typically a strap tugging at the tubing—or of clothing layers against one another or of clothing against skin can produce sound that is easily misinterpreted as cardiac. Leaving the brassiere on (Fig. 8.18), or lowering only one cup, or auscultating with the stethoscope insinuated into cleavage or under a cup represent well-meaning but utter failures to honor modesty and per-mit accurate diagnosis. If the patient is wearing a hospital gown, the examiner may erroneously reason, "the patient is so exposed already, let me not make it worse" (Fig. 8.19), or "there is no modest way to lower this to the waist and still keep the private parts covered." However, a sheet can serve the needed function. All attempts to leave the gown in place (Fig. 8.20) impair diagnosis, without which management can only be general and supportive.

Disrobing comfortably requires privacy and a degree of physical *warmth* beyond what clothed individuals need. A shivering patient experiences a miser-able contact with the medical system, and body movement can mask or mimic pathologically significant sound. Inadequate *lighting* hampers inspection and may lead to missing a clue about where to palpate or where to listen with special care.

Examiner physical discomfort. Physical discomfort for the examiner must also be avoided. Sometimes, auscultation needs to proceed for some time, and the attention of the examiner must progressively turn to her own growing backache from bending too far over a low bed or a table. There is nothing wrong with sit-ting down to settle in and focus on detailed findings: The goal is the welfare of the patient.

Patient fear. *Patient fear* is immense and too easily forgotten in the clinician's world of innumerable innocent extra sounds and murmurs. Therefore a warning in advance is sometimes comforting; e.g., "I'm a slow listener, so don't think I'm bothered. Breathe normally as though I weren't here. Feel free to nap."

Manipulation of Heart Sounds and Murmurs during Auscultation

Definitive information is scant in the massive literature on this topic. Worse, responses to individual maneuvers are not consistent enough to be pathogno-monic. Nevertheless, they can be useful.

Body position. Most sounds and murmurs become easier to hear with the patient in the *left lateral decubitus* position, perhaps simply because the heart tips toward the chest wall.

Table 8.7
Adverse Effects of Examination through Clothing

Obscures genuine diagnostic sound

Creates artifactual sound that is misconstrued as meaningful

May leave patient wondering why the clinician is diffident about performing the task (?self-confidence, ?competence)

May make patient wonder why his body is so distasteful as to be avoided or examined only cursorily

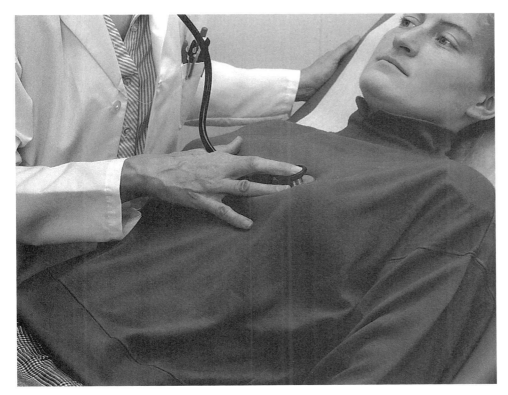

Figure 8.17   Errors in cardiac examination: auscultation through clothing. Haste or misguided modesty has led to filtering of important sound and the creation of extraneous sound.

The *standing* position reduces venous return and thus attenuates most cardiac sounds. Ideal comparison calls for listening at the site of greatest interest while the patient transfers from supine to seated to standing, a matter of considerable coordination. Once the patient is standing, have him *squat* while you keep listening. This maneuver increases venous return as the gravitational hydrostatic gradient between feet and heart is suddenly halved, but it also sharply increases afterload because of kinking of iliofemoral vessels attendant on sudden sharp flexion of the waist. In some instances you may stabilize the patient by squatting along with him. For the patient who has normal strength and balance and is in no danger of lurching or falling, however, you can remain seated throughout, reaching the stethoscope upward to the chest while the patient stands and lowering it with him when he squats. This helps you focus on the sound rather than attending to your own movements.

The *seated* position can bring out some pericardial rubs (Fig. 8.21) and some murmurs of aortic insufficiency. The legs may be dangled, and the trunk may be leaned slightly forward if necessary.

Valsalva maneuver. This is conducted as described in the Extended Examination section of Chapter 2. Reiterated briefly, the patient is instructed to push outward against a closed glottis, which in practical terms means *pushing out the abdomen* as far as possible, with a sustained effort. There should be no air movement, and the patient's face should turn red, and his veins should pop up after the maneuver has been in progress for some seconds. Once the patient has demonstrated the ability to perform the maneuver, he is told to relax again. Then the examiner auscultates the area in question, then asks the patient to perform the maneuver while the examiner listens uninterruptedly. It must be ended with the

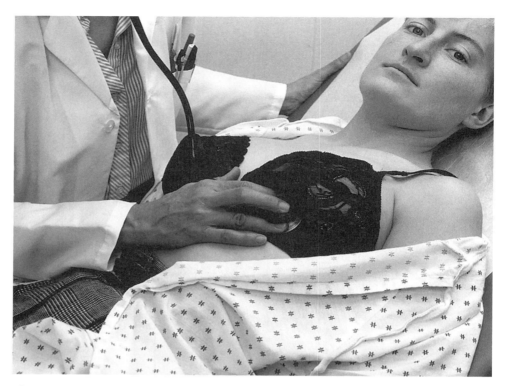

Figure 8.18   Errors in cardiac examination: auscultation through brassiere. The notion that this compromise produces a more favorable ratio of diagnostic accuracy to personal privacy is misguided.

instruction, "now breathe normally," after 15 seconds. However, auscultation continues for another 15 seconds thereafter.

Attention is paid to murmur intensity or timing of events, with comparison made to baseline at several distinct points in time: (*a*) 5–10 seconds after initiation, (*b*) immediately on release, (*c*) 1–2 heartbeats after release, and (*d*) 4–6 heartbeats after release. The opposite maneuver is called the *Müller* maneuver, and it is even more difficult for patients to perform. The patient must *inspire* against a closed glottis for this maneuver, so the instruction is, "Pull in your belly as tight as you can, and don't breathe." The timing of events and the need to auscultate continuously through the maneuver and beyond, parallel those of the Valsalva maneuver. The responses, however, are generally the opposite.

Handgrip.   The hemodynamic consequences of isometric exercise such as sustained handgrip include increases in heart rate, afterload, and blood pressure. Tell the patient, "While I listen, please grip this ball (or my fingers) as hard as you can. *Don't* stop breathing while you do so. Keep up the tight squeezing until I tell you to stop, and remember to breathe normally [Fig. 8.22]." This maneuver is contraindicated in symptomatic unstable coronary artery disease (unstable angina pectoris or acute myocardial infarction) and in symptomatic aortic stenosis, since it may precipitate serious arrhythmias in these settings. If the maneuver produces chest pain or breathlessness in any patient, the test is terminated promptly.

Passive straight-leg raising.   Unlike the preceding two maneuvers, passive straight-leg raising is feasible even if the patient cannot cooperate. Prompt straight-leg raising infuses 300–600 mL of blood from the high-capacitance leg veins into the circulating blood pool. Thus right-heart return increases almost at

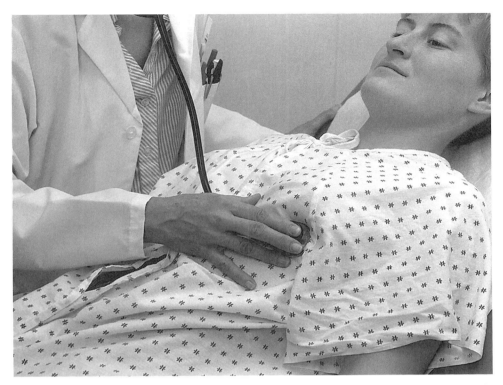

Figure 8.19   Errors in cardiac examination: auscultation through hospital gown. Same problem as in Figure 8.18.

once, and left-heart return soon afterward. While auscultating, the examiner can sometimes raise one of the patient's legs, but the two legs together are usually too heavy for the examiner, and the effort may be distracting. An assistant is most valuable. The examiner listens at the site in question, then instructs the assistant to raise both of the patient's legs and thighs, usually with knees locked, to 75° of hip flexion, and to keep them there. During continued auscultation, note the immediate effect on cardiac sound and any effect that is delayed 4–6 heartbeats, as well as corresponding changes immediately after relowering and 4–6 heartbeats after relowering.

Aortic insufficiency maneuvers. The early diastolic blowing murmur of aortic insufficiency is often hard to hear, both because of faintness and because of its high pitch. To enhance audibility and recognition of aortic insufficiency murmurs, certain special maneuvers have been developed. Three of these mechanically move the source of sound production closer to the stethoscope head by gravity:

1.   Have the seated patient lean forward, exhale deeply, and cease breathing for a few seconds (Fig. 8.23); this is the usual maneuver used to bring out or augment an aortic insufficiency murmur.
2.   Have the patient assume a knee-chest or knee-elbow (dog) position on the bed, so that the heart settles toward the anterior chest wall.
3.   Have the patient lie prone (face down) on the bed. Then have him turn his head away while you slip the diaphragm of the stethoscope between the sternum and the mattress or between the patient's breasts, with or without breath holding in expiration.

Other maneuvers rely on increasing afterload so that more backflow will occur, e.g., sustained handgrip and squatting. Any maneuver that slows the heart

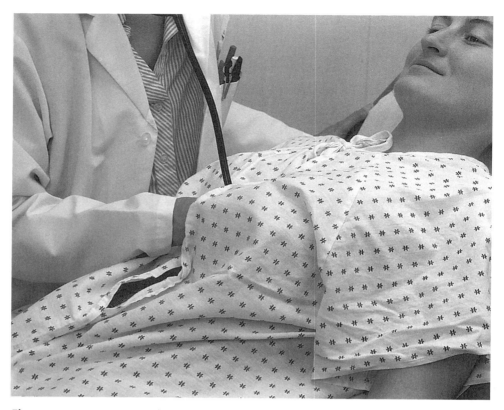

Figure 8.20   Errors in cardiac examination: auscultation around hospital gown, without proper exposure. Even if sound is not filtered, proper placement of the stethoscope is not ensured, and both inspection and palpation of the heart are hindered.

may relatively selectively lengthen diastole, so that both severity and duration of regurgitant flow tend to increase.

Postextrasystolic beat and cycle lengths.   This is not a maneuver but an experiment of nature. Postextrasystolic beats tend to have increased ventricular filling, increased stroke volume, and forceful contraction. These alterations may produce diagnostically useful changes in cardiac sound. Similarly, variations with preceding cycle length in atrial fibrillation may clarify as well as obscure diagnosis.

Respiration.   *Breath holding* allows the examiner to "subtract" dynamic respiratory phenomena from cardiac ones, but at the price of altered hemodynamics. Many patients inadvertently perform a Valsalva maneuver when asked to hold the breath, so a better wording for the request is, "Please stop breathing for a moment." Breath holding is justified in discriminating pericardial rubs from pleural rubs, but it has no role in determining splitting of the second heart sound or in seeking other acoustic phenomena that change with right-heart filling, such as murmur manipulation. For these, the Valsalva maneuver, passive straight-leg raising, and cycled respiration provide more reliable results.

Cycled respiration refers to intentionally slow, deep breathing that gives the examiner an opportunity to observe the effects of inspiration and expiration on acoustic phenomena. The patient is instructed by both words and demonstration and is reminded that for this maneuver, breathing is through the nose. (Oral breathing enhances airway sound, which confounds cardiovascular assessment.) Several breathing cycles are auscultated (Fig. 8.24). In contrast to the oral hyperp-

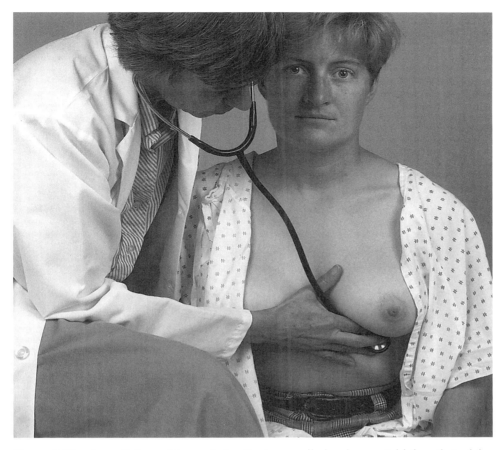

Figure 8.21   Auscultation of the seated patient generally has lower yield than that of the supine patient, but it may bring out some pericardial rubs that are inaudible with the patient in the supine position and may make a diagnosis of mitral valve prolapse more clear-cut.

nea employed for lung assessment, cycled respiration does not tire out the patient, make him dizzy, or produce alkalosis.

Transient arterial occlusion.   The systolic blood pressure is measured. Then an assistant places a sphygmomanometer around *each* upper arm and inflates both cuffs 30 torr above the systolic pressure. In the meantime, the examiner listens to the cardiac sound in question. Any change over the ensuing 30 seconds is noted, as are any changes for the 30 seconds after fully opening the valves of both cuffs so that their pressures fall to zero.

Amyl nitrite.   This pharmacologic agent is a potent, short-acting systemic vasodilator used to evaluate murmurs by manipulation. The patient is first advised of the nature of the drug and the procedure: "Any nausea, light-headedness, or racing pulse will last only briefly, after which you will return to normal." The patient is then asked to lie down (to avoid fainting), and cardiac auscultation is begun. An assistant measures the blood pressure and leaves the cuff in place. The ampule of amyl nitrite is broken, and the patient inhales the drug. (The expended ampule is dropped into a paper cup of water so that the drug is not released into the ambient air or inhaled by the examiner.) Blood pressure measurements decline sharply within 30 seconds, and there is a reflex increase in heart rate. All effects abate after a few minutes. Amyl nitrite is contraindicated in pregnancy, with hypertension, and with severe aortic stenosis.

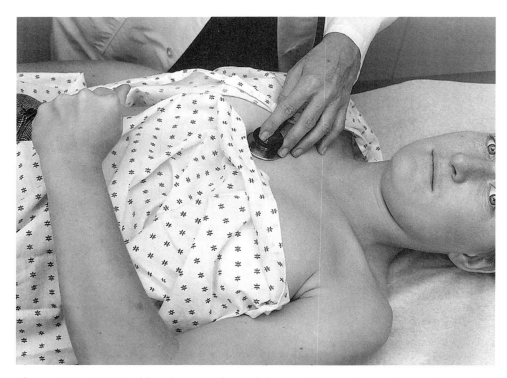

Figure 8.22 Sustained handgrip—with careful instructions *not* to perform an inadvertent Valsalva maneuver simultaneously—produces several hemodynamic changes that can help in murmur classification. *However, this maneuver is dangerous if the patient has aortic stenosis or coronary artery disease* and should be stopped at once if the patient experiences chest pain, dizziness, or breathlessness.

Abdominojugular maneuver. The patient lies supine although not necessarily flat. The trunk may be elevated with pillows for comfort. He breathes normally without straining. Pressure is applied to the midabdomen in a "trial run" to illustrate what will be done. The examiner observes for and counsels against an inadvertent Valsalva maneuver or other breath holding in response to pressure. After the demonstration, auscultation is resumed at the site of interest—typically the left lower sternal border, since tricuspid regurgitation is the usual murmur in question. While auscultation continues, firm pressure is applied with the palm and slightly spread fingers of one of the examiner's hands (Fig. 8.25). This pressure is maintained for 10 seconds at about 20 torr (20 mm Hg). Auscultation proceeds during compression and for some 10 seconds afterward. Despite the old name of "hepatojugular test," the pressure need *not* be applied to the liver. If no audible change in the murmur occurs with slow deep inspiration or with the abdominojugular maneuver alone, the two manipulations are combined. After full exhalation, unusually deep and slow inspiration is carried out for as long as possible short of breath holding, while the abdomen is pressed as before. Auscultation is continued after *sudden* release of both inspired air and abdominal pressure, in the hope that a sharp reduction in sound may be more acoustically recognizable than a slow augmentation during the maneuver.

Arteries

INTENSITY: SPECIAL FOCUS

The examiner feels paired radial, femoral, or foot arteries simultaneously, attending closely to asymmetry of force or timing. The carotids can be palpated sequen-

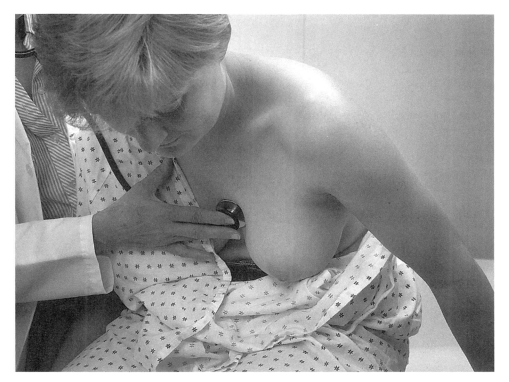

Figure 8.23   To bring out the murmur of aortic insufficiency, auscultation is performed with the patient leaning forward and holding breath in end-expiration. The effect is to bring the source of the sound waves closer to the stethoscope.

tially—not simultaneously—with attention given to the variable force of the pulse. Finally, with carotid auscultation, the examiner can pay attention to the clarity of transmission of the first heart sound (fainter) and second heart sound (loud). Normally both are audible, especially the second, and normally the intensity of heart sounds does not differ between one carotid and the other.

MURMUR IN THE CAROTID: FROM WHERE?

It commonly happens that a murmur-like sound is heard in one or both carotids during systole. If there is no systolic murmur at the right upper sternal border—the aortic valve focus—the examiner can safely infer that the sound arises from arteries and not from the heart. However, such sound may have arisen in the subclavian artery and have no adverse implications. The following sequence is recommended:

1. Listen at the right second intercostal space. If a systolic murmur is heard, inch the stethoscope slowly up, noting whether the sound intensity steadily attenuates, peaks in the supraclavicular fossa and then falls off, or reaches a nadir above the sternum and then grows louder, longer, or different in quality as you reach the carotid bifurcation.
2. If there is no cardiac murmur *or* if there is a more prominent sound in the supraclavicular fossa, reauscultate each carotid with the *shoulders hyperextended,* and note whether the carotid murmur is unchanged or greatly reduced by this maneuver.
3. If substantial suspicion of a loud sound of carotid origin persists, palpate the carotid a little longer, trying to ascertain the presence of a palpable systolic arterial *vibration*—not the pulse, but a sensation akin to a cardiac *thrill.* This is called a *shudder* in the case of the artery.

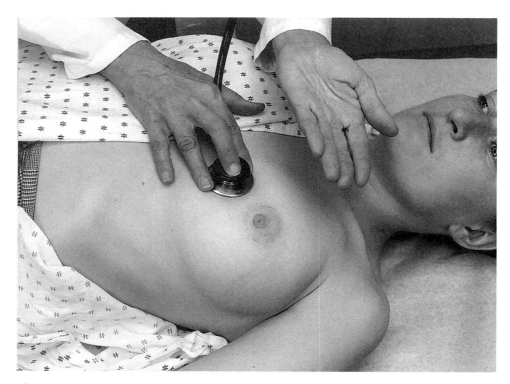

Figure 8.24   Slow deep breathing (cycled respiration) may augment recognition of hemodynamic changes related to respiratory cycle. Here the examiner indicates to the patient the need to continue inspiring, which will louden some tricuspid insufficiency murmurs.

4.   Continuous (systolic-diastolic) murmurs heard over the carotid can be presumed to have an arterial rather than a cardiac origin, but the same maneuvers to investigate the subclavian are indicated, as well as others to distinguish a cervical venous hum. These consist of listening with the patient upright (Fig. 8.26) and seeking obliteration of the sound with gentle compression of the jugular outflow at the clavicle (Fig. 8.27).

ERRORS IN CAROTID EXAMINATION

The commonest error is to listen too low (Fig. 8.28). The carotid bifurcation, the area of greatest interest, projects acoustically just below the angle of the jaw, a little higher than where the examiner usually palpates the carotid pulse. Listening too far anteriorly or posteriorly also hinders assessment. In a neck deformed by surgery, the highest point of palpable pulsation is a guide to the right spot; the anteroposterior locale at which carotid transmission of the normal second heart sound is loudest provides an independent confirmation.

Applying excess pressure to the artery is said to be able to produce arterial obstruction and devastating stroke. The incidence of this problem is unknown. Gentleness remains the watchword, whether palpating with digits or touching with the head of the stethoscope. The caveat applies to all patients, most vividly to those with suspected carotid atherosclerosis. So great is the concern, that even gentle bilateral simultaneous palpation of the carotids is discouraged.

A reversible complication of excess pressure on the carotid is creation of turbulence, with an artifactual systolic murmur or false bruit.

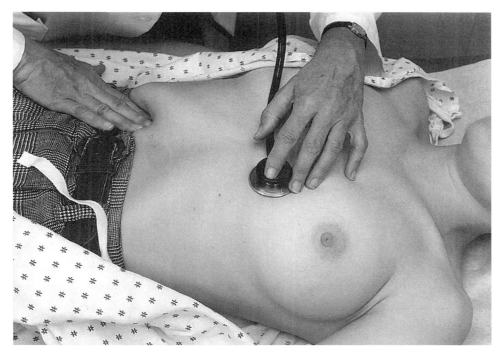

Figure 8.25 Abdominojugular test hemodynamics are also brought to bear in selective enhancement of some murmurs of right-heart origin, classically the systolic murmur of tricuspid insufficiency. By observing the jugular blood column at the same time, the examiner generates two data for the time and effort of one.

Great Veins
TECHNIQUE

The jugular venous blood columns present the most difficult part of the cardio-vascular examination to perform and interpret skillfully. Some examiners advocate looking at the *height* of the *external* jugular venous blood column and at *waveforms* in the much less distinct *internal* jugular. The latter is reflected in movements of the soft tissues of the neck slightly anterior to the external jugular and the common carotid artery. For assessment of jugular venous pressure, inspiration may render the vein more visible and prominent; raising and lowering the thorax can help, too. The normal pressure in the jugular veins ranges from 4 to 9 cm of water. For practical purposes the specific gravity of blood is considered equal to that of water, so that the column of blood aggregately filling the right atrium, superior vena cava, innominate vein, and jugular vein should extend 4–9 cm above the midpoint of the right atrium. The sternal angle of Louis lies 5 cm above the midpoint of the right atrium, whether the patient is supine, supported at 45°, or upright. Thus, in normal persons, the apex of the jugular venous blood column will lie anywhere from a point below view, to 4 cm above the angle of Louis. These simple facts have been obscured by widespread inattention to two key points:

- The *height* of the blood column, not its length, matters. The two numbers coincide only if the neck and chest are upright. Otherwise, the length of the column—the more "natural" measurement—is greater than the height. The relationship is that of the hypotenuse of a right triangle compared with a side (i.e., sine of the angle above supine × length of blood column = height of

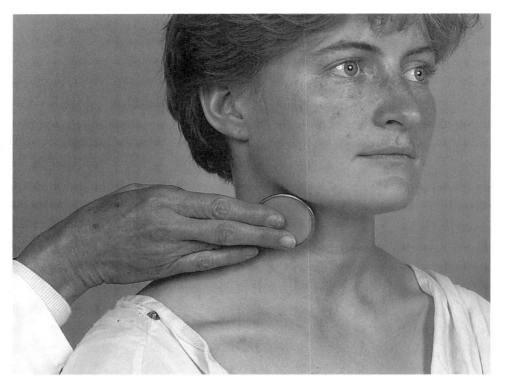

Figure 8.26   Auscultation of neck of seated patient. Discovery of a venous hum may depend on this maneuver.

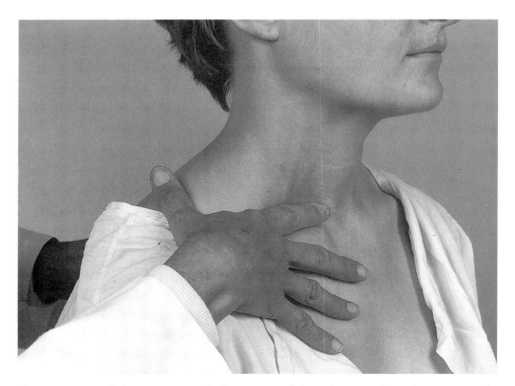

Figure 8.27   With the patient seated, the patency of this right external jugular vein is easily demonstrable by compressing the outflow against the clavicle.

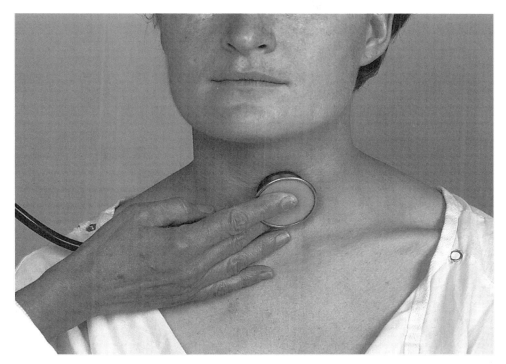

Figure 8.28 Errors in great-vessel examination: stethoscope placed too low on the neck. Real carotid bruits may be missed, and innocuous subclavian bruits may be made too much of.

blood column). This has been translated into clinical gadgets that are cumbersome and useless. If you cannot measure vertically for some reason, then measure the diagonal length of the column from the angle of Louis, and multiply the measurement by the sine of the body angle, bearing in mind that sine 30° equals 0.5 and sine 45° equals 0.71.

•   Then always remember to **add 5 cm** to estimate the central venous pressure!!

Practical examples. Four patients are seen, each with a measurable blood column 8 cm *long*. Patient A is supine, Patient B is at 30°, Patient C is at 45°, and Patient D is sitting bolt upright. What are their estimated central venous pressures (ECVPs)?

Patient A has no vertical dimension above the angle of Louis, except the width of the vein, and therefore has an ECVP = 0 + 5 cm, or 5 cm of water.

Patient B has a vertical dimension of (0.5) × (8 cm) = 4 cm above the angle of Louis + 5 cm, thus an ECVP = 9 cm of water.

Patient C has a vertical dimension of (0.71) × (8 cm) = 5.7 cm above the angle of Louis + 5 cm, therefore an ECVP = 10.7 cm of water.

Patient D has a vertical dimension of 8 cm above the angle of Louis + 5 cm, thus an ECVP = 13 cm of water.

Of course, pointing a ruler groundward from the apex of the blood column could give these answers much more easily!

The jugular veins do not have any visible filling above the clavicle in many normal persons. However, in a head-down or *Trendelenburg* position (Fig. 8.30) the angle of Louis lies *below* the level of the right atrium, and the jugular vein is always seen unless the central venous pressure is severely depressed or the vein has been obliterated. Tests for vein *patency* include gentle compression of the jugular outflow against the clavicle (Fig. 8.27), which should bring up the visibility of the blood column; observation during inspiration; and, with an easy-to-manipulate electric bed, progressively lowering the head of the bed and with it the patient's trunk, until the veins come into view (Figs. 8.29 and 8.30).

Neck vein inspection is aided by (a) relieving tension on the neck muscles, if need be by adding or removing a pillow, but in general by minimizing flexion of the neck on the chest, and (b) cross-lighting at a tangent to render the vein more visible. Some examiners advocate having the patient extend the neck a bit and rotate it slightly away from the examiner, but we often find this to be as detrimental as it is helpful.

All these maneuvers notwithstanding, many persons with fleshy necks—some without obesity—will have no assessable jugular blood columns or pulsations.

Inspiration normally *lowers jugular venous pressure.* The paradoxical elevation of venous pressure with inspiration is called *Kussmaul's sign.* Absence of any effect of inspiration on the height of the venous blood column suggests that that column is functionally uncoupled from the intrathoracic structures, e.g., that there is fibrous obliteration proximally, and therefore the examiner should instead employ the opposite jugular vein as a marker of intrathoracic events.

If *large* jugular pulsations are observed, time them with respect to audible heart sounds. An outward and/or upward bulge just before S_1 will be an "a" wave from *right* atrial contraction. Normally, this is the most prominent jugular pulsation. A bulge that coincides with S_2 will be a "v" wave, reflecting right ventricular contraction. The examiner can palpate the carotid pulse simultaneously, in which case an "a" wave should precede the carotid pulse and a "v" wave will follow it, but these are subtle distinctions that take years of practice to recognize.

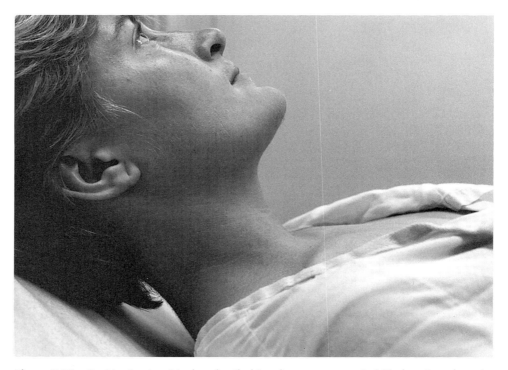

Figure 8.29   Positioning is critical to detailed jugular assessment. At 30° elevation, the vein may be invisible in many normal patients.

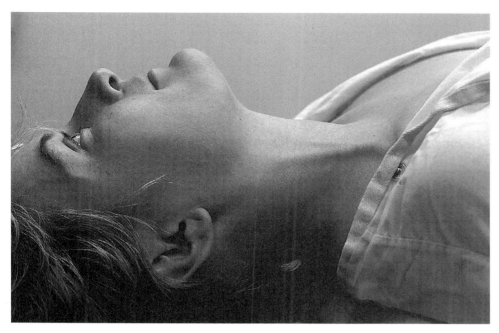

Figure 8.30 When the patient is lying flat or with head down (Trendelenburg position), the jugular veins should always be full, barring prior obliteration or severe intravascular volume depletion.

ABDOMINOJUGULAR TEST

The abdominojugular test has been described above in relation to murmur manipulation. When applied to the height of the jugular venous blood column, one precondition changes, and one new variable is measured. The **precondition** is an assessable jugular venous blood meniscus. In some patients with so much venous hypertension that the top of the jugular venous blood column cannot be seen below the angle of the jaw even with the trunk at 70°, the test cannot be performed. Nor is it feasible if a thick neck, depleted intravascular volume, or fibrous obliteration of veins prevents visualization. The **new variable** measured is not acoustic but is *visible* jugular blood column height. In performing the test, the height is measured in a position in which venous pulsations are most visible at baseline; then the jugular column is observed through 10 seconds of *Valsalva-free non-breath-holding* firm abdominal compression (Fig. 8.31), and for a few seconds after sudden release of this pressure on the abdomen. If the jugular venous pressure is unchanged throughout, the test is normal. If the pressure promptly rises 4 cm or more, then drops rapidly back to normal during abdominal compression, this too is considered negative. However, when there is a prompt rise of 4 cm or more which is sustained throughout the 10 seconds, and then a *prompt* drop of 4 cm or more on release, the result is abnormal. When a *slow* decrease toward baseline occurs during compression but a further sharp drop is observed on release, this is characterized as a positive test and is distinguished from the second type of negative largely by the drop-off on sudden release of abdominal pressure.

INTERPRETING THE FINDINGS
Heart
PALPATION

Impalpable and invisible apical impulses are common in normal people. An absent apical pulse cannot be inferred until the precordium has been searched from the fourth left costosternal junction to the sixth interspace in the anterior axillary line. Displaced apical impulses may be overlooked and are abnormal.

Medial displacement of the apical impulse occurs with reduced cardiac output, as in adrenohypocorticism (Addison's disease), and with compression of the heart by *hyperinflated lungs,* as in emphysema, asthma, or other obstructive airway disease.

Nonapical cardiac impulses, e.g., from anterior myocardial infarction with or without ventricular aneurysm formation, can be misconstrued as medial displacement of the apical beat, particularly if the apex impulse is not itself palpable. It is thus a sound practice to percuss 1 or 2 cm lateral to a suspected medially displaced apical impulse. If dullness is present, the impulse is ectopic rather than apical (or adjacent lung is consolidated). If resonance is elicited, it is apical. If the area is hyperresonant, the impulse is apical, and the reason for medial displacement is hyperinflation.

Left ventricular hypertrophy, classically from hypertensive heart disease or aortic stenosis, produces an increase in force, duration, and sometimes size of the apical impulse but does not displace it. An isolated increase in force may also reflect a hyperdynamic circulation, a common cause of hypertension in young adults and at times a transient complication of exertion or acute mental stress.

An isolated prolongation of the apex beat beyond the first third of systole may represent the effect of myocardial hypertrophy or delayed electrical activation complicated by slow mechanical contraction.

Any apical impulse exceeding 4 cm across should raise the question of dyskinesia, characteristically from left ventricular aneurysm.

Lateral displacement, with or without accompanying inferior displacement, is seen in left ventricular dilation. This may be physiologically adaptive, as in marathon runners, or it may reflect pathologic and counterproductive dilatation associated with elevated filling pressures. In the latter setting, it is associated with decompensation. This is found late in the course of hypertensive heart disease, aortic stenosis, and other conditions associated with myocardial hypertrophy.

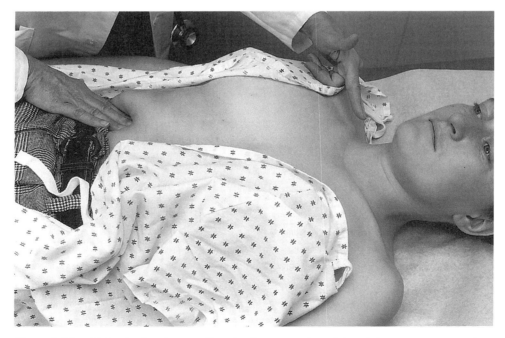

Figure 8.31   Abdominojugular test. Sustained compression of the abdomen causes a pathologic sustained elevation of the jugular venous blood column.

Apparent lateral displacement cannot be accepted as accurate if the apex beat is palpable only in the left lateral decubitus position, since this body position produces unpredictable movement of organs within the chest. By contrast, an apex beat that is unduly forceful, sustained, or enlarged in the left lateral decubitus position retains the same diagnostic meaning as if these findings appeared with the patient supine.

Palpable heart sounds and gallops have no separate significance from those that are only audible. However, whenever the pulmonic component of the second heart sound (S_2P) is palpable in an adult over 25 years of age, pulmonary hypertension is likely present.

Thrills

Thrills are nothing more than palpable murmurs, almost without exception systolic or continuous rather than diastolic. It is exceedingly rare to feel a thrill without hearing a murmur, but this can happen with very low-pitched sound. It is common, by contrast, to hear a murmur without feeling a thrill (at least in this technical sense!). In the grading of systolic murmurs, a thrill defines the murmur as grade 4/6 or above, therefore always significant diagnostically and usually significant hemodynamically and pathologically. Thrills appear to be more accurate than sound for murmur localization. There are four settings, one at each valve projection site, in which the discovery of a thrill has greatest clinical utility:

1. Consider the patient with a systolic ejection type murmur maximal at the right upper sternal border, in whom maneuvers have failed to discriminate between two or three of the following: aortic stenosis, hypertrophic cardiomyopathy, and innocuous "aortic sclerosis." Here a thrill at the right second intercostal space proves that the murmur is aortic stenosis and mandates special steps in diagnosis and management.
2. In the patient with a systolic ejection-type murmur that "ought" to arise from the aortic valve or that is associated with unexplained features presumed to reflect right-heart strain, a thrill at the second left intercostal space demonstrates pulmonic stenosis, whether in isolation or as part of a complex.
3. In the patient who has a long or holosystolic murmur that appears equal at the left lower sternal border and the apex and that will not reveal its origin with cycled respiration, the abdominojugular test, the Gooch maneuver or peripheral tests, a parasternal thrill establishes the cause as tricuspid regurgitation or ventricular septal defect, and an apical thrill establishes the cause as mitral regurgitation.
4. In the patient who has an apical systolic murmur that is not holosystolic and therefore does not obliterate both S_1 and S_2, an apical thrill proves that the murmur is mitral regurgitation, perhaps an acoustically atypical form such as occurs with mitral valve prolapse.

Right Ventricular Lift

An impulse distinct from the apex beat and not vibratory may lift the palpating hand at the left lower sternal border. This is a parasternal or right ventricular lift, the best bedside sign for right ventricular myocardial hypertrophy. (By contrast, excess jugular venous pressure or a positive abdominojugular test depends on some degree of decompensation or stiffening, and an increase in S_2P depends on audibility and on pulmonary hypertension as the cause, neither of which occurs universally.) Right ventricular lifts may rise to the hand and drop back from it a little less briskly than apex beats.

AUSCULTATION

Loud S_1

A loud first heart sound is the earliest physical sign of mitral stenosis, before the diastolic murmur, the opening snap, or atrial fibrillation appears. It is easily recognized when the first heart sound is louder than the second at the base, i.e., the second intercostal spaces. Loud S_1 sounds are also heard in tachycardia with short PR intervals, in hyperkinetic states such as anemia and thyrotoxicosis, and in any condition that enhances the force of left ventricular contraction.

Loud S_2

Since the usual dominant component of S_2 is S_2A, not S_2P, "loud S_2" not otherwise qualified refers to a loud aortic component. The determination is a judgment call. S_2 should exceed S_1 at the base, but when S_2 exceeds S_1 at the apex as well, S_2 may still (sometimes) be normal. The most common cause of a loud S_2 is systemic arterial hypertension. Along with the increased intensity of S_2 there often is heard a corresponding change in quality to a crisper, higher-pitched note. The adjective "tambouric" is often applied to this noise.

Soft S_2

All heart sounds grow softer with depression of myocardial function, as, for example, from septicemia. One author recalls obtaining emergency echocardiography, seeking pericardial effusion in a patient in the intensive care unit with *Klebsiella* septicemia whose heart sounds had become very faint. Studies revealed no effusion but a "stunned" myocardium that reversed, with normalization of heart sound intensity, after fluid resuscitation and effective antimicrobial therapy.

The differential diagnosis of global heart sound attenuation also includes anything that can mechanically alter sound *transmission* even if sound *production* is unchanged. Pericardial effusion and pneumothorax are two such problems, which can arise over hours or even less; emphysema is another, which develops over years.

Such mechanisms would *not* selectively diminish one cardiac sound in relation to others. Also, **selective** alterations in intensity do not change from day to day but change over years.

A soft aortic component of the second heart sound is described in aortic valvular stenosis. The differential diagnosis of a systolic ejection murmur, maximum at the aortic focus, includes (*a*) hemodynamically significant stenosis with a gradient and (*b*) the benign counterpart and possible precursor, so-called aortic sclerosis. The test is hampered by comorbidity in the aged. Perhaps because of the high prevalence of hypertension, with its opposite effect on S_2A, reduced amplitude of the aortic component occurs only in a minority of proven cases of aortic stenosis in the aged. Unfortunately, a decreased S_2A also does not conclusively establish aortic valvular stenosis.

Loud S_2P

In a patient above age 25, an S_2P that is louder than S_2A carries only two differential diagnoses: pulmonary hypertension or a reduced S_2A. Distinction between the two is usually very simple. If splitting of S_2, with expected respiratory variation, is audible at the cardiac **apex**, S_2P is by definition increased, and pulmonary hypertension is present, whether or not S_2A is reduced also.

If the examiner relies exclusively on the expected sequence of S_2A preceding S_2P and hears a louder second component of the second heart sound, an error can creep in: When splitting is paradoxical (see below), the pulmonic component

(S_2P) will precede the aortic (S_2A), and this splitting will occur only in *expiration,* not in inspiration. If the clinician ignores the respiratory phase in which the sound is heard, she may misinterpret the normally louder S_2A, because it comes last, as an abnormally increased S_2P.

In seeking this most important sign, bear in mind that normal inspiratory splitting of S_2 may be best heard anywhere from the first to the fourth intercostal space at the left sternal border, and may sometimes transmit to the right upper sternal border. Thus the mere presence of an audible S_2P at any of these sites, in contrast to its presence at the apex, does not prove increased intensity or pulmonary hypertension.

Single Second Heart Sound

Inspiratory splitting of the second heart sound is audible in most normal children and young adults who are examined supine, in some but not all normal middle-aged adults, and in only a few normal aged adults. Thus a single second heart sound cannot pinpoint the presence or absence of heart disease.

Audible Expiratory Splitting

Many normal young people, and some older ones as well, when examined *supine,* have a narrowly split second heart sound in expiration that splits further with inspiration, i.e., that widens physiologically. For most of these persons, moving to the seated or standing position will obliterate the audible expiratory splitting, as decreased right-heart return speeds right ventricular ejection. If there are no other indications of cardiorespiratory disease, if the aortic and pulmonic components of S_2 are individually normal in character, and if the splitting widens further with inspiration—i.e., is neither paradoxical nor fixed—*and* if sitting ablates the finding, no further investigation is needed, and the finding can be regarded as normal. If all of the above applies except that audible expiratory splitting persists when the patient is seated or standing, it is likely that the patient has a right bundle-branch block, a common stable abnormality without ominous significance. (*Acute* right bundle-branch block in clinical acute right-heart strain is another story but is clinically obvious from acute symptomatic respiratory or right-heart disease, right ventricular lift, rapid development of elevated jugular venous pressure, edema, and hepatic congestion.) Intermittent audible expiratory splitting with compensatory pauses afterward may come from premature ventricular contractions in the left ventricle.

Paradoxical Splitting

If there is audible expiratory splitting of the second heart sound but the components of the second sound *fuse on inspiration,* paradoxical splitting is present. A short differential diagnosis of etiologies applies: (*a*) Delayed electrical activation of the left ventricle, or (*b*) delayed mechanical contraction of the left ventricle, or (*c*) premature contraction of the right ventricle may be responsible. When paradoxical splitting is diagnosed, bear in mind that the sequence of components is reversed, so that as discussed above, you will hear a soft component first, then a loud one (S_2P, *then* S_2A) if the intensity of the two components is normal.

Delayed electrical activation of the left ventricle is seen in *left bundle-branch block,* an "incidental" finding with adverse prognosis. Paradoxical splitting of the second heart sound thus requires investigation, although some causes are innocuous. *Artificial pacemakers* depolarize the right ventricle first, so their effect on timing resembles that of left bundle-branch block. Hence, in the patient with a pacemaker, if both components of the second heart sound are audible, and assuming there is no antecedent left bundle-branch block, paradoxical splitting of the second heart sound is a *reassuring* finding that the artificial pacemaker is firing and capturing.

Premature contraction of the right ventricle is seen in (spontaneous) premature ventricular contractions of right-heart origin. Premature contractions of left ventricular origin are far more common than those from the right heart. On occasion, with concentration *and luck,* you can determine the ventricle of origin with the stethoscope. Compare the second heart sound in the premature contraction with that of the background regular beats in relation to phase of respiration. If the premature contraction occurs in expiration and shows wide splitting, whereas subsequent regular beats show the physiologic pattern of inspiratory splitting and expiratory fusion, right ventricular depolarization was delayed in the premature contraction, which must have been a conventional premature (left) ventricular contraction.

Delayed mechanical contraction of the left ventricle can occur with marked myocardial hypertrophy, as with hypertensive heart disease and aortic stenosis. These settings are also prone to left bundle-branch block, so that the physical finding of paradoxical splitting does *not* allow prediction of the ECG pattern. In addition, *ischemic myocardium* can sometimes display delayed or defective electromechanical coupling, with paradoxical splitting of the second sound, with or without left bundle-branch block, as its chief or sole bedside manifestation.

Fixed Splitting

Fixed splitting does not refer to dynamic splitting throughout the respiratory cycle, i.e., audible expiratory splitting. Rather, fixed splitting is continuous *static* splitting in which there is no respiratory variation in the timing of S_2P with respect to S_2A. It can be taken as evidence of equilibration of pressures between the two atria, obliterating differential timing of contraction between the two ventricles. The classical causative condition is *atrial septal defect,* but several caveats apply:

1. There are cases of atrial septal defect without this finding, so it is not a perfect indicator.
2. Persistence of the finding after successful surgical closure of atrial septal defects has been reported repeatedly and would seem to destroy the pathophysiologic explanation offered above.
3. Equally counterintuitive, fixed splitting does not occur in large *ventricular* septal defects, in which one would expect parallelism of right- and left-heart pressures.
4. The finding rarely occurs in other conditions, including pulmonary embolism.

Despite these gaps in understanding of fixed splitting, its recognition can produce lifesaving intervention in an asymptomatic host at risk of developing irreversible pulmonary vascular damage over time. If fixed splitting is present, *whether or not S_2P is increased,* especially if there is a systolic murmur at the second left intercostal space, the likelihood of atrial septal defect is high.

Third Heart Sounds

In children and healthy young adults, third heart sounds are normal and deserve no separate attention. In athletes and perhaps other normal adults up to age 40, the same appears to be true. However, above age 40, S_3 is always considered abnormal. It is seen in some cases of mitral regurgitation in the absence of heart failure, but except in this setting it signifies cardiac failure. Unfortunately, depending on the examiner's skill, the patient's individual characteristics, and the mode of examination, the sign is lacking in many patients with proven heart failure. Therefore, S_3 is "valuable only when heard," and no inference can be drawn from its absence; i.e., heart failure is not ruled out when there is no S_3. A third heart sound is sometimes the first or only physical sign of heart failure. Sometimes, early heart failure is suspected but can only be demonstrated by the presence of this sign, when the usual concomitants such as peripheral edema, pulmonary crackles, elevated jugular venous pressure, and pleural effusion are lacking.

The factors that most often prevent detection of an S_3 that is actually present include ambient noise; obesity; emphysema; failure to apply the bell precisely to the cardiac apex; excess pressure with the bell, which dampens or abates low-frequency sound; and examination with the patient in the *seated* position, because transfer to bed or examining table is considered too cumbersome or time-consuming. When an S_3 is sought vigorously, because management will be altered, all correctable items on the preceding list are reversed. Then auscultation is repeated, and still again as the patient rolls into the left lateral decubitus position and spends a few seconds in that position, and if need be, yet once more after return to the supine position. Rarely, the exertion of rolling "back into place" causes the sound to emerge. If the patient cannot move or be moved onto the left side, passive straight-leg raising may bring out a latent S_3.

If the heart rate is over 100 beats/minute, discrimination of third from fourth heart sounds is impossible, and a "galloping" triple rhythm is designated as a **summation gallop.** This may represent an S_4, an S_3, or both. Until the rate is slowed, the examiner can only guess which it is (unless there is atrial fibrillation, which precludes S_4).

A loud apical sound heard after S_2 in some cases of pericardial constriction is called a pericardial knock. Some observers consider it unique. Others designate it a high-pitched, early, and prominent variant of S_3.

Right Heart Gallops, the Clavicle, and the Supraclavicular Fossa

The preceding segment discusses gallops arising from the left heart and localizing to the apex. However, *right atrial* gallops may produce S_4 sounds. *Right ventricular* S_3 sounds are located at the left lower sternal border rather than the apex and often increase with inspiration, whereas their left-heart counterparts can soften with inspiration and increase in expiration. Sometimes, a gallop is equal at both the tricuspid focus and apex or is loudest in between. If the effect of inspiration fails to establish its origin, auscultation in the right supraclavicular fossa sometimes helps. Right-heart gallops may radiate there, whereas left-heart gallops do not. The sensitivity of this test is poor: A positive test implies right-heart origin, but the absence of supraclavicular radiation does not prove left-heart origin.

Emphysema can produce cor pulmonale and, with it, right-heart gallops. Its sound attenuation may obscure precordial audibility of a right ventricular S_3; the supraclavicular fossa may then be the best place to find the right-heart gallop. If the right fossa is silent, the left will occasionally reveal the gallop, although the right generally has a higher yield.

In deciding about chamber of origin, if passive straight-leg raising causes an S_3 to appear 4 or 5 heartbeats after the maneuver is undertaken and the gallop persists 4 or 5 heartbeats after release, consider a left ventricular origin over a right, whereas if responses occur within the first or second heartbeat, favor the right. Investigation and corroborative research are lacking, however.

Although aortic valvular murmurs are usually diminished when transmitted to the right supraclavicular fossa, empiric study shows amplification in many instances over the middle of the right clavicle (the bone). A murmur exhibiting this phenomenon is presumed to arise from the aortic valve: from stenosis or possibly sclerosis if it is systolic; and from aortic regurgitation if it is diastolic.

Responses to Maneuvers

Body position. *In general,* supine auscultation optimizes intensity and clarity of cardiac sound. However, occasional heart sounds and murmurs—sometimes unpredictably—are louder in other positions. The left lateral decubitus position not only enhances gallops, as noted above, but also can bring out the opening snap and the murmur of mitral stenosis.

Rapid *standing,* whether from a seated or squatting position, reduces venous return and therefore right ventricular filling. Left ventricular filling inevitably falls soon afterward. Thus the systolic murmurs of mitral prolapse and hypertrophic cardiomyopathy are often lengthened or loudened. By contrast, the decreased stroke volume sometimes decreases murmurs of aortic stenosis. In nonprolapse mitral regurgitation, the direction of change is unpredictable.

Squatting augments venous return but simultaneously increases afterload and has complex effects on blood pressure. Squatting has unpredictable effects on systolic murmurs including mitral regurgitation other than prolapse, and generally decreases those of hypertrophic cardiomyopathy. It increases most aortic insufficiency murmurs and brings out some that were silent before.

Sitting may disclose pericardial rubs and aortic insufficiency murmurs not heard before. When the position is chosen because of suspected aortic insufficiency, leaning forward is also included.

Valsalva and Müller maneuvers. Many patients cannot perform a Valsalva maneuver even with detailed demonstration and instruction. With others, so much extraneous noise is created from noncardiac sources that cardiac sound becomes indistinguishable.

If cardiac sound is assessable, most murmurs decrease during the strain phase, but two–thirds of hypertrophic cardiomyopathy murmurs increase. Because of a 30% rate of unexplained murmur *reduction* in hypertrophic cardiomyopathy, Valsalva response cannot be adduced as proof that a systolic murmur is *not* from this source. Some mitral prolapse murmurs also increase, but also with poor reliability.

On release of strain, resumption of normal murmur intensity within 1 or 2 heartbeats suggests a right-heart origin, whereas a delay for several additional beats implicates the left side of the heart, e.g., aortic stenosis rather than pulmonic stenosis. Intuitively, the same timing criterion should apply to "falloff" in tricuspid prolapse as compared with mitral prolapse, but data are lacking.

The Müller maneuver can augment right-heart murmurs and diminish or abate the murmur of hypertrophic cardiomyopathy, but inconsistently.

Handgrip. Sustained handgrip isometric exercise (Fig. 8.22) can be dangerous, as described above. It can also produce uninterpretable auscultatory changes if there is a simultaneous Valsalva maneuver. When these limitations do not apply, it increases murmur intensity in at least two thirds of patients with mitral regurgitation or ventricular septal defect, in a minority of those with aortic stenosis (on whom you should not perform this test!), and in still fewer with right-heart murmurs. It sometimes increases the murmur of aortic sclerosis but, again, ought not be done because of the prospect that the murmur is aortic *stenosis.* It decreases the murmur of hypertrophic cardiomyopathy very consistently but, "paradoxically," also reduces some mitral regurgitation murmurs (?from mitral prolapse). Thus the test does not display sufficiently distinctive patterns to permit systolic murmur diagnosis by itself.

Among diastolic murmurs, both mitral stenosis and aortic regurgitation are usually increased.

More useful clinically is the effect of handgrip in bringing out a ventricular gallop (S₃) that was previously occult or a latent opening snap.

Passive straight-leg raising. The suddenly increased venous return that occurs with passive straight-leg raising mimics some effects of squatting but without the change in afterload. Thus many murmurs increase, whereas most of those due to hypertrophic cardiomyopathy are reduced.

Aortic insufficiency maneuvers. Aortic insufficiency is often difficult to hear. Usually, the problem is not how to *interpret* a high-pitched diastolic murmur but rather how to *find* it at all. Depending on how vigorously you need to look and how much and how long the patient is willing to try, any subset from the top down is recommended, and then Maneuver 9 is followed:

1. Perform conventional supine auscultation with diaphragm.
2. Repeat auscultation with the patient seated and leaning forward as far as possible.
3. Add breath holding in end-expiration.
4. Delete breath holding, and add isometric handgrip if no contraindications to isometric exercise exist.
5. Repeat auscultation with the patient promptly squatting.
6. Repeat auscultation with isometric handgrip with the patient in the squatting position if there is no contraindication to isometric exercise.
7. Repeat auscultation with the patient prone or on all fours.
8. Repeat Maneuver 7 with breath held in end-expiration and/or with isometric handgrip if there is no contraindication.
9. If murmur is audible, assess (*a*) location and (*b*) effect of slow deep inspiration, to help distinguish aortic insufficiency from pulmonic insufficiency. If you are still unsure, assess slow versus quick change after release of Valsalva. If these maneuvers are unsuccessful, consider the use of amyl nitrite.

Postextrasystolic beat and cycle length in atrial fibrillation. The postextrasystolic beat or the hemodynamically analogous beat after a long cycle length in atrial fibrillation is associated with *increased* murmur intensity in aortic stenosis but not in mitral regurgitation. The constancy of mitral regurgitation murmur intensity despite variable filling does *not*, however, apply to ischemic papillary muscle dysfunction, where murmur intensity may *decrease* in the postextrasystolic beat. Other murmurs tend to increase if they are due to ventricular outflow obstruction, e.g., pulmonic stenosis, and to remain unchanged if they are not of this obstructing type. However, in hypertrophic cardiomyopathy, results are variable.

Cycled respiration. Inspiratory augmentation is highly characteristic of the right-sided systolic murmur of tricuspid regurgitation, which correspondingly, then, shows expiratory diminution. (Pulmonic stenosis murmurs, however, usually *diminish* with inspiration.) Many left-sided systolic murmurs do not change appreciably with respiratory phase. Those that do, diminish on inspiration and increase on expiration. Right-sided diastolic murmurs may be inconsistent, but if an inspiratory increase is found in a diastolic murmur, the origin is *probably* the right heart. Breath holding produces a Valsalva maneuver in most persons and alters hemodynamics in such a complex manner that it cannot be used to reproduce these manipulations. Rather, engage the patient in dynamic, ongoing respiration that is somewhat slower and deeper than normal, i.e., cycled respiration.

If tricuspid regurgitation is suspected and inspiratory augmentation of a holosystolic murmur (*Carvallo's sign*) has been negative, the abdominojugular test is performed. If there is no change with the latter, both tests are done at once as *Gooch's test*. If the murmur increases, tricuspid regurgitation is very likely. If localization, radiation, and manipulation fail to distinguish mitral from tricuspid regurgitation, amyl nitrite may discriminate between the two.

Transient arterial occlusion. In limited studies, at 20 seconds after transient arterial occlusion, most mitral regurgitation and ventricular septal defect murmurs increase, and none of them decreases, whereas other systolic murmurs remain constant or decrease. The maneuver does not discriminate between mitral regurgitation and ventricular septal defect. If there is no change in the murmur with the maneuver, no conclusion can be drawn about its origin. This method appears to be more sensitive than squatting, as sensitive as handgrip and amyl nitrite inhalation for identification of left-sided regurgitant murmurs, and more specific than both squatting and isometric handgrip for this distinction. Among diastolic murmurs, transient arterial occlusion increases aortic insufficiency, but data are scant.

Amyl nitrite. Because of decreased systemic vascular resistance, murmurs of left-sided regurgitant lesions—aortic insufficiency and mitral regurgitation—decrease with amyl nitrite inhalation or, at least, do not increase. Patent ductus arteriosus should decrease also.

Innocuous aortic flow murmurs, as well as aortic stenosis and hypertrophic cardiomyopathy murmurs, usually increase. If the issue is a forward flow murmur from the left ventricular outflow tract versus mitral regurgitation, discrimination is good. (Transient arterial occlusion may supplant this use of the drug.)

The pulmonic flow murmur associated with atrial septal defect increases with amyl nitrite inhalation, as does that of pulmonic stenosis; but the systolic murmur of the tetralogy of Fallot does not.

Tricuspid regurgitation and mitral stenosis increase as well. Pulmonic insufficiency increases or remains constant, in contrast to the diminution of aortic insufficiency. The diastolic Austin Flint murmur, which has elements of aortic insufficiency, should decrease. Its distinction from pure mitral stenosis is a chief function of amyl nitrite. The distinction between mitral and tricuspid regurgitation can be made because amyl nitrite characteristically decreases mitral regurgitation murmurs but increases tricuspid regurgitation or leaves it unchanged.

Ventricular septal defect with left-to-right shunt (i.e., without supervening Eisenmenger physiology) often decreases. However, it can increase in the setting of marked pulmonary hypertension.

In mitral prolapse both murmur and clicks respond to amyl nitrite too variably for diagnostic use.

Pericardial Rubs and Mediastinal Crunches

Pericardial rubs have up to three components that encompass portions of both systole and diastole. They are of medium pitch and often sharply localized either over the mesocardium (midprecordium) or elsewhere. They are often best heard with the diaphragm and with the patient seated and leaning forward. They are distinguished from pleural rubs by *synchrony with the cardiac cycle* rather than with the respiratory cycle. If this is inapparent, transient breath holding is undertaken. Remind the patient not to perform a Valsalva maneuver.

Pericardial rubs can be evanescent and recurrent. The examiner needs to be comfortable with this subtlety. Failure to hear a rub that somebody else has heard is *not* an auscultatory deficit but a common corollary of the nature of the sound.

Mediastinal crunches have been described not only with pneumomediastinum, and with inflammation in the mediastinum, but also in a small minority of left pneumothoraces without pneumomediastinum. If a crunchy or popping sound is heard over the precordium, radiographs directed to the discovery of extrapulmonary air are mandatory. Some mediastinal crunches are position-dependent.

Some are associated with visible subcutaneous popping, and some are perceptible to the patient's unaided ear.

Opening Snaps and Ejection Clicks

Opening snaps are sharp diastolic sounds that are best known in mitral stenosis but can also occur in mitral regurgitation, in ventricular septal defect, and rarely in high-output states. They are of medium to high pitch and sometimes tightly localized, although in other instances they radiate widely. They occur at the apex or the left lower sternal border or in between. It is suggested that they be sought, when clinically suspected, with the patient supine. The diaphragm of the stethoscope is inched from the second left intercostal space downward and then laterally. If the snap is still not found, it is resought during and after a roll of the patient into the left lateral decubitus position. A further enhancement is handgrip exercise (if not contraindicated).

When the opening snap occurs rapidly after S_2, the severity of mitral stenosis is greater than when the S_2A-OS interval is wider. However, a host of other factors affect this timing. In the present era of low prevalence of mitral stenosis, no individual examiner will gain great expertise in this assessment. However, one mnemonic is generalizable and deserves reiteration. When one says "Pa-Pa," a time span of 0.10 second, corresponding to the S_2A-OS interval in milder stenosis, is approximated. If one says "Pa-Da," this takes 0.05–0.07 second, suggesting more severe mitral stenosis. (These phrases can be applied to the timing of *any* clinical event.)

Opening snaps can mimic third heart sounds, although S_3 usually has a lower frequency and comes later. The distinction may become impossible with tachycardia.

Distinction from S_2P may be difficult when the opening snap is well heard all the way up to the left second intercostal space. However,

- If *three* sounds are heard at the end of systole in inspiration, they should be S_2A, S_2P and OS, in that order.
- If a physiologic split is heard, the later component must be S_2P, since an opening snap does not migrate with respect to S_2A during the respiratory cycle, although it may soften on inspiration.
- Standing will narrow the S_2A-S_2P interval but not an S_2A-OS interval.
- Unless there is pulmonary hypertension, manifest as an accentuated S_2P, any *sharp* sound after S_2A at the apex should be an opening snap, not S_2P.

Opening snaps can be absent in mitral stenosis, particularly when the mitral valve leaflets have become heavily calcified. Therefore, the lack of an opening snap does not militate against the diagnosis.

Ejection clicks occur in systole, usually early but sometimes at midsystole or at multiple points. They are found in aortic stenosis, in pulmonic stenosis, and sometimes in other conditions, but they are *not* found in mitral prolapse, whose clicks are not of the ejection type. Ejection clicks are sharp, high-pitched sounds, and their chief import is (*a*) to be recognized as related to the valvular lesion and not taken for some other sound such as a split S_1 or S_1 following S_4 (if the antecedent S_1 is misinterpreted as a high-pitched atrial gallop) and (*b*) to be distinguished, if possible, from the mid- to late-systolic nonejection clicks of mitral prolapse.

Systolic Ejection Murmurs

Systolic ejection murmurs are diamond-shaped murmurs that do not obscure S_1, which precedes them, or S_2, which follows them. The following are the key questions to be answered about such a murmur: Is it hemodynamically significant, and will its cause progress to a point of compromising the patient's cardiorespiratory function? Is it a regurgitant lesion (of atypical acoustic characteristics) that calls for prophylaxis against infective endocarditis when a bacteremia is anticipated? Or is it innocuous and stable?

Characteristics that *in aggregate* rather than individually increase confidence that a given systolic murmur is innocuous are

- Absence of cardiorespiratory symptoms including with exercise
- Normal, regular apical pulse rate
- Normal respiratory rate
- Normal carotid upstrokes, jugular venous pressure, and jugular waveforms
- Normal lung examination
- Normal location and *character* of apex beat
- Absence of associated thrill where maximal murmur intensity is heard, and absence of radiation to the axilla
- Normal timing and *characteristics* of first and second heart sounds, whether or not splitting of S_2 is present
- Absence of associated diastolic murmur
- Short duration, occupying one-half of systole or less, and nonharsh sound quality
- Absence of S_3 when the patient is over 40 years of age (absence of S_4 *not* necessary in this case; absence of S_3 not necessary when the patient is under 40 years of age)
- Absence of second systolic murmur elsewhere in the precordium and of ejection clicks
- Absence of augmentation by Valsalva maneuver
- If extant, normal chest x-ray, ECG, and echocardiogram

There are many patients with systolic ejection murmurs who fail one or more of these criteria but who lack heart disease. Conversely, serious pathology may occasionally slip through this net, e.g., dangerous hypertrophic cardiomyopathy in an asymptomatic young athlete whose murmur belongs to the minority that are disguised by failure to increase with the Valsalva maneuver. Hypertrophic cardiomyopathy and aortic stenosis (as sources of systolic ejection murmurs) are associated with sudden, sometimes calamitous complications rather than with the slower development of compromised circulation.

Whether this prognostic test list has or has not been passed, *location* and *radiation* remain key elements in deciding the site of origin and therefore the most likely pathology if any. When factors are present that raise cardiac output above baseline, such as fever, intravascular volume depletion, marked anemia, severe mental stress, pregnancy, or thyrotoxicosis, one additional strategy can be simple *observation*, if deemed safe, for response after alleviation of reversible factors.

Accurate timing is preeminent: Working up a systolic murmur as though it were diastolic is most futile! Although the atrioventricular valve regurgitant murmurs are often "box shaped" and overlie S_1 and S_2, exceptions exist: Mitral regurgitation remains a consideration when a "systolic ejection murmur" is loudest at the apex, lasts through the final two-thirds of systole, and increases with transient arterial occlusion. Distinction between aortic stenosis, aortic sclerosis, and hypertrophic cardiomyopathy is covered under Manipulation of Heart Sounds and Murmurs, above, and Aged Patients with Basal Systolic Murmurs, below.

Mitral Prolapse

Mitral prolapse, a diagnosis made in a far higher percentage of echocardiograms than of physical examinations, has become a "swamp." A subset of mitral prolapse patients need endocarditis prophylaxis, and a few are at risk of progressive mitral regurgitation with consequent left-heart dysfunction. Several features simplify interpretation:

- If S_1 is followed by a midsystolic click and then a mitral regurgitation-type "square" murmur occupies the latter part of systole beyond this point, mitral prolapse is present, and there is enough valvular regurgitation that endocarditis prophylaxis is indicated.

- If there is no murmur but there is a mid- or late-systolic click (or more than one click), best heard at the apex, mitral prolapse is probable. Without auscultatory evidence of mitral regurgitation, the need for prophylaxis is not agreed on.

- If there is an apical systolic murmur only, without a click, mitral regurgitation is present, and the question becomes one of distinguishing mitral prolapse from nonprolapse mitral regurgitation. In mitral prolapse, the active strain phase of the Valsalva maneuver can increase both duration and amplitude of the murmur, which does not happen in nonprolapse mitral regurgitation. Thus if the murmur begins earlier during the Valsalva strain phase and loudens, with reversal of these changes a few beats after release, mitral prolapse with mitral regurgitation can be diagnosed confidently. Failure to show these changes *does not exclude* mitral prolapse.

- Demographic features play a role. A young Caucasian woman will probably have mitral prolapse as the cause of mitral regurgitation and has little risk of progression. An older man is likely to have a nonprolapse cause. However, if mitral prolapse is proven, he will have a higher risk of progression to hemodynamic dysfunction.

- Murmurs that obliterate both S_1 and S_2 at the apex are less likely to be mitral prolapse and are more likely to be nonprolapse mitral regurgitation. *Nonholosystolic* mitral regurgitation is usually nonrheumatic but not necessarily prolapse.

- It is the (unexplained) nature of mitral prolapse to change auscultatory features from day to day. Similar variability is not characteristic of other mitral regurgitation murmurs. Thus,

  —If mitral prolapse is suspected but some features are missing or equivocal, you can relisten on other occasion(s) and/or with manipulations. The picture may become clear either because classical features emerge or because mutability itself supports the diagnosis.

  —A more prominent mitral regurgitation murmur on a second visit does *not* necessarily mean that a case of mitral prolapse is progressing. The pattern and consistency of change in physical signs, as well as associated symptoms of left-heart dysfunction or arrhythmia, must be considered in a total context, which often includes serial echocardiography as well.

  —In deciding about endocarditis prophylaxis, one instance of audible mitral regurgitation warrants prophylaxis. However, given the variability, the *absence* of the murmur on a first hearing does not exclude the need. The examiner can relisten on other days. If no murmur is ever present, many clinicians would omit prophylaxis. Alternatively, the clinician can try maneuvers to bring out the murmur. The Valsalva maneuver lengthens it and moves the click earlier, sometimes causing it to fuse with S_1. Squatting has sometimes been employed. If maneuvers fail to bring out an audible murmur, many examiners are satisfied that there is no need for prophylaxis.

  —The auscultator need not be troubled about the auscultatory competence of someone who misses mitral prolapse. As with pericardial rubs, detection depends not only on skill but also on listening when the abnormality happens to announce itself noisily.

Holosystolic Murmurs

The chief holosystolic murmurs are mitral regurgitation and tricuspid regurgitation. In addition, some cases of ventricular septal defect and of patent ductus arteriosus give rise to holosystolic murmurs. The latter two are seldom differential diagnostic problems. The murmur of ventricular septal defect is usually loudest parasternally, is often associated with a prominent parasternal thrill, and tends to have a pure *decrescendo* shape diminishing from its origin until it disappears before or with S_2, which it sometimes obscures. Since left ventricular pressure exceeds right ventricular pressure throughout most or all of the cardiac cycle (except in the case of Eisenmenger physiology), ventricular septal defects can also produce a subtle or softer diastolic murmur, rendering the murmur *continuous* although not *uniform*. A most important cause of a new ventricular septal defect murmur in the adult is *perforation of the interventricular septum from myocardial infarction* involving the septum. Such perforation characteristically calamitously worsens heart failure, producing prominent congestion of the systemic veins rather than the pulmonary vasculature. Its murmur and thrill, unlike those of mitral regurgitation, are maximal at the left lower sternal border, not the apex.

The murmur of patent ductus arteriosus is loudest at the base or over the back. It is usually continuous, not purely systolic, and its character is often described as machinery-like.

Tricuspid regurgitation should be louder at the left lower sternal border than at the apex, but mitral regurgitation is the reverse. If a thrill is palpable, it should correspond to the region of maximum acoustic intensity. Radiation to the axilla is far more typical of mitral regurgitation than of tricuspid regurgitation. Radiation to the epigastrium *slightly* favors tricuspid regurgitation. The abdominojugular test, with or without slow cycled respiration, further distinguishes these. So does the timing observed between straining and change or release and change with the Valsalva maneuver. Associated signs are also of help: giant v waves or pulsatile hepatomegaly prove tricuspid regurgitation, but these high-specificity signs are uncommon, so their absence does not rule out tricuspid regurgitation. Amyl nitrite inhalation, as described above, may settle thorny cases. Finally, tricuspid regurgitation engenders clinical humility: It can be prominent physiologically, with little or no murmur—a tendency recognized for a century!

Diastolic Murmurs

In contrast to the frequent innocence of systolic ejection murmurs, diastolic murmurs almost always signify structural heart disease. Two exceptions are severe sickle cell anemia, in which diastolic as well as systolic murmurs have been described without organic heart disease, and a diastolic murmur that can result from complete heart block. The pathophysiology of these two exceptions to the rule remains unsettled. Diastolic murmurs are graded 1–4, in contrast to the 1–6 scale of systolic murmurs. *Apparently* this is because the very loudest murmurs, those audible without the stethoscope, are exclusively systolic.

The commonest diastolic murmur, *aortic insufficiency,* begins with or just after S_2A and tails off in diastole. Patients can have remarkably well-compensated cardiovascular function despite aortic insufficiency, so the discovery of the murmur should not lead to proscriptions or gloomy prognostication. All the classical auscultatory features of aortic insufficiency relate to the chronic, slowly evolving lesion. There are different clinical, imaging and laboratory features in acute aortic insufficiency from rapid destruction of a valve leaflet by endocarditis or trauma. The peripheral signs of aortic insufficiency are discredited. When aortic insufficiency is an established diagnosis, *shortening* of the murmur over time is *not* encouraging: As valvular regurgitation progresses and, to a lesser degree, as left ventricular diastolic pressures rise, equilibration between aortic and left ventricular pressures can occur earlier in diastole, abbreviating the murmur. The examiner's instinct that a shorter murmur means decreased hemodynamic derangement is incorrect. Finally, in seeking this murmur, the examiner must constantly "reset" the ears and brain to listen for a high-pitched sound that is closer in frequency to breath sound than to other murmurs.

Pulmonic insufficiency, the Graham Steell murmur, should be loudest at the right sternal border, but it overlaps aortic insufficiency. Even experienced examiners can and do mistake either of these for the other. One clue is the presence of pulmonary hypertension, marked by an accentuated S_2P. In this setting, pulmonic insufficiency is increased in prevalence, but aortic insufficiency is not.

The murmur of *mitral stenosis* is a rumbling murmur best heard in the periods of rapid ventricular filling: early diastole and, unless atrial fibrillation is present, (ventricular) protosystole corresponding to the atrial "kick" of atrial systole. The mitral stenosis murmur is loudest at the apex or somewhat medial to this point and can be manipulated with maneuvers described above. Turning the patient into the left lateral decubitus position is a favored means of enhancing this subtle and often difficult-to-appreciate murmur.

The *Austin Flint murmur* is said, variously, to embody elements of both mitral stenosis and aortic insufficiency or to represent the anterior leaflet of the mitral valve "flapping in the breeze" as it is struck by simultaneous blood flow forward through a (?diseased) orifice and backward through a regurgitant aortic valve cusp. Today, it is enough to identify a diastolic murmur that has a confusing mixture of characteristics of aortic insufficiency and mitral stenosis and to leave conclusive anatomic localization to technologic imaging.

Aged Patients with Basal Systolic Murmurs

Valvular heart disease increases in prevalence in the elderly, but so do innocuous murmurs. Unfortunately, the criteria for innocence listed above are too rigorous, so that numerous aged persons cannot meet them because of unrelated heart disease—often coronary or hypertensive—despite the murmur that the examiner hears being innocuous. Furthermore, pathologic conditions may produce no, or deceptively minimal, physical signs. The commonest troublesome evaluation is of a grade 2/6 systolic ejection murmur, maximal at the right upper sternal border, without radiation to the neck, alteration in the carotid upstrokes, reduction of S_2A, or lowering of either the systolic blood pressure or the pulse pressure, and without the harshness ("sawing quality") found in some aortic stenoses. By classical criteria, still applicable to younger adults, this should be a functional aortic valve murmur such as "aortic sclerosis." In the aged, however, all the following apply to catheterization-proved aortic stenosis:

- The murmur is frequently neither as loud, nor as long, nor as rough (harsh) as the older textbooks would have it.
- It may not radiate to the neck.
- The carotid upstroke is seldom attenuated or delayed, because age- and atherosclerosis-related stiffening *improves* pulse propagation.
- Although the intensity of S_2A may be reduced by the process, it has been increased at baseline by hypertension so frequently that the net result appears falsely normal.
- As with S_2A intensity, the systolic blood pressure may be reduced from a baseline that was elevated, producing a summation that is deceptively normal or even high.
- The pulse pressure need not be decreased even by severe aortic stenosis in the aged. This may also relate to arterial stiffening.

Striking physical findings retain great diagnostic import and specificity in the aged, and *changing* physical findings remain very important. A paucity of findings must be interpreted with appropriate humility about the limits of physical examination so that if symptoms or other features suggest a particularly damaging and treatable process, other means of investigation will be considered.

Aortic Stenosis and Insufficiency Separately and Together

Many of the processes that deform aortic valves produce both stenosis and insufficiency, by preventing both proper excursions and normal coaptation of the cusps. Thus whenever you detect aortic stenosis, check for aortic insufficiency, and whenever you detect aortic insufficiency, check for aortic stenosis. However, increased *forward* flow across the aortic valve in aortic insufficiency encompasses both the regurgitant fraction coming forward again on the next beat and ordinary left atrial output. Thus a high-flow systolic murmur can result at the aortic valve focus. In a patient with aortic insufficiency, you would suspect that such a murmur represented coexistent aortic stenosis. Nevertheless, in some instances the murmur will relate exclusively to high blood flow across a structurally normally opening valve, i.e., an aortic valve with normal systolic function.

The *Gallavardin phenomenon,* first described in France in 1925, is an acoustic alteration whereby aortic stenosis produces a murmur that becomes louder and more musical at the apex. The frequency of this anomaly is not established, but it is worth considering when (*a*) a musical pitch or character is identified in an apical systolic murmur and (*b*) you are tempted to diagnose multiple different systolic murmurs in a single person. There certainly are individuals with two genuinely different murmurs. However, the usual combination considered, aortic stenosis and mitral regurgitation, is especially lethal: Left ventricular forward flow is impaired, while backflow is permitted. Some such patients exist, but there are also individuals with aortic stenosis *only,* whose peculiar sound propagation mimics a second process. No data are extant on the frequency of the Gallavardin phenomenon in other aortic systolic ejection murmurs, e.g., in aortic sclerosis. (One also wonders if some allegedly affected patients have not actually had hypertrophic cardiomyopathy with coexistent mitral regurgitation.)

Arteries
PULSUS PARVUS ET TARDUS

A delayed, diminished carotid upstroke has long been regarded as a hallmark of aortic stenosis. However, as described above, the noncompliant vasculature reduces the sensitivity (prevalence) of this finding, and unfortunately the specificity is reduced because of arterial disease. When the carotid pulse is diminished, aortic arch/innominate/common carotid atherosclerosis is much more likely responsible than is aortic stenosis. In trying to decide the respective contribution of each, when both pathologies are believed to be present, keep the following in mind:

- If one carotid upstroke is normal in timing and intensity, then aortic outflow tract disease cannot be invoked to explain the other. Differential signs from side to side implicate lesions distal to the common proximal pathway shared by the two vessels.
- If one side is less abnormal than the other, the degree of aortic valve obstruction explains *at most* the milder side, using the same reasoning.
- If there is a systolic ejection murmur at the right upper sternal border and symmetric delay and diminution in the carotid pulses, multiple hypotheses will account for the findings. They are
—Indeed, there is significant aortic stenosis, alone.

—There is aortic sclerosis and arterial disease that is either proximal or symmetrical.

—There is both aortic stenosis *and* arterial disease.

DECREASED CAROTID PULSE INTENSITY

The differential diagnosis includes both arterial disease and left ventricular outflow tract disease. Regarding arteries, *dissecting hematoma* ("dissecting aneurysm") as well as conventional obstructive atherosclerosis can be responsible, but dissecting hematoma is less common. A *tearing* quality to chest pain increases the likelihood of dissection, as do marked inequities of pulse strength and blood pressure from limb to limb and a history of a condition that predisposes, namely, hypertension or Marfan's syndrome. Even with all these features, asymmetry or spotty atherosclerotic stenoses may prove to be the cause of unequal carotid pulses in any given case.

Global attenuation of pulses raises the prospect of widespread vasculopathy—usually obvious from the total history and physical—versus narrow pulse pressure. The latter hypothesis is readily tested by measuring the blood pressure.

INCREASED CAROTID PULSE INTENSITY

Increased carotid pulse intensity is the mirror image of the preceding. A *wide pulse pressure* can be responsible. **Aortic insufficiency** is often the first diagnosis to come to mind, but any *high cardiac output state* can also produce *bounding pulses* (sometimes called, with a curious attachment to obsolete points of reference, water-hammer pulses or, eponymously, Corrigan's pulse). Such changes can be produced by hyperthyroidism, anemia, pregnancy, extreme anxiety, early septicemia, and the excess arteriovenous connections seen in some cases of Paget's disease of bone and in many cases of cirrhosis.

CAROTID BRUIT VERSUS TRANSMITTED MURMUR

The simplest test to distinguish between bruit and murmur is hyperextension of the shoulders. If this obliterates the noise in the neck, the noise is a *subclavian artery bruit,* which is innocuous and needs no further attention. If not, the following applies.

If there is *no* murmur over the base of the heart, the distinction is between subclavian artery, carotid artery, and venous hum. If there *is* a cardiac murmur, it must be considered as a source. *Progressive attenuation* from the second right interspace to the supraclavicular fossa to the carotid bifurcation is characteristic of an *aortic valvular murmur* with transmission (propagation). Peaking at the supraclavicular fossa sometimes corresponds to obliteration by hyperextension of the shoulders, in pointing to a subclavian source.

The same effect might reflect an aortic valvular murmur that is attenuating upward and a carotid bruit that somehow transmits downward. More commonly, however, coexistent valvular and arterial lesions produce the opposite acoustic phenomenon: loud systolic sound at the right upper sternal border, a falloff in the supraclavicular fossa, and resumption of loudness over the carotid bifurcation.

Although it is more difficult to ascertain, a murmur should be *longest* as well as loudest at the site of origin. A change in *quality* usually means two separate acoustic phenomena. If vibrations are palpable in the carotid, constituting a *shudder*, the source can be arterial or a transmitted aortic stenosis. A certain number of carotid sounds remain impossible to classify accurately by bedside examination alone.

Finally, if *partial* release of pressure on the stethoscope causes the carotid murmur to disappear, reconsider whether that murmur has been an artifact of iatrogenic turbulence via excess pressure—and never repeat the mistake, which can be hazardous as well as misleading.

Veins

ELEVATED JUGULAR VENOUS PRESSURE

The first need, beyond proper examination technique as delineated above, is clear thinking. The old term "JVD" ("jugular venous distension") sets one astray. Normal jugular veins are distended to some degree, and what is sought is the pathologic finding of *elevated jugular venous pressure.* If the abbreviation JVD were to disappear from the earth, the practice of medicine would be enhanced!

Some observers dispute the accuracy of inferring central venous pressure from jugular venous pressure because of discrepancies between measured and predicted pressures and interposed venous valves. Venous tone also plays a role in determining height, breadth, and pulsation of jugular venous blood columns. Nevertheless, a jugular venous pressure corresponding to an estimated central venous pressure over 12 cm of water is highly suggestive of right-heart failure complicated by *systemic venous hypertension,* often but not always in association with extracellular fluid volume overload. When this finding in the right external jugular accords with the total clinical picture, as in clear-cut biventricular cardiac failure, accept it at face value. When it does not, check the opposite jugular and consider the sources of jugular venous pressure elevation without central venous hypertension that are discussed below.

KUSSMAUL'S SIGN

When jugular venous pressure rises on inspiration, the differential diagnosis includes pericardial constriction (but *not* cardiac tamponade), right ventricular myocardial infarction, congestive heart failure, acute cor pulmonale, and restrictive heart disease. Despite recent work, the mechanism remains poorly understood, as does a putative relationship to the abdominojugular test. Could increased intra-abdominal pressure resulting from inspiration be transmitted via the great veins to an inelastic right heart? A host of possible confounding factors exist. For example, the effect of isolated right ventricular hypertrophy has not been assessed, nor has that of tense ascites without overt heart disease. The sign is only sought in a few settings. It is best brought out with slow deep breaths (cycled respiration) and a body angle at which the top of the jugular venous blood column lies between the clavicle and the mandible. One key distinction is between constriction and tamponade, which share many features. Kussmaul's sign will strongly favor the former; its absence, the latter. However, technology is almost certain to be employed whatever the jugular venous response to inspiration.

ABDOMINOJUGULAR TEST RESULTS

A rapid 4-cm or greater falloff in jugular venous blood column on release, after 10 seconds of Valsalva-free firm midabdominal compression, is associated with an elevated pulmonary arterial wedge pressure, i.e., *left*-heart dysfunction and increased central blood volume. This contrasts with older interpretations that inferred *right*-heart dysfunction. However, the test may also be positive in patients with a recent right ventricular myocardial infarction even without elevated pulmonary arterial wedge pressure and in patients with isolated right ventricular dysfunction. The parallelism with Kussmaul's sign is suggestive, yet interpretation of abnormal results in the two tests is widely divergent.

Despite exciting recent research, we are still struggling to understand how these signs work, *precisely* what they mean, and what they represent pathophysiologically.

UNILATERALLY ELEVATED JUGULAR VENOUS PRESSURE

When one jugular venous pressure exceeds the other by more than 1 cm, several possible explanations may be invoked:

*   The "flat" vein is nonpatent, therefore not reflective of central venous pressure.
*   There is proximal obstruction of the more distended vein.
*   Abnormal or aberrant valves are masking or mimicking central venous hypertension by local effect.
*   The patient has idiopathic jugular venous ectasia, which can look almost like a vascular malformation or neoplasm and about which we understand next to nothing.
*   Some combination of the above is true.

Proximal obstruction will usually be obvious if it is part of a superior vena cava syndrome, but it may also occur in more localized forms. An *uncoiled atherosclerotic aorta* may pinch the termination of either jugular in the respective subclavian–innominate vein complex, as may an *ectatic atherosclerotic aorta* and, more ominously, an *aortic dissecting hematoma.* This last sign is avidly sought in suspected thoracic dissection, whether the carotid pulses are unequal or not. If the disparity in jugular pressure is known to be new, imaging may be undertaken emergently in this setting.

It is imperative to decide which of the two jugular veins is the accurate marker of intrathoracic events. Variability of column height with respiratory cycle, with change in body position, and/or with the abdominojugular test suggests the accurate side, and lack of response to these tends to point to the misleading vessel. The more normal-looking jugular venous column height is not always the accurate one—there may just as well be jugular venous hypertension and one obliterated vein, as one artifactually distended and the other normal!

PERSISTENTLY FLAT JUGULAR VEINS

The differential diagnosis here is extreme *venous hypotension,* characteristically from marked intravascular volume depletion, versus *fibrous obliteration of the venous lumen.* The Trendelenburg position will usually bring out a blood column in any patent jugular, even with hypovolemia, but cannot open up a solid cord. At times, cautious intravascular volume repletion may assist this assessment. Patients at maximum risk of fibrous obliteration are the aged, in whom the phenomenon can develop spontaneously and without any clinical signs or symptoms; intravenous drug abusers, in whom endothelial damage and/or thrombosis may have contributed; and persons who have had central vascular catheters, including but not limited to internal jugular venoclyses. Such individuals need not have had clinical jugular thrombophlebitis to develop late scarring and luminal obliteration.

STRIKING JUGULAR VENOUS PULSATIONS

Normally, a single prominent pulsation is seen in the neck with each heartbeat, and that is the carotid artery. It will persist in pulsating even if light pressure is applied at the root of the neck just above the clavicle; by contrast, pulsations arising from the veins will not. A prominent outward pulsation before the carotid pulse, just before S_1 and synchronous with an S_4 if there is one, will be a *giant "a" wave* representing excessively prominent atrial contraction. This is seen in *tricus-

pid stenosis, in which a hypertrophic right atrium squeezes forcefully in order to move the cardiac output across a diastolic gradient. These, and giant "a" waves resulting from a noncompliant hypertrophic right ventricle, are **regular** and easily timed with reference to acoustic events.

Unusually forceful atrial contraction against a closed tricuspid valve during (premature right) ventricular systole can produce the same kind of pulse, but admittedly this is difficult to sort out without reference to the ECG. However, the appearance of **intermittent** "cannon a waves" is a valuable clue that the right atrium is sometimes contracting against a closed tricuspid valve and suggests that either complete heart block, or ventricular tachycardia with independent atrial activity, or *perhaps* an unusual supraventricular tachycardia is present. The patient must **not** be considered unlikely to have ventricular tachycardia simply because he is hemodynamically stable. The sequence to follow when cannon "a" waves are observed in a patient who is comfortable, with a regular pulse, is to relisten for variability in intensity of S_1 (which is likely), and to check for beat-to-beat major variations in systolic blood pressure (disappearing first Korotkoff sound that is not pulsus paradoxus or pulsus alternans). Then it is time to do an ECG promptly and to seek experienced help expeditiously.

A prominent outward pulsation after the carotid "c" wave, nearly coincident with S_2A, will be a *giant "v" wave.* These occur in tricuspid regurgitation, in which the pathologically open valve permits the superior vena cava and therefore the jugular to reflect systolic contraction of the right ventricle—from which they are otherwise protected by valve closure even in a premature ventricular contraction. Perhaps not altogether surprisingly, the abdominojugular maneuver and Gooch maneuver can bring out enlarged "v" waves in some cases of relatively mild tricuspid regurgitation.

Irregular *giant "v" waves* are sometimes seen in atrial fibrillation even without tricuspid regurgitation. By contrast, in complete heart block the timing should be such that the excess pressure generated in the right ventricle automatically snaps the valve shut, preventing the formation of giant "v" waves.

VENA CAVAL OBSTRUCTION

The features of *inferior venal caval obstruction* are listed in the Extended Examination section of Chapter 9. *Superior vena caval obstruction* is recognized at the bedside by findings of venous hypertension and congestion limited to the upper trunk, head, and neck and sometimes to the upper limbs, without involvement of abdomen, back, perineum, or lower limbs. The search is for selective plethora (redness) or cyanosis, sometimes with chemosis (conjunctival edema), facial edema, and highly dilated superficial veins throughout. The unnamed veins on the anterior chest may bulge grotesquely. The jugular veins are typically distended to the angle of the jaw. Partial and variant forms (e.g., right innominate vein obstruction) may limit abnormalities to one side of the face and the ipsilateral upper limb, for instance.

VENOUS HUM VERSUS CAROTID BRUIT

Usually, the distinction between venous hum and carotid bruit is simple. In children and young adults, cervical venous hums are common, and carotid arterial bruits are rare. Noises in older adults are often arterial; however, they can be venous, especially if there is a high-output state from exertion, anxiety, anemia, or other reasons. The venous hum is often continuous and *louder in diastole,* whereas most carotid bruits are exclusively systolic. Carotid bruits are augmented or unchanged when the patient is recumbent, whereas venous hums are best heard when the patient is seated and are reduced or absent when the patient

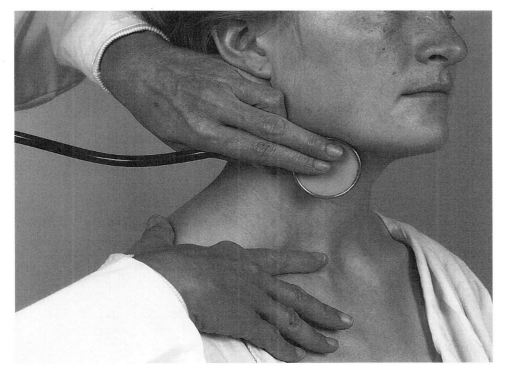

Figure 8.32 Auscultation of the neck with the jugular outflow obliterated should lead to the abatement of any noise that was of jugular origin. Thus a venous hum will disappear, and a carotid bruit will be unchanged.

is supine. Light pressure on the jugular outflow just above the clavicle should obliterate a venous hum but should have no effect on a carotid bruit (Fig. 8.32).

RECORDING THE FINDINGS

Sample Write-up

72-year old woman, generally healthy apart from marked rheumatoid arthritis of hands, seen for murmur evaluation. Is asymptomatic from cardiorespiratory point of view.

Vital signs: Pulse 86/minute and regular, no orthostatic change. Respirations 14, not labored. BP 130/74, supine and standing.

Cardiovascular system:

Arteries/veins: Carotid upstrokes normal, timing normal. Transmission of S_1 and S_2 normal, no murmur transmission. ECVP 9 cm, without prominent "v" waves.

Heart: Apex beat barely visible, not sustained, enlarged, or unduly forceful, in 5th intercostal space in anterior axillary line. No thrill here, and no lift anywhere.

S_1 normal, louder than S_2 at apex, single. S_2 physiologically split with soft S_2P, and tambouric S_2A that exceeds S_1 at the base. S_4 heard at apex only. No S_3. Long, steady, high-pitched systolic murmur maximal at apex but heard in axilla and left lower sternal border also. Grade 2–3/6, increased in left lateral decubitus, decreased with Valsalva maneuver, no inspiratory augmentation or Gooch positivity, and no change perceived with sustained handgrip. No diastolic murmur even with exercise in LLD, and no opening snap.

Impression: Mitral regurgitation, early left ventricular dilatation, reasonably compensated circulation; doubt prolapse is cause, doubt rheumatic because not holosystolic. Myocardial hypertrophy with S_4, tambouric S_2A.

BEYOND THE PHYSICAL EXAMINATION

There is some overlap, inevitably, with modalities used to assess the thorax and those employed to further assess the neck and the limbs.

Heart

Functional testing includes *exercise tolerance tests,* also known as graded exercise tests or treadmill stress tests. These are employed largely to check the consequences of possible coronary artery stenoses or to examine for reduced cardiac reserve. They have limited sensitivity and specificity. The addition of *thallium imaging* is employed to disclose reversible regional myocardial perfusion defects. Since many patients who take little exercise are deconditioned and thus unable to generate heart rates sufficient to tax the coronaries, *dipyridamole* has been added to some stress tests to increase heart rate and to precipitate "coronary steal," thus delineating less evident perfusion deficits, but the efficacy of these diagnostic modes is still debated.

Arterial blood gas measurements are useful in assessing cardiac dysfunction. In suspected intracardiac defects such as ventricular septal defect, an increase (step-up) in mixed blood oxygenation between samples from the right atrium and those from the right ventricle provides evidence of "contamination" by oxygen-enriched blood that has returned from the lungs to the left side of the heart and then crossed the defect. When Eisenmenger physiology supervenes, i.e., the right-heart pressures exceed the left, and shunting is from right to left through the defect, this step-up no longer occurs.

Electrical testing encompasses, most frequently, **electrocardiography.** The ECG is used to seek rhythm disturbances including abnormal impulse propagation, myocardial ischemia, vector attenuation as with pericardial effusion and amyloid heart disease, and a striking variety of other cardiac abnormalities.

Ambulatory electrocardiography, the so-called Holter monitor, records 24 hours or more of electrical signals from the heart and is correlated with a symptom diary kept by the patient. The lengthy record is analyzed by both human interpreter and computer. Detection of rhythm disturbances by this method is superior to detection of temporary myocardial ischemia, although the latter has improved recently.

Signal-averaged electrocardiography enhances detection of abnormalities in the heart that has sustained myocardial infarction previously, and helps predict patients at greater risk of sudden cardiac death or lethal arrhythmias.

Electrophysiologic studies are the ultimate electrical investigation of the heart and have enormous sensitivity—too much, some believe—and power to direct rational therapy for the most complex and refractory arrhythmias.

Cardiac imaging centers not on the mediastinal shadow on the plain chest radiograph but rather on the *two-dimensional transthoracic echocardiogram,* with or without simultaneous M-mode studies and color Doppler interrogation and with or without the newest advance, *transesophageal echocardiography.* Echocardiography serves well for investigation of global left ventricular contractility and regional left ventricular wall motion, as well as left atrial dimensions, and it defines or excludes pericardial effusion very well. It delineates valvular regurgitation and stenosis, especially on the left side of the heart. One now encounters, by echocardiography, acoustically silent valvular regurgitation whose significance, prognosis, and need for endocarditis prophylaxis remain undetermined. These methods also enormously assist assessment of cardiac and mediastinal masses, prominently including *intracardiac thrombi* and, less reliably, valvular vegetations of *infective endocarditis.* There are a whole array of *nuclear cardiology* techniques that address both myocardial perfusion and pump function.

Computed tomography is sometimes employed, but although dynamic techniques can minimize blurring from movement during the cardiac and respiratory cycles, neither this modality nor *magnetic resonance imaging* has yet gained wide clinical application for the heart and great vessels. *Cinefluoroscopic coronary angiography* and *left ventriculography* use injectable radiocontrast materials for detailed assessment of arterial patency and anatomical distribution. They also allow direct visualization of portions of the left ventricular walls and associated structures for contractility, filling defects, valvular regurgitation, cardiac aneurysms, and even shadowgrams of the papillary muscles.

Right-heart catheterization permits measurement of both right-sided chamber pressures and pulmonary arterial pressures throughout all phases of the cardiac cycle. The pulmonary arterial wedge pressure or pulmonary "capillary" wedge pressure can be measured as a proxy for left ventricular end-diastolic pressures. Waveform abnormalities with such a catheter mirror left-heart events, just as those in the neck veins mirror right-heart events, so that, for example, prominent v waves in a pulmonary vascular tracing bespeak *mitral regurgitation. Cardiac output* is measured with thermodilution techniques using these catheters.

When indicated, a bioptome can be employed for transvascular right ventricular *endomyocardial biopsy,* a safe and well-tolerated procedure when performed by an expert, which is used in follow-up after cardiac transplantation, as well as in native hearts for investigation of possible myocarditis, amyloid heart disease, and distinction of restrictive from constrictive heart disease. *Open-lung biopsy*— most often undertaken during operative repair of a cardiac abnormality—is an element in assessment of the effects of various *complex congenital heart diseases* on the lesser circulation.

Regarding infective endocarditis, *blood cultures* and *echocardiography* are the leading tests to establish etiology and anatomic extent, respectively. Both are subject to considerable numbers of false-positive and false-negative results.

Teichoic acid antibody tests, once touted as distinguishing staphylococcal endocarditis from bacteremia, have fallen from favor.

Arteries

The *carotid arteries* can be assessed with a variety of *ultrasound images* including duplex Doppler and even triplex measurements. Indirect measurements of systolic blood pressure in periorbital arteries by ocular plethysmography show reduction in both flow and pressure between aorta and eyes.

Digital subtraction angiography from an intra*venous* injection is sometimes favored. The goal of all these tests is to reduce the use of *carotid arteriography,* which has the highest morbidity and mortality of any purely diagnostic procedure. When carotid endarterectomy is contemplated, however, the surgeon may require the detailed database from contrast angiography, notwithstanding difficulty, cost, and invasiveness. This realm is changing rapidly, however.

When the more proximal innominate artery, or the root of a subclavian or vertebral artery, or even the aortic arch is of concern, retrograde passage of a catheter from a peripheral artery is sometimes undertaken, followed by injection of a radiocontrast agent for an *aortic arch study* or for *selective arteriography* of one area in question. Since contrast agents can wreak havoc with kidneys or heart, the minimum dose is administered, and the radiologist does not seek excuses to "take an additional peek while we're in there." Although the aorta can be injected in this way for contrast aortography, less invasive and less dangerous methods such as computed tomography and especially *transesophageal aortography* are replacing it, including for assessment of suspected *dissecting hematoma.*

Veins

Investigation of suspected *superior vena cava syndrome* by direct measurement of pressure in the superior vena caval distribution, via needle puncture of a surface vein and the use of monometry, is fraught with problems caused by valves in between the site of suspected trouble and the point of sampling. The passage of a *central venous catheter* is more rational, since with it the manometer can be placed at the site "where the action is." Other indications for such catheters have been largely supplanted by flow-directed pulmonary artery catheters (Swan-Ganz catheterizations), which provide far more data.

Plain-chest radiography is of some use in delineating a mediastinal mass. Various *ultrasound techniques* are rapidly gaining use. However, *contrast venography (phlebography)* remains the gold standard, short of direct (and unnecessary) operative visualization. When a central venous catheter is thought to be obstructed with thrombotic material, direct injection of contrast material through the catheter can provide optimal imaging. When infection of such a catheter is at issue, blood cultures are drawn through the catheter and compared with those drawn peripherally.

Consultants

The particular colleague to be called on depends almost entirely on one's assessment of the locale, etiology, and optimal management of the particular problem. Thus a refractory pericarditis could lead to consulting a cardiologist, an infectious diseases specialist, or both. If the problem were complicated by a pyopericardium needing surgical drainage, a general surgeon or cardiothoracic surgeon would be a logical choice, as might an *interventional radiologist. Vascular surgeons* are at home in the chest, but *cardiac surgeons* are even more so—at least inside the pericardium! Frequently, the clinician will ask a *cardiologist* for help with an apparently medical heart problem, and if the need is identified, a *heart surgeon* is sought in turn. Since surgery on the chest is always major, nobody—medical or surgical doctor, patient or family member, or primary physician—will opt for surgical management of a cardiovascular problem that can be taken care of with medicines. For example, a thrombus-clogged permanent superior vena caval–right atrial catheter being used for cancer chemotherapy, blood drawing, and parenteral nutritional support could be removed under anesthesia in the operating room and replaced, but all parties would prefer, when not contraindicated, if thrombolytic agents could be administered through the catheter to fragment, dissolve, and dislodge the obstructing matter and to restore luminal patency and therefore function.

RECOMMENDED READINGS

Abrams J. Precordial motion in health and disease. Mod Concepts Cardiovasc Dis 1980;49:55–60.

Benchimol A, Desser KB. The fourth heart sound in patients without demonstrable heart disease. Am Heart J 1977;93:298–301.

Cotter L, Logan RL, Poole A. Innocent systolic murmurs in healthy 40-year-old men. J R Coll Physicians Lond 1980;14:128–129.

Duthie EH, Gambert SR, Tresch D. Evaluation of the systolic murmur in the elderly. J Am Geriatr Soc 1981;29:498–502.

Horwitz LD, Groves BM. Signs and symptoms in cardiology. Philadelphia: JB Lippincott, 1985.

Hurst JW, Staton J, Hubbard D. Precordial murmurs during pregnancy and lactation. N Engl J Med 1958;259:515–517.

Napodano RJ. The functional heart murmur: a wastebasket diagnosis. J Fam Pract 1977;4:637–639.

Perloff JK. Physical examination of the heart and circulation. Philadelphia: WB Saunders, 1982.

9

Abdomen

SCREENING EXAMINATION OF THE ABDOMEN

APPROACH AND ANATOMICAL REVIEW

Approach

After completing the supine cardiac examination, the examiner moves to the abdomen. The patient remains recumbent, and the examiner conducts the examination from the patient's right side. The patient's chest should be covered with a gown folded up to the xiphoid process and a half-sheet or similar drape positioned to cover the lower extremities and groin (Fig. 9.1).

The instruments required for the abdominal examination are **warm hands** and a **warm stethoscope diaphragm.** Good lighting and complete exposure of the abdominal wall facilitate inspection. The abdominal examination begins with **inspection,** followed by **auscultation,** then **percussion,** and, lastly, **palpation.**

Anatomical Review
SURFACE LANDMARKS

The surface landmarks of the abdomen (Fig. 9.2) that are palpable and sometimes visible include the following:

*   **Costal margins.** The right and left costal margins are made up of the lower six costal cartilages and the "floating" cartilage tips of the 11th and 12th ribs.
*   **Xiphoid process.** This bony triangle is attached to the lower end of the sternum by a cartilaginous junction.
*   **Iliac crests.** The highest points of the iliac crests lie at the level of the 4th lumbar spine and 2–8 cm caudad to the cartilage of the 12th rib. The variation in distance between the iliac crest and the lowest rib is a reflection of body habitus and, in some instances, bone disease or deformity.
*   **Anterior superior iliac spine.** This portion of the iliac crest is an easily palpable anterior projection that serves as a useful landmark for location and description of anatomical findings.
*   **Pubic crest and tubercles.** These structures define the most inferior (or caudal) bony boundaries of the abdomen and pelvis.
*   **Inguinal ligament.** This fibrous band underlies the groove that marks the division between the abdomen and the thigh.
*   **Umbilicus.** The indentation is located in the midline, typically at the level of the fourth lumbar spine, although its position varies with the amount of abdominal fat.
*   **Linea alba.** This superficial mark, sometimes visible as a midline furrow, labels the groove separating the right and left **rectus abdominis muscles.** The lateral borders of the rectus muscles are often visible or palpable in muscular individuals as a curved line extending from the fifth costochondral junction to the pubic tubercle.

For convenience of description and location of organs and abnormalities, the abdomen, like the breast, is divided into quadrants. By drawing one imaginary line from the tip of the xiphoid to the midpoint of the symphysis pubis and a second line that horizontally transects the abdomen at the level of the umbilicus, the four quadrants are defined and labeled as right and left lower, right and left

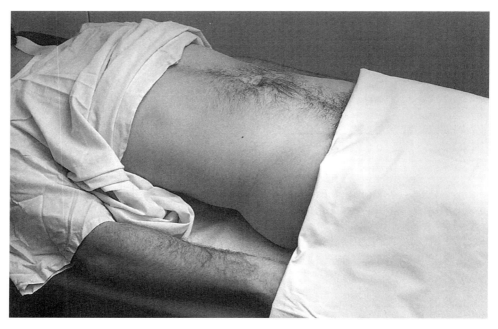

Figure 9.1 Placement of drapes for the abdominal examination.

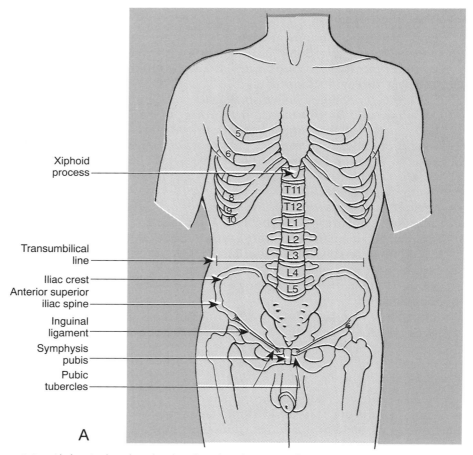

A

Figure 9.2 Abdominal surface landmarks related to internal anatomical structures.

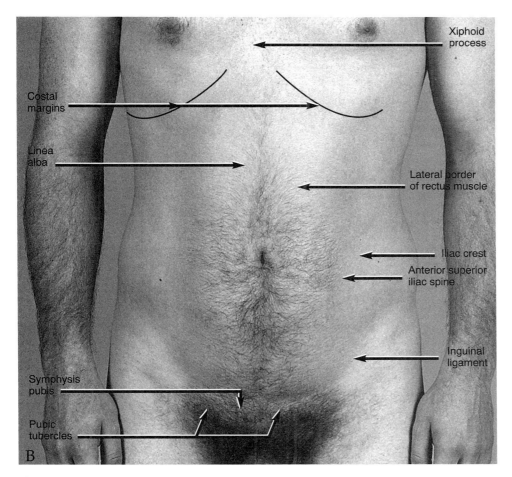

Figure 9.2   B.

upper. The right-left designations refer to the *patient's* right and left sides. An alternative approach is to divide the abdomen into nine segments. Because of the use of the segment terminology in some medical textbooks, this designation is also described here. This text, however, utilizes the quadrantic designations exclusively for anatomic localization (Fig. 9.3).

ORGANS WITHIN THE ABDOMINAL CAVITY

The organs of concern are reviewed in relation to their surface projections (Fig. 9.4). They include the following:

- **Liver.** The upper border of the liver lies under ribs 7, 8, 9, 10, and 11 on the right, curves to just below the right nipple, crosses the midline, and continues to a point near the left nipple. Its sharp lower border (the term liver **edge** is thus reserved for the lower border) crosses in front of the gastric pylorus and generally follows the margin of the right lower rib cage (right costal margin). The normal liver is palpable in some individuals, but not in all.
- **Gallbladder.** The **gallbladder** lies at the lateral border of the rectus abdominis muscle below the costal margin and is not normally palpable. Deep to the gallbladder lies the superior portion of the **duodenum.**
- **Pancreas.** The pancreas sits deep in the retroperitoneal space behind the stomach, with its head nestled in the duodenal curve and its tail extending across the left upper quadrant. It is nonpalpable even when enlarged.

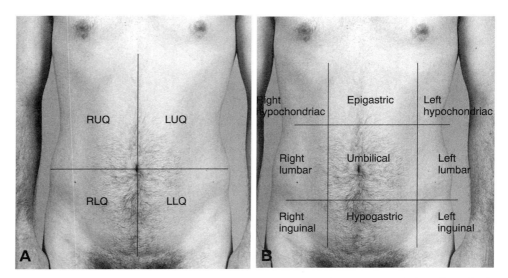

Figure 9.3   Two standards of abdominal area designations for purposes of describing findings. **A.** Quadrantic division, the most commonly used today. *RUQ,* right upper quadrant; *LUQ,* left upper quadrant; *RLQ,* right lower quadrant; *LLQ,* left lower quadrant. **B.** Regional division of abdominal wall into nine sections.

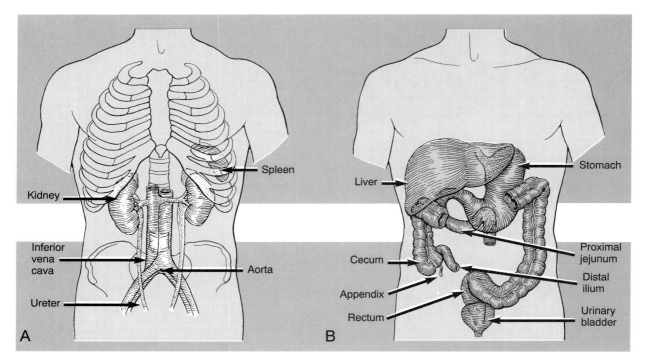

Figure 9.4   Some relationships of abdominal organs. **A.** Deep abdominal structures. **B.** Ventral (more anterior) organs.

- **Stomach.** The stomach is located, also rather deeply, mostly in the left upper quadrant. It is partially overlain by the **transverse colon,** near its splenic flexure.
- **Spleen.** The spleen lies superficially under the left rib cage parallel to ribs 9, 10, and 11. Unless enlarged to about three times normal size, it cannot be palpated in adults. Its largest dimension is directed transversely, not craniocaudally.

- **Aorta.** The aorta enters the abdomen at the level of the 12th thoracic vertebra and bifurcates into the **common iliac arteries** at the level of the navel. It follows the course of, and lies immediately anterior to and slightly to the left of, the vertebral bodies.
- **Kidney.** The lower pole of each kidney lies just above the transumbilical plane, usually deep to the hollow viscera.
- **Urinary bladder.** The urinary bladder is partly protected by the symphysis pubis, although if very full, it may project from behind the bone and become palpable through the abdominal wall.
- **Colon.** The colon commences (in continuity with the distal ileal portion of the small bowel) with the **cecum** and its **appendix** in the right lower quadrant. The ascending colon courses cephalad, becoming the transverse colon at the hepatic flexure. Its caudad course (descending colon) begins at the splenic flexure and becomes retroperitoneal as the **sigmoid** colon traverses the peritoneum in the left lower quadrant. The intestinal tract terminates in the retroperitoneal midline with the rectum and anus. The hollow of the abdominal cavity is filled by the **intestinal** loops and their mesenteric suspensions.

Note that the **adrenal glands,** lying over the upper pole of each kidney, are not palpable. Normal pelvic organs, uterus (unless pregnant), Fallopian tubes, and ovaries are not palpable on abdominal examination except as part of the bimanual pelvic examination.

TECHNIQUE

See Table 9.1 for summary of the steps in the screening abdominal examination.

Inspection

The inspection of the abdomen includes its general contour, movement, and, of course, skin. The examiner should note whether the abdomen is protuberant, i.e., bulging beyond the level of the bony landmarks, flat, or scaphoid, i.e., sunken beneath the prominence of the anterior superior iliac spines. The umbilicus is assessed for protuberance or indentation. The skin of the abdomen should be inspected for surgical or traumatic scars and for the presence of skin markings such as discoloration, local skin lesions, and venous pattern. In the thin person, an epigastric or periumbilical transmission of aortic pulsation may be visible. Observe for peristaltic movement and the normally faint rise and fall of the abdominal wall with respiration (abdomen up with inspiration, down with expiration).

Table 9.1
Steps in the Abdominal Examination

Inspection	Palpation
Contour	**Light palpation, four quadrants**
Skin	**Deep palpation, four quadrants**
Movement (peristalsis)	**Liver**
	Spleen
Auscultation	**Aorta**
Bowel sounds	**Inguinal and femoral lymph nodes**
Vascular sounds	Kidneys
	Urinary bladder, uterus
Percussion	Femoral arteries
Liver span	
Spleen	
Urinary bladder	

[a]**Boldface,** universally performed; other, selective.

Auscultation

Auscultation with the diaphragm of the stethoscope is the second step in the abdominal examination. Note that the sequence of examination differs here from that for the rest of the body in that auscultation *precedes* palpation rather than follows it. The diaphragm is placed against the skin of the abdomen to make complete contact. The first sounds to be assessed are those of **bowel gas** and may be appreciated in any one of the quadrants. Press the diaphragm against the skin and listen for the intermittent gurgles of normal bowel activity. By placing the diaphragm in the epigastrium (midline just inferior to the xiphoid) **transmitted cardiac sounds** are often heard, sometimes better than in the precordium, especially when emphysematous lung partially overlies the heart and dampens sound transmission. With the diaphragm just above the umbilicus and pressed deeply, a systolic sound may be audible in the abdominal aorta.

Percussion

After inspection and auscultation of the abdomen, percussion is performed. In the asymptomatic patient, percussion is utilized primarily to outline solid organs (liver and spleen) or fluid-filled hollow organs **(urinary bladder).**

LIVER

Percussion of the liver is a highly imperfect but widely used method of determining liver size or **span.** The liver, being a solid organ, is dull to percussion and thus may be differentiated from the resonant lung above and the even more resonant sound resulting from intraluminal bowel air inferior to the right lobe of the liver. Beginning at the right third or fourth intercostal space, the examiner percusses caudally in the midclavicular line. When the resonance of the lung changes to the dullness of the underlying liver, the upper border of the liver has been reached, and this transition level is marked. Ask any cooperative patient to place a finger at the point where percussion notes change in order to mark it. Percuss cephalad from the transumbilical plane (bowel resonance) or below, up to the dullness of the inferior border of the liver. The **percussion span** of the liver is measured from the upper border of dullness to the lower border of dullness in the right midclavicular line (Fig. 9.5).

SPLEEN

Percussion of the spleen is not routinely performed because of its subtlety (see the Extended Examination section under Spleen).

BLADDER

The urinary bladder, when very full and rising above the symphysis pubis, may be percussed as a globular dullness in this area. As with the spleen, routine bladder percussion is not useful.

In general, the abdominal hollow viscera occupying most of the cavity are resonant to percussion, since they contain gas. There is little useful information to be gained from percussing areas of the abdomen and seeking differential percussion notes unless symptoms or signs indicate an abnormal process.

Palpation

Abdominal palpation begins with a very light touch, but a touch firm enough to overcome skin sensitivity. Using the palmar surface of the approximated fingers of one or both hands, the examiner proceeds from quadrant to quadrant, pressing downward to a depth of no more than 1 cm while assessing for tenderness, cutaneous or subcutaneous masses, and unusual sensitivity. After each quadrant has been lightly palpated, deep palpation is initiated. If the patient has expressed concern or has become tense with light palpation, it is sometimes useful to ask that he flex his hips and knees a few degrees in order to facilitate the relaxation of the abdominal muscles. To monitor response to abdominal palpation the examiner should watch the patient's face continuously during the examination. Many patients will not verbally express pain but will show discomfort with facial change. It has been noted that the usual response to painful palpation includes wide opening of the eyes expressing apprehension.

If the patient has indicated an abdominal complaint during the history, begin palpation remote from the complaint, reserving deep palpation of the area in question until last. Warn the patient that you will be feeling deep in the abdomen, and ask that he let you know if there is discomfort.

Each quadrant is assessed for tenderness and for any mass or enlarged organs. The palpatory consistency of the abdomen is soft with the sensation of mobile bowel that gives way to deep prodding. The patient may experience some discomfort on deep palpation of the epigastrium and of the left lower

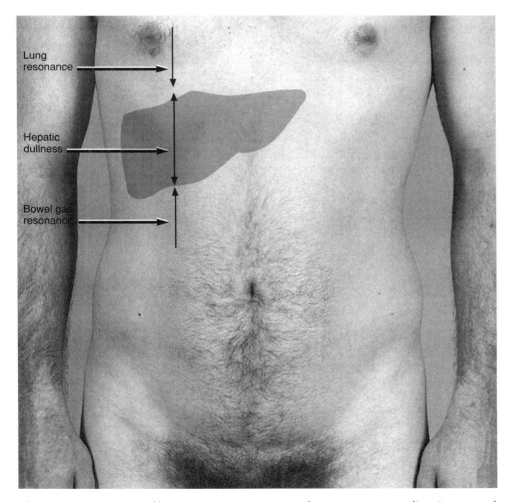

Figure 9.5   Percussion of liver span. Note transitions of percussion note as liver is traversed from the resonant lung above to the resonant bowel below in the midclavicular line.

quadrant, but normally there should be *no sharp or localized pain* elicited by this maneuver.

The specific organs to be sought by palpation include the liver, the spleen, the borders of the abdominal aorta, and, in some thin patients, the lower pole of the right kidney. The technique for assessing each of these structures is described below.

LIVER

Two methods are commonly utilized for palpating the lower margin of the *liver*. The previously percussed lower margin gives the examiner an approximate location, and palpation is guided by this information. After placing the fingers of one or both hands deep into the right upper quadrant, 1–2 cm caudad to the anticipated location of the margin, the examiner then asks the patient to inhale deeply and exhale slowly, repeating the cycle several times if necessary. The depressed diaphragm beneath expanded lung forces the liver edge to descend slightly, and as the lung is inflated, the liver edge slides over the examiner's fingers, creating the sensation of something solid, yet soft, "flipping" over the fingertips. The second technique involves curling the fingers from above over the lower rib cage margin and thus deep into the right upper quadrant and asking the patient to perform the same respiratory motions (Fig. 9.6*A* and *B*). Normal livers are frequently not palpable and are seldom felt through an obese or very muscular abdominal wall. If felt, the liver edge is assessed for consistency, clarity or "sharpness" of the margin, smoothness of contour, and the presence or absence of tenderness to palpation.

SPLEEN

Palpation for the high and well-protected spleen is facilitated by asking the patient to roll toward the examiner (into the right lateral decubitus position), which allows the organ to drop medially and inferiorly off the lateral rib cage. With the left hand pressing into the left flank from behind the lower margin of the rib cage, the right hand is pressed up and back beneath the anterior rib margins. The spleen also moves with the diaphragm, so the patient is asked to inhale, then exhale while the inferior tip of the spleen is sought (Fig. 9.7). If palpable, the organ is assessed for consistency and tenderness, and its size is estimated (see the Extended Examination section under Spleen).

AORTA

Deep palpation in the midline near the umbilicus may allow definition of the margins of the aorta in a thin person or a person with a very lax abdominal wall. By utilizing both hands and pressing deep on either side of the aorta, an estimate may be made of its lateral dimensions (Fig. 9.8).

KIDNEYS

Renal palpation is attempted by elevating the flank with the nondominant hand and pressing the dominant hand deep and upward under the rib cage. The kidneys, as retroperitoneal organs, are rarely felt unless they are enlarged or ptotic. The right kidney lies 1–2 cm more caudal than the left and thus is occasionally palpable—even when normal in size—in thin adults (Fig. 9.9).

SUPRAPUBIC AREA

If dullness to percussion has been elicited suprapubically, palpation of the pubic area may reveal a full **urinary bladder** or, in the female patient, an enlarged

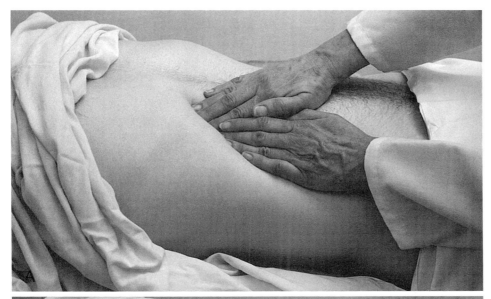

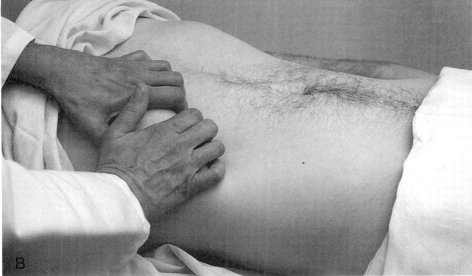

Figure 9.6 **A.** Palpation of lower margin of right lobe of liver. Note the examiner's hands pressed deeply beneath the right costal margin to capture the "flip" of the liver edge as it moves upward on expiration. **B.** Alternative "hook" method, for assessing an elusive liver margin.

uterus. The former is sometimes soft and compressible, and palpation may elicit from the patient a report of the urge to urinate. Further assessment of any other palpable mass in the suprapubic area is discussed in Chapters 13 and 14.

INGUINAL AND FEMORAL LYMPH NODES

The **inguinal nodes** are located along the inguinal ligament, are superficial, and even when normal are often palpable. They are small, soft, and freely mobile. The **femoral nodes** are located in the femoral triangle of the proximal thigh, approximately at the level of the junction of the medial and middle thirds of the inguinal ligament and 2–3 cm below the ligament. The femoral triangle is located by find-

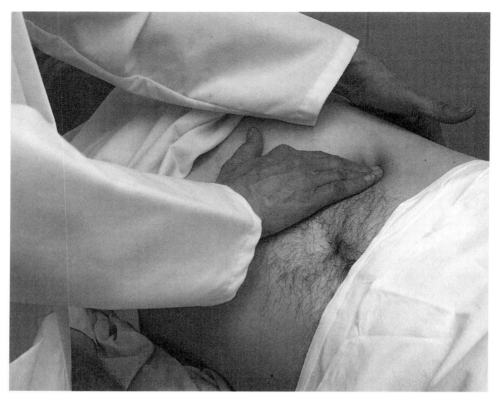

Figure 9.7　Splenic palpation. Note that patient is rolled slightly onto the right side so that the examiner's left hand may compress the posterior flank anteriorly while the examiner's right hand presses deep under the left costal margin.

ing the pulsation of the femoral artery. The nodes lie just medial to and parallel with the vessels. Normally, they are tiny or impalpable.

Palpation and Auscultation of the Femoral Arteries

In the efficient regional examination, palpation and auscultation of the femoral arteries are logically done at the conclusion of the abdominal examination. The femoral artery pulsations are best appreciated just above or below the inguinal ligament, 2–3 cm lateral to the pubic tubercle. Compression with the tips of the index and middle fingers will allow location of the femoral pulse. The magnitude of the pulsations should be equal bilaterally. If there is a difference in the amplitude of the two pulses, the bell of the stethoscope should be applied to each artery in search of a bruit (see Chapter 10 for indications and interpretations of large vessel abnormalities).

NORMAL AND COMMON VARIANTS

The variants of normal that may be anticipated by the examiner of the abdomen are discussed in the framework of the steps of the examination: inspection, auscultation, percussion, and palpation (Table 9.2).

Inspection
CONTOUR

The contour of the abdominal wall is determined by the volume of subcutaneous tissue, the development of its musculature, and the presence of distorting scars.

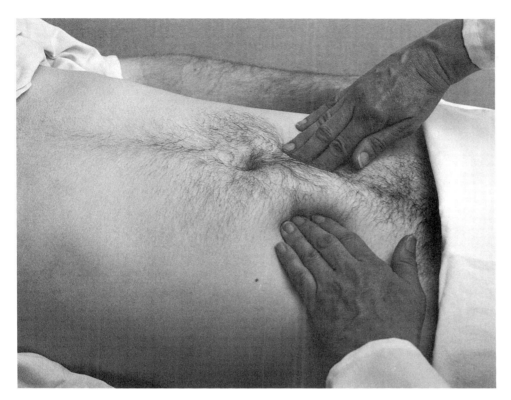

Figure 9.8   Palpation of abdominal aortic margins just below umbilicus.

The well-conditioned, nonpregnant, unconstipated adult of normal weight will have a flat or scaphoid abdomen in the supine position. The older, sedentary, or overweight person's abdomen may be protuberant as a result of increased subcutaneous fat, flaccid abdominal wall muscles, or both. Scar tissue from prior surgical procedures may distort the contour. The normal umbilicus is usually indented but may be flush with the abdominal wall or slightly protuberant.

SKIN

Skin over the abdomen is subject to the variations and lesions seen in skin elsewhere. It is common to find small hemangiomas, seborrheic keratoses, and nevi on the abdominal wall. Such lesions are noted and, if indicated, recorded (see Chapter 3 for indications to record or further assess skin findings). All surgical or traumatic scars should be inquired about and recorded by quadrant on the patient's record using a sketch. There is conventional nomenclature for describing certain surgical scars (Fig. 9.10). Striae, or "stretch marks," are white, pale tan, or slightly bluish bands of discoloration and may be seen in women who have been pregnant and persons who have had large weight gains. The venous pattern of the abdominal wall, when visible, is uniform, faint, and reticular. The veins of the abdominal wall drain cephalad from the transumbilical line and caudad below it.

MOVEMENTS

Resting abdominal movement in the supine person is minimal. The relaxed abdomen will rise slightly with inspiration as the diaphragms descend. Epigastric or midabdominal pulsations transmitted from the aorta may be visible in slender persons. Normal peristaltic waves of the intestine are rarely visible.

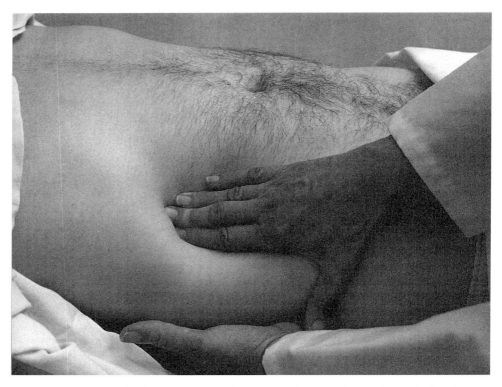

Figure 9.9   Renal palpation is attempted by pressing the posterior flank anteriorly with one hand while deeply palpating at the costal margin with the other. The inferior pole of a normal right kidney is sometimes thus compressible between the two hands.

Auscultation

BOWEL SOUNDS

Bowel sounds are audible throughout the abdomen with the diaphragm of the stethoscope lightly pressed against the skin. Peristalsis becomes more active with increased volume of the intestinal contents. Postprandially, bowel activity intensifies, and the gurgling sounds of air-fluid interfaces being propelled become more frequent. At rest, the peristaltic sounds are less frequent. Thus, the range of normal frequency and amplitude of bowel sounds is highly variable. Except under the particular circumstances discussed in the Extended Examination section of this chapter, these sounds are usually recorded as normal or present.

VASCULAR SOUNDS

Vascular sounds include transmitted cardiac sounds and murmurs in the epigastrium. A small fraction of apparently healthy persons are found to have some type of abdominal murmur. A continuous soft, low-pitched murmur with systolic accentuation has been described in the epigastrium of young, thin women. A low-intensity, high-pitched continuous hum to the right of the umbilicus has been attributed to flow in the inferior vena cava, although its differentiation from the hum of portal hypertension or from renal bruits by auscultation alone is rarely possible. Other vascular sounds such as bruits and pericardial friction rubs must be considered pathologic until proven otherwise.

Table 9.2
Normal and Common Variants Noted on Examination

Inspection	Percussion
Localized or generalized protuberance	**Air/gas variants**
Fat	Liver span range
Flatus	Urine-filled bladder
Feces	Pregnant uterus
Fetus	
Fluid (ascites)	Palpation
Neoplasms	Diastasis recti and incisional hernias
Local or small contour irregularities	Innocuous subcutaneous masses
Cutaneous or subcutaneous tumors	**Colonic feces**
Scars with retraction or puckering	Lower border of liver
Skin	**Aortic pulsation**
Nonpigmented striae	Lower pole of the right kidney
Pattern of venous flow	Urine-filled bladder
Common benign lesions	**Pregnant uterus**
Hemangiomas	**Small inguinal lymph nodes**
Seborrheic keratoses	
Nevi	
Auscultation	
Range of bowel sounds	
Normal vascular bruits	
Transmitted	
Local	

[a]**Boldface,** most common.

Percussion

Percussion notes over the abdominal viscera normally range from tympanitic over the gastric bubble in the left upper quadrant, to resonant over loops of small intestine or colon that contain some gas, to dull over solid organs such as the liver or over fluid-filled hollow organs such as the urinary bladder. The upper border of the liver as defined by percussion is located at the fourth to fifth intercostal space in the right midclavicular line. An upper border below the fifth intercostal space can be the result of downward displacement of the liver by an overinflated lung. The lower border of liver dullness is less clearly defined because of the variability of resonance in the adjacent bowel. The usual vertical span of liver dullness is 6–10 cm, commonly at the upper range in men and in tall adults and less in women and short persons. As noted earlier, a fully distended urinary bladder may sometimes be percussed as a rim of dullness extending 1–2 cm above the symphysis pubis, but physical examination is notoriously insensitive at detection of bladder enlargement.

Palpation

LIGHT PALPATION

Light palpation of the abdominal wall is used to assess extraperitoneal structures. A finger pressed into the umbilical depression will normally meet with fascial resistance, indicating full integrity of the underlying fascial support. The rectus abdominis muscles may be separated by a muscular defect large enough to admit the fingertips (**diastasis recti**), but again the underlying fascia and transversalis and oblique muscles will resist further insertion. Having the

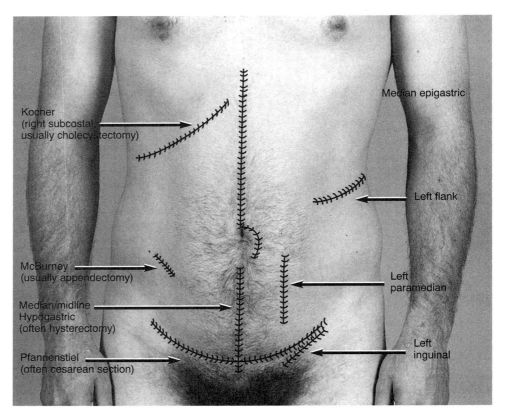

Kocher
(right subcostal,
usually cholecystectomy)

Median epigastric

Left flank

McBurney
(usually appendectomy)

Left
paramedian

Median/midline
Hypogastric
(often hysterectomy)

Pfannenstiel
(often cesarean section)

Left
inguinal

Figure 9.10   Common locations of classic abdominal surgical scars

patient raise the head from the table will accentuate any such defect, and the integrity of the underlying musculature may be determined. Innocuous subcutaneous masses such as lipomas or sebaceous cysts are usually located by light palpation. Light palpation may be uncomfortable for the patient who is ticklish and must occasionally be bypassed because of this problem. Deep palpation is better tolerated by such persons, since the firm, constant pressure tends to overcome ticklishness.

DEEP PALPATION

Deep palpation of the normal abdomen causes, at most, slight discomfort in the epigastrium and/or the left lower quadrant. Unless the examiner's hands are cold or the technique is too rapid or too deep, the abdomen should not resist palpation. Very well-developed rectus abdominis muscles may impede palpation somewhat, and it can be useful to have the patient flex the knees slightly to maximize passive rectus abdominis muscle relaxation. Except for the commonly palpable, stool-distended descending and sigmoid colon, discrete bowel segments cannot usually be distinguished by palpation. Occasionally, a normal cecum proves to be an exception.

The lower border of a normal liver should not extend more than 2–3 cm below the right costal margin. When palpable, the liver margin is distinct, smooth, soft to slightly firm, and mildly tender to deepest palpation. The normal spleen is not palpable in adults, and the lower pole of a normal kidney is occasionally barely appreciable as a firm, rounded tip deep in the flank.

RECORDING THE FINDINGS

The assessment of the abdomen is recorded in the patient's record immediately after the cardiovascular examination. It begins with a description of the contour of the abdomen and any surface markings noted. Abdominal skin lesions are usually recorded under SKIN as organ system, with the exception of local scars, which can be dealt with most rapidly and effectively via a sketch in the ABDOMEN section. The assessment of organs by palpation indicates whether any solid organ is palpable and, if so, what its characteristics are. Note that in the aged, because of the high prevalence of abundant stool and fecal impaction, a comment on fullness or diffuse firmness can be very helpful. Next, a record of the percussion measurements is made. Finally, auscultatory findings are added. Note that the *findings* are recorded in conventional order, even though the *sequence* of the examination differs from that elsewhere in the body.

Sample Write-up

Abdomen: Nondistended, symmetrical, flat, with normal respiratory movements. Well-healed, 7-cm, surgical scar, RLQ. Liver edge felt at right costal margin, smooth, soft and nontender. Spleen, kidneys, aorta, and colon not palpable. No tenderness to deep palpation; no masses felt. Liver 7 cm by percussion; remainder of abdomen normally resonant. Normal bowel sounds; no bruit or rub.

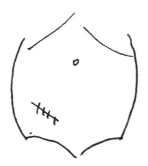

EXTENDED EXAMINATION OF THE ABDOMEN

INDICATIONS

Focus on the abdominal examination with the application of special examination maneuvers may be dictated by information acquired in the medical history or by the discovery of abnormalities on the screening physical examination. Since the abdominal cavity contains multiple organs representing several physiologic systems, the examiner must be able to think about the anatomic organ placement, as well as possible systems that might be implicated, while assessing abdominal complaints and findings. See Table 9.3.

Abdominal Symptoms

The cardinal symptom directing attention to the abdomen is **pain.** Abdominal pain may be **acute, chronic, or intermittent.** Assessment of abdominal pain by history includes details of the dimensions of any complaint, plus specific items

Table 9.3
Indications for Extended Examination

Abdominal symptoms
    Pain
    Nausea, **vomiting,** hematemesis
    Diarrhea, constipation, change in character of stool, **blood in stool,** melena
    Unexplained weight loss
    Jaundice, pruritus, dark urine
    Hematuria, back pain
    Claudication of leg, hip, or buttocks
    Change in girth or contour
    Weight loss

Abdominal signs
    On inspection
        Distension, localized or generalized
        Visible peristalsis
        Engorged abdominal wall veins or skin discoloration
        Skin lesions associated with internal disease
    On auscultation
        Absent or otherwise **abnormal bowel sounds**
        Vascular bruits
        Rubs
    On percussion
        Tympany, generalized or localized except over Traube's space
        Enlarged organs
        Unexpected areas of dullness
    On palpation
        Tenderness
        Guarding or rebound tenderness
        Organ enlargement
        Masses

[a]**Boldface,** most common.

that would otherwise be in the review of systems for gastrointestinal, reproductive, and genitourinary tract. When did the pain begin? Where is the pain? (See Figure 9.11 for visceral pain projections.) What are its qualities—sharp or dull, colicky, tearing, cramping, or continuous? What relieves the pain and what fails to relieve it? What makes it worse? What changes have occurred over time; i.e., is the pain getting worse or better, or have its characteristics altered? Have there been any other symptoms? Silen's textbook on the acute abdomen covers the details of comprehensive questioning.

From the past medical history, the clinician will learn about past occurrences of abdominal pain and any prior abdominal surgery. Pertinent questions from the review of systems embrace the systems potentially related to abdominal pain:

- **Gastrointestinal:** nausea, vomiting, hematemesis; diarrhea, constipation, change in stool habits or characteristics, bloody or tarry stools (melena); jaundice, pruritus (generalized itching), dark urine; change in abdominal contour; alcohol and medication history; prior attacks of cholecystitis or pancreatitis
- **Genitourinary:** history of renal stone, ingestion of calcium, gout; history of urinary tract infection or hematuria; flank pain or lower back pain; frequency or hesitancy; in women, a complete menstrual history, possibility of current

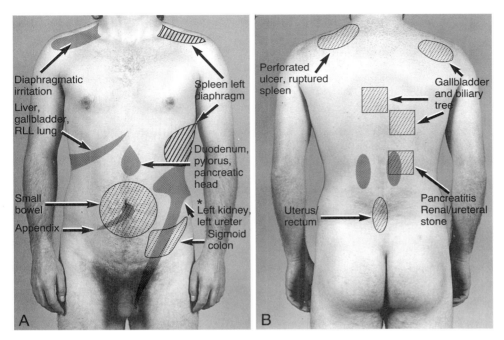

Figure 9.11 Common surface projections of visceral pain. Although not always perfectly represented, these are the clues the clinician seeks in helping to determine the organ(s) responsible for abdominal pain syndromes. **A.** Anterior. *Asterisk* indicates symmetric findings seen with involvement of opposite paired organs. **B.** Posterior.

pregnancy or recent miscarriage or therapeutic abortion; sexual activity and practices

- **Vascular:** history of chest pain or of diagnosed vascular problems such as coronary artery disease, congestive heart failure, hypercholesterolemia, known disease of the aorta, claudication, or prior vascular surgery (coronary insufficiency can present as epigastric pain); postprandial abdominal pain suggesting abdominal angina
- **Pulmonary:** pleurisy, shortness of breath, cough or expectoration, hemoptysis, chest pain (lower lobe pneumonia is a notorious cause of upper abdominal pain)
- **General:** fever, weight loss or gain, fatigue, night sweats

Any of the following symptoms elicited during the history demand special attention during extended examination of the abdomen: **nausea, vomiting, or hematemesis; weight loss, diarrhea, constipation, change in character of stool; jaundice, pruritus, or dark urine.**

Abnormalities Detected on Screening Examination

Occasionally, the clinician finds unsuspected abdominal abnormalities in the asymptomatic patient. Any of the following findings indicates a need for special maneuvers or further investigation:

- *On inspection:* generalized distension or localized bulging, visible peristalsis, engorged abdominal wall veins, jaundice
- *On auscultation:* absent or infrequent, high-pitched bowel sounds; vascular murmurs (bruits); rubs

- *On percussion:* generalized or localized tympany except over gastric air bubble, enlarged organs, or an excessive area of suprapubic dullness
- *On palpation:* tenderness, involuntary guarding, organ enlargement, mass, or sense of fecal impaction (abnormally firm texture throughout the mid-abdomen)

CONDUCTING THE EXTENDED EXAMINATION

Symptoms or signs referable to the abdomen or to systems or organs contained in the abdomen require modifications and expansions of the assessment. The particular maneuvers are dictated by the complaints of the patient and/or the findings of the examiner. The discussion of these procedures begins with the examination of the painful abdomen, then focuses on organ-specific and system-specific maneuvers. Table 9.4 is a summary of common terms used in the description or elicitation of abdominal signs.

Table 9.4
A Miniglossary of Abdominal Signs and Maneuvers

Abdominal signs
- Ascites: excess fluid in the peritoneal cavity
- Borborygmus: loud bowel "rushes" suggestive of intestinal obstruction
- Courvoisier's sign: presence of a palpable but nontender gallbladder suggestive of regional malignancy
- Cullen's sign: bluish-green to purple discoloration around the umbilicus
- Grey Turner's sign: nontraumatic ecchymoses on abdomen or flank
- Ileus: a paralysis of the peristaltic movement of the bowel
- Involuntary guarding: rigidity of the abdominal wall secondary to peritoneal irritation, which the patient cannot cause to abate
- Ladder sign: dilated loops of bowel visible on inspection of the contour of the abdominal wall
- Rebound tenderness: tenderness of the abdominal wall, which is greater on the sudden release of deep pressure than during the pressure itself; suggests peritoneal irritation
- Referred tenderness: tenderness elicited by local palpation but experienced in a different area; suggests peritoneal irritation at site where discomfort is felt by patient
- Referred rebound tenderness: discomfort on release, remote from site palpated
- Spider angiomata: superficial vascular lesions indicative of chronic liver disease

Abdominal maneuvers with interpretations
- Fluid wave: the tactile perception of free fluid moving within the abdominal cavity with ballottement
- Iliopsoas test (positive): pelvic pain produced by flexion of the thigh against resistance; suggests retroperitoneal irritation
- "Inching" the stethoscope: moving it inch by inch over the area in question to locate changes in intensity of sound
- Murphy's sign
  - Arrest of inspiration with deep palpation in the area of the gallbladder; suggests inflammation of the gallbladder
  - Tenderness on percussion of the costovertebral angle (a different Murphy's sign)
- Obturator test (positive): pelvic pain elicited by forced rotation of the flexed hip on the ipsilateral side suggests retroperitoneal irritation
- Puddle test: a method for detecting small amounts of ascites
- Scratch test: an auxiliary method of determining the location of the lower border of the liver
- Shifting dullness: change in location of percussive dullness secondary to movement of free intraperitoneal fluid with shift in body position

Painful Abdomen

Before beginning the detailed examination of the painful abdomen, flex the patient's knees slightly and passively with a small pillow or rolled sheet that will support and maintain the flexion. If possible, the patient should be fully recumbent with the abdomen exposed from just below the breasts to the symphysis pubis. During the examination the examiner should observe the patient's face for signs of discomfort, either spontaneous or inducible by the examination.

INSPECTION

Is the abdomen distended? If so, is the distension generalized, or is it localized to one area of the abdomen? Is the umbilicus everted? Is there a bulge near to or involving either the umbilicus or a surgical scar? If there is venous engorgement, in what direction does the venous blood flow? (See Figure 9.12 for a technique for assessing the direction of venous flow.) Is there bluish discoloration about the umbilicus (Cullen's sign) or apparent ecchymosis on abdomen or flank (Grey Turner's sign)? Are there spider angiomata in the superior caval distribution?

Is there visible peristalsis? Inspection of the abdomen for peristaltic movement is facilitated by shining a light horizontally or at a low transverse angle across the abdominal wall. Listen for borborygmus or intestinal sounds audible without the stethoscope, which may accompany visible peristalsis.

AUSCULTATION

Place the diaphragm of the stethoscope firmly on any abdominal quadrant. Does the stethoscope produce less pain than equal pressure exerted by palpating fingers? Are bowel sounds heard? If so, are they normal or composed of very occasional, high-pitched "tinkles?" Are there loud intermittent rushes associated with visible peristalsis and/or cramping pain noted by the patient? To be confident of the absence of bowel sounds, the examiner must hear none for a full minute.

PERCUSSION

Does percussion elicit pain, guarding, or withdrawal?

Is the abdomen tympanitic? Is the tympany generalized, or is it localized to one quadrant? Is there dullness to percussion, suggestive of an enlarged organ, a mass of solid tissue, or fluid in the peritoneal cavity?

PALPATION

If the patient has cited localized pain, begin palpation in the nonpainful quadrants and away from any visible bulges or discoloration. Skin hypersensitivity sometimes points to the pain source. If light touch elicits cutaneous hypersensitivity, consider dermatomal referral as a clue to the involved area (Fig. 9.13).

Light Palpation

Palpate lightly. Does the patient **guard?** That is, does the area that is touched immediately become tense and resistant? Is there rigidity, and is it localized or generalized? Can it be overcome by further elevating the patient's knees or asking the patient to breathe slowly and deeply? Resistance that cannot be overcome by these simple relaxation maneuvers is considered **involuntary** and *indicates peritoneal irritation.* **Voluntary guarding** is that which can be at least partially overcome by muscle relaxation.

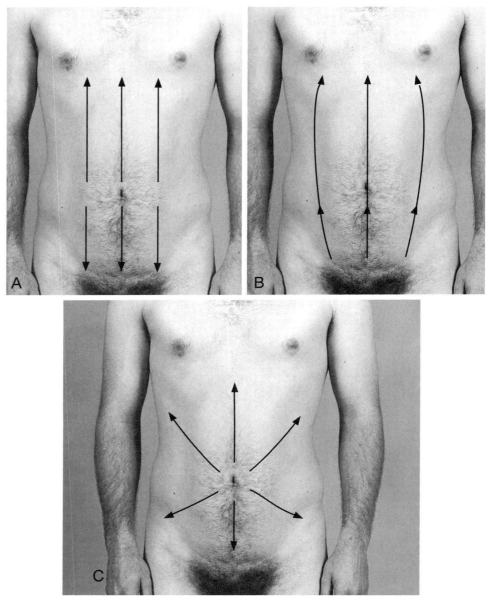

Figure 9.12   Classic patterns of abdominal wall venous flow. **A.** Normal flow up and down from transumbilical plane. **B.** Obstructed downward flow resulting from loss of inferior venal caval patency. **C.** Diverted flow with portal hypertension secondary to hepatic cirrhosis or portal vein obstruction. **D.** Technique of assessing direction of venous flow. Index fingers compress the vein; one finger moves laterally to strip the vein of its blood, and is then released, and the rapidity of filling of the stripped segment is observed. The opposite vein segment is then stripped and released. The segment that fills most rapidly indicates the direction of venous flow.

Deep Palpation

Generalized involuntary guarding may be sufficient to prevent deep palpation. In this instance, further physical evaluation of the site is not possible, and other modes of assessing the cause of the pain are required (see Beyond the Physical Examination).

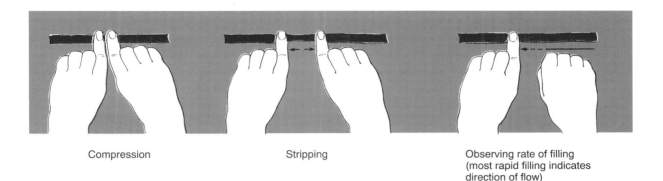

Compression   Stripping   Observing rate of filling
                                                            (most rapid filling indicates
                                                            direction of flow)

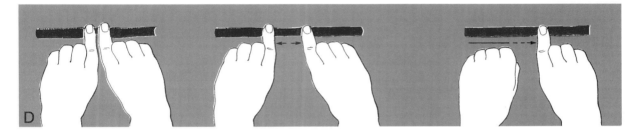

Figure 9.12 D.

In the case of regional voluntary guarding, the protected area may sometimes be assessed by palpating deeply from adjacent areas in a search for masses or enlarged organs. **Referred tenderness** is elicited by pressure on a painless, non-tender area that prompts a complaint of pain elsewhere. **Rebound tenderness** is elicited by sudden removal of palpation pressure. If the pain sensation is greatest after the pressure is released, rebound tenderness is recorded as present. Rebound, like tenderness, can be direct (present at the palpated site) or referred (produced remote from the area that is being palpated). Both signs are indicative of peritoneal irritation.

ADDITIONAL MANEUVERS

In the presence of deep abdominal or pelvic pain, two additional maneuvers can help determine the site of the pathology:

- **Iliopsoas maneuver.** The **iliopsoas test** is conducted by asking the patient to flex the thigh on the painful side, then to attempt to extend it against the resistance of the examiner's hand (Fig. 9.14*A*). Pain deep in the pelvis produced by this maneuver indicates irritation of the retroperitoneum, especially the ipsilateral iliopsoas muscle. Many variants of this test, all slightly different from one another, have been published.
- **Obturator maneuver.** To assess for irritation over the **obturator** muscle area, the patient is asked to flex the thigh on the affected side to 90°. The examiner then fixes the ankle and, with the other hand, attempts to externally rotate the hip by pulling the knee laterally against resistance. Pelvic pain produced by this maneuver indicates obturator muscle irritation (Fig. 9.14*B*).

The comprehensive assessment of abdominal pain requires that the femoral pulses be palpated for integrity and symmetric intensity. A rectal examination (see Chapters 13 and 14) is essential in every case of acute abdominal pain, to

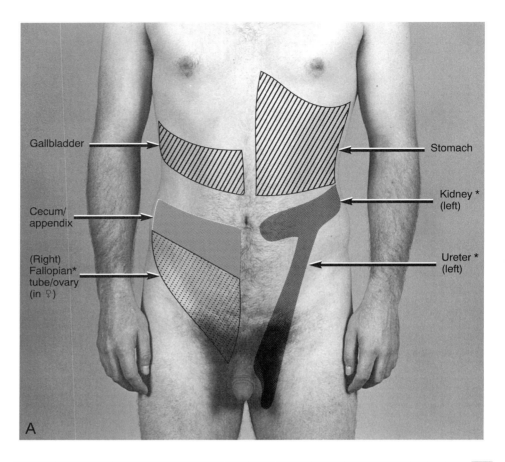

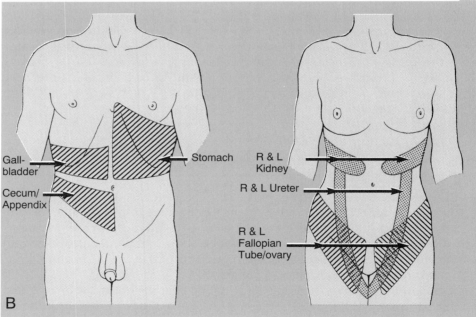

Figure 9.13 **A.** Cutaneous hypersensitivity to light touch as an indicator of the visceral source of pathology. *Asterisk* indicates symmetric findings seen with involvement of opposite paired organs. **B.** Schematic drawings of sensitive areas for male (*left*) and female (*right*) organs. Men can have renal-ureteral referral sensitivity in the same distribution as women, involving the penis and scrotum.

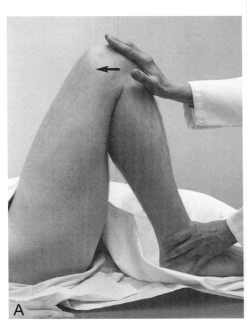

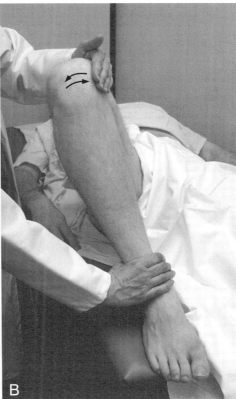

Figure 9.14 **A.** Iliopsoas maneuver for determining retroperitoneal irritation of the ipsilateral iliopsoas muscle. Note that examiner's left hand fixes the foot and ankle as the patient attempts to extend the thigh against patellar pressure. Alternatively, the patient may be asked to hyperextend the hip over the edge of the examining table. Either maneuver, in the face of inflamed iliopsoas fascia, will cause pelvic pain. **B.** Obturator maneuver to assess for irritation over the obturator muscle. External and internal rotation of the flexed hip with ankle fixed causes pain of an irritated ipsilateral obturator muscle.

seek tender sites or posterior pelvic masses and to seek pelvic tenderness. In women, a full pelvic examination (see Chapter 14) must be carried out in each case of acute abdominal pain, to determine whether uterus, ovaries, Fallopian tubes, or supporting and vascular structures are the source of the pain.

Abnormalities Discovered on Screening Examination

On occasion, physical findings with or without symptoms are noted by the examiner. These include (*a*) abnormalities of contour, (*b*) abnormalities of organ size, (*c*) masses, and (*d*) vascular abnormalities. Additional maneuvers for assessing deviations from normal are described as they might present during the course of a routine examination.

ABNORMALITIES OF CONTOUR

Localized Distension

Localized distension such as that of the upper abdomen should direct the examiner's attention to possible abnormalities of regional underlying organs. For example, an upper abdominal distension could represent dilatation of the stomach. Lower abdominal enlargement suggests cecal, urinary bladder, uterine, or ovarian abnormality. The regional localization of distension dictates the further percussion and palpation focus of the examination.

Generalized Distension

Generalized distension without pain may be secondary to obesity or to poor muscle tone; however, it could also represent **ascites** (free fluid in the peritoneal cavity). The signs suggestive of free fluid include bulging flanks, shifting dullness, and a fluid wave, although the sensitivity of physical examination alone for predicting ascites is poor. The clinician should be prepared to carry out the following techniques in an attempt to differentiate free peritoneal fluid from abdominal wall variants:

- **Shifting dullness.** This refers to the movement of the horizontal line of percussion note alteration as patient position changes. In the supine position, the air-containing (resonant) bowel "floats" to the top of a collection of ascites; when the patient rolls to one side or the other, the bowel assumes the uppermost position, and the level of the air-fluid interface will change. The principles of this assessment are illustrated schematically in Figure 9.15A.
- **Fluid wave.** Free fluid in the abdominal cavity will shift with flank ballottement. Hold one hand (the "receiving" hand) on one flank and press. Tap the other hand sharply against the opposite flank while the patient or an assistant compresses the midabdomen. The passive "receiving" hand will detect the wave of fluid driven by the ballotting hand (Fig. 9.15B). Unfortunately, false-positive as well as false-negative results can occur.
- **"Puddle" test.** This technique is sometimes used to define small amounts of free peritoneal fluid. It has the disadvantage of being uncomfortable for the patient and probably is not sufficiently productive of reliable information to be useful except in special situations. To elicit the puddle sign, the patient is asked to support himself on his knees and forearms such that the midabdomen is dependent. The examiner places the stethoscope over the most dependent portion of the abdomen and flicks one finger of the opposite hand against the flank so that the sound waves pass through puddled fluid. As the stethoscope is inched toward the opposite flank, the flicking is continued from a fixed position. An abrupt decrease in the intensity of the sound generated by the flicking finger as the stethoscope moves above the pooled fluid is considered a positive sign. If such a change is perceived, the process is repeated on the opposite side of the pool to define its margin (Fig. 9.16).

A very large **ovarian cyst** may produce several physical signs of ascites. The thin-walled, fluid-filled sac can distend the abdomen, evert the umbilicus, cause bulging of the flanks, and test positively for shifting dullness and a fluid wave. There are, however, important differences between the two that can be exploited for differentiation by physical examination. For example, the cystic mass arising from the pelvis forces the air-containing bowel toward the diaphragm such that the percussion note remains dull over the most anterior point of the abdomen, which is uppermost if the patient is supine, and the resonance of gut lies in the epigastrium. Also, some cysts transmit aortic pulsations; ascitic fluid dampens them. Thus a ruler or a sheet of paper laid on the abdominal wall below the umbilicus may sometimes be seen to move with the pulse if the distension is caused by a cyst.

Discrete **bulges** visible on the surface of the abdominal wall can represent subcutaneous masses, hernias, or intra-abdominal masses. A bulge or break in the smooth contour that arises in the extraperitoneal wall can usually be partially surrounded by the examining fingers and will be definable as subcutaneous by

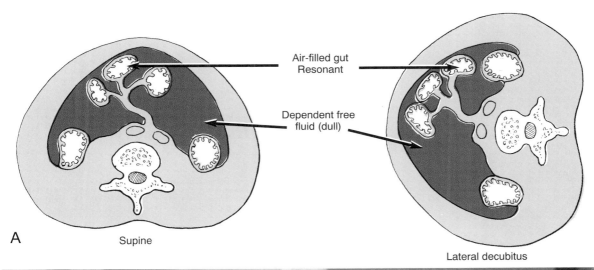

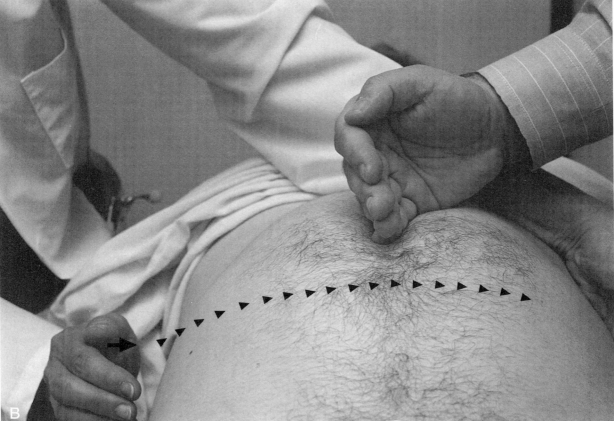

Figure 9.15   A. Shifting dullness. Schematic representation of free fluid (ascites) movement in the peritoneal cavity. Level of percussible dullness shifts with body position from supine to lateral decubitus as resonant bowel is floated upward on the shifting free fluid. **B.** Fluid wave. Assistant compresses anterior abdominal wall in midline, while examiner performs ballottement on the right flank and feels for transmitted fluid pulse in left flank.

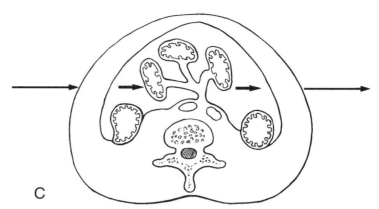

Figure 9.15   C. Schematic illustration of the method and mechanics of free peritoneal fluid wave transmission.

becoming sharper when the patient lifts his head from the table, thus tensing the muscles beneath the mass. A mass that becomes more prominent with this maneuver (which also increases intra-abdominal pressure) represents either a *superficial structure* or *herniation* of a preperitoneal or intraperitoneal structure through a wall defect. Such **hernias** are most common in the midline above the umbilicus, around the umbilicus itself, at the site of a surgical scar, or at the margins of the abdominal muscle layers. If such a bulge is present, use the fingertips to define the rim of the defect through which it protrudes. Determine by pressing gently against it whether or not it is tender and can be reduced easily back into the abdominal cavity. *Do not force reduction of a painful, tender, or resistant herniation.*

ABNORMAL ORGAN SIZE

If one of the abdominal organs is found to be enlarged or otherwise abnormal to examination, special techniques may be indicated. The liver, spleen, and kidneys are the primary organs to be considered.

Liver

If the liver span is found to be greater than 12 cm on percussion at the midclavicular line on the right or if the edge is palpable more than 2 cm below the right costal margin in the absence of pulmonary hyperinflation, enlargement of the organ is suspected. When the examiner has difficulty defining the lower border of the liver, the **scratch test** is useful as an adjunct. The diaphragm of the stethoscope is placed over the liver just above the costal margin in the midclavicular line. One finger, scratching gently against the skin, is zigzagged progressively cephalad along the midclavicular line toward the right upper quadrant. When the scratching finger crosses above the liver edge, its sound is transmitted more clearly through the solid organ (Fig. 9.17). Once the liver margin is identified, it should be palpated laterally and medially, and irregularities of contour or variations in consistency should be observed.

If there is tenderness to palpation of the liver or caudal to its margin, attempt to elicit a **Murphy's sign.** This is accomplished by asking the patient to inspire deeply while the examiner's fingers are pressed deeply below the liver edge (or the ribcage, if the liver is impalpable). An abrupt arrest of respiration when the examining fingers contact the gallbladder region indicates probable gallbladder inflammation and constitutes a positive Murphy's sign.

Tenderness to a *light* punch just above the right costal margin, 5 cm lateral to the midclavicular line, is a test for hepatic inflammation.

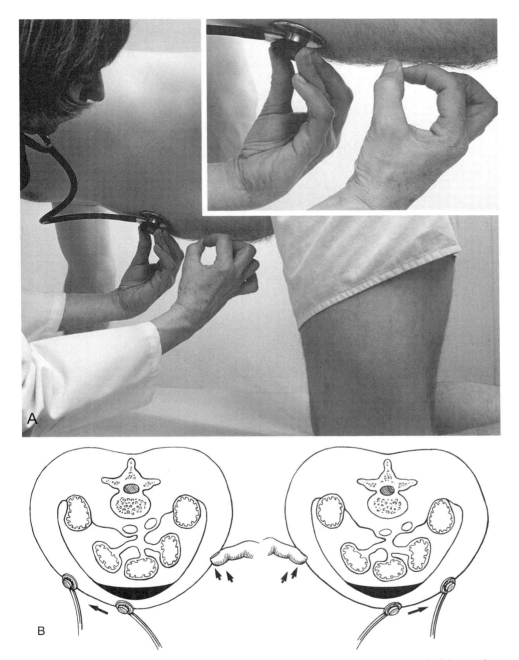

Figure 9.16   Puddle sign elicitation. **A.** Note the position of the patient and of the stethoscope and the examiner's flicking finger. As the stethoscope is moved toward the opposite flank, the examiner listens for an increase in intensity of sound produced by flicking, which indicates a puddle of free fluid in the dependent abdomen. **B.** Schematic representation of dynamics of the puddle sign test.

Spleen

If **splenic** enlargement is suspected, percussion of the area is conducted by moving to the patient's left side and assisting the patient into a right lateral decubitus position. Percuss over the lowest intercostal space in the midaxillary line while asking the patient to inhale and exhale slowly and deeply. Resonance to percus-

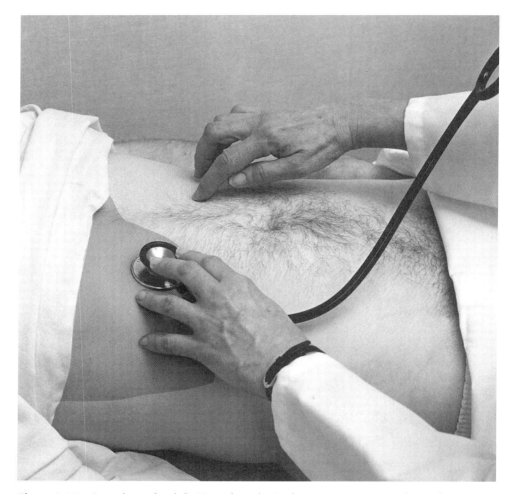

Figure 9.17   Scratch test for definition of an elusive liver margin. See text for explanation.

sion during expiration, which is replaced by *dullness in deep inspiration,* suggests splenomegaly, as the organ descends with the diaphragm.

While the patient is still in the right decubitus position, feel for the tip of the spleen. Use your left hand to press the flank anteriorly from behind while you press your right hand beneath the cartilage of ribs 9–11 (see Fig. 9.7). A palpable spleen on deep inhalation indicates enlargement of 2–3 times normal size or more. The amount of spleen felt below the rib margin is measured in order to estimate organ size. A palpable spleen should be *gently* assessed for tenderness and consistency. It is normally somewhat soft but, when enlarged, is more commonly quite firm.

An alternative method of palpating for the spleen, especially when a rib tip is causing confusion, is conducted from the left side of the table with the patient in right lateral decubitus position. Place both hands on the left costal border and curl the fingers around the costal margin at the top of ribs 9–11, "hooking" the fingertips into the subcostal tissue. On deep inspiration, the edge of an enlarged spleen may tap the tips of the your flexed fingers (Fig. 9.18).

Kidneys

When an enlarged kidney is suspected, attempt to "capture" it by standing on the side to be examined and placing your left hand posteriorly in the flank, par-

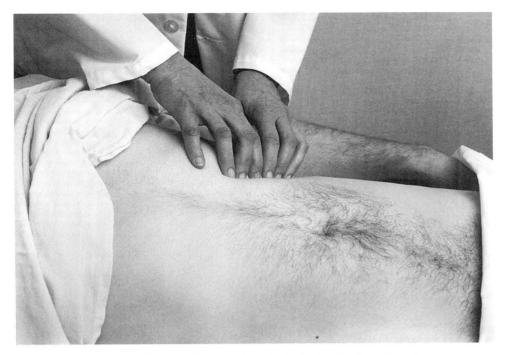

Figure 9.18 "Hook" technique, the second method of palpation for spleen tip.

allel to the plane of the table, and palpating deeply anteriorly under the rib margins with your right hand, in a parallel plane. Ask the patient to inhale deeply, and press your hands toward each other. As the patient exhales, reduce the inward pressure and feel the kidney slip between your hands. A readily palpable left kidney must be considered abnormal. Either it is enlarged, or there is a retroperitoneal mass. Assess the palpable kidney for irregularity of contour and for tenderness.

MASSES

When a **mass** is discovered on abdominal examination, the examiner must attempt several determinations. Is the mass solid or cystic? Is it inside the peritoneal cavity? Is it part of or separate from abdominal organs?

Light palpation with a maneuver such as asking the patient to raise his head from the table should define the mass as extraperitoneal or intraperitoneal, as discussed above. In general, the first step in palpating an apparent abdominal mass is to use this maneuver to tense the abdominal wall muscles. The contracted muscles will cloak an intraperitoneal or retroperitoneal structure, which therefore "disappears" with this maneuver. Unchanged or enhanced palpability with abdominal contraction localizes the mass to the abdominal wall.

Deep palpation is used to determine the size, mobility, and attachments of the mass. Is it hard and fixed to the abdominal wall or to other abdominal organs? In which quadrant or quadrants does it reside? Does it move with deep respiration (indicative of lying on the diaphragm or freely mobile within the peritoneal cavity)? What is the contour of the mass? Is it tender to palpation?

A mass in the lower abdomen requires pelvic and rectal examinations to further define its extent and site of origin once a distended urinary bladder has been ruled out. Auscultatory percussion may help delineate bladder distension: Using your nondominant hand, hold the bell of the stethoscope in the midline immediately above the symphysis pubis. Then, using a finger of your dominant hand, percuss (no pleximeter) the symphysis in a midline vertical plane beginning just below the umbilicus. When your percussing finger reaches the upper border of a urine-filled bladder, you will notice an abrupt increase in intensity of the transmitted sound heard through the bell. The procedure may be repeated to define the lateral margins of an overfilled urinary bladder.

VASCULAR ABNORMALITIES

Vascular abnormalities may be discovered on auscultation or palpation. The presence of bruits, which are murmurs heard over large vessels, usually indicates luminal narrowing that results in turbulent, noisy blood flow. A systolic bruit over the aorta can be a sign of partial obstruction or, on occasion, of aneurysm, although it is not a sensitive indicator of either. Flank bruits suggest renal artery narrowing, but lateralize poorly. A continuous (systolic-diastolic), or to-and-fro murmur may signal an arteriovenous fistula or a highly vascular tumor. When a murmur is heard, inch the stethoscope over the abdominal wall to determine its point of greatest intensity, any systolic and diastolic components, and direction(s) and extent of radiation.

When a difference in the amplitude of femoral artery pulsation is noted by palpation, listen over the vessels for bruits. If on palpation of the aorta the normally anterior pulsation appears to be lateral, the possibility of aneurysm should be considered. If you are unable to feel the aortic pulsation on routine palpation, an alternative method is suggested. Place the palmar surfaces of both hands along the abdomen just left of the midline with the midpalm at the umbilical level. Then press deeply inward to locate the lateral borders of the aorta and to assess the vessel for width and direction of pulsation. When a paramedian pulsatile mass is felt, palpate it bimanually, sliding inferiorly to bring the fingertips just below the umbilicus to determine its mobility. Since the aorta is fixed proximally and distally, an aneurysm can typically be moved side to side but not longitudinally, whereas a mass overlying the aorta and transmitting pulsations from it may be mobile in the cephalad or caudad direction. Having said this, we acknowledge that (a) aortic pulsations are impalpable in many normal thin persons and most normal obese persons; (b) an overdiagnosis of aortic aneurysm is often made because of striking pulsations; (c) many large aortic aneurysms are impalpable; and (d) ultrasonography plays an enormous role in refining both diagnosis and exclusion of aneurysm when the aorta feels abnormal on palpation.

INTERPRETING THE FINDINGS

Symptoms and signs referable to the abdomen may arise from several physiologic systems and may implicate a number of organs. For detailed discussion of diseases of the abdominal organs, the reader is referred to textbooks of medicine and surgery as well as the selected articles and texts listed in the Bibliography. The following overview will be confined to broadly categorized abnormalities as they present in the medical history and the physical examination.

Painful Abdomen

The approach to the patient with abdominal pain varies enormously, as does the level of urgency dictated by the patient's general condition. Severe pain, especially if accompanied by fever, chills, signs or symptoms of shock, or evidence of intestinal obstruction or rupture of an intra-abdominal viscus, is a medical emergency. Chronic or intermittent pain without systemic signs of sepsis or vascular collapse warrants a less pressured diagnostic approach.

ACUTE ABDOMINAL PAIN

In the physical assessment of the patient with a complaint of acute abdominal pain, certain signs are suggestive of specific pathophysiologic processes (Table 9.5). **Generalized distension** of the abdomen is suggestive of **ileus,** a disruption of normal bowel motility. Ileus may be either mechanically or metabolically induced. An obstructed bowel will eventually dilate, become edematous, and cease its normal peristaltic and absorptive function. Inflammation of the bowel (as in peritonitis), ischemia of the bowel (as in mesenteric vascular insufficiency), and lack of chemical substrates and/or mediators for electromechanical coupling (as in hypokalemia) will all present as ileus. The *nonfunctional small bowel is silent* or nearly silent to auscultation (conducted for a full minute). When the next phase, gas accumulation, supervenes, it becomes tympanitic to percussion. Thus, the generally distended, silent, and tympanitic abdomen signals ileus; the underlying cause of the ileus becomes the diagnostic dilemma. Note that a normally functioning bowel may be silent in the patient on a respirator as a result of lack of air swallowing in this situation.

In the presence of ileus, a rigid abdomen means **peritonitis.** Peritonitis, or inflammation of the serosal surfaces of the abdomen and its organs, may be induced by infection or by leakage of bowel contents, bile, or blood into the peritoneal cavity. Ileus without peritoneal signs such as rigidity or involuntary guarding is suggestive of mechanical obstruction without perforation of viscus or of a metabolic or electrolyte derangement, including narcotic-induced and bed rest-induced pseudo-obstruction (Ogilvie's syndrome).

Other important signs of some differential diagnostic significance in the painful and guarded abdomen include (*a*) periumbilical blue-purple to greenish-yellow discoloration (Cullen's sign) or flank ecchymoses (Grey Turner's sign), either of which indicates seepage of blood along tissue planes from intraperitoneal or retroperitoneal hemorrhage classically in hemorrhagic pancreatitis but also in diverse other settings; (*b*) loops of visibly dilated small intestine (ladder sign) in the setting of volvulus or ileocecal obstruction; and (*c*) visible contour of distended large bowel in the case of distal colonic obstruction. A mass obstructing the finger on rectal examination announces a dramatic cause. The presence of jaundice, spider angiomata, and engorged abdominal wall veins in a distended, painful, and tender abdomen raises the question of spontaneous bacterial peritonitis secondary to infected ascitic fluid.

Visible peristalsis, with or without borborygmi, in the nondistended abdomen suggests early intestinal obstruction in the stage preceding ileus. Stethoscope auscultation will reveal loud rushes of bowel sounds separated by periods of silence, or generalized hyperactive bowel sounds.

If the patient has indicated localized pain, consult Figure 9.11 for the most commonly represented processes. Local guarding, rebound tenderness, and referred pain may help to pinpoint the site of pathology, although exceptions can occur. Positive iliopsoas or obturator tests suggest retroperitoneal irritation, the location of which may be further defined by rectal or pelvic examination. The importance of these techniques and of checking routinely for *incarcerated inguinal and femoral hernias* in every case of acute abdominal pain requires strong emphasis.

A complaint of intense steady or colicky pain in one flank, especially with radiation to the groin and vulva or penis and scrotum, is indicative of *ureteral calculus.* In the classic situation, the patient's discomfort is so intense that lying still is difficult; yet the examination of the abdomen is surprisingly normal, with minimal tenderness and no evidence of ileus or peritonitis. Apart from this situation, patients with an acute abdomen and very little in the way of localizing signs, most particularly if they also have hypotension, are likely to have a vascular cata-

Table 9.5
The Acutely Painful Abdomen

Symptoms and Signs	Considerations	Other Evidence
Central pain only	**Early appendicitis** **Small bowel obstruction** Acute pancreatitis [Acute myocardial infarction] [Pericarditis] [Herpes zoster]	
Central pain with vascular collapse	Acute pancreatitis Acute mesenteric ischemia Ruptured aortic aneurysm Dissecting aortic hematoma [Myocardial infarct] Intra-abdominal hemorrhage	Back and bilateral flank pain; vomiting; rigidity Symptoms and signs of vascular disease; blood in stool Shock; radiation of pain to groin/perineum; pulsatile mass Often begins in chest and back; absent femoral pulses [see Chapter 8] Abdominal distension; shortness of breath with shallow respirations
Pain, vomiting, and distension	**Small bowel obstruction** Early peritonitis	Visible peristalsis Increasing rigidity
Severe pain, shock, and general rigidity	Perforated viscus Dissecting hematoma	Board-like rigidity, vomiting, distension, shoulder pain (if periphery of diaphragm is irritated)
Left upper quadrant pain and rigidity	Pancreatitis Perforated gastric ulcer Splenic rupture Perinephritis Acute upper urinary, process (stone, infection) [LLL pneumonia]	Vomiting Sometimes dysuria and back pain See Chapter 7
Right upper quadrant pain and rigidity	[RLL pneumonia] [Pleurisy] **Acute cholecystitis** Leaking duodenal ulcer Perforated/penetrating ulcer Pancreatitis Subphrenic appendix with appendicitis	See Chapter 7
Left lower quadrant pain, tenderness, guarding	**Diverticulitis** Pyelonephritis Pelvic peritonitis (often secondary to salpingitis) Ruptured ectopic pregnancy	
Right lower quadrant pain and rigidity	**Appendicitis** Regional enteritis Meckel's diverticulitis Pyelonephritis Pelvic peritonitis Ruptured ectopic pregnancy	

[a]**Boldface,** common; [. . .], extraabdominal etiologies; RLL, right lower lobe.

strophe such as acute mesenteric ischemia, aortic aneurysm, or dissecting hematoma of the aorta.

The complaint of chronic or intermittent abdominal pain without current evidence of acute illness should be assessed by systematic observations and approached as discussed below.

ABNORMALITIES OF CONTOUR
Localized Distension

Localized distension of the upper abdomen can be caused by gastric dilation resulting from outlet obstruction, aperistalsis (gastroparesis) secondary to trauma, autonomic neuropathy (usually diabetic), or surgical manipulation. An enlarged liver or a tumor of the upper abdominal organs can change the surface contour. Isolated distension of the lower abdomen may be seen with a greatly overdistended bladder in mechanical or neurogenic outlet obstruction. A uterus enlarged by pregnancy or neoplasm may distort the lower abdominal contour, as may a huge ovarian mass. In the thin patient, a large accumulation of feces in the sigmoid colon is sometimes visible in the left lower quadrant and may represent impaction or megacolon.

Discrete **bulges** disrupting the normal contour of the abdominal wall characterize *hernias*. The defect in the integrity of the wall may admit preperitoneal fat only, segments of small bowel with or without omentum, or, uncommonly, portions of solid organs. The common sites for abdominal hernias are the linea alba in the epigastrium, the umbilical ring, a surgical scar (incisional hernia), or the linea semilunaris (Spigelian hernia) (Fig. 9.19). Inguinal and femoral hernias are discussed in Chapter 13.

Generalized Distension

The formal differential diagnosis of abdominal distension is sixfold: obesity, ascites, fecal impaction, flatus, neoplasia, and pregnancy

Generalized distension in the absence of peritonitis or ileus suggests ascites. Large accumulations of free fluid in the peritoneal cavity may be indicative of any one of a number of pathophysiologic conditions. Portal hypertension, with reduction of portal flow through the liver as the result of hepatic scarring, leads to fluid transudation in the tributary capillaries of the portal bed. Similar pathophysiology applies with neoplastic or thrombotic obstruction of the hepatic veins (Budd-Chiari syndrome) and portal vein. Right-sided heart failure and nephrotic syndrome may eventually result in ascites, although the liver sinusoids partially protect the portal system from elevated caval pressure. Several diverse conditions such as myxedema can cause ascites. Neoplastic or tuberculous implants on the peritoneal surface directly increase capillary permeability by way of inflammation. Chylous ascites accumulates from obstruction of the lymphatic drainage of the abdomen, usually by tumor or rarely from disruption of the thoracic duct; it can also be seen in conventional cirrhosis; the mechanism is unclear.

Intra-abdominal Masses

Masses palpable within the peritoneal cavity or in the retroperitoneal space represent either organ enlargement or neoplasia. To evaluate possible sources of a mass, it is useful for the examiner to consider the abdomen by region, keeping in mind that a mass arising in any given quadrant may extend well beyond its origin (Table 9.6).

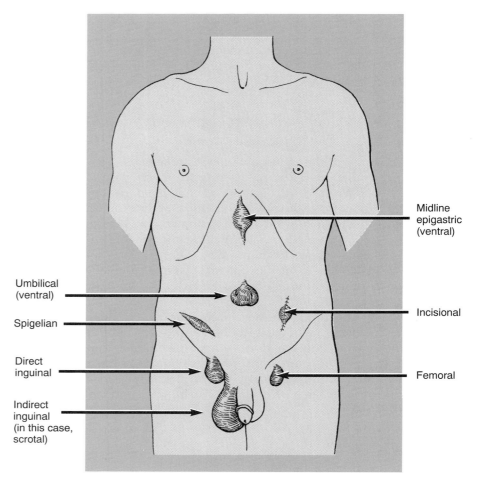

Midline
epigastric
(ventral)

Umbilical
(ventral)

Spigelian

Direct
inguinal

Indirect
inguinal
(in this case,
scrotal)

Incisional

Femoral

Figure 9.19 Sites of presentation of common abdominal and groin hernias.

RIGHT UPPER QUADRANT MASSES

The dominant organ of the **right upper quadrant (RUQ)** is the liver. An enlarged, but smooth and nontender liver can be caused by fatty infiltration, hepatic venous obstruction (which often produces tenderness), lymphoma or leukemia, displacement of normal hepatic tissue by amyloid or active hematopoiesis, primary or metastatic carcinoma, or parasitic infestation. If the enlarged, smooth liver is tender, consider hepatitis (viral, microbial, toxic, or medication-induced), congestive heart failure, or bacterial or parasitic infection. A very hard liver suggests neoplastic infiltration and is a rather specific, albeit insensitive, indicator. Surface nodularity is found in metastatic carcinoma and in some forms of cirrhosis. The massively enlarged organ raises the question of myeloid metaplasia or chronic myelogenous leukemia.

Tumors of the liver, either primary or metastatic, can present as diffuse enlargement of the organ or as discrete masses contiguous with normal-feeling liver tissue. The combination of a hepatic rub and bruit is more specific than either alone for primary or metastatic liver cancer. Definitive diagnosis of hepatic tumors requires imaging procedures and histologic study.

If a mass is palpated on the inferior surface of the liver, enlargement of the gallbladder should be considered. The acutely inflamed enlargement of cholecys-

Table 9.6
Abdominal Masses

Superficial and subcutaneous masses
    Fibromas, **lipomas,** and other innocuous masses
    Hernias

Intra-abdominal masses
    Right upper quadrant masses
        Infiltrative diseases of the liver (steatosis, amyloid, etc.)
        Tumors of the liver (primary, metastatic, or hematologic)
        Inflammatory enlargement of the liver
        Inflammation of the biliary tree
        Obstruction of the gallbladder
        Tumors of the right kidney
    Left upper quadrant masses
        Infiltrative disease of the spleen
        Inflammation or vascular congestion of the spleen
        Hematoma of the spleen (including subcapsular)
        Tumors of the left kidney
        Feces in the left colon
    Epigastric masses
        Pancreatic cyst or tumor
        Neoplasm or infection of stomach, omentum, transverse colon, left lobe of liver
        Gastric outlet obstruction or gastroparesis
        Aortic aneurysm
    Right lower quadrant masses
        Inflammation, abscess, or neoplasm of the cecum, distal ileum, or appendix
        Inflammation or tumor of the right salpinx and/or ovary
    Left lower quadrant masses
        Inflammation or tumor of the sigmoid colon including **diverticular abscess**
        Fecal impaction of the sigmoid colon
        Inflammation or tumor of the left salpinx and/or ovary
    Midline lower abdominal masses
        Aortoiliac enlargement
        Bladder distension
        Enlargement of the uterus from pregnancy or tumor

[a]**Boldface,** most common.

titis or gallbladder empyema is rarely palpated because of extreme tenderness and guarding in this situation. Occasionally, hydrops, or noninflammatory enlargement in the face of cystic duct obstruction, or painless distension secondary to carcinomatous obstruction of the ampulla of Vater will render the gallbladder palpable. A palpable nontender gallbladder suggests regional malignancy; the eponym Courvoisier's sign is used for this condition.

A polycystic right kidney, hydronephrosis, single large renal cyst, or renal tumor can occasionally be appreciated as a RUQ mass. Depending on the degree of enlargement, this may be difficult or impossible to distinguish from hydrops of the gallbladder or a pancreatic pseudocyst. Finally, a mass from the hepatic flexure of the colon may present here.

LEFT UPPER QUADRANT MASSES

Left upper quadrant (LUQ) masses may be renal, analogous to those noted above, or, more commonly, related to splenic enlargement. The spleen may harbor diverse infiltrative, infectious, hematologic, and neoplastic diseases. The reader is referred to a textbook of medicine for the differentiating features of the diseases that enlarge the spleen. In the setting of a history of upper abdominal or flank trauma and a tender, palpable spleen, the examiner should consider subcapsular hematoma of this highly vascular organ. Tumors of the splenic flexure of the colon can produce LUQ masses.

An upper midabdominal (**epigastric**) mass that is distinguishable from the liver raises the possibility of pancreatic cancer or pseudocyst or of involvement of the stomach, omentum, left lobe of the liver, or the transverse colon by neoplasm or infection. Usually, it is impossible to discriminate among these by physical examination alone.

RIGHT LOWER QUADRANT MASSES

The **right lower quadrant (RLQ)** contains the cecum, distal ileum, and vermiform appendix and, in females, the right Fallopian tube and ovary. If a firm mass is felt in the ileocecal region, consider Crohn's disease, periappendiceal abscess, cecal carcinoma, and, rarely, granulomatous disease. Reproductive organ differential diagnoses are considered in Chapters 13 and 14.

LEFT LOWER QUADRANT MASSES

Masses confined to the **left lower quadrant (LLQ)** are related to the pelvic organs, as indicated previously, or to the sigmoid colon. The latter may be a tender inflammatory mass from diverticulitis with abscess formation, a nontender cancer, or distension with feces as a result of obstruction or, more commonly, severe constipation. A diagonal "sausage" shape and a mass that retains an indentation from a palpating finger strongly suggest distension by excess feces.

Suprapubic Zone

The **midabdomen** contains the urinary bladder and uterus (see Chapters 13 and 14), aorta, inferior vena cava, and proximal iliac vessels, the periaortic lymph nodes, and overlying loops of small bowel. A pulsatile mass in this area suggests aortic aneurysm, although solid tumors may also transmit normal aortoiliac pulsations. As in the epigastrium, definitive differentiation of the organs or tissue primarily involved in masses in this area usually requires imaging.

Vascular Abnormalities

Since abdominal bruits are not rare in healthy individuals, interpretation of such sounds must be made with caution. The majority of normal bruits occur in systole and are heard in the midline between the xiphoid and the umbilicus, without radiation to the sides. They have low intensity and pitch. Pathologic bruits have certain characteristics that help to differentiate them. A bruit occasionally found in pancreatic carcinoma is usually sharply localized in the left upper quadrant, presumably because it is caused by fixation and external compression of the splenic vein by the enlarging mass. The murmurs of hepatic tumors are often loud and harsh and located directly over the liver. The murmur of renal artery stenosis may be audible in the midline, but it often radiates to or is best heard laterally, in a flank, or even posteriorly. Authorities disagree on whether renal bruits are best heard anteriorly or posteriorly over the flanks. The continuous murmur of an arteriovenous fistula is also well localized. Differentiation between the normal venous hum of the inferior vena cava and the venous hum of portal hypertension is difficult, and such hums should be interpreted in the light of other clinical signs.

Absence or diminution of pulse or presence of a bruit in either or both femoral arteries—especially with a history suggestive of claudication or signs such as cool leg temperature, reduced color, or hair loss in the lower limb—point to obstructive disease in the aortoiliofemoral arterial system. Total bilateral absence of femoral pulsations with **hip and buttock claudication** is found with occlusion of the aortic bifurcation (Leriche's syndrome). In this setting, vascular impotence is a nearly constant cosymptom. The more common situation is that of asymmetrical involvement of the arteries with resultant asymmetry of physical findings.

RECORDING THE FINDINGS

Abnormalities discovered on the examination are recorded in the patient's chart with accompanying sketch, when indicated, for clarity. Skin lesions or scars are described by quadrant and location, length (and, sometimes, width), and significant characteristics (especially abnormalities). Organ abnormalities are recorded as to location, the organ involved if this can be determined, and the nature of the abnormality (i.e., enlargement, abnormality of contour and/or consistency, tenderness). Masses are located by quadrant; measured (if possible) or estimated dimensions; contour, consistency, fixation and/or immobility (including reducibility of any hernia); presence or absence of pulsation, tenderness; percussion note; and overlying auscultatory findings. Abnormal sounds such as vascular bruits are located and described as to intensity, phase of cardiac cycle, pitch, and radiation. Bruits can be recorded, with a further systematic approach, under ARTERIES instead, whereas the venous and angiomatous findings belong under ABDOMEN rather than under SKIN or VEINS.

Sample Write-up

Abdomen: Moderately distended, with bulging flanks and protuberant umbilicus. Skin icteric. Venous pattern prominent, with flow radiating from umbilicus but without frank caput medusae. Right hypogastric paramedian scar, well-healed, with easily reducible small central herniation. Bowel sounds present, slightly diminished. Fluid wave and shifting dullness both present. Liver span 14 cm. Nontender, firm, and smooth liver edge 4 cm below right costal margin, no nodules. Spleen tip barely palpable, firm. No tenderness to deep palpation, and no masses are appreciated. Aortic pulsation not felt, but both femoral arteries palpable equally and without bruits. No rubs nor bruits heard, including over liver.

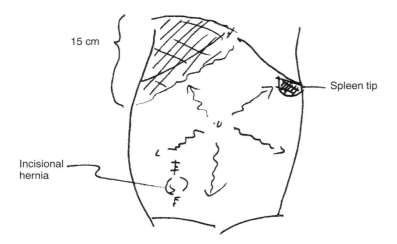

BEYOND THE PHYSICAL EXAMINATION

After the history, physical examination including abdominal examination, genital and rectal examination, and assessment of the general condition of the patient are completed, the clinician considers which laboratory tests, imaging, and/or special procedures are indicated to refine further the diagnostic hypotheses and to determine the situations in which consultation is needed.

The management of the acutely painful abdomen with signs of ileus and/or peritonitis is very often a surgical emergency, and the assistance of a surgeon is essential and thus routinely sought early in the workup. A **complete blood count (CBC)** with differential cell count is indicated to determine the amount and detail of the patient's leukocytic response and "baseline" hematocrit. A urinalysis for blood or evidence of infection is required. The urine specific gravity also assists assessment of intravascular fluid volume. With a history of vomiting or diarrhea, physical evidence of depleted blood volume (orthostatic hypotension, tachycardia, etc.), ileus, or intra-abdominal free air or fluid, serum electrolytes are determined along with renal function indices. A plain radiograph of the abdomen may define isolated areas of entrapped air or air-fluid levels in the intestine pointing to the location of an obstruction. Radiopaque calculi visible in the gallbladder, distal ileum (gallstone ileus), or ureter help to confirm a diagnosis suspected by history or physical examination, whereas their absence does not mean anything, since many stones are radiolucent. When perforation of a viscus is suspected, an upright chest or abdominal radiograph may reveal free air in the peritoneal cavity, but the patient has to stay upright before the film for 20 minutes to optimize yield. In the patient who has no evidence of an acute surgical abdomen, diagnostic studies are dictated by the history of symptoms and the physical examination findings. Stool specimens need to be examined for white cells and blood, Gram-stained, and cultured when diarrhea is a major symptom. If melena or blood in the stool has been described or observed by the clinician, proctoscopy, sigmoidoscopy, or colonoscopy are often indicated. Vomiting, epigastric pain, or hematemesis sometimes requires consultation for consideration of upper gastrointestinal endoscopy.

When physical examination suggests ascites, the etiology of which is not clear, abdominal paracentesis through analysis and culture of the ascitic specimen aspirated will often provide diagnostic clarification. A history of blood in the urine may require renal ultrasonography and/or excretory or retrograde urography.

The capability for noninvasive diagnostic study of abdominal masses and organ enlargement has been markedly enhanced by the development of ultrasonography, computed tomography, and magnetic resonance imaging. The rapidly progressive refinement of these technologies demands that the clinician continue to keep abreast of the indications and preferences for selection among them.

Ultrasonography is useful in determining the location and size of vascular aneurysms, but invasive arteriography is sometimes needed to evaluate the extent of vascular abnormalities and, in particular, obstructions. See Table 9.7 for a summary of additional procedures indicated by specific historical information or examination findings.

RECOMMENDED READINGS

Cattau EL, Benjamin SB, Knuff TE, Castell DO. The accuracy of the physical examination in the diagnosis of suspected ascites. JAMA 1982;247:1164–1166.

Collin J, Gray DWR. The eyes closed sign. Br Med J 1987;295:1656.

Cummings S, Papadakis M, Melnick J, Gooding GAW, Tierney LM Jr. The predictive value of physical examinations for ascites. West J Med 1985;142:633–636.

Eicher ER, Whitfield CL. Splenomegaly: an algorithmic approach to diagnosis. JAMA 1981;246: 2858–2861.

Fuller GN, Hargreaves MR, King DM. Scratch test in clinical examination of liver. Lancet 1988;1:181.

Gray DWR, Seabrook G, Dixon JM, Collins J. Is abdominal wall tenderness a useful sign in the diagnosis of non-specific abdominal pain? Ann R Coll Surg Engl 1988;70:230–231.

Guarino JR. Auscultatory percussion of the urinary bladder. Arch Intern Med 1985;145:1823–1825.

Hegde BM. How to detect early splenic enlargement. Practitioner 1985;229:857.

Heinz GJ, Zavala DC. Slipping rib syndrome. JAMA 1977;237:794–795.

Mellinkoff SM. "Stethoscope sign." N Engl J Med 1964;271:630.

Perloff JK. Physical examination of the heart and circulation. Philadelphia: WB Saunders, 1982:248.

Rivin AU. Abdominal vascular sounds. JAMA 1972;221:688–690.

Sherman HL, Hardison JE. The importance of a coexistent hepatic rub and bruit. JAMA 1979;241:1495.

Silen W, ed. Cope's early diagnosis of the acute abdomen. 18th ed. New York: Oxford University Press, 1991.

Simel DL, Halvorsen RA, Feussner JR. Quantitating bedside diagnosis: clinical evaluation of ascites. J Gen Intern Med 1988;3:423–427.

Sullivan S, Krasner N, Williams R. The clinical estimation of liver size: a comparison of techniques and an analysis of the sources of error. Br Med J 1976;2:1042–1043.

Verghese A, Dison C, Berk SL. Courvoisier's "law"—an eponym in evolution. Am J Gastroenterol 1987;82:248–250.

Zhang B, Lewis SM. A study of the reliability of clinical palpation of the spleen. Clin Lab Haemat 1989;11:7–10.

Table 9.7
Beyond the Physical Examination[a]

Major Sign or Symptom	Possible Additional Procedures
The "acute abdomen"	Request **surgical consultation** **WBC with differential** **Urinalysis** with Gram stain **Serum electrolytes, BUN, and creatinine** Plain abdominal film ("flat plate") Ultrasonography [contrast imaging]
Perforation suspected	All of the above plus upright abdominal film
Vomiting, hematemesis	Hemoglobin, prothrombin time, platelet count Upper gastrointestinal endoscopy
Diarrhea	**Stool test for blood** **Stool smear for WBC** **Stool for cultures** [Stool for ova and parasites] [Stool for fat content] Proctosigmoidoscopy [mucosal biopsy]
Melena or blood in stool	**Confirm blood by stool test** **Hemoglobin, prothombin time, platelet count** Proctosigmoidoscopy [colonoscopy]
Unexplained peritoneal fluid	Diagnostic **paracentesis** with full studies of fluid specimen
Masses or enlarged organs	Urinalysis, stool test for blood Ultrasonography, imaging procedures
Vascular abnormalities	Ultrasonography, imaging procedures [Arteriography]

[a]**Boldface,** most vital tests; [. . .], second-level diagnostic procedures dependent on the specifics of the case; WBC, white blood cell count; BUN, blood-urea-nitrogen.

10

Limbs

SCREENING EXAMINATION OF THE LIMBS

APPROACH AND ANATOMICAL REVIEW

The regional examination of the upper and lower limbs requires the crossover of several physiologic systems. The peripheral vascular, musculoskeletal, and the sensorimotor components of the central and peripheral nervous systems are examined as integral parts of each limb. The joints cannot move without their muscles, the muscles cannot perform without motor nerve supply, and these systems require blood supply. The functional anatomy of each limb is reviewed with this multisystem integration in mind. In addition, the limbs provide clues to other systemic malfunctions, such as cyanosis or clubbing secondary to cardiac or pulmonary disease, the edema of renal impairment, venous or lymphatic obstruction, or that reflecting cardiac failure.

Peripheral Vasculature

The **arteries** to be assessed are the major branches of the **femoral artery** in the lower limb and the **brachial artery** in the upper limb. On the "venous side," the leg is drained by the **saphenous** system into the **femoral vein** and the arm by the branches of the **brachial veins** (deep) and the **basilic and cephalic veins** (superficial) into the **axillary vein** (Fig. 10.1*A* and *B*).

Bones, Joints, Muscles, and Nerves
LOWER LIMB
Bones and Joints

The **hip** joint is the ball-and-socket articulation between the head of the femur and the acetabulum of the ilium. Heavy ligaments surround the joint capsule, and a series of bursae guard against friction (Fig. 10.2*A*). The **knee** is a complex hinge joint, permitting movement of the **tibia** on the distal femur. This articulation also contains the head of the **fibula**, the **patella**, the cartilaginous lateral and medial menisci, a series of **ligaments** that stabilize joint movement, and several bursae (Fig. 10.2*B*).

The **ankle** joint articulates the distal tibia and fibula with the **talus** of the foot. This hinge joint allows only flexion and extension of the foot on the long bones of the leg. Rotation of the foot occurs at the transverse tarsal joint and the subtalar articulation.

The **condyloid** joints of the foot are the **tarsometatarsal, metatarsophalangeal,** and **interphalangeal** articulations, all of which permit movement in two planes (flexion and extension, as well as side to side), but without rotation (Fig. 10.2*C* and *D*).

Muscles

The muscles of the lower limb control the movements of the limb as a whole and each joint individually. For illustration of the major muscles, see Figure 10.3. Each joint movement is carried out by a muscle or, more often, a group of muscles. Understanding of the physical examination of the joints and muscles requires an awareness of these muscle functions. For convenience, they are summarized in Table 10.1.

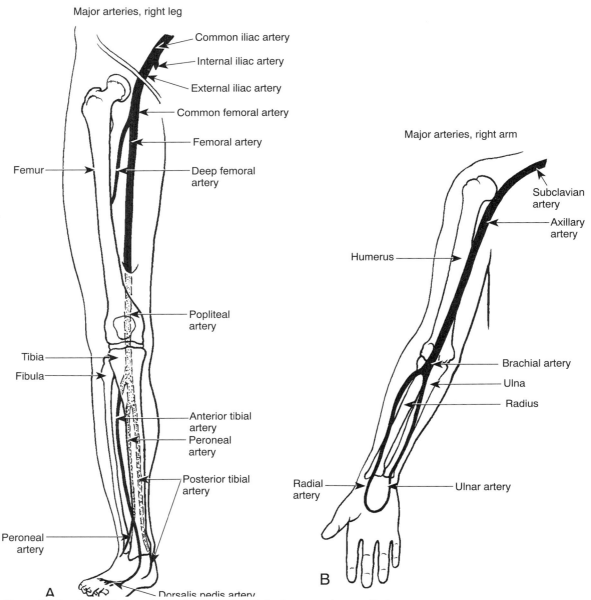

Figure 10.1   **A** and **B.** Drawings of the arteries of the lower and upper limbs.

Nerves

Each muscle or group of muscles is innervated by a **peripheral nerve** that is made up of motor fibers from the spinal cord. The gray matter of the motor cortex of the brain contains the **neurons** of the descending motor nerves. The **pyramidal tract** conveys the messages of tone, inhibition, and facilitation to the muscles of the body. The pyramidal motor pathway decussates (crosses sides) in the medulla of the brain such that the right cerebral cortex controls the muscles of the left-sided limbs and left cerebral cortex controls the muscles of the right-sided limbs. The motor nerves to the lower limb begin their exits from the spinal canal at the level of thoracic vertebra 12 (T12) and continue to exit through the sacral segments. Table 10.1 summarizes the innervation of muscle groups in terms of

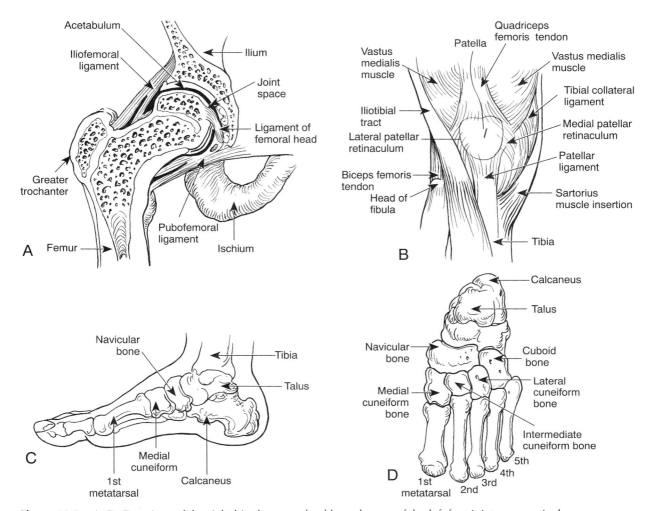

Figure 10.2   A–D. Drawings of the right hip, knee, and ankle and some of the left foot joints, respectively.

both the peripheral nerve involved and the vertebral segments from which its components leave the spinal canal (which are not always identical with the level at which they exit the substance of the spinal cord).

UPPER LIMB

Bones and Joints

The articulation of the head of the **humerus** with the **scapula** occurs at the **glenoid fossa** and is an incomplete ball-and-socket joint. It permits movement of the arm in many planes and is protected by the coracoid and acromion, bony processes and fibrous ligaments (Fig. 10.4*A*).

The **elbow,** a hinge joint, permits movement of the proximal radius and ulna on the distal humerus in one plane only, flexion and extension. A large bursa overlies the olecranon of the ulna (Fig. 10.4*B*).

At the **wrist,** the distal radius articulates with the carpal bones of the hand. The radiocarpal joint, as well as the metacarpophalangeal joints of the hand, are condyloid. As in the foot, corresponding to each digit, there are articulations between the carpal bones of the wrist and each metacarpal that will lead to a phalanx, and between the metacarpal and proximal phalanx as well as between the proximal and distal phalanx (Fig. 10.4*C* and *D*).

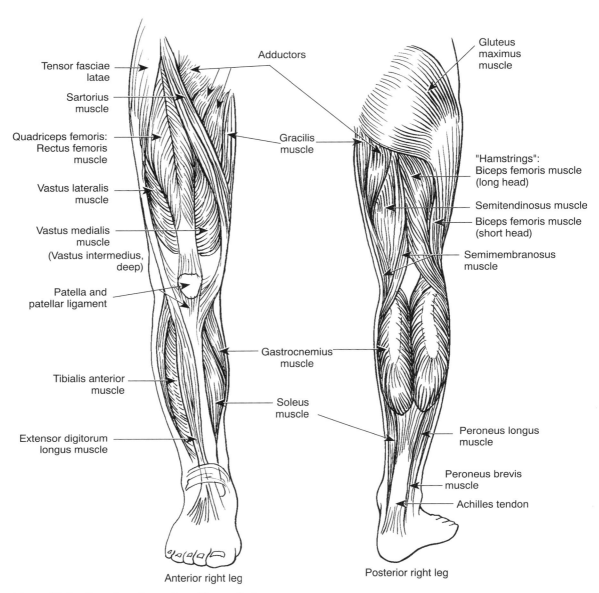

Tensor fasciae latae

Sartorius muscle

Quadriceps femoris: Rectus femoris muscle

Vastus lateralis muscle

Vastus medialis muscle (Vastus intermedius, deep)

Patella and patellar ligament

Tibialis anterior muscle

Extensor digitorum longus muscle

Adductors

Gracilis muscle

Gastrocnemius muscle

Soleus muscle

Anterior right leg

Gluteus maximus muscle

"Hamstrings": Biceps femoris muscle (long head)

Semitendinosus muscle

Biceps femoris muscle (short head)

Semimembranosus muscle

Peroneus longus muscle

Peroneus brevis muscle

Achilles tendon

Posterior right leg

Figure 10.3   Drawing of muscles of lower limb.

Muscles and Nerves

General comments about the relationships among the joints, their muscles, and the nervous system that were made about the lower limb apply also to the upper limb. The **motor** nerves of the upper limb derive from fibers exiting the corticospinal tract at the mid to low **cervical and upper thoracic levels.** The muscle group actions on each joint of the upper limb and the peripheral and spinal-segmental innervation sources are summarized in Table 10.2.

TECHNIQUE

Formal examination of the limbs begins after completion of the abdominal examination. The patient remains in the supine position for the initial inspection and palpation of the anterior lower limbs and for some assessment of the hip joint. Then he is asked to sit for the remainder of the lower limb examination and all of

Table 10.1
Muscle and Nerve Control of Lower Limb Joint Motion[a]

	Motion	Muscles	Innervation	
			Nerve	Vertebral Exit
Hip	**Flexion**	Iliopsoas	Lumbar branches, femoral	T12–L4
	Extension	Gluteus maximus	Inferior gluteal,	L5–S2
		"Hamstrings"[b]	sciatic branches	L4–S3
	External rotation	Obturator	Obturator	L2–L4
		Quadratus femoris		
	Internal rotation	Gluteus medius	Superior gluteal	L4–S1
		Gluteus minimus		
	Abduction	Gluteus medius	Superior gluteal	L4–S1
		Gluteus minimus		
	Adduction	Adductors	Obturator	L2–L4
		Gracilis		
Knee	Flexion	"Hamstrings"[b]	Sciatic branches	L4–S3
	Extension	Quadriceps femoris	Femoral	L2–L4
Ankle	**Dorsiflexion**	Tibialis anterior	Deep peroneal	L4–S1
	Plantar flexion	Gastrocnemius	Tibial	L5–S2
		Soleus		
	Supination of foot	Tibialis anterior	Deep peroneal	L4–S1
		Tibialis posterior	Tibial	
	Pronation of foot	Long extensor of digits	Deep and superficial peroneal	L4–S1
Toes	**Flexion**	Flexor hallucis longus and brevis	Tibial	L5–S2
		Flexor digitorum longus		
	Extension	Extensor hallucis longus, extensor digitorum longus	Deep peroneal	L4–S1

[a]**Boldface** indicates routinely assessed.
[b]Semimembranosus and semitendinosus.

the upper limb examination. Consult Table 10.3 for the sequence of the limb examination.

For the supine portion of the examination, the patient's thorax and abdomen should be covered by a gown. A half-sheet is manipulated to provide genital coverage unless the patient has been asked to wear underpants for the abdominal examination. In the sitting position, the sheet is used to cover the patient's lap during assessment of the leg and the upper limb.

Some *general principles* of the limb examination deserve consideration before beginning the maneuvers:

1. As the examination of each limb proceeds, it is efficient and systematic to work from proximal to distal in order to maintain a routine that facilitates completion of all components.

2. For efficiency, the joint range of motion and the neuromuscular assessments are combined by region. For example, as the knee is being examined for function of the joint and periarticular structures, it is simultaneously or sequentially assessed for the integrity of muscles and their motor nerve supply.

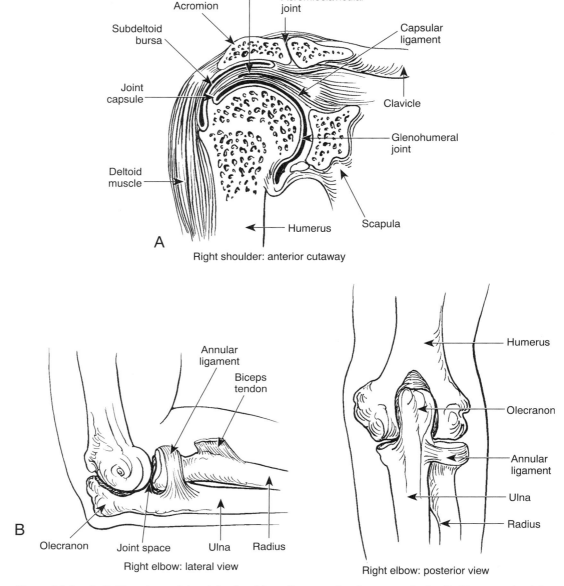

Figure 10.4   A–C. Drawings of the right shoulder, elbow, and wrist, respectively. **D.** Photograph of the right hand showing palmar landmarks.

3. If the patient cannot **actively** perform any particular limb movement described below, the examiner attempts the motion **passively,** i.e., moves the joint in question with her hands. For example, if the ankle cannot be moved voluntarily by the patient, the examiner attempts flexion, extension, inversion, and eversion. If neither patient nor examiner can put the joint through normal range of motion, the stiffness suggests joint or periarticular disease; if, on the other hand, the patient cannot actively perform the movement, but the examiner can freely maneuver the joint, this incriminates muscle or nerve and exonerates the joint.

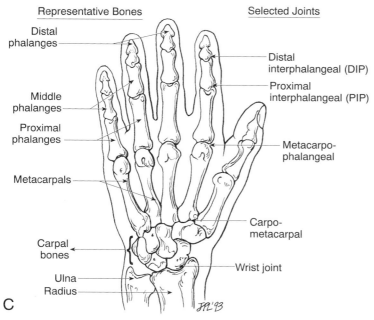

Representative Bones   Selected Joints

Distal phalanges

Distal interphalangeal (DIP)

Proximal interphalangeal (PIP)

Middle phalanges

Proximal phalanges

Metacarpo-phalangeal

Metacarpals

Carpo-metacarpal

Carpal bones

Wrist joint

Ulna

Radius

C

Figure 10.4   C.

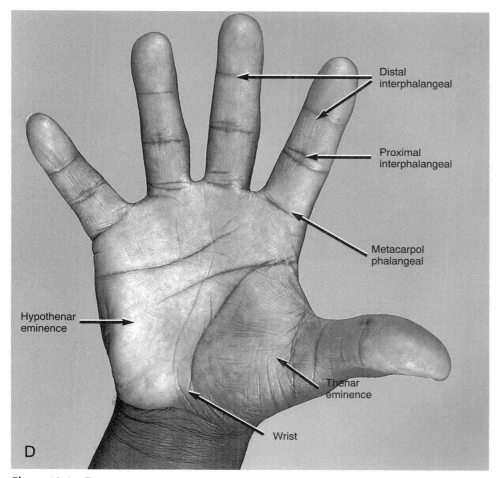

Distal interphalangeal

Proximal interphalangeal

Metacarpol phalangeal

Hypothenar eminence

Thenar eminence

Wrist

D

Figure 10.4   D.

Table 10.2
Muscle and Nerve Control of Upper Limb Joint Motion[a]

	Motion	Muscles	Innervation	
			Nerve	Cord Segment
Shoulder	**Elevation**	Levator scapulae		C3–C5
		Trapezius	Cranial nerve XI	
	Abduction	Deltoid	Axillary	C5–C6
		Supraspinatus	Suprascapular	C4–C6
	Adduction	Pectoralis major	Medial and lateral pectoral	C5–T1
	Flexion	Coracobrachialis	Musculocutaneous	C6–C7
		Anterior deltoid	Axillary	C5–C6
	Extension	Latissimus dorsi	Subscapular	C5–C8
		Teres major		
	External rotation	Infraspinatus	Suprascapular	C5–C6
	Internal rotation	Subscapularis	Subscapular	C5–C8
		Teres major		
		Latissimus dorsi		
Elbow	**Flexion**	Biceps, brachialis	Musculocutaneous	C5–C6
	Extension	Triceps	Radial	C6–T1
	Supination of forearm	Biceps, supinator	Radial	C5–C7
	Pronation of forearm	Pronator teres	Median	C6–C7
Wrist	Flexion	Flexor carpi radialis	Median	C6–C8
		Flexor carpi ulnaris	Ulnar	C7–T1
	Extension	Extensor carpi radialis longus	Radial	C5–C8
		Extensor carpi ulnaris	Radial	C6–C8
Fingers	**Flexion**	PIP joints: flexor digitorum superficialis, profundus[b]	Median	C7–T1
		MCP joints: flexor pollicis brevis, lumbricals[b]	Median / Ulnar	C6–T1 / C8–T1
		Distal phalanges: flexor digitorum profundus	Median / Ulnar	C7–T1 / C8–T1
	Extension	Extensor digitorum extensors to individual fingers	Radial	C6–C8
	Abduction	First dorsal interosseous, abductor digiti	Ulnar	C8–T1
	Adduction	Palmar interossei	Ulnar	C8–T1
Thumb	**Abduction**	Abductor pollicis brevis	Median	C6–T1
	Adduction	Adductor pollicis	Ulnar	C8–T1
	Flexion	Flexor pollicis brevis	Median	C8–T1
	Extension	Extensor pollicis longus and brevis	Radial	C6–C8
	Opposition of thumb and 5th finger	Opponens pollicis	Median	C6–T1
		Opponens digiti minimi	Ulnar	C8–T1

[a]**Boldface,** routinely assessed.
[b]PIP, proximal interphalangeal; and MCP, metacarpophalangeal.

Table 10.3
Sequence of the Limb Examination[a]

Patient supine: lower limb
  Inspection
    Anterior lower limb
    Soles of feet
  Palpation
    Skin temperature
    Peripheral arteries
      Dorsalis pedis
      Posterior tibial
      (Popliteal)
      Femoral, if not done with abdominal examination
    Joints and muscles (Hip range of motion and muscle strength)
        (Flexion, with knee extended)
        (Flexion, with knee flexed (also indicates knee range of motion))
        (External rotation)
        (Internal rotation)
        (Abduction)
        (Adduction)
Patient seated: lower limb
  Palpation
    Joints and muscles
      (Knee range of motion and muscle strength)
        (Extension)
        (Flexion—for strength of knee flexors)
      (Ankle and foot range of motion and muscle strength)
        (Dorsiflexion of the ankle)
        (Plantar flexion of the ankle)
        (Inversion and eversion of the ankle)
        (Abduction and adduction of the ankle)
        (Plantar flexion of the toes)
        (Extension of the great toes)
Patient seated: upper limb
  Inspection
    Both upper limbs, anterior (and posterior)
  Palpation
    Arteries of the upper limb
      Radial, if not done while doing vital signs
      (Ulnar)
      (Brachial)
    Epitrochlear lymph nodes
    Joints and muscles
      (Shoulder range of motion and muscle strength)
      Elevation (obtained "free" during breast inspection)
      (Abduction)
      (Adduction)
      (Flexion)
      (Hyperextension)
      (Internal rotation)
      (External rotation)
    (Elbow range of motion and muscle strength)
      (Flexion)
      (Extension)
      (Supination of forearm)
      (Pronation of forearm)
    Wrist and hands range of motion and muscle strength
      (Extension of wrist)
      (Flexion of wrist)
      Abduction and adduction of fingers ("finger spread")
      Flexion curl of phalangeal joints (form a fist)
      Grip strength

[a]Parentheses indicate an assessment not done on all routine examinations.

4. Continuous conscious observation is made not only for range of motion of each joint but also for the tone, strength, and symmetry of each muscle group. The muscle mass is palpated briefly to corroborate a visual impression of normality, atrophy, or hypertrophy and is observed for abnormal involuntary movement (twitches or fasciculations—see Chapter 11).

5. Each description of maneuvers of a given joint or complex of joints and muscles is cross-referenced to (a) the appropriate table of muscle groups and their innervations that act on the joint and (b) a figure illustrating the technique of the maneuver(s).

6. In the narrative description of the maneuvers a star (☆) is used to indicate that the test is for **joint range of motion** and a triangle (Δ) is used to indicate that the maneuver tests **muscle strength.**

Examination of the Lower Limb

INSPECTION

The posterior surface is assessed with the patient standing, during the back examination (see Chapter 12). The limbs are assessed generally for symmetry of length and diameter, color, and contour. Observe for localized or generalized swelling of one or both limbs. The skin of the limb is inspected for color, texture, hair distribution, venous pattern, and lesions. **Do not forget to inspect the soles of the feet.**

PALPATION

Place your hands on corresponding points of each of the patient's lower limbs, e.g., each midthigh, midcalf, and dorsum of the foot, to determine the symmetry of skin **temperature.**

The **peripheral arterial supply of the lower limb** is palpated as follows (Fig. 10.5):

*   The **dorsalis pedis pulse** is located across the arch of the dorsum of the foot. Palpate both simultaneously for equality of force. If they are hard to find or are faint, seek each individually, assess it on its own, mark the spot, and compare side to side at the end.

*   The **posterior tibial pulse** may be found behind and inferior to the medial malleolus of the tibia. Again, palpate the two pulses simultaneously for symmetry, after preparation similar to that described for the dorsalis pedis is made.

*   The **popliteal pulse** is best located by slightly passively flexing the knee and placing the fingers of both hands deep in the popliteal space. The pulse is usually located slightly medially in the space. In a significant minority of patients this pulse cannot be felt, especially in a very muscular or very obese leg. If the foot pulses are normal, by inference the popliteal artery is patent; it is sought, then, only when the foot pulses are diminished or the patient has symptoms suggestive of compromised arterial blood supply to the leg or foot (see the Extended Examination section).

For palpation of the **femoral artery,** see Chapter 9.

JOINTS AND MUSCLES

Before beginning the maneuvers of range of motion and muscle strength, each joint is inspected for *swelling, discoloration, or misalignment* and is palpated for *heat or tenderness.* The joint and muscle examination is described for one limb; repeat all maneuvers on the opposite limb.

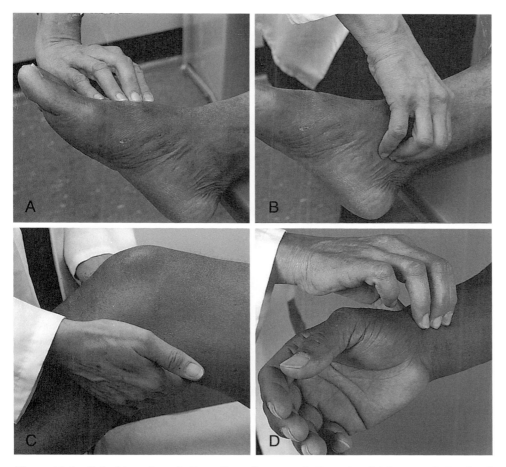

Figure 10.5   Palpable pulses. **A.** Dorsalis pedis artery. **B.** Posterior tibial artery. **C.** Popliteal artery, very deep in popliteal fossa. **D.** Radial artery.

Hips

The patient remains in the supine position for the hip maneuvers (refer also to Table 10.1 and Fig. 10.6).

1. Flexion.
   a. With knee extended.
      △☆ Ask the patient to elevate the leg as far as possible off the table, *or*
   b. With knee flexed.
      ☆ Ask the patient to bring the knee up onto the abdominal wall.
      △ With the knee flexed onto the abdomen, ask the patient to resist your attempts to return the thigh to its supine resting position.
2. Extension (see Chapter 12 for this maneuver, which is done with the patient standing for the lower back examination)
3. External rotation (for internal and external rotation testing, the knee *must* be flexed, or the other joints will contribute to movement and strength that appear to arise from the hip, vitiating all interpretations).
   ☆ With the knee flexed at 45°, rotate the patient's hip externally (laterally).
   △ With the hip externally rotated, ask the patient to maintain the position against your attempt to return the limb to midline.

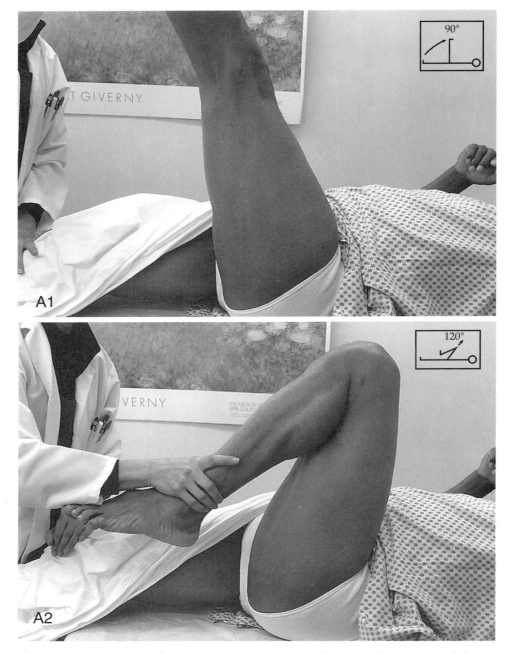

Figure 10.6   Hip range of motion, patient supine. **A1.** Flexion with knee extended. **A2.** Flexion with knee flexed. **B.** External rotation. **C.** Internal rotation. See page 400 for **D** and **E.**

4. Internal rotation.
    ☆With the knee flexed at 40°, rotate the patient's hip internally (medially).
    Δ With the hip internally rotated, ask the patient to maintain the position against your attempt to externally rotate the hip.
5. Abduction (lateral movement from the midline).
    ☆With the limb straight and patient supine, ask the patient to move the limb laterally.

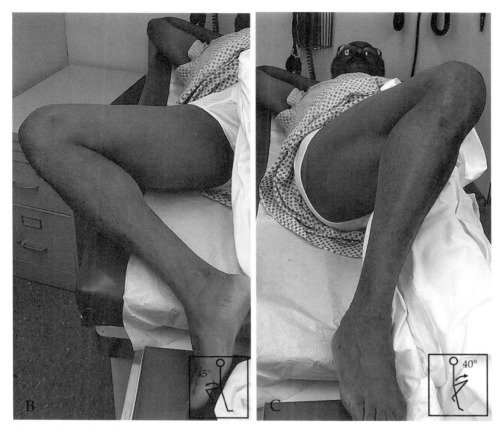

Figure 10.6   B and C.

Δ With the limb abducted, ask the patient to resist your attempt to return it to midline.
6.   Adduction (medial movement across the midline).
☆ With the limb straight, ask the patient to cross it medially over the opposite lower limb.
Δ With the limb in the midline, ask the patient to resist your attempt to forcibly abduct it.

The patient is now returned to the sitting position for the remainder of the limb examination; legs should be dangling over the end of the table or bed.

Knee

For examination of the knee, refer also to Table 10.1 and Figure 10.7.

1. Flexion.
☆ Flexion of the knee has been observed during the hip examination (Step 1b above).
Δ Ask the patient to resist your attempt to straighten the flexed knee.
2.   Extension.
Δ☆ Ask the patient to straighten his leg (Fig. 10.7B).
Δ With the knee just barely flexed (170°), place one palm on the patient's thigh, and ask the patient to resist your attempt to flex the knee further. This position is used to avoid the "locking" of the joint, independent of

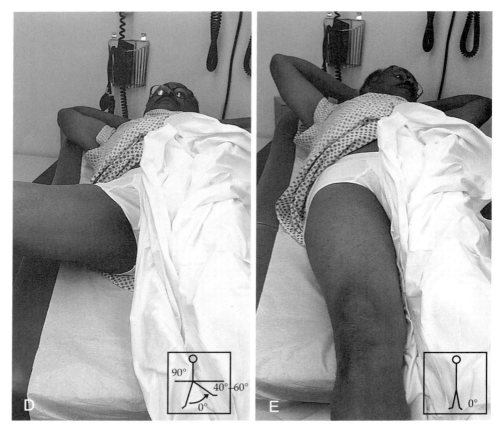

Figure 10.6   D. Abduction. **E.** Adduction. Note that the adducted hip is in a rest or baseline position.

power, which can occur with full extension and can lead to overestimation of quadriceps femoris strength.

Ankle and Foot

For examination of the ankle and foot, refer also to Table 10.1 and Figure 10.8.

1. Dorsiflexion of the foot.
   ☆ Ask the patient to point both feet toward the ceiling or back up at his head.
   Δ Ask the patient to maintain dorsiflexion against your attempt to force the forefoot toward the floor.
2. Plantar flexion of the foot.
   ☆ Ask the patient to point the foot toward the floor ("step on the gas pedal").
   Δ Ask the patient to maintain plantar flexion against your attempt to dorsiflex the foot.
3. Inversion and eversion of the foot.
   ☆ΔStabilize the patient's leg above the ankle, and ask the patient to rotate the sole of the foot away from the other foot (eversion) and then toward the other foot (inversion).
4. Plantar flexion of the toes.
   ☆ Ask the patient to curl the toes toward the sole of the foot.
   Δ With the toes curled, ask the patient to resist your attempt to straighten them.
5. Extension of the great toe.

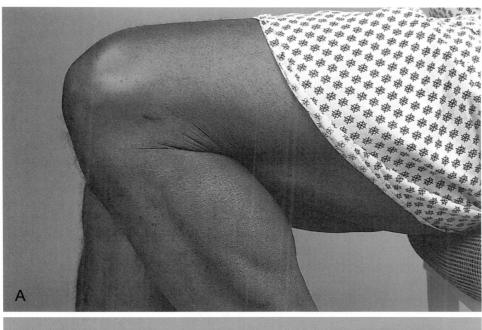

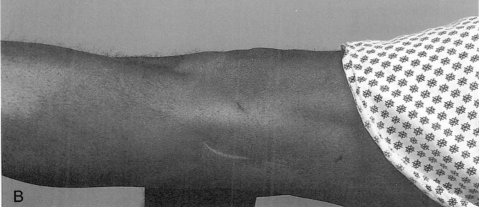

Figure 10.7   Range of motion of the knee, patient seated. **A.** Flexion. Note the similarity at this joint to the posture in Figure 10.6*A2*. **B.** Extension.

☆While you stabilize the foot in moderate plantar flexion, ask the patient to extend the great toe toward the ceiling or toward his chin.

Δ Ask the patient to resist your attempt to flex the extended great toe.

Examination of the Upper Limb

Now the examiner moves to the inspection and palpation of the upper limbs. General inspection of contour and symmetry and of the skin is as described for the lower limb. The **radial arteries** may now be palpated for symmetry of pulsation. If both are present and normal, the brachial artery need not be assessed except to determine stethoscope placement for sphygmomanometry.

Just proximal to the medial epicondyle of the humerus lies a small cluster of lymph nodes that drain the hand and forearm. These **epitrochlear** nodes should be sought during the palpation of the elbow (Fig. 10.9); they are found between the tendons of biceps and triceps and are most easily felt with the forearm supinated.

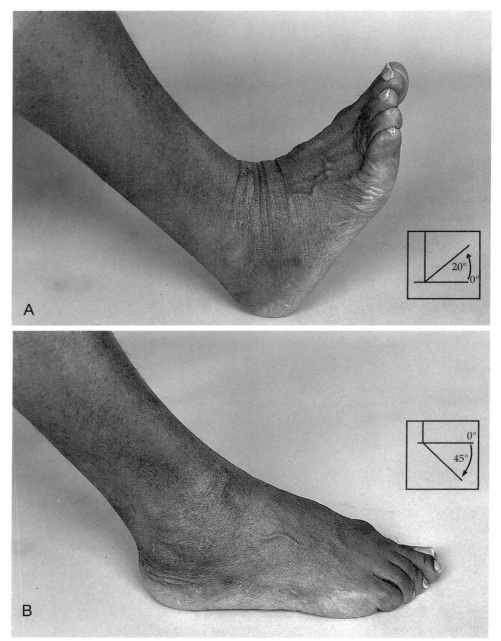

Figure 10.8.   Ankle and foot. **A.** Dorsiflexion of foot. **B.** Plantar flexion of foot. **C.** Inversion of foot. **D.** Eversion of foot. **E.** Plantar flexion of toes. **F.** Extension of the great toe (hallux).

JOINTS

Shoulder

For examination of the shoulder, refer also to Table 10.2 and Figure 10.10.

1. Elevation ("the shoulder shrug" was assessed as part of the cranial nerve XI assessment (see Chapter 4)).
2. Abduction.
   ☆ Ask the patient to raise his arms laterally until his fingers touch above his head.

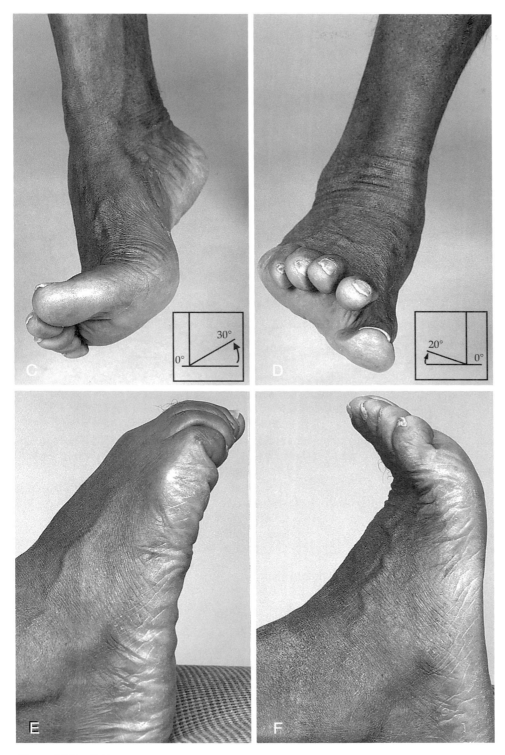

Figure 10.8   C–F.

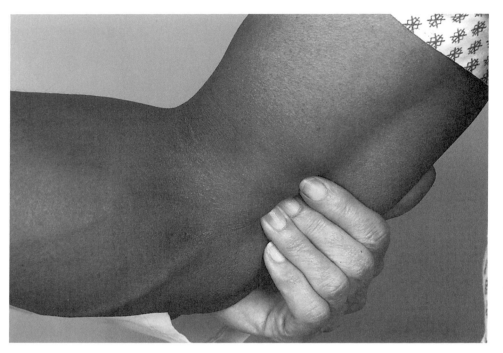

Figure 10.9   Palpation for epitrochlear lymph nodes.

Δ Ask the patient to return his arms straight out laterally and resist your attempt to force them to the sides of the trunk.
3.   Adduction.
     ☆Ask the patient to move each arm across the front of his body as far as possible (this position also facilitates testing of the triceps reflex (see Chapter 11)).
4.   Flexion.
     ☆Ask the patient to raise both arms, parallel to the trunk—"reach for the basket"—as far anterosuperiorly as possible.
5.   Internal rotation.
     ☆Ask the patient to clasp his hands together behind his *lower back*.
6.   External rotation.
     ☆Ask the patient to clasp his hands together behind his *head*.

Elbow

For examination of the elbow, refer also to Table 10.2 and Figure 10.11.

1.   Flexion.
     ☆Ask the patient to bend his elbow maximally.
     Δ Ask the patient to resist your attempt to extend his flexed elbow ("don't let me straighten your arm").
2.   Extension.
     ☆Ask the patient to fully straighten his elbow, with his arm at his side
     Δ Ask the patient to resist your attempt to further flex the almost fully extended elbow ("don't let me bend your arm"). Once again, *complete extension is avoided to preclude a confounding contribution from "locking."*
3.   Supination.
     ☆With his forearms resting in his lap, ask the patient to turn the palms of his hands toward the ceiling.

4. Pronation.
    ☆With his forearms resting in his lap at the end of the prior maneuver, ask the patient to turn the palms of his hands toward his lap.

Wrist and Hand

Inspect the two wrists for swelling, redness, or visible asymmetry. Examine the dorsum and the palm of each hand, looking at the skin and comparing the **thenar and hypothenar eminences** for bilateral symmetry. Observe for swelling or deformity of the metacarpophalangeal and the proximal and distal interphalangeal joints of each digit (except the thumb, which has only a single interphalangeal joint). **Palpate** any joint that appears swollen or otherwise distorted for synovial bogginess, tenderness, or warmth, and look carefully at it for erythema. The maneuvers to be used in range of motion and muscle testing follow (refer also to Table 10.2 and Fig. 10.12).

1. Extension of the wrist.
    ☆Ask the patient to elevate the back of his hand toward the wrist, i.e., to hyperextend the wrist.
    Δ With the wrist thus hyperextended, ask the patient to resist attempts to return it to the neutral position.
2. Flexion of the wrist.
    ☆Ask the patient to bend the palm toward the wrist.
    Δ With the wrist thus flexed, ask the patient to resist an attempt to return it to the neutral position.

Fingers

Unless the patient has specific complaints or the hand appears abnormal on inspection, the functional movements of the joints and the integrity of the muscles and nerves of the hand and fingers can be screened with the following maneuvers:

    ☆ΔAsk the patient, with wrists in neutral position, to spread his fingers apart and then bring them back together.
    ☆ΔAsk the patient to make a fist such that you can observe the flexion curl of each set of metacarpophalangeal joints and each group of interphalangeal joints.
    ☆ΔAsk the patient to grasp, squeeze, and hold the first two fingers of your hands in his grip.

See the Extended Examination section for more detailed hand muscle assessment when history or screening examination calls for further investigation.

NORMAL AND COMMON VARIANTS

In this portion of the examination, there are few common variants that are not considered pathologic. The expected range of joint motion is presented below, as well as the occasional situation in which a vascular or joint deviation from normal falls within the acceptable common variant range. Any other finding should be considered abnormal, and directions for further physical examination assessment should be sought in the Extended Examination section of this chapter.

Lower Limb

The lower limbs are equal partners, of symmetrical contour, length, and color. On inspection, small veins and telangiectases, sometimes stellate, are often visi-

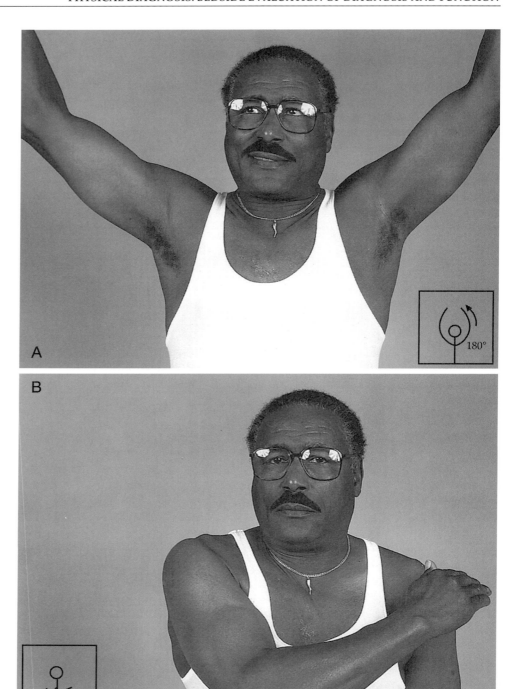

Figure 10.10 Range of motion of shoulder. **A.** Abduction (arms raised from the sides). **B.** Adduction, verging on hyperadduction. **C.** Flexion. Note similarity of endpoint of this maneuver, achieved with the arms pointing forward the whole time, to endpoint of abduction in *A*. **D.** Extension. **E.** Internal rotation. Hands are clasped behind the *back,* with the elbows flexed. **F.** External rotation. Hands are clasped behind the *head,* with the elbows flexed.

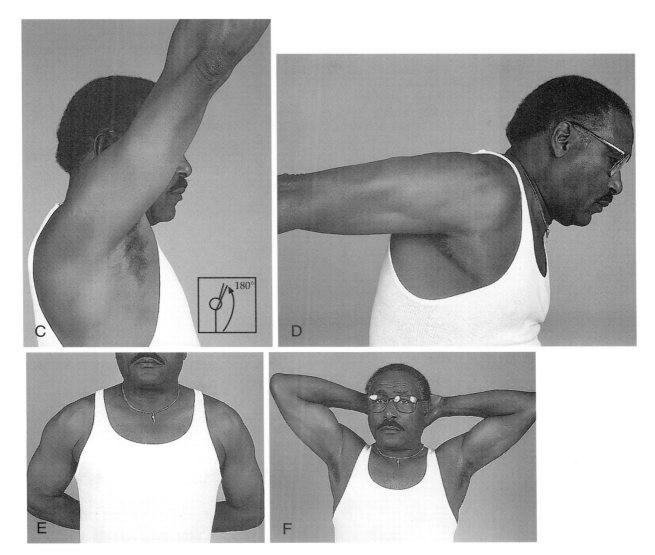

Figure 10.10. C–F.

ble at the skin surface, especially on the thighs and about the ankles and feet. Superficial varicosities, or dilated networks of larger veins, become increasingly apparent with aging. The line between normal surface venous pattern and significant **varicose veins** is more a matter of the presence of symptoms than of appearance.

Normally, there is **hair** apparent on the leg and on the dorsum of the feet and toes. Men who have long worn snug hose may have bilaterally symmetrical thinning of hair below the "sock-top" level as an artifact of civilization. A clear asymmetric absence of leg and foot hair is suggestive of vascular impairment. Since legs are shaved or depilated for diverse reasons, an inquiry may settle the cause at once.

On palpation, the skin temperature should be symmetrical from one limb to the other. The limbs, however, are often normally progressively cooler to touch as the examining fingers move distally.

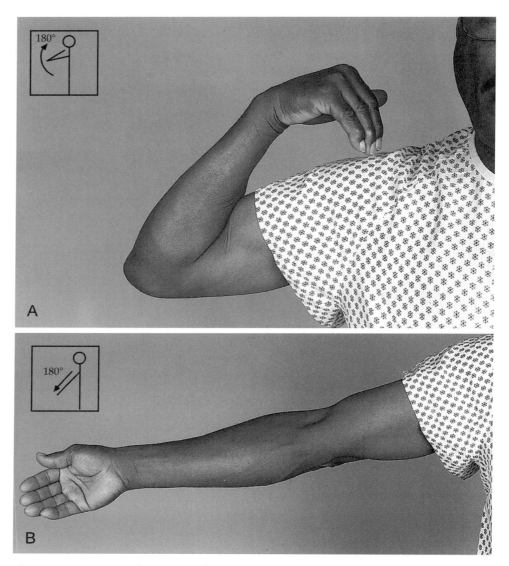

Figure 10.11   Range of motion of elbow. **A.** Flexion. **B.** Extension. **C.** Supination. **D.** Pronation. The hands in the lap wind up palm downward.

PULSES

The arterial pulses are assessed for presence, amplitude, and symmetry, especially the pulses of the foot. It has been demonstrated that a significant minority of healthy adults and even children have congenitally nonpalpable dorsalis pedis pulses, and a smaller number, no locatable posterior tibial pulsation. The anomaly is usually bilateral and should not be confusing if there is normal foot warmth, skin color, and hair distribution.

If the foot pulses are normal, it is not necessary to attempt to locate the popliteal pulse, which is the most difficult pulse to feel. Recall that the femoral arterial pulse should be easily palpable, equal in amplitude bilaterally, and free of bruit on auscultation (although femoral bruits have poor positive predictive value for symptomatic vascular disease).

With aging, the tortuosity of both veins and arteries increases. The amplitude of the arterial pulsations, however, should remain full and equal from side to side.

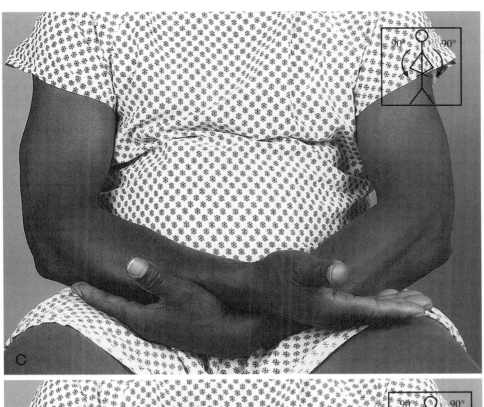

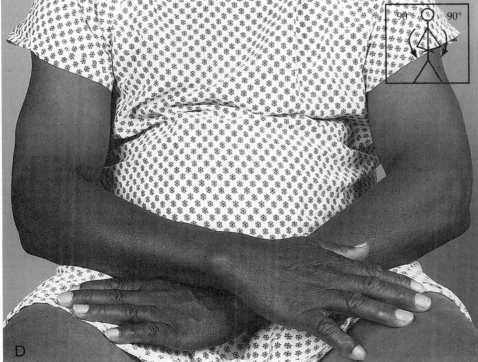

Figure 10.11   C   and D.

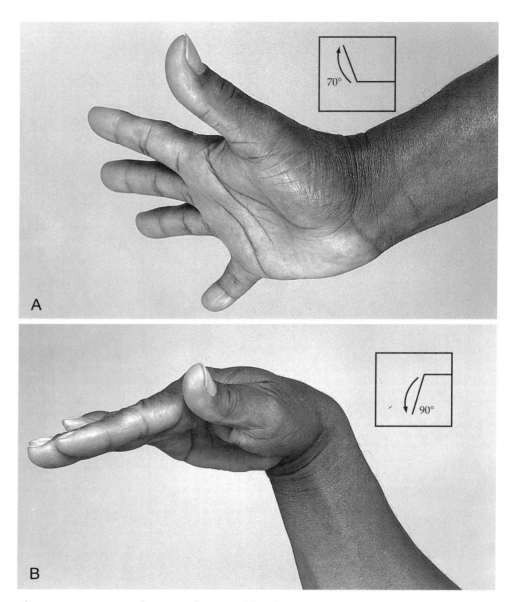

Figure 10.12   Range of motion of wrist and hand. **A.** Extension of wrist. **B.** Flexion of wrist. **C.** Full range of finger-spreading. **D.** Side view of fist, showing normal degree of flexion of both metacarpophalangeal and interphalangeal joints. **E.** Gripping examiner's fingers, which tests both joint mobility and strength.

BONES, JOINTS, MUSCLES, AND NERVE SUPPLY

For expected normal range of motion of the lower limb joints, see Figures 10.6–10.8. Any deviation from this degree of motion implies articular or periarticular pathology.

Muscle strength is quite variable from individual to individual and dependent on age, gender, and physical conditioning. Except for conditions of enforced muscle disuse of one limb or muscle group (such as following casting for a fracture or immobility secondary to trauma), the mass, tone, and strength of each group tested should match that of its counterpart on the opposite limb. Any deviation from symmetry is considered abnormal and must be further assessed.

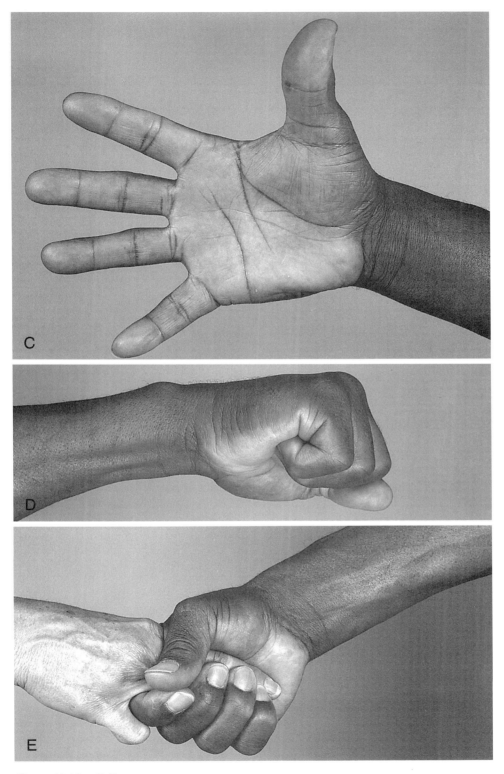

Figure 10.12   C–E.

The knee is the most vulnerable to trauma of the large peripheral joints. There are no normal variants in knee function. Refined assessment of a knee that does not move normally is discussed in the Extended Examination section.

The foot, having long resided in shoes that do not always fit well, often demonstrates the ravages of pressure. These induced signs of chronic trauma are so common as to be considered variants of the normal. Examples include corns, thickly keratinized tissue overlying the dorsum of one or more distal phalanges, and calluses, pads of heaped-up keratin found on the soles or over the lateral protuberances of the distal foot.

Deviations of the toes over time may lead to deformities of the foot. Examples include the **hallux valgus deformity** in which the great toe is laterally deviated, often resulting in the compensatory formation of a bursa at the medial pressure point. If inflamed and painful, this protuberant bursa is called a **bunion.** The normally flat toes may have been chronically deformed at the distal interphalangeal joint by ill-fitting shoes, resulting in the **hammertoe deformity.**

The arch of the foot varies widely and is congenitally determined. **Pes planus** is the term used to describe a very flat arch (flatfoot), and **pes cavus** is the term used to describe an unusually high instep arch. There should be no symptoms associated with these variants.

Upper Limb

General considerations regarding the **vasculature** of the lower limb apply also to that of the upper limb. The patency and amplitude of the brachial artery was assessed during blood pressure determination; the radial pulses were felt at the same point in the early examination.

The epitrochlear lymph nodes are not normally palpable. The presence of appreciable nodes in this location suggests distal infection (hand or forearm) or a systemic nodal disorder.

JOINTS, MUSCLES, AND NERVES

For anticipated range of motion of joints of the upper limb, see Figures 10.10–10.12. Any deviation from the expected implies articular or periarticular disease (see the Extended Examination section). The principles applied to musculature of the upper limb are analogous to those of the lower limb.

There is one common anomaly of the hands that, although considered abnormal, is seen with great frequency. For reasons not understood, the palmar fascia of one or several fingers begins to contract and forms a firm, palpable "tunnel" that pulls the affected finger(s) into varying degrees of fixed flexion. This phenomenon, called Dupuytren's contracture, has a hereditary component, tends to be bilateral, and increases in incidence with age.

RECORDING THE FINDINGS

Because of the multiple systems involved, the findings of the limb examination are, by convention, recorded by system: the peripheral pulses with the CARDIOVASCULAR system, the epitrochlear nodes with LYMPH NODES, skin findings under SKIN, joint range of motion with MUSCULOSKELETAL, and the muscle strength testing under the NEUROLOGIC system, motor section. If an entry on LIMBS is included, it usually mentions only those features that do not fit neatly into another system, e.g., "LIMBS—no cyanosis, clubbing, edema, or asymmetry." A typical record of the limb examination might look like the following:

Skin: Legs tan, with scattered patches of vitiligo on each shin. Nails normal and well groomed. Symmetrical hair both lower legs, skin temperature normal. Skin and appendages on the upper limbs normal.

Lymph nodes: No palpable epitrochlear nodes.

Cardiovascular: Peripheral pulses:

	Femoral	D. Pedis	Post Tibial	Radial
Right	2+	2+	2+	2+
Left	2 +	2+	2+	2+

Joints: No swelling, tenderness, or limitation of motion of any.

Neurologic:

Motor: Muscle groups in all limbs normal and symmetrical bilaterally.

EXTENDED EXAMINATION OF THE LIMBS

INDICATIONS

Advanced examination of the limbs encompasses an enormous diversity of organ systems and considerations. Never does one routinely perform detailed assessment of all four limbs and all systems. Rather, workup is geared to the particulars at hand. Therefore, both for the reader's convenience and to render the material comprehensible, we subdivide the discussion that follows into four systems of concern: (*a*) peripheral vasculature; (*b*) lymphatic system; (*c*) musculoskeletal system, including joints; and (*d*) (peripheral) neural system.

In some instances the examiner may check all of these carefully, e.g., after major trauma to a limb or with a deep primary neoplasm of the limb. Many other settings call for only a subset.

History

Problems that lead to extended evaluation of a limb are *pain, trauma,* unexplained loss of any *functional capacity* whether from *weakness, stiffness, abnormal involuntary movements* or any other cause, and the special case of *falls,* which require increased attention to the lower limbs.

Physical Examination

Limb abnormalities noted on the screening examination are followed by focused assessment. For example, limb *edema* will prompt extended examination of the venous and lymphatic systems; *loss of function,* of the musculoskeletal system and relevant peripheral nerves; *gait instability,* of musculoskeletal, neural, and some selected central nervous system function.

Laboratory and Imaging

Diabetes mellitus will heighten interest in the foot and lead to a search for diabetic foot ulcers. *Hyperuricemia* will provoke examination for gouty deformities. A positive serology for *antibodies to HIV* may prompt looking for lymphatic or cutaneous complications or for hyperalgesic thrombophlebitis. If thyroid function tests are abnormal, a hunt for *pretibial myxedema* may be made.

CONDUCTING THE EXTENDED EXAMINATION
Peripheral Vasculature
CAPILLARY
Blood Leakage Tests

The **Rumpel-Leede test** is fully described in the Extended Examination section of Chapter 3. The examiner draws a circle 2.5 cm across on the forearm, inflates a blood-pressure cuff above systolic blood pressure, watches the circle, and leaves the sphygmomanometer at this pressure for 5 minutes or until 10 petechiae appear, whichever comes first, then promptly and completely deflates the cuff.

Pinch purpura is sought by making a firm pinch on the arm or other locale that has mobile skin and a cosmetically acceptable location for a bruise, remote from any site recently used for a Rumpel-Leede test.

Capillary Refill

The capillary refill consists of milking the blood color out of a region of skin with strokes of the examiner's fingertip pushed along the skin surface, indenting the skin a few millimeters throughout the course, and then timing how long it takes for normal color to return. The palm and the dorsum of the foot are common sites used, although any spot can be employed.

Osler Nodes and Janeway Lesions

Osler nodes and Janeway lesions are much discussed but are seldom seen. The search for them consists of inspecting the hands, wrists, ankles, and feet, with adequate exposure and lighting. If any unexplained macules or, less commonly, papules or pustules are located in these zones, ask whether they are painful, and check for tenderness with a *gloved* finger.

ARTERIAL
Brachial and Radial Arteries

Detection of the *brachial pulse* is often surprisingly difficult. The examiner often has to push the lower body and tendon of the biceps laterally to uncover the pulsation (Fig. 10.13). This is true in skinny people as well as in the obese and the weight lifter. The rule is, "To find a brachial, push laterally, not deeper."

Bilateral simultaneous palpation of radial pulses (Fig. 10.14) may disclose inequality of timing or force. Either can be a valuable clue to differential arterial pathology. Closely related is measurement of *bilateral upper limb blood pressures,* since inequalities on sphygmomanometry may be present even without differences in pulse intensity. In the search for *subclavian-steal syndrome,* the examiner can have the patient exercise one arm or both arms, e.g., by repeatedly lifting this book, and observing for symptoms of vertebrobasilar insufficiency.

Brachioradial delay and variants. Simultaneous palpation of the brachial and radial arteries is employed in evaluating cardiac function, not arterial function. The *brachioradial delay test* consists of feeling the brachial artery pulse with one hand and the ipsilateral radial artery pulse with the other hand, then attending to whether there is a perceptible time lag between the proximal brachial and the distal radial (Fig. 10.15).

The examiner can also seek delay between carotid and radial arteries by palpating both at once (Fig. 10.16) or can feel the radial and femoral pulses or the carotid and femoral pulses simultaneously. In these settings, however, slight palpable delay may correspond to normal propagation of the pulse wave.

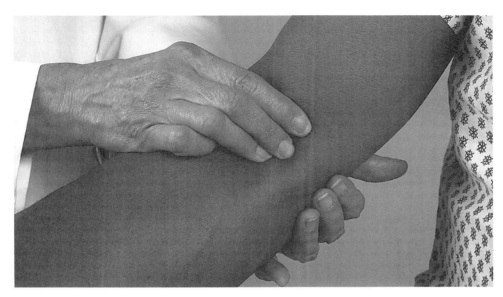

Figure 10.13   Pushing the biceps muscle laterally to uncover the often elusive brachial pulse.

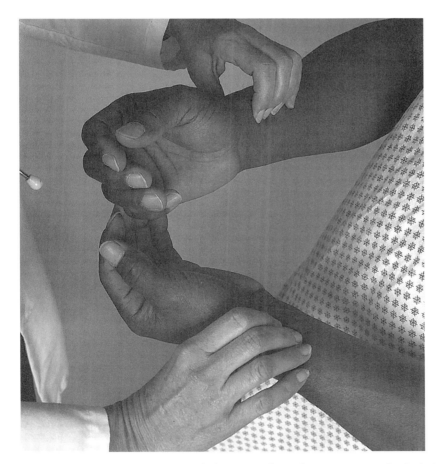

Figure 10.14   Bilateral simultaneous radial artery pulse palpation assesses both timing— normally synchronous—and relative force of the left- and right-sided systems, which are normally equal.

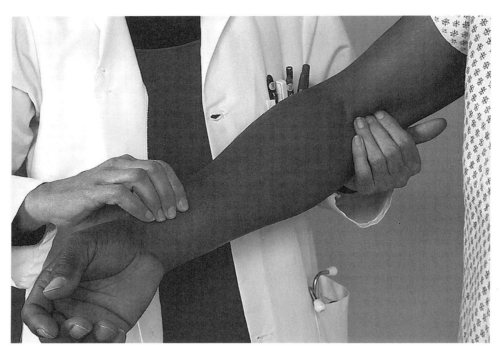

Figure 10.15 Technique of examining for brachioradial delay. See the text for full particulars.

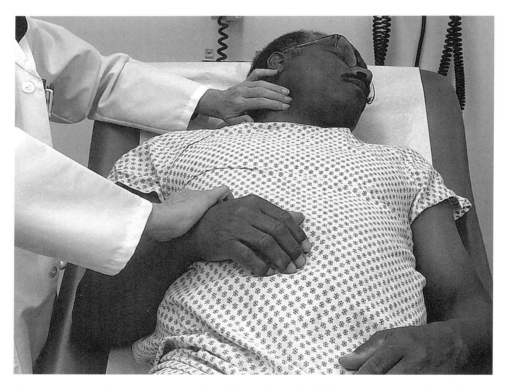

Figure 10.16 Palpating one carotid and the ipsilateral radial artery, to search for midaortic delay in pulse propagation.

Ulnar Pulse

The ulnar pulse is palpable in most normal persons on the lateral (radial) aspect of the ulna, just proximal to the wrist (Fig. 10.17). The key points are

• Don't seek the pulse "outside" the bone as with the radial pulse, but rather seek it in between the ulna and the radius.
• If it is difficult to find, gently passively flex the patient's wrist a bit to bring it out.

Allen's Test

Allen's test studies the *functional patency of the radial and ulnar arteries* (and palmar arch) by examining refilling of the capillary bed of the palm. First, identify the radial and ulnar pulses, then have the patient make a tight fist to squeeze blood out of the palm. Now press *very firmly* on both arteries, using both thumbs (Fig. 10.18). Wait a few seconds while doing so. If the whitened palm "pinks up" during continued pressing, the pressure applied has been insufficient, and the test must be started again. If, however, it stays pale, release *only the ulnar artery* (Fig. 10.19), then measure the time needed for recoloring of the palm. The test is repeated, this time with *only the radial artery* being released, recording the time needed to restore palmar color through the radial artery.

If the patient is paralyzed or comatose and therefore unable to make a tight fist on command, have an assistant apply external pressure over the whole hand to blanch it for the start of this test.

More on Lower-Limb Pulses

The **popliteal pulse** is notoriously difficult to feel. If the patient can assume a prone position, the pulse is most easily felt with the knee *passively flexed*—usually part way (Fig. 10.20). With the popliteal artery, you will feel pulsation that is transmitted, not the arterial wall, in contrast to the radial and even foot pulses.

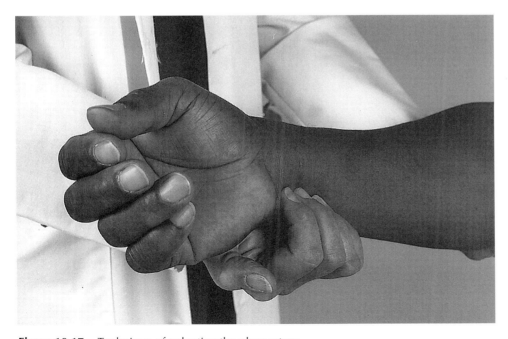

Figure 10.17   Technique of palpating the ulnar artery.

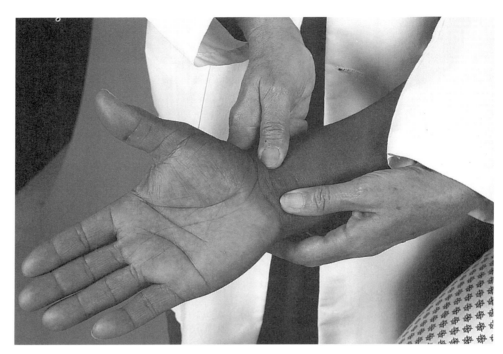

Figure 10.18　Early phase of Allen's test: sustained firm pressure on both the radial and ulnar arteries.

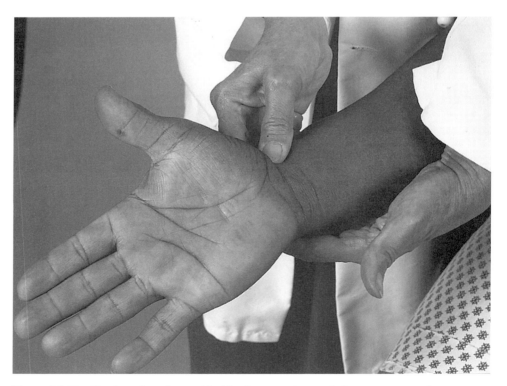

Figure 10.19　Testing ulnar flow with Allen's test: release of ulnar pressure only, to assess timing of blood flow into the emptied arteries and arterioles of the palm proper, i.e., recoloration as an indicator of integrity of the palmar arch.

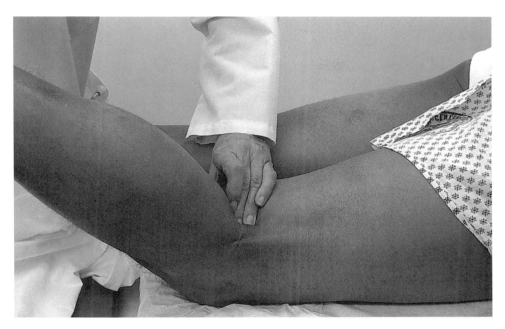

Figure 10.20   The popliteal pulse can sometimes be revealed with the patient prone and all tension taken off the posterior knee joint via gentle passive flexion of the knee.

You may have to probe very deeply in the obese or heavily muscled patient and to be wide-ranging about mediolateral localization. Beyond a learning period, make the effort only when indicated by absent foot pulses, symptomatic distal limb ischemia, or an ischemic ulcer.

When the posterior tibial pulse is difficult to feel, it can sometimes be found by searching more widely, throughout the space behind the medial malleolus and anterior to the tendo Achillis. More often, *passive dorsiflexion* of the ankle, using the opposite hand, will be of help (Fig. 10.21).

Discrepancies between pulses and symptoms call for special interpretation and sometimes for maneuvers. When there is claudication but the pulses are normal at rest, repalpate them after exercise, i.e., after having the patient walk, to see if they become reduced or absent.

Gastrocnemius Compression Sign

To elicit the gastrocnemius compression sign, the belly of the calf is squeezed firmly, but not suddenly or harshly, with both of the examiner's hands. The patient is asked to report any sensation. The test is always performed bilaterally.

Dependent Rubor and Variants

In seeking subtle arterial insufficiency, passively raise the supine patient's leg just as for straight-leg-raising tests, and observe for *blanching on elevation,* especially on the sole of the foot. This **Buerger's test** is usually followed by reactive erythema over the dorsum of the foot—and sometimes over the whole leg—when the foot is lowered again. This erythema is akin to *dependent rubor,* a prominent reddening of the foot, ankle, and shin when the legs hang over the edge of bed or chair (Fig. 10.22). For research purposes, the leg is elevated to 60° for 2 minutes, and then the patient sits up, and his legs are permitted to hang vertically from the examining table for 2 minutes. In practice, neither assessment is given more than 30 seconds.

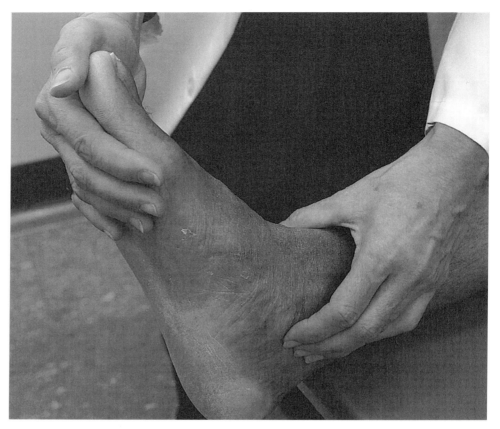

Figure 10.21   Slight and gentle passive flexion of the ankle can render a previously impalpable posterior tibial pulse detectable.

Additional Red Limbs

In seeking to explain a leg with erythema, positional or otherwise, that does not fit the above pattern, inquire about previous injury to the area, about pain brought on by warmth or dependency and relieved by elevation and/or removal of coverings, and about medicines in use. Then observe both the color of the limb in question and of its opposite in three positions: dependent, supine, and elevated. Also check for edema.

Cyanosis Evaluation and Differential Cyanosis

When cyanosis is observed in a limb, the first task is to determine whether there is also central (oral or perioral) cyanosis and whether the patient is gravely ill. Central cyanosis *sometimes* bespeaks critical illness needing immediate intervention.

When *normal vasoconstriction* is suspected as the cause of cyanosis localized to *cold feet,* the feet are warmed, whether with water or warm ambient air, and then reinspected.

Apart from these extremes, systematically review the four limbs and the trunk to establish (*a*) *localization* of cyanosis to one limb or group of limbs and (*b*) whether the finding is confined to the **acra** (fingertips and/or toes) or extends proximally. Check whether other acra, such as the tip of the nose, the nipples, or the tip of the penis, are involved. Compare the two hands against the two feet, ideally by having the patient sit on the bed or floor and place the pronated hands (dorsa up) atop the dorsa of the feet. Simultaneously observe for clubbing of the nails on all four limbs. If there is uncertainty about where or whether

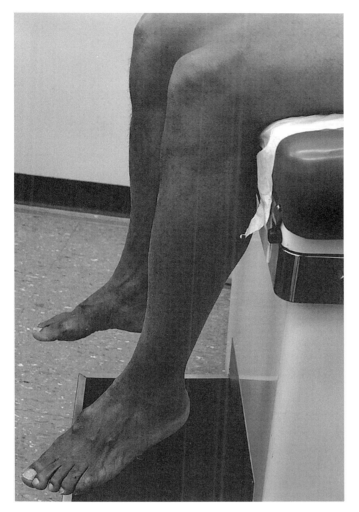

Figure 10.22   Ideal position for seeking dependent rubor. Gravitational pressure on arteries is substantial, yet the limb is not bearing weight. For seeking venous insufficiency, full standing is preferred.

cyanosis is seen, the patient can walk about for a few minutes and then resume the initial position or can be reobserved after immersing both hands and both feet in warm water.

VENOUS

Testing for Varicose Veins

With all other factors being equal, veins fill best when subjected to maximal hydrostatic pressure by gravity. Ask the patient to stand upright for a full minute, or observe veins right after testing the gait. For the weak patient, active stance is bypassed by having him rest his buttocks against a table with hips minimally flexed. Ectatic veins are often most prominent on the medial aspect of the thigh and leg. This saphenous territory is hidden if looked at from the side, unless the patient stands with one foot forward, exposing the medial portion of the far limb (Fig. 10.23). If the patient is leaning back against a table, external rotation of the hip will accomplish the same end.

It is a mistake *not* to recheck upright after varicosities are seen with the patient seated or supine. Often, much more severe venous insufficiency becomes

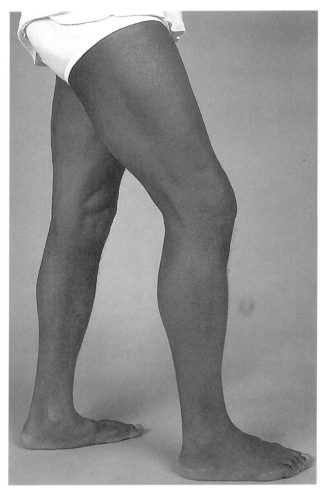

Figure 10.23 Inspection of medial surface of leg and thigh for venous distension is optimal with the patient standing, nearer foot forward, as the examiner checks from each side in turn.

noticeable with the patient in the upright position. Assessment of *severity* and *functional impact* requires the maneuver.

Edema

In the ambulatory patient, the usual first site for accumulation of edema due to heart failure or hypoalbuminemia is just *anterior to and about the medial malleolus*. This localization incorporates both gravity and areolar tissue that favors fluid extravasation. The sole of the foot, the most dependent area, has tight planes and may be "pumped dry" more regularly by muscular action. In the wheelchair-bound patient, first accumulation is also around the malleolus. However, for the patient who is bed-bound for a day or more, the sacral zone (not the intergluteal area) is the usual site. The search for edema in these areas means exposing and looking. The presacrum is exposed by having the patient sit on the bed and *lean very far forward* or, if not feasible, *lie on one side*. Assessment must be visual as well as tactile, to turn up incipient *pressure sores (bed sores)*. You cannot merely reach under the elastic at the top of underclothing and feel for pitting edema; you must lower the briefs so as to see and to palpate simultaneously.

Variants on edema. In considering the cause of an edematous limb, note key associated features listed in Table 10.4.

Venous Thrombosis and Variants

For superficial thrombophlebitis, seek cord-like superficial veins that are hard, tender, and slightly reddened. Sometimes, a broader erythema adjoins such veins, particularly when thrombosis and inflammation have arisen from an intravenous catheter and the puncture that has been made in its placement. When this is the source, feel for fluctuance at the site, which is difficult to distinguish from the "give" of a patent vein but not from the woody character of uncomplicated superficial phlebothrombosis, and attempt to express pus from the hole in the skin.

There is no physical sign diagnostic of *deep venous thrombosis,* nor is there any sign whose absence excludes deep venous thrombosis. Check for edema and erythema, and feel for a palpable venous "cord" by probing *deeply* in the calf. Is there a gastrocnemius compression sign? Homan's sign is neither specific nor sensitive enough to employ. There are times to be humble about the limits of physical diagnosis, and deep venous thrombosis leads the list.

Lymphatic System
SPECIAL LYMPH NODES

When there is a special need to detect lymphadenopathy, search the conventional chains of the head and neck, axillae, groin, and periclavicular zones. In addition, consider the epitrochlear lymph nodes, described in the Screening Examination section of this chapter, and a few fine points:

- *Subhumeral lymph nodes* are an axillary subgroup that is easy to miss, because they lie superiorly, not on or near the chest wall as do the other axillary chains. Rather, they hug the inferior surface of the proximal humerus at the superolateral aspect of the axilla. They are sought by pressing firmly but not painfully high in the axilla against this bone, and sweeping back to front for "BBs," "jelly beans," or larger nodes that glide or pop under the fingertips.
- *Popliteal lymph nodes* can enlarge with inflammation of the feet. Foot infection is so common that you would expect to find popliteal lymphadenopathy commonly, but it is rare. Perhaps the depth of the nodes within the popliteal fossa explains their usual impalpability. Passively flex the knee with the patient prone to probe for these nodes.
- *Inguinofemoral lymph nodes* form two palpable chains: a diagonal group, which follows the inguinal ligament inferomedially; and a vertical group, which

Table 10.4
Issues in Edema

Chronic venous insufficiency?
Lymphadenopathy at apex of limb (groin, axilla)?
Symmetry?
Inflammatory features (erythema, marked tenderness, *heat*)? Red streaks at proximal margin?
Known stimulus, e.g., bee sting?
Smooth or highly bumpy?
Gravitational?
Effect of use of the limb?
"Pitting" type, i.e., retains indentations made by a prodding fingertip applied for 10 seconds?
Most proximal point of pitting (separate from most proximal point of visible swelling)?
Measured circumference of the limb and its mate?
Skin shiny (usual with tense edema), atrophic, hyperkeratotic, scaly?

---

contains both deep and surprisingly superficial elements, with the latter usually palpable in normal hosts. This femoral group runs down the medial border of the quadriceps femoris muscle just medial to the femoral vein.

LYMPHANGITIC STREAKING

Minute red streaks proximal to an area of inflammation strongly suggest local lymphangitis. They are sought by scrutinizing the lymphatic course between the affected part and the limb's lymph node drainage at groin or axilla, using wide exposure and good lighting.

CELLULITIS EVALUATION

Bacterial infection of skin and soft tissue is common not only in normal persons but especially in diabetics with peripheral arterial insufficiency, intravenous drug abusers at sites of nonsterile injection, and patients with intravenous catheters. *Suppurative thrombophlebitis* is discussed elsewhere. The most ominous cellulitides are associated with maximal systemic reactions—high fever, white count, and bandemia—and those associated with *tissue necrosis* in the limb of origin. Ominous bedside signs of cellulitis are given in Table 10.5.

CHRONICALLY SWOLLEN LIMB

The history is very helpful, as with the differentiation of the kinds of edema outlined above. Seek a history of *deep venous thrombosis* with known *postphlebitic syndrome;* of *immobility* of the limb, usually a leg; of onset from childhood; of *trauma* to the limb or to its lymphatic drainage, whether iatrogenic or otherwise, especially from a motor vehicle crash; and of disabling *claudication* relieved only when the leg is dependent.

On examination, look for indicators of venous insufficiency, including using *upright* position to bring out *substantial* varicose veins. Look for massive enlargement of the whole limb or selective swelling of the affected calf and ankle, with relative sparing of the foot. Look for a squared-off appearance of the toes. Check pulses if the history so indicates. Compare motor function of the limb to what is expected from the history.

Musculoskeletal System Including Joints

UPPER LIMB

Shoulder

The simplest extended examination is a hard look at the two shoulders, individually and then together, from front and then back (Figs. 10.24 and 10.25), fully exposed, to assess contour, symmetry, and height relative to each other. Note whether the usual rounding in the frontal plane has been reduced or rendered concave, with the greater tuberosity of the humerus becoming more prominent.

Table 10.5
Ominous Clinical Features in Cellulitis

Blackened skin or devitalization
Ulcer that develops de novo or enlarges during the course of cellulitis
Brown or foul discharge, whether thin or viscous, scant or copious
Softening of affected area (inflammation alone should indurate both skin and deep tissue)
Sloughing of skin
Palpable gas, i.e., crepitus
Suppuration (softening or spontaneous drainage through the skin) of lymph nodes

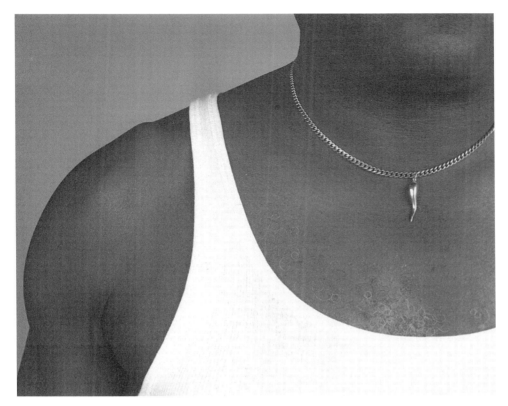

Figure 10.24 Anterior view of normal male shoulder contour. Examination would have been more productive if the patient had removed his undershirt: Pectoral musculature, clavicle, and male breast would be assessed simultaneously.

Look for shoulder enlargement as if by shoulder pads. If found, the enlargement is palpated to determine its texture. The symmetry of the clavicles is assessed by inspection.

Functional tests include the *Apley scratch test,* in which active range of motion is assessed by observing three activities for any limitation of motion, asymmetry, or discomfort (Table 10.6).

The functional *drop-arm test* has the patient abduct the shoulders, i.e., put both arms out as far to the sides as possible. Then he is asked to lower both arms slowly to the sides and is observed for inability to complete the action smoothly. The arm may drop at some point. Asymmetry of performance may show the nondominant side performing less well, but this can be overcome with practice. If you wish to increase sensitivity, perhaps at the cost of specificity—degree unknown—after a negative drop-arm test, the *drop-arm stress test* adds a gentle tap on the dorsum of the forearm to precipitate dropping of the abducted arm to the side.

Elbow

Look at the *carrying angle* of the elbow, which is normally about 10° lateral (valgus) to the long axis of the upper arm when the whole limb is held in anatomic position (Fig. 10.26*B*). In other positions, the angle cannot be assessed (Fig. 10.26*A*). The angle may be emphasized by having the patient carry a heavy weight in the hand.

Special *palpation for effusion* in the elbow consists of feeling for somewhat indistinct soft-tissue fullness between the lateral epicondyle, the proximal end of

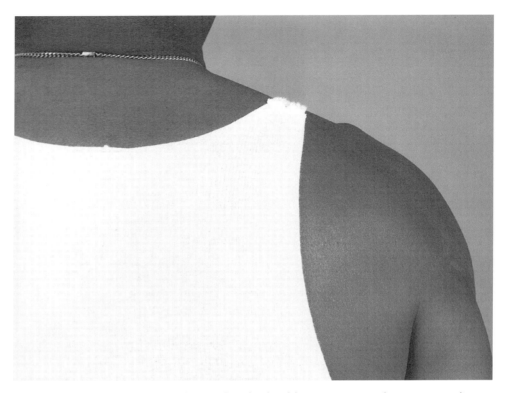

Figure 10.25   Posterior view of normal male shoulder contour. Similar caveat applies to upper spine and scapulae when exposure is limited by clothing.

the radius, and the olecranon. If found, this has to be distinguished from a more superficial fluid-filled bursal swelling directly over the olecranon and from sub-cutaneous solid masses.

In seeking lateral epicondylitis or radiohumeral bursitis (*tennis elbow*), hold the proximal forearm, then have the patient make a fist and extend his wrist against your flexing pressure. Inquire about sudden severe pain. If the patient says "yes," ask where it is experienced, being careful not to direct by suggestion. This is **Coen's test.**

Rheumatoid Nodules

Painless, nontender subcutaneous nodules can be sought near bony prominences, tendons, and joint capsules, especially on extensor surfaces and particularly over the elbow and back of the forearm. Fingers and knees are less common sites, and ankles and occiput are less common still. Whenever an apparent rheumatoid nodule is discovered, palpate to determine whether it is cystic. If so, look for a surface *pore.* Finally, test whether indentation or "squishing" occurs with pressure, especially if the lesion abuts the extensor aspect of the wrist.

Myoedema

Myoedema is not simple swelling of a muscle but rather is a striking deformity of a muscle body as a result of contraction immediately after the part is struck firmly with a reflex hammer. The appearance may occasionally be that of a ridge. It lasts about 5 seconds, abating thereafter. It is conventionally sought by tapping the biceps. Presumably, this reflects inappropriate posttraumatic muscular contraction, which is somewhat delayed in both onset and relaxation.

Table 10.6
Apley Scratch Test

A. Patient reaches his hand behind his head and touches ("scratches") the superomedial angle of the opposite scapula (lost with *defective abduction and external rotation*)
B. Patient reaches in front of his chest to rest his hand on the opposite shoulder (lost with *decreased internal rotation and adduction*)
C. Patient reaches behind his back to touch the inferior angle of the opposite scapula (lost with *decreased internal rotation and adduction*)

The Hand, Ulnar Deviation, and Rheumatoid Arthritis

Observe the hand in motion as, for example, the patient undoes his coat, shakes your hand, and gestures during the history. Observe the rest position, which normally shows slight flexion of all joints beyond the wrist.

To see ulnar deviation and the hand deformities characteristic of osteoarthrosis and rheumatoid arthritis, ask the patient to lay both hands flat, palms down, next to each other on a horizontal plane or in his lap, with the fingers pointing toward the examiner. Are the hands as a whole (or any digits) deviated "valgus-fashion" to the ulnar side? Ascertain whether any of the metacarpophalangeal joints are selectively enlarged and whether any interphalangeal joints are held in abnormal flexion or hyperextension.

Arachnodactyly

"Spider fingers," the literal translation of arachnodactyly, are sought more often than their diagnostic importance warrants. Inspect the hands, spread out on the table as for the previous examination, to see whether the fingers are unduly elongated. Have the patient fold the thumb as far as possible into the palm, then close the other digits over it, to seek *Steinberg's thumb sign* (protrusion of the thumb past the fifth finger). A follow-up test is the *wrist sign.* This sign is elicited by having the patient enclose one wrist, just proximal to the ulnar styloid, between his contralateral thumb and fifth finger; measure how much overlap of these two digits occurs.

Trigger Fingers, Discordant Fingers, and Contractures

Look for any finger that remains fully extended while the others are in rest position (slightly flexed). Any finger that is kept markedly more flexed than the others is also noted. With the latter, palpate the palmar fascia for thickenings or nodules, most commonly found in the ulnar half of the palm proximal to the fourth and fifth metacarpophalangeal joints. If reduced mobility is most marked in one digit or a digit pops with movement and no arthritic explanation is found, have the patient flex and extend the fingers rapidly, and seek a palpable and audible popping motion in one digit. The point in the cycle of flexion and extension where the phenomenon occurs varies from one case to another.

Knuckles, Finger Joints, and the Big Picture

A sophisticated screening test to exclude important hand arthritis, barring symptoms, is given in Table 10.7. If the chosen test is completed without functional defect, pain, or visible deformity, further evaluation is unnecessary.

If the screen is positive, observe whether the knuckles stand out from adjacent soft tissue at rest or when the patient makes a fist. (If pain limits fist-making, a very loose fist serves for this assessment.) Palpate the dorsolateral aspect of one metacarpophalangeal joint at a time, with the hand in rest position. Recall that the joint is 1.5 cm distal to the bend of the knuckle. (The knuckle, which we falsely

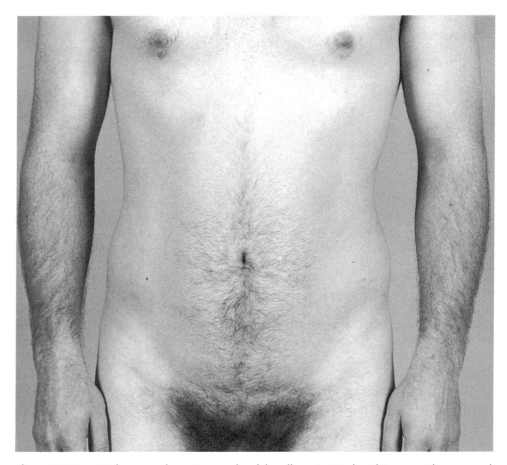

Figure 10.26   A. The normal carrying angle of the elbow is 10°, but this cannot be assessed here because the palms are not forward; i.e., the arms are not in anatomic position. **B.** Carrying angle with arms properly positioned.

regard as the joint, is actually the junction of the dorsal and distal aspects of the metacarpal bone.) Examine by pressing the joint at the bottom of the normal "slide" onto the dorsum of the proximal phalanx—with a finger from each of your own hands—on the two sides in search of palpable *enlargement*. Confirm metacarpophalangeal joint inflammation by noting *tenderness on compression* or *warmth*. A wince on handshake signifies metacarpophalangeal inflammation, too.

Inspect the proximal and distal interphalangeal joints for deformity; feel them to determine whether fluid, synovial proliferation, or bone enlargement is responsible. Look at and feel each joint in rest position (Fig. 10.27) for a more diffuse swelling of entire fingers, a *dactylitis*. Check for erythematous scaly skin changes over the metacarpophalangeal joints and for violet or normal-colored thickenings of the dorsa of the interphalangeal joints.

Finally, inspect the hand as a whole. If functional deficits are suspected, ask the patient to write his name (and keep this specimen of handwriting in the chart) or have him button a shirt or pick up a paper clip. Such *functional testing* has more predictive value than does an etiologic diagnosis.

Finkelstein's Test

Finkelstein's test is for *chronic stenosing tenosynovitis* of the abductor longus and extensor brevis tendons of the thumb, at the wrist. The patient folds the sympto-

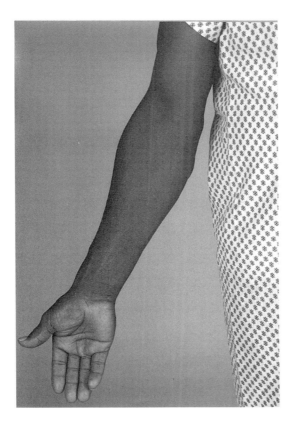

Figure 10.26 B.

Table 10.7
Advanced Hand Screen (Done on Each Hand Separately)

Make a tight fist
Pick up a small object from a flat surface
Squeeze two of the examiner's fingers as firmly as possible

matic thumb into its palm and then curls the ipsilateral fingers around as for Steinberg's test. The examiner stabilizes this forearm with one hand and pushes it toward its ulnar side to stretch the tendon in question. The patient is asked nondirectively about symptoms produced by the maneuver.

Tophi

With known gout or with an arthritis that might be either rheumatoid or gouty, look and feel for nodules in the helix of the external ears, on the feet and ankles—especially near the first metatarsophalangeal joint and at the Achilles' tendon—and in the forearms, wrists, and hands. Nodules are assessed for tenderness, contour, surface ulcers, and extruded material. Search for induration or grittiness in the fingertip pads.

LOWER LIMB

Simian Stance

Two bedside tests help differentiate claudication from the *pseudoclaudication* of spinal stenosis: stance and the bicycle test.

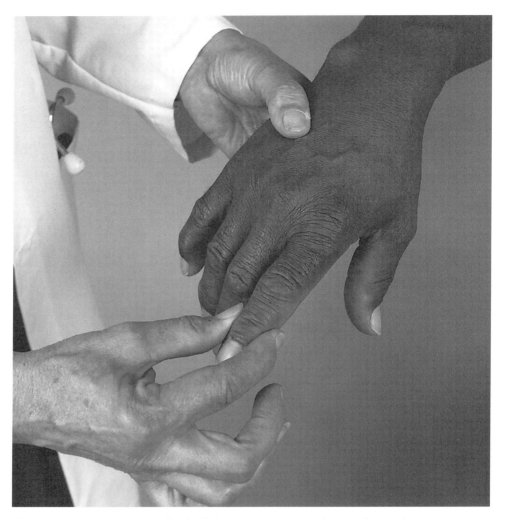

Figure 10.27 Squeezing individual distal interphalangeal joints for tenderness or previously unrecognized boggy hyperplastic synovium.

Stance. If the patient stands with both the hips and the knees slightly flexed, so that the stance resembles that of a simian, *lumbar spinal stenosis* is likely. Observe the patient without his knowing that his posture is under study. More normal erect posture tends to be assumed, despite pain, when the patient realizes he is being watched.

Bicycle test. If the patient can exercise in a seated position without producing leg, back, or buttock pain that would occur with a comparable level of walking, the bicycle test is positive. The history may not point clearly to pseudoclaudication, so in difficult cases you may need to have the patient use a stationary bicycle.

Abnormal Gait

Observe the gait, particularly for *antalgic gait,* also known as *favoring one leg,* to minimize pain from moving some structure in that leg. The appearance has been compared to stepping on a tack as the host tries to abbreviate weight bearing on the limb as much as possible. Another abnormal gait is the **lurching gait** associated with gluteus medius muscle weakness. *Gait and stance are the best functional* *tests of* **hip extensor power:** The downward pull of the body's weight, opposed by these antigravity muscles, exceeds most extrinsic forces applied by examiners in any of the numerous tests of this critical function.

Hip Tests

Gait and range of motion are critical functional tests for the hip. Because of the importance of the hip and the frequency of disease involving it, particularly osteoarthrosis, many other tests have been developed.

Trendelenburg test. This test consists of observing the patient from behind and looking at the dimples over the posterior superior iliac spines. With normal weight bearing evenly distributed to both legs, the two spines and the two buttocks should be at the same level. Then have the patient stand on just one leg, and observe for normal elevation of the opposite hemipelvis (Fig. 10.28). Failure to elevate or actual lowering of the buttock on the unsupported side constitutes a positive test.

Leg length discrepancy. If the legs appear unequal and the pelvis does not seem tilted, test for *leg-length discrepancy.* Use bony landmarks so that the mea-

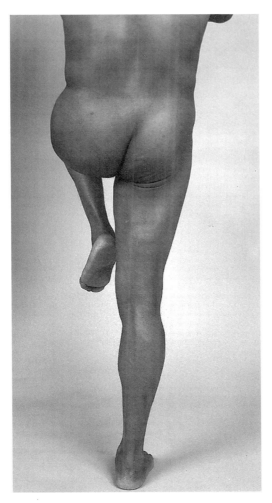

Figure 10.28   Normal Trendelenburg test result. Buttock does not sag with ipsilateral hip flexion.

surements of the two sides are comparable. The patient lies supine, with each leg abducted exactly as far from the midline as the other. Measure from the concavity just inferior to the anterior superior iliac spine, to the ipsilateral medial malleolus. The measuring tape crosses the anterior patella at its midpoint. (The iliac spine itself is not used because the tape measure may slip off it.) Tape measures of paper or metal are preferred to cloth, for cloth may stretch, introducing an additional source of error.

If the lengths are unequal, have the patient lie supine and flex both knees to 90° (if possible), with both feet *flat on the table.* Then look for one knee that is higher than the other or one that projects farther distally (toward the foot) than the other.

If the leg length measurements are equal, reconsider the causes of an **apparent** *inequality of leg length* that is not real, notably *pelvic obliquity and flexion contracture of the hip.* With the patient upright, check for pelvic tilt by comparing the heights of the anterior superior iliac spines and then of the posterior superior iliac spines: Unevenness despite equal-length limbs proves pelvic tilt.

Thomas' test. Thomas' test unmasks occult flexion contracture of the hip that was compensated and hidden by local increase in lumbar lordosis. Have the patient lie supine, with both legs adducted to the midline. Inspect for an excessive hollow between the superior aspect of either buttock and the small of the back. Then the hip *contralateral* to the suspected contracture is flexed fully up onto the trunk. This flattens the lumbar spine and stabilizes the pelvis, eliminating compensatory lordosis and bringing out hidden flexion contracture contralaterally. Record the degree of involuntary flexion of the involved side for serial evaluation by measuring the angle made by the limb's long axis with the table.

Workup of the flexion-contracted hip. When a flexion contracture of the hip is present, consider diagnoses other than the usual cause, namely osteoarthrosis. Depending on acuity versus stable chronicity, check for other prospects. Does the patient have fever, rheumatoid deformities of other joints, a bulging, tender hip joint capsule on palpation, an abdominal, flank, iliac fossa, or groin mass or a mass that is pointing in the upper medial thigh, or a positive psoas sign (see the Extended Examination section of Chapter 9)? If psoas abscess is being considered along with septic arthritis of the hip, check the effect on tenderness of testing external rotation with the hip *flexed* versus with the hip *extended.*

Fractured hips. Fixed external rotation, especially with shortening, is characteristic of *hip fracture,* but some cases fail to show this sign. Any movement of the joint is painful, as is direct pressure. Range of motion is decreased, especially flexion and (further) external rotation. However, the presence of pain, spasm, and guarding is of help only if they not have been chronically present from preexisting osteoarthrosis. *Auscultatory percussion* has been used for fracture evaluation. For this test, the patient is kept supine, if possible, with symmetric minimal abduction of both hips, and the legs are kept flat, i.e., no flexion at hip or knee. If one leg is shortened and externally rotated to begin with, then the opposite limb is placed in the same position so that error due to variable position is omitted. Place the stethoscope on each anterior iliac crest in sequence, and auscultate the sound made by percussing the ipsilateral patella with moderate force, using one finger (directly—no pleximeter). The force employed for each side must be equal if sound transmission is to be compared meaningfully.

Other hip-related issues. **Forceful adduction** is sought in patients with reduced gait and dementing illnesses or mental retardation. This is sometimes fixed, more often voluntary. Attempt abduction with gentle explanation and discussion, and if this fails, with distraction from an assistant or relative.

Look for tenderness on internal rotation during range of motion testing. Pain over the greater trochanter or its bursa is sought by pressing on these structures.

Also observe both *fully exposed* thighs in the search for inequality that is seen with *quadriceps atrophy.*

Straight-leg-raising test. The straight-leg-raising test is discussed in detail in the Extended Examination section of Chapter 12 but needs brief review here. Have the patient lie supine, with both legs adducted. Scoop up the painful leg from beneath the heel, using your opposite hand to keep the knee straight, and raise the leg until pain is produced. If it is, the patient tells whether pain is felt only in the back, only in the posterior thigh, or all the way down the leg—or in the opposite leg. Then lower the heel 4 or 5 cm, so the pain is relieved, and then passively but maximally *dorsiflex the foot* of this leg. Again the patient is asked if this produces pain and, if so, where. The test is then repeated on the unaffected (painless) side.

Patrick's test. In seeking hip or sacroiliac joint pathology, Patrick's test, also known as *Fabere's test,* is employed. Have the patient lie supine and place the foot of the symptomatic side on the opposite knee to achieve flexion, abduction, and external rotation of the hip and fixation of the femur to the pelvis. Then ask the open-ended question, "What sensation has this produced or reproduced?" Then press downward on the anterior superior iliac spine in question and on the flexed knee, "as though opening a book," during which the same inquiry is repeated.

Functional Testing

Mobility disorders in the aged are more consistently identified by a simple functional test than by neuromuscular evaluation. Ask the patient to sit in a hard, armless chair. Then tell the patient to perform each step in the **Tinetti functional test.** That is, have the patient *arise, walk* along a straight path (indicated by pointing), *turn* around, *return,* and *be seated* again in the chair.

The patient is dressed and wears shoes as well as any hearing aid or eyeglasses that are normally employed. He also uses any cane or walker employed in daily life.

The longest available pathway that is free of obstacles and rugs is used for the test. Observe the patient's ability to arise from a chair, the step height, the smoothness and ease of turning, and the patient's ability to sit down again smoothly and on target.

Knee Effusions

The knee and its disorders are complex. For the nonorthopedist, key issues are stance, gait, and effusion. Many derangements of the knee cause excess fluid to accumulate. Detection of this fluid may lead to localization but seldom to specific etiologic diagnosis.

All bedside methods unless specified otherwise employ inspection with *the knee fully extended and with the quadriceps muscle relaxed.*

The simplest means of detecting effusion in the knee is inspection for *deformity.* This method is insensitive. Observation for obliteration of the normal indentations just medial and lateral to the patella at rest has been advocated, but these may also be lost from obesity.

Ballottement. For *ballottement of the knee,* press the suprapatellar pouch with one hand, and push the patella sharply posteriorly into the trochlear groove, the track on the front of the femur in which the patella sits, with your other hand; then quickly release. A *click* may be heard as the patella taps the femur. With effusion, the fluid wave rebounds from the edges of the joint cavity, and the patella pops back up against the examining fingers. This method, sometimes called the *tap test,* can detect substantial effusions.

Bulge test and variant. The *bulge or stroke test* may demonstrate smaller accumulations, perhaps as little as 4 mL. For this, squeeze the suprapatellar pouch and milk the fluid out of it and out of the medial part of the cavity by pressing just medial to the patella and creating a small concavity there. Finally, briskly stroke or tap the lateral aspect (Fig. 10.29), causing a fullness to bulge outward promptly—not merely as tissue displacement—on the medial side. If the expected reaction is not accomplished, repeat the test 1–2 cm up or down or with the knee very slightly flexed. Consensus is lacking on whether the medial approach is preferable to the lateral.

For the *fluctuation test,* squeeze the suprapatellar pouch and rock or fluctuate fluid from medial to lateral and back again.

Mann's test. Mann's test, perhaps the most sensitive for small effusions, relies on observing hollows to either side of the *patellar ligament.* This midline structure, you remember, extends from the bottom of the patella—level with the bottom of the femur—to the prominent tibial tuberosity immediately inferior to and at the anterosuperior extremity of the tibia. (Feel the patellar ligament on yourself. It's the firm but nonosseous band that constitutes a defect in bony continuity between the patellofemoral unit above and the tibiofibular one below.) In the normal slightly flexed knee observed from the side, a hollow is seen just lateral to this ligament. With further flexion, the hollow fills in. If excess fluid is present in the knee joint, the *point of filling in is reached sooner.* The side that fills in first should be the one with effusion. At the (premature) point of filling in, you can press the thumb on one side of the ligament, with the index finger on the other, and rock the intra-articular fluid back and forth as in the fluctuation test. For serial observation, record the flexion angle at which the hollow disappears on the normal side and, sequentially over time, on the affected side. With accumulation of additional fluid, the angle at which the hollow is lost approaches 180° (extended knee). With resolution, it returns toward normal.

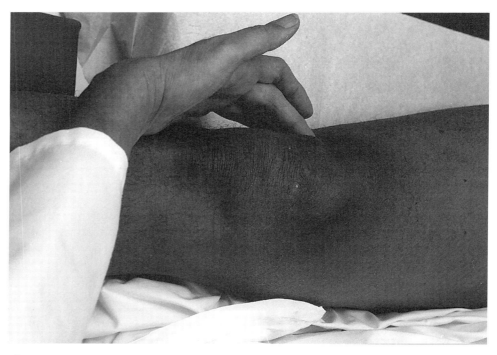

Figure 10.29 Technique of "pushing" small knee effusion from lateral aspect, to produce a bulge on the medial side of the knee.

Other Deformities

Observe the patient standing in rest position, first anteriorly and then from the side, noting the angulation of the tibia with respect to the femur in both planes. Normally, the tibia is slightly lateral (valgus) in the frontal plane and straight in the parasagittal plane viewed from the side.

When *bowlegs* (a *genu varum* deformity) are diagnosed, note whether the shins are curved and, if so, whether they are curved symmetrically or unilaterally. If the time of onset of bowlegs is known, it will help determine etiology.

Knee Draw(er) Tests

Knee draw(er) tests ascertain **integrity of cruciate ligaments,** which tether the tibia to the femoral condyles, by showing how slight is the mobility of the tibia on the femur. Have the patient lie supine, with knees flexed to 90° and feet flat on the examination table. Stabilize the foot on the side being tested by sitting on it sidesaddle, and then place both hands around the knee in question, fingers in the popliteal fossa and thumbs on the medial and lateral sides of the knee joint. Draw the tibia forward, noting if it budges forward more than a few degrees from under the femur or more than on the opposite side. Then push the tibia back not only to base position, but if it will go, backward under the femur. Do it bilaterally every time: Side-to-side comparison is requisite.

Charcot's Joints: Ankle and Other

Charcot's joints have *neuropathic arthropathy,* reflecting failure of protective action against repetitive trauma in activities of daily living as a result of reduced sensation. The most common scenario in 1994 is the *ankle with diabetic peripheral neuropathy.* Marked *joint deformity* incorporates enlargement and displacement. *Laxity with increased* (not restricted) *passive range of motion* contrasts with joints damaged by other processes. The proprioceptive and other sensory deficits in the affected area and the lack of tenderness on firm palpation are distinctive. Distortion of the joint may be extraordinary. Sometimes, palpation or passive range of motion testing produces coarse bone-on-bone crepitation. With weight bearing, instability of the joint is emphasized more clearly. The joint often feels like "a bag of bones."

Ankle Arthritis versus Dependent Edema

The distinction between ankle arthritis and dependent edema can be particularly difficult if the two processes coexist. Both can fill in the hollows (sulci) anterior to the medial and lateral malleoli. Compare the two ankles for symmetry, check for pitting in the skin, assess tenderness on palpation and during passive range of motion, and assess active and passive range of motion. Finally, search for pre-existent venous disease and for presacral edema, both at presentation and, if need be, after therapeutic elevation, compressive hose, or diuretics.

Foot Examination Technique

For foot examination, *adequate exposure* must be reiterated. Socks and shoes must be off and, despite the greater inconvenience, so too must panty hose. The feet can be neither inspected nor palpated adequately even through thin transparent nylon. *Shoes* are examined for uneven wear, for evidence of tilted weight bearing, and for abnormally diagonal folds at the toes.

A pillowcase or paper towel is placed on the ground for the patient to stand on. Then inspect with the patient's feet parallel to one another and bearing weight equally. Look from in front, from each side, and from the back. If the patient is mobile and has good balance, have him make a "right face" 4 times in succession. Recheck gait with bare feet, looking for antalgic gait and for excess impact on heels or ankles. Thereafter, with both you and the patient sitting, examine the foot elevated onto an examining stool or onto the seated examiner's anterior thigh. Proper visualization of the *sole* requires that the patient lie supine and the examiner look from the foot of the table. The heel is most difficult to expose; to see the posterior and inferior surfaces in continuity, neither seated nor supine positioning is effective. However, alternatives exist (Table 10.8).

Minor pressure markings over the metatarsophalangeal joints represent normal variation, as does minor flat-footedness (pes planus, flattening of the longitudinal arch of the foot), and perhaps even minimal clawtoe (hinted at in Fig. 10.30).

Table 10.8
Alternative Methods for Bringing the Heel into View (in Descending Order of Patient Strength)

Have the patient kneel backward in a chair, hands on the chair back
Have the patient lie prone on the examining table and flex the knee (or lie flat-out prone); look on from the head of the table
Put the patient into the lateral decubitus position

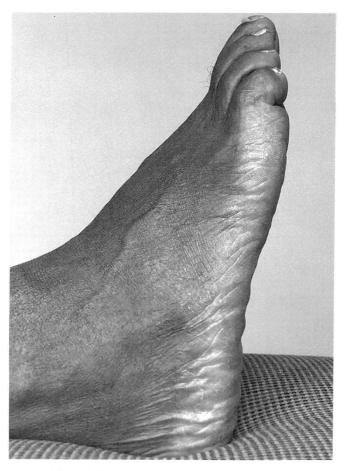

Figure 10.30   Normal lateral foot contour. The subject has slightly flexed metatarsophalangeal and interphalangeal joints, but the resultant "deformity" is of no importance.

Hindfoot. Inspection and palpation proceed from proximal to distal. The Achilles tendon is inspected for contracture, which produces a **pes equinus deformity** whereby the patient stands and walks on toes and forefoot rather than having the broader use of the foot. The Achilles tendon can be palpated for *xanthomas,* if indicated. The *ankle mortise* is palpated with both thumbs pressing just anterior to the malleoli, and all eight fingers curled around the back of the ankle and heel. Tenderness and deformity are sought. A finger or two sweeps the heel for palpable bone spurs if localized pain suggests one.

Midfoot and forefoot. Squeeze all five metatarsophalangeal joints at the base of the toes, using a single hand, to seek tenderness. If tenderness is present, check each metatarsophalangeal joint by pressing with the pads (not tips or nails) of your second and third fingers on the plantar surface, your thumb on the dorsum, and gently rocking the toe through passive flexion and extension while palpating the joint through the plantar surface, seeking tenderness or evidence of joint deformity, expansion, or reduced range of motion. If in doubt about mild tenderness, apply equal pressure over the head of the respective metatarsal bone for comparison.

For intrinsic toe (interphalangeal) joints, techniques and interpretation are closely analogous. On the *sole,* inspect the *transverse arch* just posterior to the metatarsal heads, and look for *callosities* under the metatarsal heads. Then assess for *flatfeet* or its opposite, excess longitudinal arch height *(pes cavus).* The findings are correlated with any *callosities over the head of the talus.*

Gout

The usual site attacked by both gout and bunion is the medial aspect of the first metatarsophalangeal joint, i.e., the medial border of the foot at that point. During an *acute gout attack,* this will be red, hot, swollen, and extraordinarily tender. The only realistic differential diagnosis at that moment is **septic arthritis.** Later, urate deposition may lead to a *tophus* at this site, with characteristics described previously. When a reddened but only mildly tender focus is found over the head of the first metatarsal, the differential diagnosis is a **bunion,** which should mean a history of no *agonizing* pain. With bunions, there is usually an underlying *hallux valgus* deformity and sometimes an etiologically related *pes planus.* Marked reduction in passive range of motion of the metatarsophalangeal joint suggests articular or synovial damage, i.e., gout.

Diabetes

Diabetic foot ulcers reflect diminished sensation as a result of neuropathy and coexistent arterial insufficiency: The host is unaware of minor trauma, and repair is defective. The feet are "the end of the line" for neural transmission and for blood supply. Any condition compromising both predisposes the host to ulcers from even trivial injury. Since the feet are often moist from sweat and are kept in confining socks and shoes that reduce air-drying, their cutaneous bacterial counts are high. An unhealed wound becomes a portal of entry for microbes that perpetuate and amplify tissue injury. The most common area affected is the sole, particularly the weight-bearing areas over the metatarsal heads. Any part of the diabetic foot and ankle can be affected. With marked venous insufficiency, the premalleolar zones are predisposed also. Diabetic foot ulcers often have unsuspected complicating *osteomyelitis* in the bone beneath and frequently augur amputation, usually for gangrene. Some principles of diabetic foot examination are listed in Table 10.9.

If an ulcer is shallow and white-pink *dermis* is seen in the base, with or without white fibrinous exudate or bits of yellow pus, osteomyelitis is less likely but

Table 10.9
Principles of Diabetic Foot Examination

Insist on *podiatric consultation* for routine toenail care in this population, but do *not* relegate foot examination to the podiatrist
Take a good look at the diabetic foot at every opportunity
Characterize ulcers rapidly and thoroughly, document in detail, and refer appropriately

not excluded. If fat, tendon, bone, or a base obscured by exudate is seen, the outlook is worse. If white, solid tissue of uncertain nature is seen, put on a sterile glove or finger cot. Place this in the base of the wound. (Neuropathy has rendered the area hypesthetic.) Feel for bony hardness. Try to move the base anteriorly or inferiorly over subjacent bone. If this can be done, and you are not simply pushing exudate about in the wound, then the base is not bone. If it is not rock-hard, see if moving your finger, pressed firmly against the skin, brings skin at the edge of the wound along with it. If so, it must be dermis, since subcutis tethers to skin only after severe inflammation.

Toes

Inspect the toes with the patient standing, looking for discoloration (dependent rubor) or venous disease. With the patient supine, look at and between the toes for maceration and soft corns. Check the first toe to see whether it is deviated laterally (**hallux valgus**) and, if so, whether it overlaps the second toe. The associated first metatarsophalangeal joint is checked for bunion as detailed above.

Hallux rigidus is suspected when a protective gait is seen: oblique foot-strike off the four lateral toes. Oblique shoe creases over the toes (rather than normal transverse creases) corroborate this. With passive-range-of-motion testing, such a hallux moves minimally on attempted extension, and the patient complains that the maneuver is very painful.

Check the dorsa of the toes for callosities.

Clawtoes and hammertoes. Check for clawtoes and hammertoes with the patient supine.

Clawtoes usually affect all five toes on a foot and are frequently associated with *pes cavus*. They result from hyperextension of metatarsophalangeal joints and flexion of interphalangeal joints. (They do not precisely parallel either swanneck or boutonnière finger deformities.) Because of abnormal weight bearing, they often lead to callosities on the *plantar* aspects of some metatarsal heads and of some or all toe tips and, from pressure against the uppers of shoes, on the *dorsa* of the affected toes.

Hammertoes are usually solitary, most often on the second toe. They involve hyperextension of the metatarsophalangeal joint, flexion of the proximal interphalangeal joint, and hyperextension of the distal interphalangeal joint, analogous to boutonnière deformities. They tend to produce callosity on the dorsum of the flexed proximal interphalangeal joint from pressure against shoe uppers. Plantar callosities are uncommon with hammertoes.

Interphalangeal toe joints. In checking for *arthritis of interphalangeal joints* of the toes, place your left thumb and index finger on the dorsal and plantar surfaces of the joint and your right thumb and index finger on the medial and lateral surfaces, and then note whether compression in either plane distends the other—akin to the fluctuation test of the knee. If tenderness of a toe joint is equivocal, compare pressure effects on the normally more sensitive midphalanx *bone*.

Toenails. At the toenails, look for (*a*) macerated, softened, irregular nails, (*b*) hard, thickened, ridged, yellowed nails, (*c*) erythema and tenderness where the lateral margin of nail undermines the lateral nail bed, with or without pus expressible at the line of juncture and with or without erythema and fluctuance of immediately adjacent skin, (*d*) uniform whitening of nails, and (*e*) long recurved uncut nails that may actually come back and touch the skin at some distance away.

Neurologic System

LIMB TREMOR

Tremor is more often spotted in the hands than in the legs, feet, trunk, or face and is described in the Extended Examination section of Chapter 11. When tremor is identified, an examination sequence is pursued (Table 10.10).

CHEST AND SHOULDER

To detect *weakness of the serratus anterior* muscle in a patient with *trouble reaching forward* or fully elevating the arm, observe the scapula at rest and with the *push-off test.* The patient stands facing a wall at a distance of about 30 cm. Have him place both hands flat against the wall, elbows outward, and attempt to push himself away from the wall. Watch for scapular "winging," i.e., movement of the medial half of the scapula posteriorly, away from the chest wall, so that it stands out "angel-wing style." (Occasionally, the patient or a trainer may have observed this phenomenon during a push-up.)

Although testing cranial nerve XI and the trapezius muscle is described in Chapter 11, two more signs may disclose subtle trapezius dysfunction. Observe the patient in rest position from in front, his chest and shoulders bared, for a hump or point in the shoulder contour between the neck and the tip of the shoulder. This *scapular hump* signifies trapezius weakness. A *crease over pectoralis major muscle,* inferior to the normal crease where the arm joins the breast in the anterior axillary line, has similar significance, usually coexists with the hump, and is called *oblique pectoral crease.* It is further distinguished from the normal crease by superomedial orientation toward the sternoclavicular joint, whereas the normal crease tips just medial to the vertical.

CARPAL TUNNEL SYNDROME AND TINEL'S AND PHELAN'S SIGNS

In the patient with weakness or sensory changes in the distribution of the median nerve, *carpal tunnel syndrome* is commonly considered. Sensory abnormalities in the median nerve distribution (see below) are sometimes found, and support the diagnosis. So does thenar wasting or weakness. Other physical signs include pro-

Table 10.10
Tremor Evaluation

Most proximal point of spontaneous occurrence?
Symmetrical?
Do other limbs, trunk, jaw, lips, tongue, cheeks, and facial muscles show abnormal involuntary movements?
Does purposeful movement abolish tremor?
Romberg sign? Nystagmus?
Do amplitude, frequency, duration, and force change with emotion?
Have the patient bring the hands close to the face.
Family history? Gait? Mental status?
Cogwheeling?
Facies?
Speech?

duction of electric-shock pain or abnormal tingling in the median nerve distribution by exerting pressure on the flexor retinaculum at the wrist. *Tinel's sign* is elicited by sharply tapping the midvolar wrist (volar carpal ligament) with one finger to reproduce the abnormal sensation. For *Phelan's sign (inverted prayer attitude),* the wrists are maximally *flexed* for one full minute—the asymptomatic side serving as a control and as a bolster to keep the symptomatic one fully bent.

INTRINSIC HAND MUSCLES

Innumerable signs correspond to the complexity and functional importance of the hand. Three are described here:

- *Interosseous atrophy* is recognized by visible reduction in tissue between the bones.
- *Abduction of the fingers* is powered by the dorsal interosseous muscles and the abductor digiti minimi, both innervated by the ulnar nerve (spinal roots C8 and T1). A global test of this function is to have the patient's wrist and metacarpal joints extended but not hyperextended. Abduct his four fingers very slightly. Then encircle the four fingers between your thumb and index finger, and ask the patient to break the hold. Should a localization of weakness be needed, squeeze each adjacent pair of fingers together between your thumb and index fingers, and ask the patient to spread apart, in turn, the fifth and ring fingers, the ring and middle fingers, and the middle and index fingers.
- The *pinch mechanism* employs many joints, nerves, and muscles, including the lumbrical and interossei muscles. Begin as in *abduction of the fingers* above, and have the patient make an "O" from the flexed index finger and thumb and hold it against resistance. Then hook or curl your index finger just inside the circle, at the junction of the two fingertips that close the circle, and pull forcefully to try to separate these two fingertips or to distort the circle. In a variant, make an "O" inside the patient's "O," and try to pull yours through his.

MYELOPATHY HAND

Direct the patient to hold his hands out with fingers forward and palms down. Check for *involuntary abduction of the fifth finger,* at baseline or after 30 seconds. If abduction is found, then check whether abduction has also developed with the fourth (ring) finger and, if so, with the third finger also. If so, look for reduced extension at the interphalangeal joints and, ultimately, at the metacarpophalangeal joints of the involved fingers. The whole sequence is the *finger escape sign.* Exclude ulnar neuropathy as the cause by establishing normal forceful abduction of the fifth finger. Rule out amyotrophic lateral sclerosis as the cause by showing normal flexion and extension of the ipsilateral wrist against resistance—something lost when motor neuron disease affects the digits.

Then have the patient grip (flex) and release (extend) all fingers together, with the arm, wrist, and metacarpophalangeal joints in rest position, as rapidly as possible. Count repetitions for 10 seconds, and watch for *slow, incomplete finger extension,* for failure of coordination with unsought wrist flexion during attempted finger extension, and for dyssynergic wrist extension with finger flexion.

RADIAL, ULNAR, AND MEDIAN NERVES AND SPINAL DERMATOMES

A few points deserve reemphasis. The *radial nerve* derives components from C5 through T1. It is sensory to much of the proximal dorsum of the hand on the radial aspect. The most consistently radial-supplied skin, and therefore the place to test sensation if radial neuropathy is suspected, is the web space between thumb and index finger, dorsal aspect. Two motor functions of the nerve are *thumb extension and wrist extension.* Ability to keep the wrist extended against resistance shows that radial motor function is intact. A wrist-drop shows that it is not.

The *median nerve,* with fibers from C5 to T1, innervates the palmar skin of the hand. The "purest" median territory is the *radial half of the tip of the index finger* (palmar aspect, not the fingernail-bearing dorsum). Muscle actions include *thumb-pinching, opposition, and abduction of the thumb.*

The *ulnar nerve,* with fibers from C8 and T1, supplies the ulnar *palmar skin,* with the most reliable site being the *tip of the fifth finger.* Its limited motor function is *abduction of the fifth finger.*

The spinal dermatomes are simple on the palmar aspect: C6 is the thumb and index finger; C7, the middle finger; and C8, the fourth and fifth.

The *flexor digiti superficialis muscle* is tested by having the patient supinate the hand and extend all fingers except the one being tested. He is then asked to flex that finger at the proximal interphalangeal joint. If he can, the median nerve is working.

ASTERIXIS

Asterixis is a *variably rhythmic* failure to maintain voluntary muscular contraction. Its elicitation requires cooperation, so it cannot be done in the patient who is comatose or stuporous. Have the patient pronate the forearms, extend the elbows, spread the fingers slightly, and hyperextend both wrists, "as though you are a cop stopping traffic. Keep that traffic stopped for a full minute." Multiple reinforcing verbal reminders are usually needed. After a few seconds to a minute, the abnormal response is a "flap" of both hands, whereby hyperextension is involuntarily lost and quickly involuntarily regained. Asymmetry of asterixis is rare.

Patients with disordered attention—a hallmark of delirium—usually cannot cooperate. Therefore variants have been devised. For example, ask the patient to maintain a steady squeezing with each hand, on two fingers from each of your hands. Alternatively, ask the patient to keep the mercury level of a half-inflated sphygmomanometer steady. A third method involves partially externally rotating the patient's half-flexed hip or abducting his extended hip; the examiner observes for repetitive *small, quickly corrected movements* as the patient returns the limb to resting position.

COMMON PERONEAL NERVE

The common peroneal nerve runs superficially around the lateral neck of the fibula and is susceptible to trauma. The nerve can be palpated *gently* with a fingertip as it crosses the bone a bit below the insertion of the biceps femoris tendon. The nerve is usually difficult to distinguish from adjacent tissue. Injudicious examining pressure can injure the nerve, so caution is the watchword.

When *foot-drop* results from damage to this nerve, the knees are raised higher to keep the foot from scraping the floor with each step, because the foot does not dorsiflex properly. Less frequently, compensatory efforts fail and the foot does hit the ground (and the patient may fall). The high-knee gait is a *steppage gait.* Failure to dorsiflex properly is highlighted by having the patient walk on his heels. Often, an *equinovarus* deformity of the foot accompanies common peroneal nerve palsy. There may also be hypesthesia over the dorsum of the foot and contiguous anterior shin.

HOOVER'S TEST

In attempting to move a paralyzed limb, there is normally an opposed involuntary or unconscious movement of its mate downward to gain leverage. This is the basis for *Hoover's test for psychogenic monoparalysis or malingering.* With *paraplegia,* the test will not work, since there has to be a strong, intact limb contralateral to the weak one. Have the patient lie supine. Stand at the foot of the bed and cup your hands around both heels. Then ask the patient to raise the weak leg off the bed. There should be marked downward pressure (hip extension) from the sound side. With poor effort *or with bilateral disease,* this response is lacking.

INTERPRETING THE FINDINGS
Peripheral Vasculature
CAPILLARY
Blood Leakage Tests

A positive *Rumpel-Leede test* consists of ten or more petechiae appearing within the circle within 5 minutes or less. Discussion is found in Chapter 3.

Pinch purpura is detected if ecchymosis—not just petechiae—develops at the site of pinching. If the pinch has not been harsh, arteriolar fragility is demonstrated. *Amyloid microangiopathy* may be the cause. If only a few petechiae follow the pinch, consider *"cardiologist's purpura,"* whereby chronic low-dose aspirin therapy renders platelets less functional and therefore homeostatic coagulation less efficient.

Capillary Refill

Although the **capillary refill test** has been employed to assess cardiac output, peripheral vascular resistance, skin and tissue perfusion, and regional arterial obstruction, with times over 3 seconds representing abnormal cardiac and vascular status, results are inconsistent. The test is only a very broad guide to regional perfusion.

Osler Nodes and Janeway Lesions

Classically, **Osler nodes** are papular, and **Janeway lesions** are flatter. Both tend to be red-purple, presumably from erythrocyte extravasation within the lesion. Osler nodes are more often painful and tender. The dichotomy between these lesions may misrepresent a continuum or a unitary process.

ARTERIAL
Brachial and Radial Arteries

A diminished radial pulse suggests (*a*) arterial stenosis proximal to the site palpated, (*b*) remote arterial thrombosis (classically from radial artery catheterization in a critical care unit), or (*c*) acutely, a **dissecting hematoma** that has involved just one subclavian artery. The discovery prompts bilateral blood pressure measurement.

Mildly discordant blood pressures from side to side, without differences in radial pulse intensity, require only repeating the measurements twice, on subsequent visits, to ascertain whether the differences are consistent. If they are, the *higher-reading side* is used for blood pressure monitoring because it is believed that this more accurately reflects intra-arterial pressure. A 20-torr gradient in systolic blood pressure between one arm and the other carries a 90% association with **subclavian artery stenosis.** If such patients have internal mammary artery coronary bypass grafts, they can develop lethal **coronary artery steal syndrome.** If *in any patient* arm exercise precipitates brainstem symptoms such as dizziness, vertigo, diplopia, or nausea that are not regarded as psychosomatic or hyperventilatory, the *subclavian steal syndrome* is suspected. Bilateral arm blood pressures are checked both at rest and after arm exercise, and a neurologist or vascular specialist is consulted.

Brachioradial delay and variants. *Brachioradial delay* correlates with trans-aortic valvular systolic pressure gradient, *not* with heart failure from other causes. Since the diagnosis of aortic stenosis is difficult, brachioradial delay is worth trying in order to further characterize systolic ejection murmurs maximal at the right upper sternal border. Further research is needed to establish false-positive and false-negative rates. An early report suggests that the test becomes abnormal before classic symptoms of aortic stenosis appear.

Marked delay between carotid and radial, radial and femoral, or carotid and femoral pulses suggests **obliterative aortic atherosclerosis** in between the origin of one vessel and the other in the aorta or more peripherally. Discrimination from the normal, barely perceptible lag may be difficult.

Ulnar Pulse

An absent ulnar pulse calls for Allen's test to determine functional significance *if* there are symptoms of hand ischemia or *if* the brachial or radial artery is to be subjected to arterial blood gas sampling or catheterization. If in doubt about whether you are feeling your own digital pulsations or the patient's ulnar pulse, palpate your own radial or carotid pulse simultaneously. If it is synchronous with the "ulnar," both are yours; if it is not, you really have the patient's ulnar in hand.

Allen's Test

If color returns in less than 5 seconds, the palmar arch is intact. If it has *not* returned in 15 seconds, the tested artery ought not be cannulated, and probably neither should the other artery on that side: The frequency of iatrogenic thrombosis with arterial lines is substantial. Rather than the confusing terms "negative" and "positive," results are recorded with the first letter of the side and artery involved and the time in seconds for color restoration; e.g., RR 5, RU 4 means that color returned to the palm 5 seconds after releasing the right radial and then 4 seconds after releasing the right ulnar. Rarely, gangrene occurs despite a normal test; conversely, uncomplicated cannulation may follow an abnormal Allen's test. However, test results should guide decisions. If results are normal in one hand and abnormal in the other, the normal side is preferable for arterial puncture or cannulation.

More on Lower-Limb Pulses

No dorsalis pedis pulse is found in one-seventh of normal persons. If the posterior tibial pulse is strong and there are no symptoms, record the absence of dorsalis pedis pulse but do not investigate. Isolated absence of the posterior tibial pulse is also well known and occasionally associated with a palpable peroneal pulse adjacent to the *lateral* malleolus. In the aged patient, both foot pulses are frequently impalpable, but without claudication, ulcer, or trophic change, no action is needed even if the foot is cool: "If no symptoms, one good pulse per foot is always enough, and sometimes zero!"

In the setting of ischemic ulcers, the presence of one or more palpable pulses per foot predicts that an ischemic ulcer on the foot will heal. Palpable pulses also correlate with an ankle/arm systolic blood pressure ratio above 0.5, typical of noncritical lower limb ischemia.

When there is evidence of foot ischemia despite normal foot pulses, then pulse attenuation/ablation by exercise can show reduced reserve, i.e., flow sufficient for resting oxygen need but not for increased utilization with muscular exercise. If the pulses stay normal even after exercise, but there is a blue toe, *atheroembolic disease* is suspected.

Gastrocnemius Compression Sign

Asymmetric tenderness is more reliable and less subject to symptom amplification, which can cloud bilateral pain responses on squeezing. Bilateral pain can also signify bilateral disease. The test is abnormal in both **arterial insufficiency and venous thrombosis.** It does not discriminate between the two.

Buerger's Test and Variants

Blanching on elevation—a positive Buerger's test—indicates **major arterial stenosis.** It correlates with absent arterial pulses. Its presence suggests more severe ischemia and more distal limb artery disease involving the lower femoral and the popliteal arteries or their branches (anterior tibial artery, etc.) than in claudicators with negative Buerger's tests.

    Dependent rubor sounds venous but, in fact, reflects arterial disease. Arterial insufficiency produces ischemia of the veins, impairing their tone and predisposing to blood stasis. (Edema in the same setting, without cardiac failure, prior venous disease, or hypoalbuminemia, may have a similar pathophysiology.)

    Permanent distal erythema over the feet and ankles in arterial insufficiency is termed *chronic erythromelia.*

Reflex Sympathetic Dystrophy

A unilateral reddened limb can reflect local inflammation (cellulitis, gout, etc.) or venous disease but can also occur with local vasomotor defects. The posttraumatic prototype of regional autonomic dyscontrol is *reflex sympathetic dystrophy* in which pain (causalgia), erythema, blanching, edema, smooth shiny skin, and a variety of other alterations may follow injury even after a long delay. Settings include patients with strikingly unilateral findings, a prior fracture, gunshot wound, or motor vehicle crash. The last three also predispose to venous injury, cellulitis, and osteomyelitis. Any limb may be affected.

Erythromelalgia

The lower limbs are the chief site of an idiopathic vasomotor disorder known as *erythromelalgia* (erythermalgia). In this condition, skin appears normal at baseline but turns deep red and very painful with *warming or dependency.* Differentiation from peripheral arterial disease is by history: Most patients with obstructive arterial disease experience relief with the legs hanging, but this is the most uncomfortable of all in erythromelalgia. Skin warmth and the absence of claudication support erythromelalgia, as does a negative Buerger's test.

Erythema Medicamentosa

Some *vasodilators* can precipitate *erythematous edema,* notably nifedipine—more so than other calcium channel blockers. The mechanism may be selective overactivity in vessels subjected to maximal gravitational hydrostatic pressure, namely those of the feet and ankles, producing both a standing red flush and fluid transudation into the extravascular compartment.

Cyanosis

Central cyanosis suggests profound decarboxyhemoglobinemia of 5 g/dL or more of unsaturated hemoglobin in capillary (**not arterial**) blood. Such a situation implies either a toxin or, more frequently, marked cardiorespiratory dysfunction causing failure to oxygenate the blood. Several caveats apply:

* *Capillary blood, not arterial blood,* determines cyanosis. Arterial blood is always better oxygenated. Thus if the hemoglobin level is 15 g/dL and an arterial

blood gas measurement shows 80% saturation, one might calculate 20% × 15 g/dL = 3 g/dL of unsaturated hemoglobin and not expect cyanosis. However, there might be 5 g/dL *in the capillaries,* producing cyanosis.

- There is a *range* of decarboxyhemoglobinemia thresholds for the sign, not a single figure. Cyanosis becomes recognizable in some dark-pigmented persons at 6 g/dL, whereas it may appear at 4 g/dL in some light-skinned or pale individuals.

- Anemia obscures the sign, and erythrocytosis accentuates it. In the extreme case, for example, a patient with pernicious anemia and a total hemoglobin of 5 g/dL would have to have 100% unsaturated hemoglobin before cyanosis could develop!

- When the picture does not add up, consider *toxic medicines and methemoglobinemia.* This complication can even come from overuse of a commercial topical anesthetic used for mouth pain. Consider *poisons,* e.g., sodium nitrite, the inadvertent agent in the famous Berton Roueché story "Eleven Blue Men." The patient who is bluish all over but is in no distress may have some deoxyhemoglobin-independent pigment such as *argyria* after years of using Argyrol (silver nitrate) on the throat or skin, or blue discoloration can follow years of taking chlorpromazine.

Simple warming clears up nonpathologic vasoconstrictive cyanosis in cold feet, but this often worsens central cyanosis and *perhaps* some pathologic types of peripheral cyanosis.

Acrocyanosis can complicate pathologic vascular reactivity in **Raynaud's disease and systemic lupus erythematosus.** Ulcerations on tips of digits favors the most malevolent of these in terms of actual ischemic necrosis of acra, namely, **systemic sclerosis.** Acrocyanosis also occurs in low-flow states with extremely high peripheral vascular resistance from any cause, including poisons, such as *ergotism.* It can also occur when excess local metabolism extracts too much oxygen from arterial blood, with *thyrotoxicosis* being cited, although this manifestation is rare.

Differential Cyanosis

In congenital heart disease, cyanosis and clubbing run together when the whole body is uniformly exposed to hypoxemia. *Differential cyanosis* refers to cyanosis and clubbing in the feet but not the hands or to cyanosis that is markedly *worse in the feet.* The mechanism is reversed flow through a patent ductus arteriosus, contaminating *distal aortic arch* blood with deoxygenated pulmonary arterial blood, thus exposing the foot to more hypoxia than the hands. *Reversed differential cyanosis* is worse in hands than feet and reflects "ventricular reversal" on top of the previous, i.e., partial transposition of great arteries with right ventricular origin of the aorta, a left ventricular contribution to pulmonary arterial flow, and reversed flow through a patent ductus arteriosus that *improves* oxygenation of aortic blood reaching the feet.

VENOUS

Varicose Veins

Varicose veins produce soft bulges just under the skin that are variably mobile and usually nontender. They are compressible unless secondarily thrombosed. They are often bluish, depending on the thickness and color of overlying skin. Usually multiple, they often collapse when the limb is elevated above the level of the heart. Edema sometimes accompanies them, but not always. There may be an associated rusty spotting from microhemorrhages followed by polymerization of hemoglobin released from extravasated red cells to create **hemosiderin.** Rusty change may occur without large distended veins. When the skin is scaly, thickened, and erythematous as well as brown-flecked, the term *dermatitis venosa* is used. When to this is added induration, the condition is called *dermatoliposclerosis.*

Edema

In the ambulatory patient, if the ankles are not swollen and the clinician cannot produce pitting by 10 seconds of digital pressure just above the medial malleolus, there is no *systemic* edema. In the *bed-bound* patient, however, the examiner has to *check the presacrum* instead.

Inflammatory edema localizes to its stimulus, not to gravity. Any edema that does not follow dependency is presumed inflammatory, not hypoalbuminemic or venous-hypertensive.

Much leg edema reflects *local venous insufficiency,* not a systemic cause.

Edema due to venous disease is common in adults with more or less symmetric leg involvement. Since it takes years to develop brown legs, their absence supports a nonvenous cause only if the process is longstanding.

Lymphedema. Lymphedema is sometimes wrongly said not to "pit." Lymphedema pits just as do venous and other transudative edemas. Exudative edemas of acute inflammation also pit on pressure, but then the patient cries out in pain! Nonpitting reflects secondary fibrosis, from chronicity and/or duration or from a noxious process that stimulated edema in the first place, e.g., local radiotherapy. The term *"brawny edema"* is sometimes applied to longstanding edema that is palpably indurated, overlain by rough skin, and pits poorly or not at all.

Adipose pseudoedema. If "edema" in a person with wide ankles does not pit but compresses, consider whether *adipose tissue (fat pads)* may have been misdesignated as edema.

Myxedema. Edematous *anterior shins,* especially those that show a rough corrugated surface, suggest *pretibial myxedema,* a feature of *hyperthyroidism,* particularly as a result of autoimmune thyroidopathies of Graves and Hashimoto. Although *hypothyroidism* causes widespread myxedema, isolated pretibial myxedema is not part of hypothyroidism.

Pelvic connections. Lymphadenopathy at the point of drainage of a limb, if sufficiently severe, may cause both lymphatic obstruction and extrinsic compression of veins. Venous edema and lymphedema can *coexist* in this situation. Because veins and lymphatic channels are normally mobile, the process usually needs not only to enlarge the lymph nodes but also to permeate the lymphatics or to produce tissue adhesions that mat down the nodes and prevent their being pushed out of the way by an expanding mass. In the tightly packed pelvis, the channels are then subject to compression. Therefore when unexplained *bilateral* lower limb edema is found, especially if there is also vulvar, penile, or scrotal edema implicating proximal obstruction, evaluation includes deep palpation of the lowest portion of the abdomen and evaluation of the pelvis per rectum in both sexes and per vagina in women.

Other forms of edema. **Angioedema** can occur anywhere on the body and does not favor dependent regions. The history is of help: With or without known stimulus such as a wasp sting, the onset is very rapid. Erythema is variable, pitting is common, and there may or may not be systemic features of intravascular volume depletion resulting from rapid fluid shift, depending on the size of the affected region and the previous volume status of the host.

Idiopathic edema of the legs and ankles in young women in the upright position entails major fluid shifts from abnormally leaky capillaries. Marked nocturnal diuresis follows when the feet are put up—just as in many other kinds of edema. Idiopathic edema may also occur in the hands and periorbital region.

Use of the muscular pump of a limb reduces edema from some causes. However, edema from heart failure and idiopathic edema can worsen with muscular exercise. Edema from venous insufficiency may also worsen as gravity outweighs muscular pumping. Lymphedema and myxedema should be unaffected by exercise. Angioedema may worsen if movement pumps more toxin from an embedded stinger into the circulation.

Timed pitting. Rapid pitting when a finger is pressed in—deep depression within 1 or 2 seconds—with visible recovery within 2–3 seconds after release of pressure characterizes hypoalbuminemic edema. Slower responses are seen in congestive edemas. This provides a first rapid branch-point in bedside assessment of edema. However, it does *not* distinguish venous disease from heart failure, which is often the key bedside question. Research is needed to investigate the differentiation of capillary edemas from vasculitis and idiopathic edema, which should have the slowest responses and recoveries because they have the highest protein content in the edema fluid.

Venous Thrombosis and Variants

If fluctuance of an inflamed vein is found or if pus can be expressed or aspirated from the vein, the diagnosis is *suppurative thrombophlebitis,* a potentially lethal iatrogenic disease that calls for immediate consultation with a surgeon.

In the patient at risk, new unilateral edema raises consideration of *deep venous thrombosis.* No combination of signs can prove its presence, nor does a normal examination rule it out. Noninvasive technologic testing is standard practice in 1994. Where this is not available, empiric therapy is common. Marked diffuse erythema suggests *cellulitis,* but cellulitis can in turn precipitate deep venous thrombosis. A palpable cord may represent a thrombosed vein—or a deep tendon or spastic portion of a muscle. *Superficial thrombophlebitis* causes tender, indurated superficial veins that do not empty when "stripped" upward or downward because they are thrombosed. Often, the immediately adjacent skin is erythematous because of secondary inflammation. Superficial thrombophlebitis gives no guidance about cellulitis versus deep thrombosis.

The **gastrocnemius compression sign** is positive in arterial as well as venous disease. It may also be present in local irritations and perhaps in highly anxious persons.

In the acutely painful leg with new or increased swelling, several points noted in Table 10.11 are useful in the differential diagnosis.

Lymphatic System
SPECIAL LYMPH NODES

Popliteal lymphadenopathy resulting from suppuration of the foot is a differential diagnosis of a mass at the back of the knee. Isolated popliteal lymphadenopathy should prompt a careful look at the feet for infection.

If *lymphoid atrophy resulting from chemotherapy* is suspected, seek palpable lymph nodes, especially the femorals. They are slow and late to involute under lympholytic therapy. This may reflect ongoing antigenic stimulation from subclinical foot injuries. It may also reflect the tendency of inguinofemoral lymph nodes to develop both scarring and capsular thickening. (The same tendency can compromise their use to reflect ongoing lymphoid function.)

Nonmalignant causes of *inguinal node enlargement* are common enough that one oncologist remarked, "I pay attention to inguinal nodes only if I can see them

Table 10.11
Features in Assessing Acutely Painful, Swollen Leg

Finding	Suspect
Crescent of extravasated blood near the medial malleolus	*Ruptured Baker's cyst,* especially if there is known arthritis of the knee
Onset during vigorous exercise	*Ruptured plantaris longus tendon*
Prior deep venous thrombosis in the same limb	*Recurrent thrombosis* or flare-up of *postphlebitic syndrome*
Therapeutically or supratherapeutically anticoagulated	*Hemorrhage into the calf*—look for faint blue-purple to greenish discoloration visible through the skin
HIV seropositivity, especially with Kaposi's sarcoma	*Hyperalgesic pseudothrombophlebitis*

across the room!" The inguinal groups above and below the inguinal ligament are especially well illustrated by the *sign of the crease* in lymphogranuloma venereum. Here, rows of nodes enlarge above and below the ligament, which then forms a linear depression between the chains.

LYMPHANGITIC STREAKING

Lymphangitic streaking is specific for virulent streptococcal, staphylococcal, and other *bacterial cellulitides and lymphangitides* but is not sensitive. Thus the sign has value when present, but its absence offers no help. Even in frank *erysipelas,* characterized histopathologically by lymphangitis, small lymphangitic streaks are not seen clinically, and erythematous affected skin appears sharply demarcated from normal skin. Lymphangitic streaking is not seen when cancer cells ascend from a primary tumor on a limb (e.g., melanoma) to the regional lymph nodes.

CELLULITIS

Cellulitis can be fatal even in a normal host. At diagnosis, careful evaluation for ominous features is requisite. A clear written account of these features is supplemented by a drawing in the chart or marks on the patient's skin to show proximal and distal borders of erythema. Should erythema progress (expand) despite appropriate antimicrobials, prompt consultation is essential. If gas is detected, *gas gangrene* is present, and amputation is often indicated in an attempt to preserve life. Here the physical finding makes the examiner bring in the proper specialist posthaste.

CHRONICALLY SWOLLEN LIMB

Chronic immobilization and dependency, whether from paralysis or severe claudication can produce *dependent edema.* Trauma of any type can impair both venous and lymphatic drainage. A massively enlarged limb dating from childhood likely has *congenital lymphedema (Milroy's disease)* from lymphatic hypoplasia or atrophy. Against all intuition and known venous anatomy, relative sparing of the foot by edema suggests venous rather than lymphatic disease! Squared-off toes are characteristic of lymphedema, as is thickened, scaly skin without hemosiderin spots.

Minor varicose veins—seen when the patient is upright—are usually not etiologically important in edema. In the morbidly obese patient, multifactorial edema is common. In all patients, lymphedema can be a difficult bedside diagnosis.

Musculoskeletal System Including Joints

UPPER LIMB

Shoulder

A *unilateral dropped shoulder* may be *dislocated,* whereby the humeral tuberosity is displaced forward and an indentation is seen just beneath. Alternatively, it may have *reduced abductor tone.* Loss of convexity of the shoulder implies *atrophy of the deltoid muscle.* and should be accompanied by prominence of the humerus. Prominent, *symmetric enlarged shoulders* resembling football shoulder-pads, which feel *rubbery* rather than bony or fluid-filled, constitute the *shoulder-pad sign of amyloid arthropathy.* Its positive predictive value is yet unknown. A *unilateral prominent clavicle* is common with Paget's disease of bone and may be misinterpreted as dislocation, bone neoplasm, or supraclavicular lymphadenopathy. Tender sternoclavicular and acromioclavicular joints are common in **polymyalgia rheumatica.**

Apley scratch test deficits are reviewed in Table 10.6. Tests B and C should be congruent.

A normal *drop-arm test* and/or stress test excludes significant rotator cuff tears. Tears that involve the supraspinatus muscle usually cause the arm to fall from about 90°, either spontaneously or with the added stress of the examiner's tap on the forearm.

Elbow

An *increased carrying angle* can occur from old epicondylar fracture or, more frequently, from asymptomatic flexion contracture of the elbow in rheumatoid arthritis.

Effusion in the elbow joint can be seen in any inflammatory arthritis. More superficial, distinct, and localized **olecranon bursitis** fluid accumulations are easier to find and are common in gout. Subcutaneous rheumatoid nodules feel firmer than these fluid collections, with less "give." Rheumatoid nodules are most often found over the olecranon and the ulnar shaft and can be found in gout, too.

A positive *tennis elbow test* consists of pain over the lateral epicondyle. This is where the wrist extensors, which are being forcefully contracted, have their origin. Traction on this area will be uncomfortable with local inflammation.

Rheumatoid Nodules

Over a quarter of **rheumatoid arthritis** patients develop subcutaneous nodules at some point. Clinically similar subcutaneous nodules are reported in other conditions including **gout, systemic lupus erythematosus,** acute **rheumatic fever, and sarcoidosis.** In sarcoidosis, however, intracutaneous nodules outnumber subcutaneous ones. **Rheumatic fever nodules** are said to be more mobile. Subcutaneous **xanthomas** are sometimes larger than rheumatoid nodules but can share a predilection for extensor surfaces including the Achilles tendon, rendering distinction difficult on occasion. The correlation between xanthoma and xanthelasma is insufficient to adduce the presence or absence of xanthelasma as evidence for or against subcutaneous nodules being xanthomatous. **Epidermal inclusion cysts** (sebaceous cysts, wens) also produce nodules, but these should indent (partially pit), show an overlying pore, and feel somewhat "squishy." At the dorsum of the wrist, similar findings without the pore suggest a **ganglion**

cyst, which is usually tender. **Neoplasms** are at the bottom of the list of differential diagnoses, except with abnormal overlying epithelium.

Myoedema and Myotonia

Myoedema is best known in hypothyroidism. Its mechanism, prevalence, and relation to hypothyroid myopathy are unknown. It is also seen in **paralytic rabies,** but it is not the sole sign in either condition. In areas of high prevalence of rabies, examiners might gain additional expertise in eliciting and interpreting the sign. Myoedema is *not* seen with tetany, a prototype of neuromuscular irritability. Attempts to correlate myoedema with hypoalbuminemia have failed. Although it has been claimed that an extremely firm hammer blow on the biceps can produce myoedema in normal persons, data are lacking. Myoedema is not expected in normal persons struck with a reflex hammer with usual force.

Myotonia is a sustained muscular contraction after light stimulation. It usually does not require a hammer blow to be elicited. It lasts far longer than myoedema.

Ulnar Deviation and Rheumatoid Arthritis

A hand that is kept still may be *painful or paretic,* so inquire about both, palpate for tenderness, and assess grip strength by handshake. Cultural factors or shyness make some normal persons shake hands "like a dead fish," so that weakness cannot be inferred from this observation alone.

Ulnar deviation of the hand results from many factors including displacement of extensor tendons to the ulnar side of the metacarpophalangeal joints. Ulnar deviation is highly characteristic of rheumatoid arthritis. If only selected digits are affected, the fourth and fifth fingers are more difficult to interpret: They can deviate in normal older persons, whereas the index and middle fingers do not. The process may be asymmetrical and is often accompanied by other rheumatoid signs.

Certain patterns in joint enlargement are highly characteristic of rheumatoid arthritis (Table 10.12).

With these deformities, both active range of motion and passive range of motion of the affected joints are diminished, as is hand strength. If the patient can shake hands firmly and make a normally formed tight fist and if the hands lying flat on a table look normal, significant hand arthritis is unlikely.

Table 10.12
Finger Deformities

Deformity	Pattern
Swan-neck	Hyperextension of the proximal interphalangeal and flexion of the distal interphalangeal joint. Apparent flexion contracture of the metacarpophalangeal joints also contributes to this lesion. Analogous process in thumb lacks the "swan's head" because there is one less joint, one less phalanx.
Boutonnière	Opposite pattern, flexion of proximal interphalangeal, hyperextension of the distal interphalangeal. Resembles knuckle protruding through collar buttonhole. Mechanism incorporates avulsion of extensor tendon from insertion in the middle phalanx.
Metacarpophalangeal arthritis	Soft tissue diffusely swollen over the dorsum of the hand? If so, different process
Dorsal knuckle pads	Thickening of dorsum of proximal interphalangeal joints

Arachnodactyly

Arachnodactyly is associated with **Marfan's syndrome** but is not a formal diagnostic criterion. Its specificity is low; it may be impossible to distinguish from constitutional extreme height with proportional digits. A positive *thumb sign* is protrusion of the thumb tip, folded inside the flexed fingers, beyond the hypothenar eminence. Positives are seen in **Marfan's syndrome,** in some cases of **Ehlers-Danlos syndrome,** and perhaps in other conditions characterized by both joint laxity and elongation of the thumb.

Measurement on a normal will show that a normal-length thumb cannot cross the whole palm, no matter how loosely tethered.

An overlap between thumb and fifth finger of 1.5 cm or more constitutes a positive *wrist sign,* with significance and sources of false-positive results similar to those of the thumb sign.

Trigger Fingers, Discordant Fingers, and Contractures

A finger that remains extended when its mates are not must have *damaged or disrupted flexor tendons,* which are evaluated fully by an expert. One that is more flexed than the others likely has a *flexion contracture.* When there is an associated palmar nodule—often strikingly hard and protuberant—the diagnosis is **Dupuytren's contracture,** one of the **fibromatoses.** Although this lesion is often adduced as evidence of alcoholism, the association is questionable. Interphalangeal contractures as well as metacarpophalangeal contractures may occur with Dupuytren's contracture, and there is occasionally a "spillover" phenomenon to an adjacent digit.

A snapping with finger movement indicates a *trigger finger,* which most often results from a nonspecific fibrous nodule in the flexor tendon. The nodule hangs up on an adjacent structure near a metacarpal head and moves aside suddenly with a pop when traction becomes too great. The same phenomenon can cause *trigger thumb.*

Knuckles

A normal "advanced screen" (Table 10.7) is reassuring *unless* there are symptoms. An abnormal hand joint screening test is nonspecific about etiology and localization. Inability to make a tight fist may be a result of decreased range of motion of the metacarpophalangeal joints, which are normally able to achieve 90° of flexion.

Large, unduly prominent knuckles are usually partly exposed by subluxation and partly formed by large metacarpal heads in rheumatoid arthritis or, less frequently, in gout.

Knuckle pads can be seen with and even without any arthritis. However, erythematous cutaneous thickening over the dorsum of the metacarpophalangeal joints is *Gottron's sign,* diagnostic for **dermatomyositis.**

Knuckles that fail to stand out normally constitute a *knuckle sign.* This indicates metacarpophalangeal arthritis unless there is diffuse swelling of the entire dorsum of the hand that thus encompasses but is not limited to the periarticular area. With a knuckle sign, think of **rheumatoid arthritis and gouty arthritis.** Rock-hard "joint" enlargement usually means abnormal exposure of bone as a result of movement of bone on bone (*subluxation*) or alterations in vectors of tendon-muscle tension. Soft swellings that give in readily are usually fluid, i.e., *joint effusion,* whereas intermediate consistency, almost invariably termed *boggy,* means fluid and/or overgrowth of synovial tissue. Occasionally, the examiner may discern bits of soft solid matter within a joint space. Usually, this is hyperplastic synovium rather than loose joint bodies (so-called joint mice).

Interphalangeal Joints

Fusiform swellings of proximal interphalangeal joints are usually symmetric and usually represent **rheumatoid arthritis.** However, particularly when the swellings are confined to the third and fourth fingers, the differential diagnosis includes **hemochromatosis arthropathy.** Proximal interphalangeal (PIP) joint bony enlargement can reflect **rheumatoid arthritis, osteoarthrosis, posttraumatic change, or infection.** Enlarged PIP joints are called *Bouchard's nodes.*

At the distal interphalangeal joint, a similar enlargement is a *Heberden's node,* usually from **osteoarthrosis.** Heberden's nodes are extremely common in asymptomatic elderly persons as well as those with hand pain. Heberden's nodes do not exclude rheumatoid arthritis, which commonly coexists with osteoarthrosis. Besides bony change, osteoarthrosis may produce some joint space enlargement and even scant effusion. Distal interphalangeal joint arthritis and deformity also occur in *psoriatic arthritis.* Prominent pitting in the fingernails adjacent to such nodes supports psoriasis. Both psoriatic arthritis and osteoarthrosis can produce considerable subluxation deformity of the distal phalanx on the middle phalanx.

A more diffuse swelling or *dactylitis* involving the entire digit is more characteristic of *gout or sarcoidosis* than of plain arthritis. Rheumatoid arthritis occasionally produces dactylitis.

Very warm joints suggest inflammatory arthritis—rheumatoid arthritis and acute gouty arthritis being two common types—and the medical emergency, **septic arthritis.** Preexistent rheumatoid arthritis is a risk factor for local septic arthritis, not only after arthrocentesis.

Violaceous thickening over the dorsum of the interphalangeal joints (*Gottron's papules*) is akin to Gottron's sign.

When the whole hand is arthritically deformed—almost always by rheumatoid disease—and there has been resorption of phalangeal bone such that the fingers shorten, the skin overlying the damaged joints wrinkles prominently, mobility *increases* as a result of laxity and bone loss, and the appearance is of *telescoping of the digits,* the term *opera-glass hand* (*la main en lorgnette*) is used. The hand is severely functionally impaired. Preservation of even partial function in activities of daily living such as writing, dressing, and cleaning despite such deformity testifies to the determination, effort, and creativity of patients.

Finkelstein's Test

A positive Finkelstein's test consists of sharp pain in the *radial* aspect of the wrist and dorsal forearm at the radial border of the anatomic snuff box, i.e., the radial base of the thenar eminence. It correlates with chronic stenosing tenosynovitis of two thumb abductors and extensors, from inflammation of the synovial lining of a tunnel that they traverse. Risk factors are repetitive motion such as that which occurs for a staple-gun operator and also direct trauma. The symptoms are *pain during pinch grasping* and *pain on movement of thumb and wrist.* Confirmatory signs include tenderness and swelling over the radial styloid.

Tophi

Localization and context distinguish tophi from their mimics. Gout increases the pretest probability and therefore the likelihood of interpreting a mass as a tophus. Individual lesional characteristics suggesting tophi are listed in Table 10.13.

Small, hard tophaceous deposits are occasionally found exclusively in fingertips. Since very few conditions produce hard matter in the fingertips, tophi are likely when such "sand grains" are found. Sharp localization and the absence of involvement of adjacent skin, as well as a gritty rather than *horny character,*

Table 10.13
Tophus Characteristics

Usually painless and *nontender*
Hard and irregular, not smooth as are cysts
If *ulcerated, chalky* or thick *milky matter* on adjacent skin and inside ulcer; ulceration is not
   a sensitive indicator but is highly specific, especially when chalky material is present

distinguish these "tophettes" from the usual cause of fingertip induration—skin calluses.

LOWER LIMB

Simian Stance and Bicycle Test

Simian stance appears to be specific but insensitive. The precise predictive values of positive and negative tests remain unknown. A *positive bicycle test* strongly suggests *spinal stenosis.* Early reproduction of pain on a stationary bicycle is more difficult to interpret: Ordinary claudication remains a possibility, but if the *back* rather than the *leg or buttock* becomes painful, the differential diagnosis will also include a musculoskeletal, nonvascular disorder. Many patients in whom the question arises will be so deconditioned, stiff, or clumsy that they cannot complete the bicycle test at all.

Abnormal Gait

Antalgic gait is seen in many conditions including fracture, osteomyelitis, muscular overuse, thrombophlebitis, the arthritides, and foot disorders. *Lurching gait,* in the absence of cerebellar dysfunction, can occur with *weakness of gluteus medius:* The pelvis falls when it is expected to rise.

Hip Tests

Trendelenburg test. An abnormal Trendelenburg test, with failure of elevation (or even sagging) of the unsupported buttock, suggests *weakness of the ipsilateral gluteus medius muscle.* Frequently, the gait will reflect this with a peculiar lurch. Causes include **trochanteric fracture, congenital dislocation of the hip, poliomyelitis, and spinal nerve root lesions** with secondary muscular atrophy in the gluteus medius muscle. Associated weakness of hip abduction may or may not be evident on resistance testing and may or may not produce enough gluteal atrophy to show a unilateral *flattened atrophic buttock contour.*

Leg length discrepancy. *Unequal leg lengths* are often silent with a disparity of 1 cm or less. Above this level, the effect on gait is variable. The inequity cannot be automatically blamed as the cause of a gait disorder if one is present. Among the differential diagnoses of shortening are *remote poliomyelitis* and old traumatic disruption of a growth plate by a *childhood fracture.* In subcategorizing limb inequality, a higher knee on the bent-knee test corresponds to a longer tibia, whereas a more distal knee corresponds to a longer femur. The requirement that the foot stay flat on the table helps to prevent false positives.

Thomas' test. An enlarged "hollow" at the small of the back supports the accuracy of *Thomas' test.* An abnormal Thomas test consists of revelation of involuntary flexion of one hip when the other is maximally flexed. This can be quantified with a goniometer or assessed by eyeball estimate of the angle between the table and the contracted hip.

The flexion-contracted hip. Reduced extension of the hip as a result of **severe degenerative joint disease** with associated weakness is one cause of the flexion-contracted hip. Observation of gait and of overhead reaching motions from a standing position correlates with reduced extension but may not illuminate the cause.

For the chronically flexed hip, **rheumatoid arthritis** is another differential diagnosis. When flexion and associated gait impairment are acute or subacute, however, the differential diagnosis of **septic hip arthritis** is supported by a history of open trauma to the joint and by findings of fever, a tender bulging joint, and constancy of tenderness on external rotation whether the hip is flexed or not. *Psoas abscess* is supported by a positive psoas sign, a mass in the iliac fossa or upper thigh, and reduction in the tenderness of external rotation when the hip is kept flexed.

Hip fractures. New *rest position of the leg* with *shortening and external rotation* indicates **hip fracture.** Muscle spasm and guarding in the absence of a new position may reflect severe osteoarthrosis of the joint without superimposed fracture. With *auscultatory percussion,* the intact side gives a clearer, sharper, higher pitched, and louder note: Intact bone transmits vibrations from percussion of the patella better than does disrupted bone, tissue, and hematoma. False-positive and false-negative auscopercussive results are rare. In general, the *fractured hip yields a softer auscopercussion note.*

Other hip-related issues. *Forceful hip adduction* may reflect weak opposing abductor forces, particularly with a positive Trendelenburg test and a gait abnormality. When these tests are negative, consider *excess protection of modesty* that may persist in the retarded or demented despite all gentle reassurances of propriety, from habits ingrained for decades or from prior violations of personal space. Distraction usually fails to diminish such voluntary self-protection.

Increased tenderness on internal rotation suggests intra-abdominal (pelvic or retroperitoneal) inflammation or trochanteric bursitis. Direct tenderness over the trochanteric bursa also characterizes trochanteric bursitis.

Unilateral thigh atrophy often bespeaks disuse from painful hip arthritis and may correlate with other indicators, such as a positive Thomas test'. A neurologic lesion might also denervate the thigh muscles. The history will help, especially if pain preceded weakness.

Straight-leg-raising test. Normal persons can have the hip passively flexed to 80° without back or leg pain. Pain confined to the posterior thigh that develops earlier can come from tight posterior thigh (hamstring) muscles. This is not reproduced with foot dorsiflexion, which stretches the sciatic nerve more than the hamstrings. When sciatic nerve irritation is the cause, pain may travel far down the leg, corresponding to sciatic territory (see Fig. 11.5), and up the lumbar spine. Passive foot dorsiflexion usually reinstates pain by stretching the nerve. If pain spreads to the "well" leg on testing the painful one or occurs exclusively on the painful side when testing the other, there is a positive *crossed straight-leg-raising test* suggesting sciatic irritation and perhaps a herniated lumbar intervertebral disc or other mass.

Patrick's test. If the patient is malingering, stiff-jointed, or tense, pain may be everywhere. The examiner must *not* disclose where the pain is being sought. If the patient *spontaneously* complains of *groin pain* on the affected side, an abnormality of that hip or surrounding tissue is supported. If the pain increases with the downward pressure, which stresses the sacroiliac joint, then **sacroiliac pathology** is likely—except for the patient who finds every stimulus agonizing and for the sophisticated malingerer.

Tinetti's Functional Test

Abnormal arising from a chair is recognized when the movement is hesitant or subdivided into portions. The patient who has to push off with the arms or who has to shuffle the buttocks forward to arise is also abnormal, as are those who exhibit unsteadiness on first standing. *Decreased knee extension*—from *arthritis or weakness*—is a major determinant of this abnormality. Others are *poor propriocep-tive and cerebellar functions,* so that many patients with normal knee extension have trouble arising.

Problems with step height (raising the foot while stepping) are (*a*) scraping or shuffling or (*b*) excess raising of the foot, with the tip of the toe lifted more than 5 cm (2 inches) above the floor in midstride to avert this. The usual causes are *decreased hip or knee strength, reduced near vision, or proprioceptive deficit at the proxi-mal interphalangeal joints of the toes.* Frontal lobe dysfunction is also a risk factor. Yet concordance between these risks and abnormal step height is poor.

Turning deficits include stopping completely before turning, staggering, swaying, and grabbing an object for support. Underlying conditions are the same as for step-height deficits except that poor coordination supplants frontal lobe dysfunction. Again, standard assessments frequently fail to predict functional deficits.

Sitting down in a chair is abnormal if the subject plops or lands off center. Here the (imperfect) correlates are decreased hip flexion and decreased knee flexion.

This simple four-part functional gait and balance "advanced screening test" is easier, quicker, and better correlated with functional deficits than conventional testing of joints and muscles.

Knee Effusion Detection

All effusion tests work best when the synovium is thin and not hyperplastic. Changes in the lining can obscure true positives and produce false positives. It is common to miss knee effusions and to infer one erroneously, no matter which method is employed.

Ballottement. The significance of clicking is debated, but rebounding upward is proof of effusion. This test, surprisingly, can be positive when more sensitive ones are not!

Bulge test. There is no consensus about whether the examiner should try to produce a *bulge* on the medial or the lateral aspect. The medial-side bulge appears slightly favored. Although the midpatella level is advocated for this test, this remains to be defined, and unexpectedly negative tests are often repeated 1–2 cm away.

Mann's test and other knee information. *Mann's test* needs corroborative replication in other clinics.

A bluish-purple tinge over a knee (or other joint) suggests *hemarthrosis,* espe-cially in a hemophiliac. The sign is insensitive, and cutaneous or subcutaneous ecchymosis can produce false-positive results.

Knock-knees and Related Deformities

Knock-knees are called *genu valgum.* The "l" in valgum—mnemonic "**l** for lat-eral"—refers to the position of the bone distal to the joint. The opposite defor-mity, *bowlegs,* is *genu varum.* These Latin terms are so thoroughly confused that Sapira wisely advocates abandoning them and returning to the familiar English. The effect of either deformity on musculoskeletal function is variable.

In patients with curved shins, there are three differential diagnoses: **Paget's disease of bone, congenital syphilis (saber shins), and rickets.** If the condition is unilateral, it has to be Paget's disease, since the other two cannot affect develop-ment asymmetrically. Onset in or after middle age has to be caused by Paget's disease.

Minimal symmetric hyperextension of the knee is normal. However, *genu recurvatum,* the bent-back knee, creates inefficient gait and exerts a high energy toll for ambulation.

Fixed knee flexion at rest can be part of a simian stance (see "Simian Stance" above) or other disorders. It is not diagnosed, however, unless the patient fails to straighten the weight-bearing knee on command.

Knee Draw(er) Tests

Excess mobility of the tibia on the femur signifies a *cruciate ligament tear.* If the tibia can be drawn forward more than a few degrees or more than its mate, there is an *anterior draw sign* of a torn anterior cruciate ligament. If it can be pushed backward behind rest position, there is a *posterior draw sign* from the uncommon torn posterior cruciate ligament.

Charcot's Joint: Ankle and Other

Although a pure proprioceptive deficit without loss of pain sensitivity should not produce this finding, it can do so. However, vitamin B_{12} deficiency, a known cause of posterior column loss, is not cited as a cause. Diabetes, by contrast, is common.

When the shoulder is involved, consider **syringomyelia.** When the knee is involved, think of **tabes dorsalis** from neurosyphilis.

Loose bodies are common in Charcot's joints, but they do not assist the diagnosis or exclude it. Charcot's joints are suspected in several settings (Table 10.14).

Ankle Arthritis versus Dependent Edema

Bilaterality favors edema. Unilaterality is harder to interpret. If the individual always lies on the same side or has more venous disease on that side, then dependent edema may falsely localize and mimic ankle effusion. Pitting in the skin suggests edema, but localized skin edema can overlie inflammatory arthritis. Red, warm, tender pitting skin may reflect arthritis or cellulitis. Tenderness is much more common with inflammation but is also found with tense edema, which is recognized by loss of skin creases and wrinkles and a shiny, atrophic look. Edema can restrict range of joint motion, so decreased motion does not prove effusion or arthritis. If limitation of motion exceeds that expected for the degree of swelling, especially if there is marked tenderness with motion, ankle arthritis becomes more likely. A Charcot's joint, large and lax, is easy to distinguish from both edema and effusion. Prompt disappearance after elevation, compression, or diuretics favors edema over arthritis: These measures should cause no resorption of ankle effusion.

Foot and Ankle Contour

Unexpectedly *abnormal shoes* in a patient without gait disturbance or foot pain make one suspect that they were previously owned by someone else.

Table 10.14
Features of Charcot's Joints

Grotesque deformity
Unexplained deformity with known neuropathy
Deformity but preserved or increased passive range of motion
Slippage when deformed joint bears weight
Lack of tenderness on manipulation
Feel like "bag of bones" on palpation

Pes planus—flatfeet—can interfere with gait. Flatfeet often lead to callosities over the head of the talus, where the skin presses against the sidewall of the shoe. *Pes cavus* can bespeak common peroneal nerve damage and weak dorsiflexion of the foot. It is associated with familial disorders such as Charcot-Marie-Tooth syndrome via common peroneal nerve dysfunction. *Pes equinus* can result from disease and probably from chronic use of high-heeled shoes with consequent reduction in length and function of the Achilles tendon and attached calf muscles.

At the ankle, some bone spurs are palpable. Many others are not, so negative physical examination does not dismiss this diagnosis.

Midfoot and forefoot examination. Metatarsophalangeal joint arthritis, with tenderness and sometimes effusion, is common in rheumatoid arthritis. At the first metatarsophalangeal joint, consider gouty arthritis also. The metatarsal *bone* is normally slightly tender, whereas the *joint* is not; equal sensitivity to pressure in the two structures, unless the patient has generalized hyperesthesia, suggests joint inflammation. *Greater* sensitivity in joint than bone clinches this.

Callosities under the metatarsal heads suggest (*a*) intrinsic disease of the foot, (*b*) abnormality of any muscle inserted in it, (*c*) abnormal stance and gait, or (*d*) effects of ill-fitting footwear. Some distinctions require the podiatrist's insight.

Gout

Distinction between gout and rheumatoid arthritis at the first metatarsophalangeal joint relies on the history and on the pattern of joint involvement. A monoarticular arthritis is likely to be gout; if there is a tophus, the diagnosis is settled. Widespread symptoms or findings mean rheumatoid arthritis. History and context also help distinguish *bunion* from *gout*. Synovial fluid analysis is needed to distinguish *acute gout* from *septic arthritis*, hence the common practice of aspirating first episodes of acute metatarsophalangeal arthritis.

Diabetes

Diabetic foot ulcers can occur despite meticulous foot hygiene. Note the deepest tissue layer involved, and measure *with a ruler* in two dimensions. Record in a sketch. If firm white tissue at the ulcer base can be slid over deeper bone, that tissue is tendon or is indurated, scarred, inflamed subcutis. *Description rather than labeling* prevents injecting error about lesion depth. If bone or periosteum is found in the base, osteomyelitis is likely. Unfortunately, osteomyelitis is frequent even when a diabetic foot ulcer appears shallow.

Toes

Maceration or cracking between the toes is commonly associated with **superficial mycosis.** It is often unclear which process preceded the other. Although many superficial mycoses are innocent, cracks can be a portal of bacterial entry. Antifungal therapy may promote healing and prevent bacterial cellulitis.

Corns between the toes are soft because they are usually steeped in sweat. Those elsewhere are typically hard.

Hallux valgus can lead to bunion formation. In considering **gout,** recall that hallux valgus and gout frequently coexist. Thus a red tender swelling at the medial side of a hallux valgus can be gout as well as bunion.

Hallux rigidus can complicate various arthritides and can stress the patient's gait further. It is suspected when oblique *protective gait* is seen, using only the four lateral toes to step off and land. Even without this finding, oblique toe creases in the shoes suggest hallux rigidus.

Normal toes lie flat on the floor when bearing weight. *Clawtoes and hammertoes* are diagnosed by observing their deformities. Clawtoes are usually multiple and produce more extensive secondary callosities not only on the involved dorsa but also on the plantar surfaces of the metatarsal heads.

Interphalangeal toe joints. **Interphalangeal arthritis,** with or without effusion or synovial proliferation, can occur in rheumatoid arthritis and, less frequently, in osteoarthrosis. As with metatarsophalangeal joints, bone is normally somewhat tender to firm palpation, but joints are not. A joint that is more sensitive than the adjacent phalanx has to be arthritic.

Toenails. Softened irregular nails are usually infected. Responsible pathogens vary. When *ingrowing toenails* cause inflammation or when infection enters the skin adjoining a toenail margin—usually lateral or medial—the term *paronychia* applies. Erythema is universal in these cases, as is tenderness unless neuropathy has rendered the toe anesthetic; fluctuance and expressible pus are common.

Thick ridged yellow nails constitute *onychauxis,* which may reflect chronic ischemia, nail dystrophy, or fungal infection.

Long uncut nails are *ram's horn nails (onychogryphosis).* Such nails can interfere with gait and with the wearing of shoes. They reflect years of neglect, and foster poor self-image. Their discovery is seldom the sole evidence of such problems. However, onychogryphosis may be the most vivid or concrete manifestation of psychosocial difficulties. The physical finding calls for cutting by a podiatrist or orthopedist, *never* by patient, family member, nurse, physician's assistant, or general physician. It also signifies a need for psychosocial intervention.

Neurologic System

LIMB TREMOR

Among causes of limb tremor to consider, a short list must include parkinsonism, drug-induced parkinsonism (extrapyramidal syndrome from neuroleptics), cerebellar disease, and essential tremor.

Unilateral tremor can be the sole finding in stage 1 Parkinson's disease, so that asymmetry does not rule out this condition. Nor does the absence of associated features such as masked facies, festinating gait, cogwheel rigidity, or bradykinesia.

Abnormal oral movements are especially common in tardive dyskinesia. *Rest tremor* occurs in noncerebellar disease, whereas *intention tremor* is characteristic of cerebellar disease. Nystagmus or a positive Romberg test supports a cerebellar origin. Emotional exacerbation of tremor does not implicate a psychosomatic component.

Festinating gait or *markedly* diminished associated arm movements suggest Parkinson's disease. *Dementia* may occur late in Parkinson's disease. However, established dementia at the onset of tremor can suggest Alzheimer's disease, which can also produce prominent stiffness and rigidity. Alternatively, **alcoholic dementia** may coexist with alcoholic cerebellopathy in the demented tremulous patient. *Scanning (cerebellar) speech* suggests that a tremor is cerebellar but does not establish etiology.

To bring out *cogwheel rigidity,* ask the patient to draw a circle in the air with the hand whose wrist is not being passively flexed and extended by the examiner. Often this accentuates cogwheeling or elicits it. The rate of false-positive tests has not been established.

CHEST AND SHOULDER

The *winged scapula* demonstrates *serratus anterior muscle weakness.* This, in turn, can reflect cervical myelopathy at C5-C7, typically from **poliomyelitis,** which also produces other motor deficits. Alternatively, the lesion may result from brachial plexus injury, with other abnormal signs present. A winged scapula that occurs in isolation indicates injury to the *long thoracic nerve* on the chest wall or axilla. This nerve may be damaged by trauma, mastectomy, or axillary surgery. Excessive weight lifting can traumatize the nerve, especially when the amount is increased too rapidly. In this case, sensation is intact, as are reflexes. Since the serratus is prominent in shoulder protraction (reaching), the symptom is usually weakness in reaching up or forward.

The mechanism of *scapular hump* is weakness and atrophy of trapezius, with reduction or flattening of shoulder mass. There is elevation of the superior angle of the scapula so that it becomes visible from the front. The same muscular abnormality displaces the shoulder inferoanteriorly, producing oblique pectoral crease. There are no data on normals, let alone on persons with trapezius weakness or eleventh nerve palsies, to permit calculation of sensitivity and specificity of these signs.

CARPAL TUNNEL SYNDROME AND TINEL'S AND PHELAN'S SIGNS

Positive Tinel's and Phelan's signs consist of reproduction of electric pain and/or sensation or tingling with either maneuver.

Tinel's sign, initially described in axonal regeneration after trauma, has been alleged to represent carpal tunnel syndrome. A striking number of persons with electromyographically proven normal median nerves (29%) display a positive Tinel sign! Thus the predictive value of a positive test does not aid clinical decision-making. The false-negative rate also exceeds 50%! Therefore the predictive value of a negative test lacks clinical utility, and the test should be abandoned. The description above is included to show that there are signs to discard, whatever their honorable history, because they fail to earn their keep as clinical aids. The best way to "clean house" of worthless signs is via careful studies of true- and false-positive and true- and false-negative rates in well-characterized subjects— i.e., with modern physical diagnosis research.

Phelan's sign, although decades old, has not yet been subjected to such analysis. Its positive and negative predictive values remain to be established.

INTRINSIC HAND MUSCLES

Interosseous muscle atrophy is seen in several settings (Table 10.15).

Since the interossei have roots at C8 and T1, a spinal cord process or polyradiculopathy might also conceivably produce this finding.

Defective finger abduction, apart from generalized weakness, is seen in ulnar neuropathy and more proximal lesions. Since the fourth and fifth finger lumbricals are supplied by the ulnar nerve, but the second and third are supplied by the median nerve, and since only the second lumbrical accompanies the interossei in pinching, the examiner can rightfully expect a weak pinch mechanism in median neuropathy but not with isolated ulnar palsy. Deformity of the "O" as well as breaking open implies weakness of the pinch mechanism.

Table 10.15
Settings of Interosseous Muscle Atrophy

Cachexia
Neurologic disorders, e.g., peripheral neuropathy
Musculoskeletal disorders, e.g., rheumatoid arthritis
Neurodegenerative disorders

MYELOPATHY HAND

Abnormal finger escape is graded 1–4, as indicated Table 10.16.

Patients with these abnormalities often show lower limb spasticity confirming myelopathy (rather than merely root disease). Curiously, the upper rather than the lower cervical cord is characteristically affected. With a grade 1 sign, a differential diagnosis is the *digiti quinti sign* of mild hemiparesis (see the Extended Examination section of Chapter 11). Hemiparesis is excluded by absence of other features implicating representation craniad to the cervical cord: (*a*) upper motor neuron paresis, however slight; and (*b*) facial palsy. Myelopathy is confirmed if the sensory abnormalities described below or a spastic paraparesis rather than the monoparesis expected after a stroke is found.

In the grip-and-release test, myelopathy causes a decrement from the normal 20 repetitions in 10 seconds, often with failure of coordination in addition. Radiculopathy does not. When the finger escape sign is grade 1, but the grip-and-release sign is normal, radiculopathy is possible. When both signs are abnormal, however, myelopathy is present. Abnormal tests for myelopathy hand correlate with low scores on an activities-of-daily-living index, inversely to the grade of the finger escape sign.

There may be a nondermatomal sensory abnormality in this group, with hypalgesia or analgesia in the affected areas extending up the wrist and to the dorsum of the ipsilateral forearm. If a patient has spastic paraplegia and *no* myelopathy hand, place the responsible lesion at the T1 cord or below.

Normal finger abduction against resistance excludes ulnar neuropathy. Although finger abduction may be lost with progressive myelopathy and worsening finger extensor tests, check baseline flexion (not against resistance) of the metacarpophalangeal joints, which is lost in ulnar palsy.

RADIAL, ULNAR, AND MEDIAN NERVES AND SPINAL DERMATOMES

Distinction between neuropathy and radiculopathy depends on recollection of cord levels and on logical inference. For example, reduced sensation over the web space between thumb and index finger might represent C6 radiculopathy or radial neuropathy. If the tip of the index finger is affected, it must be C6, since this is *median nerve* territory and therefore would be spared with radial nerve disease. Correspondingly, the ipsilateral brachioradialis reflex should be abnormal, since this reflects C6 segment integrity. An isolated median neuropathy could not be invoked for the above-described deficit, since the web space is radial nerve territory.

If there is decreased sensation of the tip of the fifth finger, C8 radiculopathy and ulnar neuropathy are considered. Sensory findings cannot discriminate between these two, since the dermatomes are congruent. However, *finger flexion* is a C8 function, while flexion at the proximal interphalangeal joint is a function of the median nerve. Thus preserved flexion at the proximal interphalangeal joint in this setting implicates *ulnar* neuropathy, while weakness shows C8 root dis-

Table 10.16
Grading the Finger Escape Sign

Grade	Sign
1	Fifth finger drifts outward (fails to remain adducted on 30 seconds of observation)
2	Fifth (and, sometimes, fourth) finger not adducted even at rest
3	Fifth and fourth fingers not adducted and cannot be fully extended
4	Fifth, fourth, and third fingers not adducted and cannot be fully extended

ease. If proximal interphalangeal joint flexion is defective, either the tendon is disrupted or the C8–median nerve complex must be affected—which excludes ulnar neuropathy.

ASTERIXIS

The abnormal response is *loss of position* and quick regaining of it. This may appear rhythmic or more random, but it is *slower than tremor.* The two might be diagnosed together if the patient is observed for abnormal involuntary movements before asterixis testing. Asterixis correlates with metabolic encephalopathy, e.g., from cirrhosis with impending liver failure, uremia, or ventilatory failure with hypercarbia. It is seen in several electrolyte imbalances, iatrogenic overdoses, and several kinds of poisoning and even rarely in heart failure and septicemia. If you consider it something of a peripheral counterpart of delirium, the length of this list is less surprising. Like delirium, it marks increased short-term mortality.

The sphygmomanometer technique for detecting asterixis may suffer from inattention and poor hand-eye coordination producing wide fluctuations of meniscus height even without asterixis. The hip variant can be clouded by protective adduction of thighs.

Unilateral asterixis is rarely seen in disorders of the midbrain. Unilateral asterixis is a curiosity, but if it is encountered, do not go through the metabolic differential diagnosis, nor take it as a sure sign of malingering.

COMMON PERONEAL NERVE
Foot-drop

Foot-drop is easy to recognize. If the whole foot is paralyzed because of dysfunction of all muscles below the knee, the sciatic nerve is implicated. Ability to dorsiflex the foot while standing excludes common peroneal palsy and therefore rules out sciatic dysfunction. In the patient who is bed-bound, check hyperextension (dorsiflexion) of the hallux against resistance to confirm common peroneal palsy. Metatarsophalangeal *arthritis* can produce a false-positive test, as can hallux rigidus. Normal sensation in the dorsal web between the hallux and the second toe—analogous to radial nerve territory in the hand—demonstrates preserved *tibial nerve* function. With foot-drop, consider trauma near the fibula, sciatic nerve injury, and peroneal muscular atrophy of *Charcot-Marie-Tooth syndrome.*

Hoover's Test

In bilateral disease—paraparesis or worse—the test is invalid. However, in unilateral weakness, downward pushing on the intact side is characteristic of true weakness. Failure of downward pressure by the "good" heel means poor effort from somatization, conversion, or malingering.

RECORDING THE FINDINGS
Sample Write-up

82-year-old man suffered tearing and crush injury of dorsum of right forearm when a large box fell on it. Skin lacerations now sutured, patient here for follow-up.

Physical examination, right forearm and hand
Skin: Two clean, sutured, linear lacerations, each 10.5 cm long, with adjoining broad fresh ecchymoses and mild local edema but no erythema, tenderness, or pus. Neatly sutured, intact.

Arteries: Hand warm, normally colored, well perfused. Radial and ulnar pulses each 1+. Allen's test RRA and RUA 4 seconds.

Veins/lymphatics: No edema in or distal to injured zones. No erythema or bluish discoloration. Veins of hand and forearm not unduly prominent.

Musculoskeletal: Knuckle sign negative. Mobility at wrist and fingers normal. Heberden's nodes prominent at distal interphalangeal joints. Picks up penny with this hand readily, although complains of pain at laceration sites with movement.

Peripheral nervous system: Sensation intact over tips of fingers, and in web space between thumb and index finger. Grip strength and wrist power intact. Pinch normal. Phelan's sign negative.

Assessment: No evidence of neuromuscular or circulatory compromise from recent injury.

BEYOND THE PHYSICAL EXAMINATION

Bloodwork

Bloodwork varies with the disorder being sought. A few representative samples follow. The white blood count and differential are pertinent to systemic inflammatory disorders such as cellulitis with bacteremia. Platelet count and coagulation studies help work up an abnormal Rumpel-Leede test. The blood ammonia and the arterial pCO_2 can assist in evaluating asterixis. A rheumatoid factor is of use apropos rheumatoid arthritis. Blood cultures can confirm infective endocarditis that is suspected because of peripheral stigmata. Thyroid hormone levels can clarify myoedema.

Aspirates

Joint fluid analysis is mandatory in distinguishing *acute gout* with its negatively birefringent crystals, *septic arthritis* with stainable or cultivable organisms, and *calcium pyrophosphate deposition disease (**pseudogout**),* which shows positively birefringent crystals. Characteristic joint fluid profiles of several arthritides exist.

Aspiration of tissue fluid is *sometimes* undertaken to evaluate cellulitis.

Imaging and Functional Tests

Plain radiographs can be useful for *selected* disorders of bones and joints. Alas, they are often obtained needlessly.

Doppler ultrasound examination is used for determination of arterial flow and venous patency. "Noninvasive" techniques for detection of *deep venous thrombosis* include duplex and triplex *scans and impedance plethysmography.* One hopes these will unthrone the "gold standard," *phlebography,* which is expensive, painful, and sometimes thrombogenic! Other imaging techniques such as *computed tomography (CT) and magnetic resonance imaging (MRI)* are used in limb disorders. Occasionally, *angiography, lymphangiography,* or *nuclear medicine lymphatic scintiscans* are appropriate. Neuromuscular tests include *electromyography, nerve conduction velocity studies, and nerve and muscle biopsy.*

Laboratory and/or imaging evaluation of the *neck* can illuminate upper and lower limb neuromuscular disorders. Back studies can lead to diagnosis of some apparent lower limb problems.

Arthroscopy and arthrography are widely applied to large-joint disorders, especially of the knee. So are *CT* and *MRI.*

Bone scans are of help in *metabolic bone disease* and in primary and secondary bone neoplasms. *Bone densitometry* and, sometimes, *bone biopsy* are also useful for ostoporosis and osteomalacia. For osteomyelitis, plain radiographs and bone scans show defective test characteristics and are being increasingly supplanted by *tagged white blood cell scans,* although these, too, are not perfect.

Surgical exploration is an ultimate diagnostic and therapeutic intervention in, for example, median nerve exploration and flexor retinaculum decompression. Less drastic alternatives are always preferred when feasible.

Consultants

Depending on the involved system(s), a neurologist, neurosurgeon, orthopedic surgeon, rheumatologist, vascular surgeon, general surgeon, geriatrician, physical medicine specialist, or even a hematologist may be the most helpful consultant.

For *any* foot problem, regardless of system, the *podiatrist* offers expert help.

Key nonphysician consultants who serve major *diagnostic* as well as *therapeutic* roles are the *rehabilitative therapy* staff: *physical therapists* for large muscle groups of the lower limb and grosser upper limb functions such as lifting, throwing, and reaching; and *occupational therapists* for fine motor functions such as writing, dressing, and cooking.

RECOMMENDED READINGS

Carter SA. Arterial auscultation in peripheral vascular disease. JAMA 1981;246:1682–1686.

Christensen JH, Freundlich M, Jacobsen BA, Falstie-Jensen N. Clinical relevance of pedal pulse palpation in patients suspected of peripheral arterial insufficiency. J Intern Med 1989;226:95–99.

Hardison JE. Legs. Arch Intern Med 1983;143:1014.

Hoppenfeld S. Physical examination of the spine and extremities. 1st ed. Norwalk, Connecticut: Appleton-Century-Crofts, 1976.

Mann G, Finsterbush A, Frankl U, Yarom J, Matan Y. A method of diagnosing small amounts of fluid in the knee. J Bone Joint Surg (Br) 1991;73B:B346–B347.

Polley HF, Hunder GG. Rheumatologic interviewing and physical examination of the joints. 2nd ed. Philadelphia: WB Saunders, 1978.

Reilly DT, Wolfe JHN. The swollen leg. Br Med J 1991;303:1462–1465.

Shmerling RH, Stern SH, Gravallese EM, Kantrowitz FG. Tophaceous deposition in the finger pads without gouty arthritis. Arch Intern Med 1988;148:1830–1832.

Simkin PA. Simian stance: a sign of spinal stenosis. Lancet 1982;2:652–653.

Tinetti ME, Ginter SF. Identifying mobility dysfunctions in elderly patients: standard neuromuscular examination or direct assessment? JAMA 1988;259:1190–1193.

11

Neurologic Examination

APPROACH AND ANATOMICAL REVIEW

As every student of human function knows, the nervous system is the most complex and least well understood system of the human body. The beginner who attempts to integrate the anatomy of the cells, the tracts, the nuclei, and their interconnections with manifestions of brain and spinal cord function in the history and physical examination will quickly be overwhelmed. Any attempt to simplify these integrations will cut corners, leave out details, and mislead reasoning. The student must bring a certain trust (or suspension of disbelief) to the first attempts at consolidating these materials into a cogent whole.

Since the purpose of this text is the conduct and interpretation of the primary data base—patient history and physical examination—a working understanding of neuroanatomy and neurophysiology is presumed as prerequisite knowledge. The following review of anatomy and function is designed to assist in the localization of specific neurologic functions as they are reflected in the physical examination.

For purposes of anatomical review, the brain and spinal cord are presented in the most pragmatic terms: how they relate to the clinical assessment of the living patient. The student blessed with extra curiosity is referred to textbooks of neuroanatomy, physiology, and pathology for the answers to sophisticated "how" and "why" questions.

The key anatomical elements of the central and peripheral nervous systems as they relate to the physical examination are four: **brain and meninges, spinal cord, peripheral nerves, and autonomic centers and nerves.**

Brain and Meninges

Three layers of **meninges**—the pia mater, arachnoid, and dura mater—surround the brain and cord. The **pia mater** is adherent to the neural tissue surfaces and is separated from the **arachnoid** by a thin cushion of circulating **cerebrospinal fluid**; aggregately, these form the leptomeninges. The tough **dura mater** is adherent to the inner layer of the bony vaults (cranium and spinal canal of the vertebral column).

For purposes of this discussion, the brain is anatomically divided into the primitive components, the **forebrain, midbrain, and hindbrain.**

COMPONENTS

Forebrain

The **forebrain** is made up of the **cerebral cortex** with its separate **lobes** (including subcortical white matter) and the **diencephalon,** which contains such structures as the **thalamus, hypothalamus, and pituitary gland.** In the **cortex** of the **forebrain** reside the highest intellectual functions: thought, memory, and cognition, as well as integrative motor skills, sensory interpretation (as distinct from mere sensation), speech and hearing integration, visual association, and social behavior with its moral and ethical components. The cortical locations related to these functions are illustrated in Figure 11.1, insofar as they can be localized.

The **diencephalon,** in which the "conduits" of information flow, includes the thalamus, hypothalamus, and pituitary gland.

• **Thalamus**—conveys sensory information to and from the cortex, integrates voluntary movements of the motor systems based on information passing between the cortex and the periphery, and affects consciousness via the axons of the nuclei of the reticular activating system.
• **Hypothalamus**—processes stimuli to the autonomic nervous system and maintains control of body temperature, neuroendocrine action, serum osmolality and water balance, sexual drive, and hunger and satiety.
• **Pituitary gland**—controls, by hormonal secretions in response to feedback systems, growth, metabolism, lactation, gonadal function, glucocorticoid release from the adrenal, and the secretion of thyroid hormone.

Midbrain

The **midbrain** is responsible for some reflex **head and eye movement** and contains the nuclei of cranial nerve roots III and IV. The **corticospinal tract** (motor control) and the **auditory** pathways both traverse the midbrain (Fig. 11.2).

Hindbrain

Hindbrain includes the **pons, medulla oblongata, and cerebellum.** From the **pons** arise the nuclei of cranial nerves V–VIII as well as the contributors to voluntary muscle control. The **medulla** contains the nuclei of cranial nerves IX–XII, the respiratory center, a vomiting center, important contributions to vasomotor and circulatory control, and the nuclei of the reticular activating system. Within the medulla lie the great pyramidal decussations of the long (corticospinal) motor tracts passing between the cortex of each hemisphere and the opposite side of the spinal cord.

The **cerebellum** is the integrator of balance for the body. Through it the vestibular system of the inner ear and the eighth cranial nerve play into proprio-

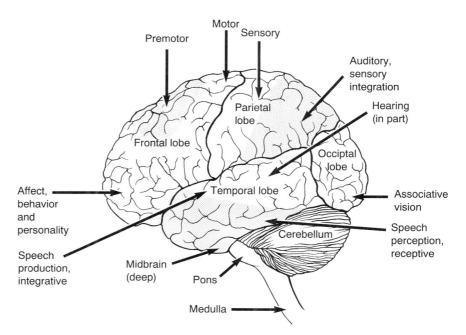

Figure 11.1 Drawing of cerebral landmarks in relation to neurologic functions.

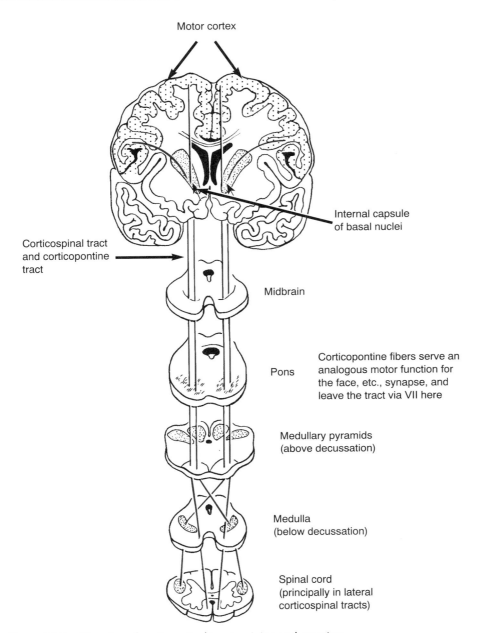

Figure 11.2 Drawing of corticospinal tract, origins and crossing.

ceptive (sensory) and musculoskeletal control from the cerebral cortex (motor). Cerebellar balance is not vision-dependent. Balance problems that occur when the patient's eyes are closed and that are corrected when he opens them are judged to arise in the dorsal column of the spinal cord, the vestibular apparatus, or the cerebellum itself.

Spinal Cord

At the foramen magnum, the inferior continuation of the medulla becomes the **spinal cord.** Long nerve tracts course through the cord carrying motor (descending ventral and lateral columns), pain and temperature (ascending lateral spinothalamic tracts), and vibratory and proprioceptive fibers (dorsal columns)

between the cerebral cortex and the periphery of the body. Within the spinal cord, at segmental levels, each spinal nerve divides into a ventral (motor) and a dorsal (sensory) root (Fig. 11.3). The former carries motor messages to the periphery either in response to the latter's sensory signals, after they have been interpreted and integrated by the cerebral cortex or lower centers, or in response to other sources of efferent cerebral impulses.

A fully functional nervous system requires integrity of (*a*) sensory receptors at the periphery, (*b*) dorsal nerve roots into the cord (afferent), (*c*) lateral spinothalamic tracts to the cortex, (*d*) cortical interpretation, (*e*) pyramidal (corticospinal) tracts back to the nerve roots, (*f*) ventral divisions of the nerve root at each spinal segment, (*g*) motor segment conduction to the muscles, and (*h*) muscles, as well as the input of modulators such as the cerebellum.

Peripheral Nerves

Before entry into and after exit from the spinal segments, nerve fibers are reorganized into **peripheral nerves.** The examiner must have an understanding of this rearrangement of nerve fibers in order to interpret abnormalities of peripheral sensory and motor function. In most instances, a peripheral nerve serving an area of skin sensitivity represents more than one spinal segment, and most muscles are innervated from multiple segments via a single nerve. As a result, peripheral nerve distribution must be learned and interpreted as anatomically different from spinal segments. For convenience, Figure 11.4 illustrates the spinal segment (dermatomal) distribution of sensory function, while Figure 11.5 shows the sensory distribution of the major peripheral nerves. For the summary of spinal segments and peripheral nerve representation of **motor** function, see Tables 10.1 and 10.2.

Autonomic Nervous System

The autonomic nervous system of nonvolitional homeostasis operates from a series of spinal ganglia with some input from central nuclei. Physiologically, it has two divisions: the **sympathetic,** which reacts to external stimuli and results in such responses as vasoconstriction, pupillary dilatation, and piloerection; and the **parasympathetic,** which moderates the sympathetic and is also involved in maintenance functions of such organs as the bowel and bladder. Only occasionally does the clinician specifically test autonomic nerve function, i.e., when particular suspicion of problems occurs. However, autonomic dysfunction may be manifest in a variety of clinical situations. For example, the clammy, cold skin surface of a patient in shock from intravascular fluid volume depletion represents an intact autonomic vasoconstrictive attempt to shunt the contracted blood volume away from the skin and to vital organs. By contrast, orthostatic hypotension with dizziness in a diabetic person with peripheral neuropathy often reflects coexistent

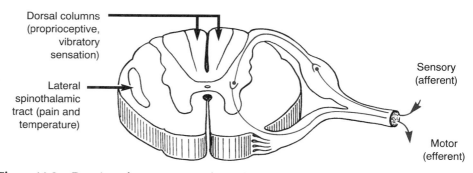

Figure 11.3 Drawing of cross-section of spinal cord and nerve root.

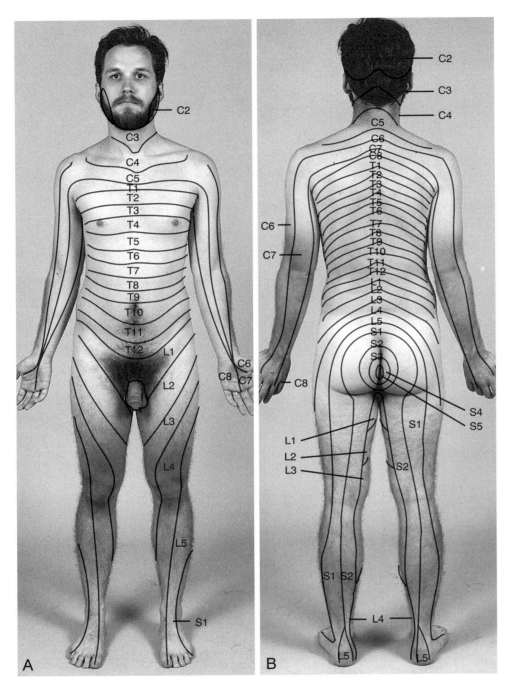

Figure 11.4   Dermatomes. **A.** Anterior view. **B.** Posterior view.

autonomic neuropathy, with failure to vasoconstrict and increase cardiac rate in response to gravity-dependent venous pooling on standing upright.

TECHNIQUE

The clinician begins neurologic evaluation of a patient at the moment the two meet one another. The behavior and mood of the patient during the medical history taking provide clues to neurologic and emotional health and function.

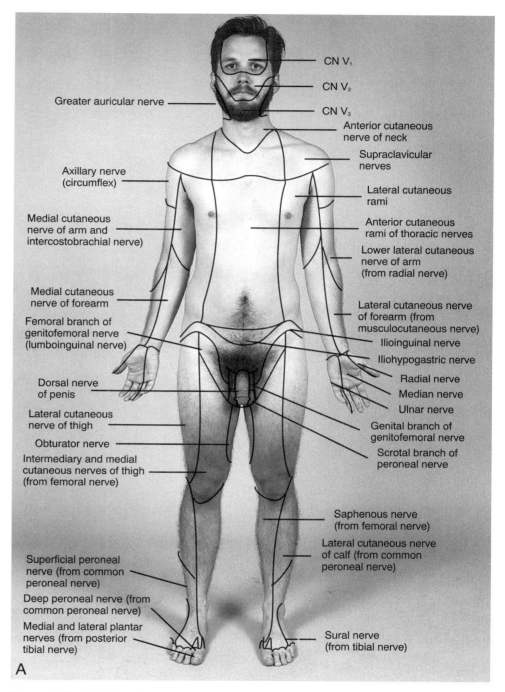

CN V₁

CN V₂

Greater auricular nerve

CN V₃

Anterior cutaneous nerve of neck

Supraclavicular nerves

Axillary nerve (circumflex)

Lateral cutaneous rami

Medial cutaneous nerve of arm and intercostobrachial nerve)

Anterior cutaneous rami of thoracic nerves

Lower lateral cutaneous nerve of arm (from radial nerve)

Medial cutaneous nerve of forearm

Lateral cutaneous nerve of forearm (from musculocutaneous nerve)

Femoral branch of genitofemoral nerve (lumboinguinal nerve)

Ilioinguinal nerve

Iliohypogastric nerve

Radial nerve

Dorsal nerve of penis

Median nerve

Ulnar nerve

Lateral cutaneous nerve of thigh

Genital branch of genitofemoral nerve

Obturator nerve

Scrotal branch of peroneal nerve

Intermediary and medial cutaneous nerves of thigh (from femoral nerve)

Saphenous nerve (from femoral nerve)

Lateral cutaneous nerve of calf (from common peroneal nerve)

Superficial peroneal nerve (from common peroneal nerve)

Deep peroneal nerve (from common peroneal nerve)

Medial and lateral plantar nerves (from posterior tibial nerve)

Sural nerve (from tibial nerve)

A

Figure 11.5 Peripheral nerve representations in cutaneous innervation. **A.** Anterior view. **B.** Posterior view.

Speech and hearing are evaluated throughout the interview. The gross movements of body position changes and the fine motor skills required of the patient during the routine physical examination provide the observant examiner with important data.

The proper detail of a formal **mental status examination** is dictated by these observations of general appearance and of affect and cognitive interaction during

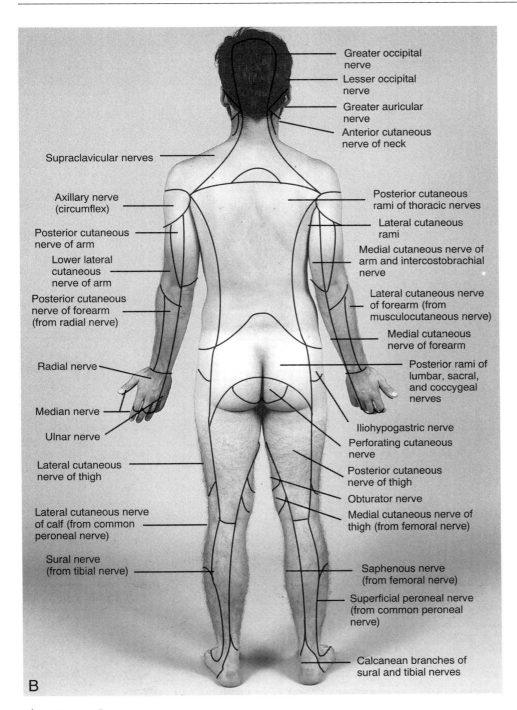

Greater occipital nerve

Lesser occipital nerve

Greater auricular nerve

Anterior cutaneous nerve of neck

Supraclavicular nerves

Axillary nerve (circumflex)

Posterior cutaneous nerve of arm

Lower lateral cutaneous nerve of arm

Posterior cutaneous nerve of forearm (from radial nerve)

Radial nerve

Median nerve

Ulnar nerve

Lateral cutaneous nerve of thigh

Lateral cutaneous nerve of calf (from common peroneal nerve)

Sural nerve (from tibial nerve)

Posterior cutaneous rami of thoracic nerves

Lateral cutaneous rami

Medial cutaneous nerve of arm and intercostobrachial nerve

Lateral cutaneous nerve of forearm (from musculocutaneous nerve)

Medial cutaneous nerve of forearm

Posterior rami of lumbar, sacral, and coccygeal nerves

Iliohypogastric nerve

Perforating cutaneous nerve

Posterior cutaneous nerve of thigh

Obturator nerve

Medial cutaneous nerve of thigh (from femoral nerve)

Saphenous nerve (from femoral nerve)

Superficial peroneal nerve (from common peroneal nerve)

Calcanean branches of sural and tibial nerves

B

Figure 11.5   B.

the medical interview. The decision to perform an extended neurologic assessment is made on the basis of these general observations, as well as on symptoms provided during the history or abnormalities detected on the screening examination. The maneuvers described below constitute a basic assessment to be carried out as a part of every general physical examination. Indications for moving beyond the basics described in this section are further delineated in the Extended Examination section.

Portions of the formal neurologic examination are completed as part of regional assessment: cranial nerves II–XII during the head examination (Chapter 4) and muscle strength, tone, and group functions during examination of the limbs (Chapter 10). The remaining components are done after the patient has been brought to a sitting position for muscle strength and joint motion testing. For tabular summaries of the equipment required and the steps of the screening neurologic examination, see Tables 11.1. and 11.2.

Cortical Function

The clinician who has been observing higher brain functions throughout the medical history develops a clear picture of **level of consciousness, speech pattern, mood and affect, concentration ability, short-term memory, and orientation.** However, since every good observer is misled now and again by seemingly capable conversationalists and can miss blatant brain dysfunction if the patient's social grace is preserved, it is important to formally test higher cortical function.

Table 11.1
Supplies and Equipment for the Neurologic Examination

Reflex hammer
Tuning fork, low frequency (128 Hz)
Cotton wisp or fluffed cotton swab
Pointed instrument: broken swab-stick, small key
Stethoscope[a]
Ophthalmoscope[a]
Snellen chart[a]

[a]Although used to conduct the neurologic examination, these instruments are traditionally used during other parts of the physical examination. Their use is described elsewhere, namely with vital signs (Chapter 2), funduscopy (Chapter 4), and visual acuity testing (Chapter 4).

Table 11.2
Sequence of the Screening Neurologic Examination (Performed with the Patient Seated)[a, b]

Higher cortical function	**Sensation**
Orientation to	**Light touch**
Person	**Superficial pain**
Time	**Joint position sense**
Place	Vibration sense
Speech pattern	
Mood and affect	**Rapid alternating movements**
Concentration	**Upper limb**
	Lower limb
Reflexes	Equilibrium
Muscle stretch reflexes	**Stance**
Triceps	**Romberg**
Biceps	**Gait**
Brachioradialis	
Patellar (knee jerk)	
Achilles (ankle jerk)	
Plantar reflex	

[a]Most motor evaluation, although legitimately part of the neurologic evaluation, is assigned to the limbs (Chapter 10) in the regional conduct of the physical examination.
[b]**Boldfaced** indicates modalities directly tested at this time.

ORIENTATION

The patient is asked to state his name (**person**), the calendar date and day of the week, the month, and the year (**time**), and where (town, name of institution) the encounter is occurring (**place**). This is the absolute minimum screen; if observations of the behaviors noted above do not raise suspicion and the patient is totally oriented in these three spheres, cortical function is assumed to be intact—sometimes erroneously.

Reflexes

The **muscle stretch reflexes (MSRs),** sometimes referred to as deep tendon reflexes (DTRs), necessary for basic assessment are five. Adequate elicitation of a stretch reflex requires: (*a*) a well-relaxed muscle group, (*b*) aversion of the patient's gaze from the tendon to avoid anticipatory muscle tensing, (*c*) a **reflex hammer,** (*d*) accurate localization of the tendon to be tapped, and (*e*) a loose, swinging motion of the hammer from the examiner's wrist to facilitate a sudden displacement, producing bouncing rebound from the stimulated tendon. Failure to adhere to these principles leads to inadequate reflex testing and, in some instances, to costly misinterpretation of a reflex that appears to be absent but that in fact has been incorrectly sought.

Careful instructions from the examiner to the patient before attempting a stretch reflex will help to avoid error: "I am going to tap on some spots. Your job is to resist watching this hammer." Do not ask the patient to "relax" a muscle group or limb. This is almost impossible to achieve on command, but be explicit: "Let your legs swing loose (patellar reflex)," or "I am going to hold your arm up; let me do all the work (triceps reflex)."

If you are surprised by an absent reflex, do not consider it abnormal until you have attempted **reinforcement.** This technique creates a diversionary spinal arc at a level above the reflex being tested and blocks cortical suppression. For example, if you are having trouble getting a lower limb reflex, ask the patient to place his hands in position to clasp one another on command, raise his eyes toward the ceiling, and await the verbal command to "clasp," as is demonstrated by the woman in Figure 11.6. With the patient thus positioned in readiness, the examiner (*a*) locates the tendon site to be tested, (*b*) positions the hammer, (*c*) asks the patient to clasp the hands and pull them one against another, and (*d*) simultaneously strikes the tendon and observes for the stretch response. This *Jendrassik maneuver* can bring out latent reflexes. For reinforcement of upper limb reflexes, the patient is asked to clench the teeth (to create an arc above the cervical spine).

Routine testing of the following stretch reflexes is described here and illustrated in Figure 11.7. Note that bilateral symmetry of response is key to interpretation of stretch reflexes; therefore, each reflex must be tested in each limb, and the two sides must be compared for magnitude of response.

UPPER LIMBS

The arm reflexes are called the **triceps, biceps, and brachioradialis** for the muscle–tendon complexes involved.

Triceps Reflex (C6, *C7*, C8)

For testing the triceps reflex, follow these steps:

1. Place the patient's upper arm in the palm of your hand such that the forearm swings loosely with the elbow bent and the upper arm hyperadducted onto the thorax, as demonstrated on the woman patient in Figure 11.7*A1.*

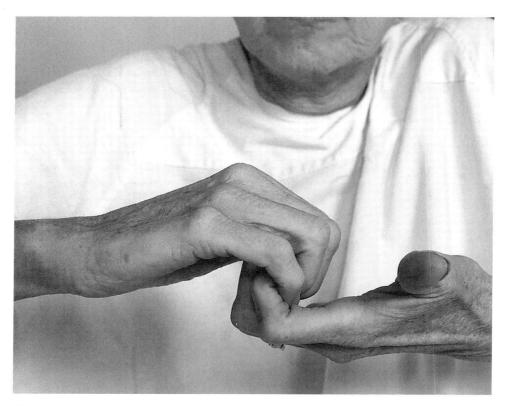

Figure 11.6   Reinforcement of reflexes with hand-tugging (Jendrassik maneuver).

2. Visualize the triceps tendon as it attaches to the olecranon on the extensor surface of the distal arm.
3. Strike the tendon sharply with the broad side of the triangular rubber reflex hammer.
4. Observe for visible contraction of the triceps muscle, which will tend to extend the elbow.

Biceps Reflex (*C5,* C6)

For testing the biceps reflex, follow these steps:

1. Ask the patient to rest the arm in her lap, which will force it into moderate flexion at the elbow.
2. Place the thumb of your nondominant hand over the prominent biceps tendon while curling the remainder of the fingers around the distal upper arm.
3. Strike your **thumb** with the point of the rubber triangle, transmitting a stimulus to the tendon that your thumb is retaining.
4. Observe the biceps muscle for contraction, which results in further flexion of the forearm (Fig. 11.7*A*2).

Brachioradialis Reflex (C5, *C6*)

For testing the brachioradialis reflex, follow these steps: With the patient's arm still resting in the lap, (*a*) palpate for the brachioradialis muscle, which can be felt on the radial surface of the mid to upper forearm; and (*b*) strike the tendon lightly along the course of the radius until a radial deviation of the wrist and the thumb or an extension of the wrist, index finger, or middle finger is noted (Fig. 11.7*A*3).

LOWER LIMBS

Patellar (Knee) Reflex (L2, L3, *L4*)

The patient should be seated with legs dangling free. Locate the tendon just distal to the patella, and with the hammer strike the tendon once, observing for quadriceps contraction and/or resultant extension of the knee (Fig. 11.7*B1* and *B2*).

Achilles (Ankle) Reflex (*S1*, S2)

To test for the Achilles reflex, with the patient's feet free and eyes averted, follow these steps:

1. Locate the easily palpated Achilles tendon at the level of the metatarsals.
2. Place the palm of the nondominant hand on the sole of the patient's foot, applying the slightest upward pressure in order to appreciate the plantar flexion response against the palm.
3. Tap the tendon briskly with the broad base of the hammer.
4. Observe for a plantar flexion response, felt as a push against the palm of your hand.

The Achilles reflex is usually the most difficult to elicit. If the reflex appears to be absent, try reinforcement; if this is unsuccessful, ask the patient to kneel on a chair seat, with feet free over the edge of the seat, and repeat the maneuvers above with the advantage of full, free view of the tendon (Fig. 11.7*C*). To reinforce in this position, have the patient grip the chair back as you strike the tendon.

Plantar Response (L4, L5, S1, S2)

With a pointed object (swab-stick, small door key), stroke the sole of the foot on its lateral aspect, beginning near the heel and crossing the ball of the foot to the base of the great toe (Fig. 11.8). The motion should be firm and continuous, noxious but not painful or ticklish. Observe the response of the toes: Do they curl under, dorsiflex, or fan out?

Sensation

Screening covers the major sensory modalities as they are represented in peripheral nerves and grouped in the spinal cord tracts: superficial pain and touch, vibration, and joint position sense. A successful sensory examination requires full concentration, comprehension of the task, and cooperation from the patient. It is the examiner's responsibility to give clear instructions and use appropriate stimuli. All maneuvers should be performed with the patient's eyes closed or averted to avoid visual cuing. The observations of each function include its (*a*) symmetry, (*b*) consistency (if initial response is incorrect) on repetition, and (*c*) patient's ability to determine which side of the body (right or left) and which part (foot, upper arm, etc.) is being stimulated. The steps of each sensory test are indicated below.

LIGHT TOUCH

- **Stimulus:** Fingertip or cotton wisp.
- **Instructions to patient:** "Tell me each time you feel this (demonstrate, using the stimulus) and where you feel it. We'll test with your eyes closed, so please close them now." (See Figure 11.9*A1*.)

SUPERFICIAL PAIN

- **Stimulus:** A sharp point such as a broken swab-stick or tongue blade alternating with a small dull object such as the blunt end of an unbroken swab-

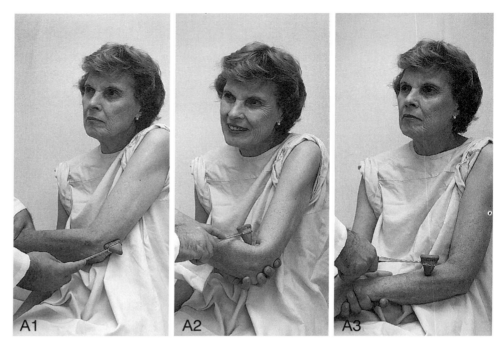

Figure 11.7 Muscle stretch reflexes. **A1.** Triceps reflex. Note passive hyperadduction of arm being tested. **A2.** Biceps reflex. Note the examiner strikes own thumb held against patient's tendon. **A3.** Brachioradialis reflex. **B1.** Patellar (knee) reflex, patient seated. **B2.** Patellar (knee) reflex, patient supine. Examiner has passively flexed the hip and knee a few degrees. **C.** Achilles (ankle) reflex, patient kneeling.

stick. The dull stimulus must be of the same material as the sharp point, or the patient may infer correct answers from texture or temperature.

- **Instructions to patient:** "With your eyes closed, tell me, each time I touch you, whether what you feel is sharp or dull and where you feel it."
- **Maneuver:** The examiner applies one or the other of the stimuli (sharp or dull) to skin surfaces after determining that the two stimuli are different enough to be discriminated and that the patient understands the task (Fig. 11.9*A*2).

JOINT POSITION SENSE

Screening for joint position is carried out at the periphery only, for if toe joint position sense is intact, proximal position sense is assumed to be normal.

- **Stimulus:** Passive movement of joint.
- **Instructions to patient:** "I will be moving your toe; each time I move it, tell me whether it has moved toward the floor or the ceiling."
- **Maneuver:** The metacarpophalangeal joint of each great toe is tested. Grasp the digit distal to the joint on its medial and lateral surfaces and move it through a range of upward and downward, stopping for the patient's interpretation of position (Fig. 11.9*B*).

VIBRATION

As with joint position, vibratory sense screening begins at the periphery and stops there if vibratory sense is normal.

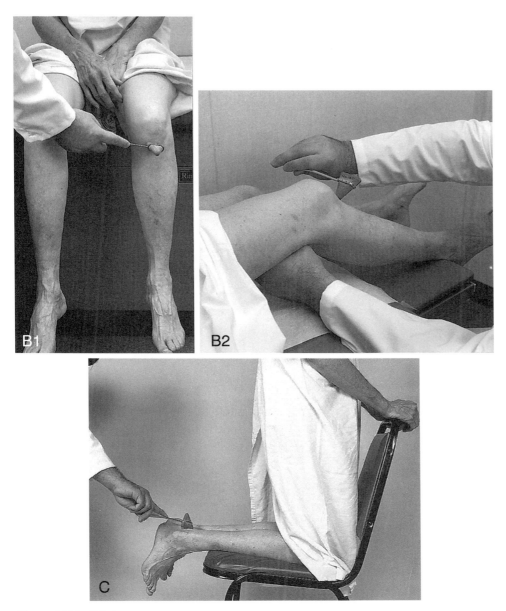

Figure 11.7   B1–C.

- **Stimulus:** A vibrating low-frequency tuning fork (128 Hz).
- **Instructions to patient:** "Close your eyes. I'm going to touch you with an object. I want you to describe what you feel, where you feel it, and when the sensation stops."
- **Maneuvers:** Place the stem of the vibrating tuning fork against the bony prominence to be assessed, as demonstrated on the patient in Figure 11.9C. When you are satisfied that the patient perceives vibration and not merely the touch of the tuning fork and when the patient has told you the vibrations have stopped, you may either damp them or, preferably, let the vibrations fade. If the patient ceases feeling the vibrations before they have stopped, repeat the test, touching the stem of the fork to a comparable site on your own body when the patient indicates that it has stopped. If you, as control, feel continu-

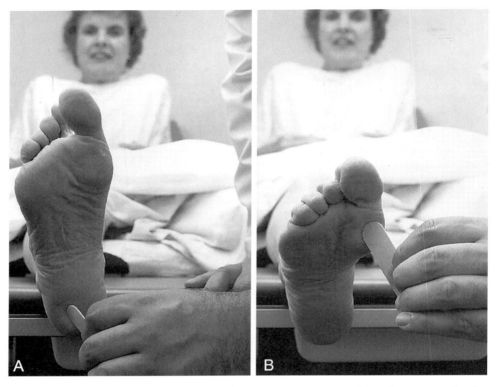

Figure 11.8   Plantar response. **A.** Stimulation begins at posterolateral extreme of sole. **B.** Stimulus applied constantly to completion just under hallux. Physiologic response, namely flexion of toes, is shown.

ing vibration, then your patient may have compromised vibratory sense. The screening is usually done at either the proximal phalanx of the great toes or the medial malleolus of the ankle (Fig. 11.9C).

Rapid Alternating Movements

The ability to perform accurate and symmetrical rapid movements requires motor control, position sense, and cerebellar mediation. Thus the following are employed to screen for dysfunction, unilateral or bilateral, of any of these portions of the integrated nervous system.

Upper limb testing is accomplished by using ONE of the following maneuvers demonstrated with the patient in Figure 11.10:

1. Ask the patient to touch sequentially the tip of each of the four fingers with the thumb of the same hand, progressively picking up speed. Test the two hands simultaneously (Fig. 11.10*A1* and *A2*).
2. Ask the patient to slap the backs and then the palms of both hands against her knees, i.e., alternately supinating and pronating, and progressively picking up to maximal speed attainable. Test both limbs simultaneously.
3. Finger-to-nose-to-finger maneuver. Ask the patient to touch her nose with the tip of her index finger, then extend the finger to touch your fingertip, and continue the motion back and forth between her nose and your finger (which you move within her field of vision, explaining, "I'm giving you a moving target; I want you to look at it") (Fig. 11.10*B*). Observe for accu-

racy, speed, and symmetry as you test each side. "Overshooting" is called **past-pointing.**

Lower limb function in this realm is usually tested by the **heel-to-shin maneuver** (Fig. 11.10C1 and C2). Instruct the patient: "Place the heel of your right foot just below your left knee, and run it straight down your shin to the ankle and back up again, repeatedly, as quickly and as accurately as you can." Then, have the patient repeat the maneuver using the left heel. Observe for accuracy of heel placement, and note if the heel is moved easily down the shin without wavering. Ability to perform this maneuver may be limited by joint disease or other non-neurologic disability, so the test must be interpreted in context.

Equilibrium

Equilibrium of the total body is a test of the combined function of the cerebellum, the motor system, the sensory proprioceptive status, and the vestibular apparatus (cochlea and vestibular branch of the eighth cranial nerve). A combined screen for these neurologic functions is shown in Figure 11.11.

ROMBERG TEST

The Romberg test was devised to assess body balance. Ask the patient to stand erect with feet together, arms extended forward, first with the eyes open (cerebellar and visual input) and then with the eyes closed (cerebellar and dorsal column proprioception). Stand near enough to catch the patient and prevent a fall, should the patient lose balance, and observe for loss of balance. If the patient loses balance and sways dangerously with the eyes open, the test is not taken to the second step.

TEST FOR DRIFT

Once the patient has "passed" the Romberg test, i.e., does not lose balance in the open-eyes and then the closed-eyes stance, ask her to turn her palms upward, close her eyes, and maintain this position. Watch for a downward drift of either arm or for *pronator drift,* a palm-down rotation of the affected arm-hand unit (Fig. 11.12).

GAIT TEST

Every patient who is not bed- or wheelchair-bound is asked to **walk,** if necessary with usual assist devices (cane, walker, or crutches) or with assistants for support and prevention of falls. The feet should be bare or stockinged only. Observe the patient for smoothness of gait, placement of feet (broad-based or normal), symmetry of leg and arm movement, step height (normal or shuffling), step length (normal or shortened), staggering, or uncertainty. Watch the patient turn around, and note the number of steps required to achieve this. As the patient returns, observe from a frontal angle. Additional useful maneuvers, if there is suspicion of a gait abnormality based on the history or screening observation, include **tandem walking** (heel to toe, Fig. 11.13A) or **hopping** on one foot and then the other, walking on toes only (Fig. 11.13B), and walking on heels only (Fig. 11.13C).

NORMAL AND COMMON VARIANTS

The range of normal neurologic function is quite narrow. Most variations indicate pathologic disturbance, and those discussed here are selected because they usually DO NOT require further detailed examination or special testing.

Cortical Function

The normally neurologically integrated adult (except when psychiatrically impaired) is appropriately dressed and groomed, is interactive with and responsive to

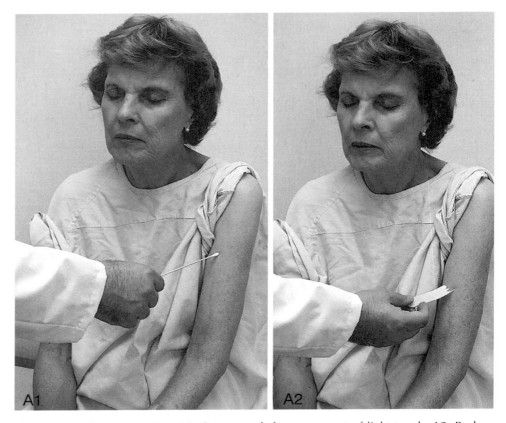

Figure 11.9 Sensory testing. **A1.** Cotton swab for assessment of light touch. **A2.** Broken throat-stick for pain. **B.** Passive extension of hallux as part of position sense testing. **C.** Testing vibration sense at the ankle.

the examiner's words and actions, is able to carry out the tasks stipulated (unless nonneurologically physically impaired, as for instance by severe arthritis), and displays normal speech patterns consistent with language background and education.

Orientation to person, time, and place is accurate, taking into consideration that we are all occasionally transiently unclear about the day of the month. Remember that the institutionalized patient may have been out of touch with world events and may be confused as to the precise date or day of the week; however, the patient should know the year and the season. If there is question about orientation to time, correct the patient's misinterpretation and reask the question later. The elderly, but neurologically normal patient should be fully oriented in all spheres. All patients over the age of 65 should have a Folstein minimental status examination to provide a baseline data set concerning higher cortical function (see the Extended Examination section). Hearing impairment, so common in the elderly, may give rise to inaccuracies in responses to questions. When in doubt about the contribution of deafness, ask the patient to respond to written questions.

Reflexes

The range of stretch reflex responses is listed in Table 11.3. In the normal individual, all stretch reflex responses should be in the +2 range (often the Achilles response is the least active) and always bilaterally symmetrical. An occasional healthy adult will have absent paired reflexes. A significant minority of elderly

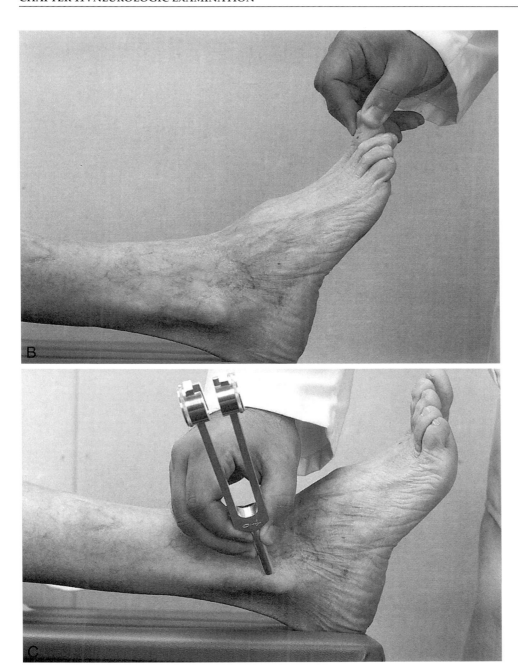

Figure 11.9   B and C.

patients lose some peripheral stretch reflexes, particularly in the lower limbs and especially at the ankles. The designation of "normal variant" in this situation depends on the remainder of the neurologic examination, the medical history, and the general physical assessment. Thus, normal individuals may have responses of 0, 1, 2, or, rarely, 3. The only grade that is *always* abnormal is 4, although any of the others may be suspicious if out of step with other findings or if asymmetric.

After the age of 2 years, the normal response to **plantar** stroking is a flexion of the toes toward the sole of the foot. Note that the initial movement in response

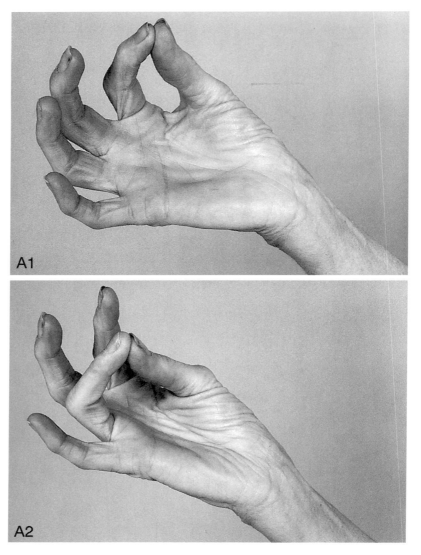

Figure 11.10   Cerebellar tests. **A1.** Beginning of rapid sequential touching of each finger against the thumb. **A2.** Later phase of same test. **B.** Finger-to-nose testing. **C1.** Beginning of a cycle of the heel-to-shin touching test. **C2.** End position in heel-to-shin touching test.

to the stimulus is the most important. An individual with ticklish soles may withdraw the foot or flare the toes when stimulated. If this response is bilateral, it is probably normal; confirmation may be obtained by applying the stimulus to the superolateral side of the foot, avoiding the sole (*Chaddock maneuver,* see Fig. 11.14). This alternative maneuver elicits a plantar flexion response or no response in the normal individual. Elderly patients, like others, may have no plantar flexion response but should not dorsiflex the great toe or flare all toes (*Babinski response*); *a Babinski response in any person beyond the age of myelination is pathologic.*

Sensation

The greatest "normal" variations in sensory response have to do with the nature of the stimulus and body location. A light touch stimulus must be perceptible; when in doubt, check the stimulus on your own skin. Discrimination between "sharp" and "dull" depends on the clarity of the stimuli. Can you tell the differ-

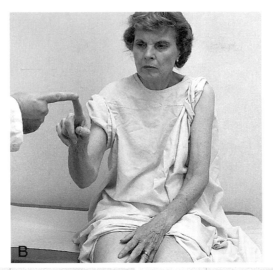

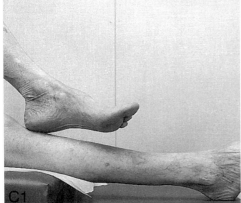
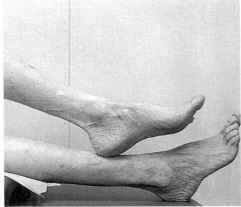

Figure 11.10   B–C2.

ence between the two on the dorsum of your own hand? When the stimuli are adequate, responses should be clear and symmetrical bilaterally in the normal patient. Recall that calloused surfaces, such as portions of the soles of the feet, have sensory endings entombed in abundant keratin matter and thus are protected from sensation; they should not be tested for light touch or superficial pain. More pressure may be required over the buttocks, less on the face, because of the varying densities of nerve endings.

The elderly patient may show diminution in response to vibration. Again, the decision as to whether a dampened sensory response is due to normal aging or secondary to a cord or peripheral nerve abnormality depends on the total context and more extended testing (see the Extended Examination section). Specifically, joint position sense does **not** suffer such a normal age-related decline; thus, it makes sense to test this modality instead of vibration in aged persons and to infer integrity of the posterior columns of the cord—in which proprioceptive and vibratory fibers run together—if joint position sense is unimpaired.

Rapid Alternating Movements

Normally, any of the rapid alternating movement tests should be performed accurately and as swiftly as the examiner is able to do them. There may be slow-

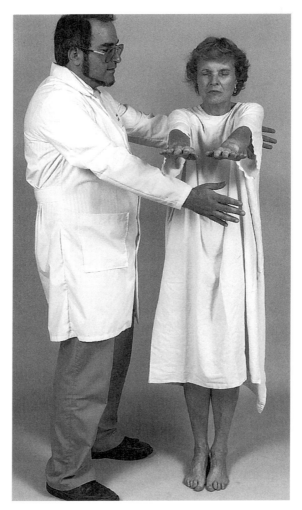

Figure 11.11   Romberg test. The examiner stands ready to catch the patient, should falling occur.

ing or slight clumsiness in the nondominant hand, but if a substantial difference in speed is noted, more extended testing is indicated. Performance of all of these maneuvers should be as accurate and swift with the eyes closed as with the eyes open. Inaccuracy with eyes open *and* closed suggests cerebellar or motor dysfunction; inaccuracy only with the eyes closed indicates proprioceptive (sensory) problems. Joint or primary muscular disease may affect these maneuvers, and the aged patient may perform them more slowly but still with accuracy. In the confused or demented elder, and even in the mentally intact old person, the rapid alternating movements in the nondominant hand may lag considerably behind those of the other hand, even in the absence of disease.

Equilibrium

Unless there is a structural musculoskeletal problem, the neurologically intact person should be able to stand in the Romberg position for 15 seconds without falling, retropulsion, or significant swaying, even with eyes closed. Extended and pronated arms should remain stable for the same length of time. Any variation is considered pathologic until proven otherwise.

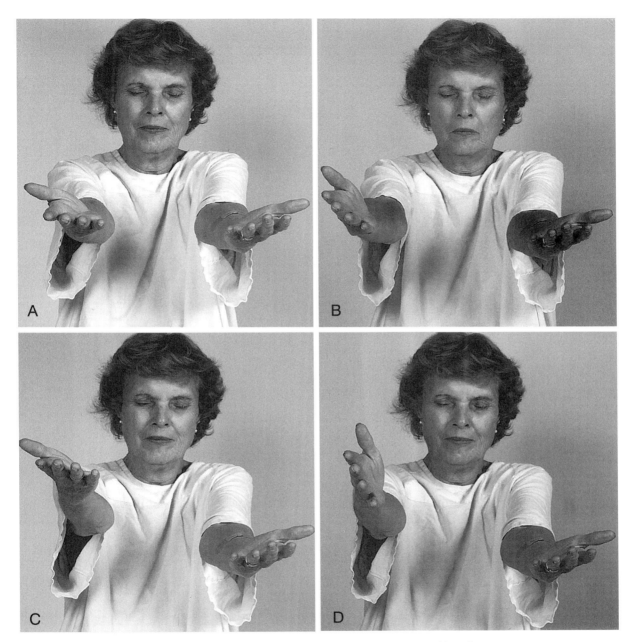

Figure 11.12   Test for pronator drift. **A.** Patient is instructed to maintain arm and hand position as placed at start, with eyes closed, as shown here. **B.** Abnormal test result: the right arm has pronated. **C.** Abnormal test result: the right arm has drifted upward. **D.** Abnormal test result: the right arm has drifted upward, and the right hand has pronated.

Gait is an integrated function of posture, bones, tendons, and muscles as well as motor, sensory, vestibular, visual, and cerebellar function. A healthy adult walks confidently with coordinated arm swing and full equal strides and is able to put one foot in front of the other (tandem) accurately, although some persons are better coordinated in this contrived maneuver than others. If the joints and muscles of the feet and legs are normal, any person should be able to heel-walk and toe-walk for short distances.

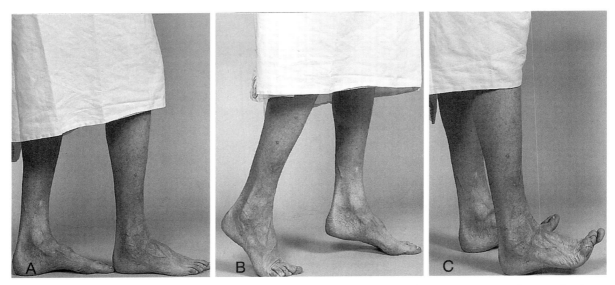

Figure 11.13   Gait evaluation. **A.** Tandem gait. **B.** Walking on toes. **C.** Walking on heels.

Table 11.3
Range of Stretch Reflex Responses

Grade	Response
0	No response elicited, even with reinforcing maneuvers
+1	Response only with reinforcement (Jendrassik or other)
+2	Moderate response without reinforcement
+3	Brisk response, with 1–3 beats of clonus (brief terminal jerking of the muscle following the initial response)
+4	Exaggerated response with sustained clonus

With aging, the gait slows and becomes less sure, sometimes slightly "shuffling." These variants must be individually judged based on the patient's general state of health, joint and bone integrity, and eyesight. More refined testing of possible neurologic bases for gait abnormalities is discussed in the Extended Examination section.

RECORDING THE FINDINGS

Although the neurologic examination is partially integrated with body regions, it is usually recorded as a single unit. Exceptions may be made for the funduscopic examination, and sometimes the cranial nerves, which can be recorded with the region (HEENT), and the assessment of muscle strength (LIMBS). An example of a normal neurologic examination record follows.

Neurological examination:
Mental status: Oriented × 3, conversationally apt and appropriate; affect and speech content normal.
Cranial nerves: II–XII normal.

	BJ	TJ	BR	KJ	AJ
R	2+	2+	2+	3+	1+
L	2+	2+	2+	3+	1+

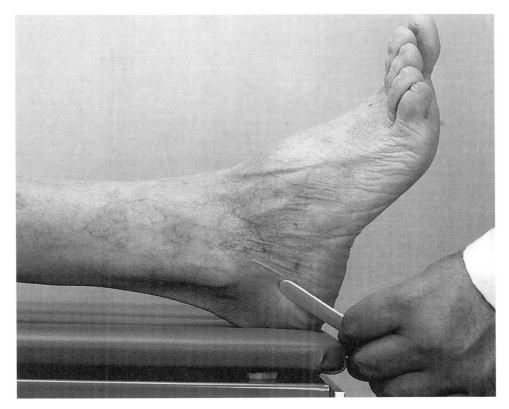

Figure 11.14   Chaddock test, a variant of plantar stimulation.

Muscle stretch reflexes:
Plantars: Downgoing.
Sensation: to pinprick and light touch, normal on trunk, feet, hands; vibratory
   sense and joint position normal in feet.
Cerebellar: Finger-to-nose, heel-to-shin performed accurately bilaterally.
Motor: All muscle groups symmetrical in tone and strength; no pronator drift.
   Normal gait including tandem, heel and toe walking. Turns easily in two steps.
Romberg: Position held well for 30 seconds.

EXTENDED NEUROLOGIC EXAMINATION

INDICATIONS

The presenting problem, clues in the routine medical history, or abnormalities
detected on the screening physical examination may call for a more extensive or
focused neurologic assessment.

Indications from the Medical History

Although the nervous system could be implicated in a vast range of complaints,
there are clusters of symptoms that point insistently toward a particular cause.
These complaints are organized here into those specific to the nervous system
and those in which the nervous system must be considered along with other systems as potentially involved.

COMPLAINTS REQUIRING EXTENDED NEUROLOGIC EVALUATION

The recent and/or unexplained appearance of any of the following symptoms warrants an extension of one or more realms of the neurologic examination:

- Change in mental function or behavior as reported by the patient, the family, or other informants
- Change in level of consciousness
- New seizure or change in frequency or nature of established seizure disorder
- Onset of involuntary movements including those that do not appear to be seizures
- Reduction or loss of function in muscle group(s) or limb(s)
- Falling or incoordination
- Loss or diminution of sensation in nerve root or peripheral nerve distribution
- Pain in nerve root or peripheral nerve distribution
- Acute onset of headache, fever, and stiff neck
- Onset of unintelligible speech, or inability to carry out verbal commands or to respond cogently to questions

COMPLAINTS THAT MAY CALL FOR EXTENDED NEUROLOGIC EVALUATION

Details of the history further guide the clinician in determining the system(s) that may be implicated. The following symptoms, although not specific to the nervous system, may direct the examiner to expand beyond the routine neurologic screening:

- Chronic headache
- "Dizziness" (recall that this symptom means different things to different people, such as true vertigo, lightheadedness, headache, malaise, etc.)
- Visual disturbance (again, obtain the specifics of the symptom)
- Change in bladder or bowel function, especially incontinence or urinary retention
- Generalized weakness
- Numbness or tingling, generalized or localized
- Syncope (fainting)

Abnormalities Detected on the Screening Physical Examination

Occasionally, an unexpected abnormality will be detected on the screening neurologic examination without a clue from the history. For the most part, before beginning the physical examination the clinician will know that expansion of the neurologic assessment is indicated. The extended tests and maneuvers described on the following pages may be indicated by either history or screening examination or both.

CONDUCTING THE EXTENDED EXAMINATION

The maneuvers for conducting the extended examination are grouped by the nervous system function to be tested.

Cortical Function

The specific indications for expanding the cortical function examination are

- History of memory loss or behavioral change
- Disorientation in any of the three spheres of person, place, or time
- Inappropriate affect, grooming, responses to medical history questions and examination instructions, or behavior during the interview or physical examination

- Abnormal level of consciousness or concentration ability.

Expanded assessment is carried out with the following maneuvers.

MEMORY

Memory testing is divided into three components:

1. Immediate memory.
    a. Ask the patient to repeat to you a series of three to five numbers.
    b. Ask the patient to repeat to you a series of three to five objects, e.g., pen, tree, apple, table, house.
2. Recent memory.
    a. Give the patient a list of three objects with the task of storing them mentally for a few minutes. Move on in the examination, but in 2–5 minutes, ask the patient to recall the items you asked him to remember.
    b. Ask the patient to recall what he had for lunch (meaningful only if you have independent access to the correct answer) or, alternatively, to repeat something that he told you earlier in this interview.
3. Remote memory.
    a. Ask the patient to give you the dates of major life events such as wedding, birth of children, age of retirement. Assessment of accuracy demands that you know the correct responses.
    b. Ask the patient to describe the home in which he grew up; this, too, may require checking on your part for accuracy.
    c. Ask the patient to name the United States presidents, starting in the present and going backward as far as possible.

CALCULATIONS

When asking the patient to calculate answers, take into consideration the educational level of the patient in choosing tasks and interpreting the responses.

a. Ask the patient to subtract 7 from 100, 7 from the answer, then 7 from that result, and so on for a total of five repetitions (serial sevens).
b. Ask the patient to indicate the amount of change expected from $1 if the purchase is X cents, Y cents, etc.

GENERAL KNOWLEDGE

Again, when questioning the patient, consider the patient's education, nationality, and cultural history when selecting the subject matter for these questions.

a. Ask the patient to cite the names of the capital cities of states in the region or of the nation. (Any American citizen or long-time resident should be able to do so.)
b. Ask for directions to a common destination in the area of the hospital (or other site) of the interview.
c. Additional questions may be tailored to the patient's profession, business, or special interests; e.g., an English professor is expected to be able to name a dozen of Shakespeare's plays, a farmer should readily tell planting dates for seasonal crops, and a tennis player should be able to describe game scoring.

REASONING

Ask the patient to describe what he would do if he found a stamped, addressed letter lying on the sidewalk. (If he says anything other than, "Put it in the nearest mailbox," ask him to explain this alternative in order to follow his reasoning.)

ABSTRACTIONS

Ask the patient to interpret any proverb, looking for ability to move beyond the concrete; e.g., "What does the following mean? 'A stitch in time saves nine.'"

THE FOLSTEIN MINI-MENTAL STATUS EXAMINATION

The standardized Folstein mini-mental status examination (Fig. 11.15) is a widely used formal test that is effective even with the diminished attention span of moderately cognitively impaired patients. It takes about 5 minutes to administer and does not require extensive training to administer or interpret. Its questions and commands test **attention, registration, memory, and praxis.** Serial repetition of the examination can be of help in assessing recovery from or progression of cognitive deficits.

Interpretation is generally straightforward. Scores of 23 or less commonly represent symptomatic dysfunction, and in the original report, scores below 20 were found only in psychosis, delirium (acute brain failure), and dementia (chronic brain failure), including psychotic depression with secondary cognitive impairment. The mean score of persons with dementia is about 12. Sources of **false-positive** tests include **inattention** as a result of distraction, **depression or other psychiatric disease, sensory loss, motor impairment** preventing writing or copying, **linguistic difficulty, or low educational level. False-negative tests** may result from the inherent insensitivity of the instrument. Certain highly educated persons may be able to disguise deficits until dementia is far advanced.

LANGUAGE AND SPEECH

The specific indications for conducting expanded language function testing are

- Unintelligible speech
- Inability to carry out verbal commands
- Inability to respond cogently to questions

Unintelligible speech may be due to motor dysfunction, hearing loss (insufficient feedback), or cerebral impairment. **Dysarthria,** or the inability to articulate, can occur with disease of any of the components of phonation: tongue, palate, jaw, lips, pharynx; **dysphonia** is the term for voice change, most commonly hoarseness, which occurs with vocal cord pathology. Pure dysarthria or dysphonia is not a language dysfunction.

APHASIAS

Accurate testing for aphasia, the inability to use language properly, requires that the patient be able to hear and to comprehend instructions and, for some of the tests described, to have functional sight as well as intact muscles of phonation. The tests are divided into clusters, depending on the specific language function they are designed to assess.

1. Tests for **verbal expression** (abnormality is called **expressive, anterior, or Broca's aphasia**).
   a. Does the patient use enough words to make complete sentences (apart from the interruptions of an eager interviewer)?
   b. Does the patient understand requests but have difficulty "getting out" or finding the words of response?
   c. Does the patient respond to every question with the same few words or repetitive "stock" phrases?
   d. Does the patient use incorrect word substitutes, such as "bat" for "ball" (**paraphasias**), or does he create meaningless words (**neologisms**)?

Mini-Mental Status Examination (MMSE)

Add points for each correct response.

		Score	Points
Orientation			
1. What is the:	Year	_____	1
	Season	_____	1
	Date	_____	1
	Day	_____	1
	Month	_____	1
2. Where are we?	State	_____	1
	County	_____	1
	Town or city	_____	1
	Hospital	_____	1
	Floor	_____	1

Registration

3. Name three objects, taking one second to say each. Then ask   _____   3
   the patient to repeat all three after you have said them.
   Give one point for each correct answer. Repeat the answers
   until patient learns all three.

Attention and calculation

4. Serial sevens. Give one point for each correct answer. Stop   _____   5
   after five answers.
   Alternate: Spell WORLD backwards.

Recall

5. Ask for names of three objects learned in question 3.   _____   3
   Give one point for each correct answer.

Language

6. Point to a pencil and a watch. Have the patient name them   _____   2
   as you point.
7. Have the patient repeat "No ifs, ands, or buts."   _____   1
8. Have the patient follow a three-stage command: "Take a   _____   3
   paper in your right hand. Fold the paper in half. Put the
   paper on the floor."
9. Have the patient read and obey the following: "CLOSE   _____   1
   YOUR EYES." (Print it in large letters.)
10. Have the patient write a sentence of his or her choice.   _____   1
    (The sentence should contain a subject and an object and
    should make sense. Ignore spelling errors when scoring.)
11. Have the patient copy the design. (Give one point if all   _____   <u>1</u>
    sides and angles are preserved and if the intersecting sides
    form a quadrangle.)

                                                      _____   Total 30

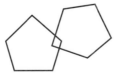

Figure 11.15   Folstein mini-mental status examination form.

    e. Does the patient struggle *excessively* to find the right word, often failing altogether (**anomia**)?

2. Tests for **written expression** (abnormality is called **agraphia**).
    a. Can the patient write his own name and address?
    b. Can he write a simple sentence?
    c. Can he copy a written sentence?

3. Tests for **comprehension of spoken language.**
    a. Ask the patient to pick common objects from a group: "Point to the penny, point to the key, etc."
    b. Ask the patient to carry out several simple maneuvers: "Pick up the key; touch your nose with one finger, etc." (Note that this requires that the patient not be apraxic.)

4. Tests for **comprehension of written language.**
    a. Give the patient written instructions to carry out a simple maneuver: "Draw a circle on the paper, clap hands, etc."
    b. Signal the patient to match the written names of simple objects to the objects themselves (key, coin, pencil, etc.).

5. Tests for **recognition of sense stimuli** (abnormality is called **agnosia**).
    a. **Tactile:** recognition of objects or symbols by touch.
       Ask the patient to identify, with eyes closed, numbers drawn by a blunt object in the palm of the hand (Fig. 11.16A). This is **graphesthesia,** and the patient can only be meaningfully tested if primary sensory modalities (e.g., light touch) are known to be intact at the sites tested (e.g., the hands). Ask the patient to identify, with eyes closed, common objects placed in his hand (key, pencil, coin, etc.), i.e., **stereognosis** (Fig. 11.16B).
    b. **Visual:** recognition of objects and symbols by sight.
       Ask the patient to name each of several objects as you point to them.
       Ask the patient to name each of several drawn symbols as you point to them: rectangle, triangle, square, etc.

6. Tests of ability to carry out purposeful movement (abnormality is called **apraxia**).
    a. Ask the patient to show you how to use some object such as a pencil, key, spoon, in the usual manner.
    b. Ask the patient to walk across the room to a given destination. (Note that some apraxias are act-specific, such as the gait apraxia of normal-pressure hydrocephalus.)

Motor Function

The specific indications for conducting an expanded examination of motor function are

- Symptoms or signs of weakness of any muscle group
- Absence or asymmetry of stretch reflexes
- Symptoms or signs of involuntary movement

WEAKNESS

Loss of strength in any muscle group calls for the following systematic assessment.

1. Define the **distribution of the weakness. Is it
    a. Served by the motor cortex **above the pyramidal decussation?** (Cortico-bulbar involvement of the face and upper and lower limbs of one side of the body is called **hemiparesis (weakness) or hemiplegia (total paralysis),** depending on the degree of the impairment.)

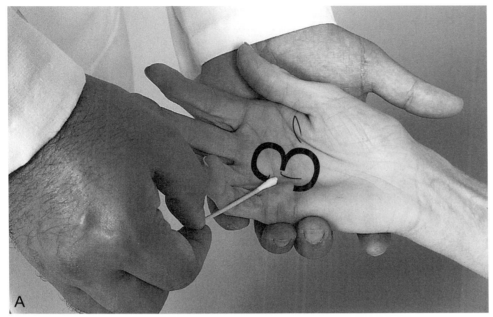

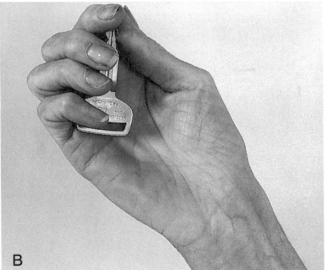

Figure 11.16   Higher integrative function testing is possible if there is no deficit in primary sensory modalities. **A.** Testing graphesthesia. **B.** Stereognosis testing.

    b.   Served by long tracts **below the pyramidal decussation** but **above the thoracic cord?** (Corticospinal involvement of the arm and leg on one side is called **hemiparesis/hemiplegia,** and that of both arms and both legs is called **quadriparesis/quadriplegia.** In either case, the face is spared.)

    c.   Served by the corticospinal tract(s) **in or below the thoracic cord?** (Involvement of both legs is called **paraparesis/paraplegia,** and that of one entire leg is called **monoparesis/monoplegia.** In each case, the face and arms are spared.)

    d.   Served by a single or several adjacent spinal segments, unilateral or bilateral (see also Chapters 5 and 10)?

    e.   Served by a **peripheral nerve** (see Fig. 11.5)?

2. Define the **degree of weakness.**
    a. Muscle group strength is quantitated as indicated in Table 11.4.
    b. Is there atrophy—decreased muscle mass—in the area under question?
3. Define the **tone** of the muscles in question. Tone is assessed by passive movement of the joints served by the muscles being evaluated and, in part, by palpating (see Step 4 below). The results are classified as follows:
    a. Absent or decreased resistance to passive movement (**atonia** or **hypotonia**).
    b. Increased resistance (**spasticity**). If spasticity is noted on initial rapid extension but disappears as extension is continued, this is called "**clasp-knife phenomenon.**"
    c. A repeated ratcheting, catch-release response as examiner extends the joint (**cogwheel rigidity**), characteristic of disease of the basal nuclei.
4. Palpate the bodies of the muscles in question.
    a. Are the muscles lax (**flaccid**) or rigid (**spastic**)?
    b. Are the muscles **tender** to palpation?
5. Observe the muscle bodies for intrinsic movement.
    a. Are there **fasciculations** (fine, random **spontaneous** twitches visible at skin surface over the muscle)? These are distinguished from tremor by the regularity of tremors (see below).

INVOLUNTARY MOVEMENTS

Most of the movement disorders described here accompany specific congenital disorders, although some are related to degenerative disease and others are related to drug side effects. Of particular importance to the care of persons taking neuroleptic drugs is assessment for **dyskinesias** created by these chemicals. Although beyond the scope of this text, the details of the Abnormal Involuntary Movement Scale (AIMS) protocol for following patients who are being treated with drugs that predispose to tardive dyskinesis are sufficiently important to require notation.

When specific **involuntary movements** are complained of or noted on the primary examination, the following extended observations are made:

1. **Tremor:** observe for
    a. Precise location (fingers, arms, legs, etc.).
    b. Laterality (unilateral, symmetric, or asymmetric bilateral).
    c. Quality (fine or coarse, rhythmic or erratic).
    d. Effect of movement on tremor (present only at rest (**resting tremor**), present only with or exacerbated by purposeful movement such as reaching for something (**intention tremor**), present only when muscles are stretched

Table 11.4
Muscle Group Strength

Score	Interpretation
5	Normal
4	Overcome by examiner's resistance more readily than average normal control patients (note that this definition allows for the large range of strength of examiners)
3	Can move against gravity but not with added examiner resistance
2	Can move only if gravity is eliminated, i.e., sideways or on a surface
1	Only a trace of contraction
0	No muscular contraction

and extended as with spreading fingers (**postural tremor**)). For additional components of tremor evaluation, see Table 10.10.

2. **Chorea:** rapid, jerky, purposeless contractions of random muscle groups.
   a. Ask the patient to extend the arms in pronation in front of the body; observe for **hyperpronation** and for **"dishing"** (hyperextension at the metacarpophalangeal joints with flexion at the wrist).
   b. Ask the patient to grasp your fingers in his grip; observe for a "milking" motion caused by the involuntary muscle spasms.
   c. If such movements are found, ask the patient to walk about the room; observe for exaggeration of the movements.
3. **Other movement disorders** are labeled by virtue of the following characteristics:
   a. **Athetosis:** slow, writhing irregular movements that begin randomly in one muscle group and spread to adjoining groups.
   b. **Dystonia:** parts of the body are held in abnormal postures for longer periods of time than would be observed in ordinary daily life.
   c. **Hemiballism:** abrupt, unilateral violent flinging motion at proximal joints.
   d. **Tic:** a spastic, regular or irregular twitching of small muscle groups.
   e. **Asterixis** (see the Extended Examination section of Chapter 10).

MUSCLE STRETCH REFLEXES

If abnormalities of **stretch reflexes** (either hypoactive or hyperactive) are noted, the following additional observations are made.

1. If one or more reflexes are **absent** on one or both sides, the affected limb(s) are evaluated for
   a. Motor function.
   b. Sensory function.
2. If one or more **hyperactive (+4)** reflexes are found on one or both sides, the affected limb(s) are evaluated for
   a. Motor function.
   b. Sensory function.
   c. **Clonus (ankle clonus** is sought—if it was not noted earlier with tapping for the ankle reflex—by sharply dorsiflexing the ankle, observing for sustained jerking of the foot; **patellar clonus** is sought by sharply moving the patella distally and observing for sustained jerky movement).
3. A clear-cut **Babinski** response to plantar stroking (dorsiflexion of the great toe and fanning of the other toes) requires no confirmation. On the other hand, an equivocal response, such as dorsiflexion followed immediately by plantar flexion or no response to stimulation, should be retested by using one of the alternative methods.
   a. **Chaddock maneuver:** The lateral aspect of the foot is stimulated with a blunt point in an arc from the malleolus toward the base of the hallux (Fig. 11.14).
   b. **Oppenheim maneuver:** Pressure with the thumb and index finger is applied over the anterior surface of the tibia in a downward sweep from the infrapatellar region to the foot.
   c. **Gordon's sign:** Application of deep pressure to the calf muscle results in dorsiflexion of the great toe and fanning of the other toes (if corticospinal tract disease is present).
   d. **Schaefer's sign:** Deep pressure on the Achilles tendon causes a dorsiflexor response (if corticospinal tract disease is present).

The clinician should note that these alternative maneuvers and signs are less consistently reliable than the plantar stroke response and have the potential for local trauma if not conducted carefully; they should be used only when the traditional Babinski response is uninterpretable.

If the Babinski response is **unilaterally** positive, the motor and sensory function of the affected side should be carefully examined. **Bilateral** upgoing toes demand full detailed assessment of motor and sensory modalities of all four limbs and a search for other evidence of diffuse cerebral dysfunction, such as the so-called cortical release signs.

CORTICAL (FRONTAL) RELEASE SIGNS

The specificity or localizing significance of the following primitive frontal lobe signs has been called into question recently. They may be most useful in confirming a suspicion of diffuse cerebral dysfunction and should be interpreted with caution.

1. **Glabellar sign:** The forehead between the eyebrows is tapped gently with a finger; normally there is no response or a single initial blink. A positive sign consists of exaggerated eye blinking and upper facial grimacing, especially if these do not abate with repetition.
2. **Snout reflex:** Place a finger vertically over the patient's lips and tap it lightly with a reflex hammer. A positive response is puckering movement of the lips.
3. **Sucking (rooting) reflex:** Lightly stimulate the corners of the patient's mouth with a finger or tongue blade. A positive response is an attempt to grasp the stimulating object with the lips and suck it.
4. **Grasp reflex:** Lightly stroke the palm of the patient's hand with a finger. Normally, there will be no response; in the case of frontal lobe disease, the patient may involuntarily grasp and have difficulty releasing the stroking fingers.
5. **Palmomental reflex:** The palm of the hand is lightly stroked, and the patient's face is observed for a twitch of the chin in response. It has been estimated that 3–5% of normal adults will have a positive palmomental reflex.

SUPERFICIAL REFLEXES

The following reflexes are sought if there is question about a lesion affecting a spinal cord level or a subtle unilateral corticospinal or cortical lesion:

1. **Abdominal:** With the patient supine, four quadrants of the abdominal skin are stroked (Fig. 11.17), observing the movement of the umbilicus in response to the stimulus. Normally, the umbilicus "winks," i.e., is pulled slightly toward the quadrant being stimulated. The two upper quadrants test T7–T9, and the lower two test T11–L1.
2. **Cremasteric:** With the patient supine and thighs slightly spread, the proximal inner thigh is stroked lightly. Normally, the scrotum or labium on the stimulated side will contract cephalad. Observe for unilateral or bilateral absence of response, which suggests disease of spinal segments L1 and L2.

Sensory Function

If the patient comprehends instructions and is alert and cooperative, the sensory examination can provide very important localizing data. If level of consciousness or concentration is impaired, it can be used only in the most gross determinations such as ability to withdraw from painful stimuli. When a sensory loss is claimed by history or discovered on screening examination of a patient who comprehends in the interview, the following maneuvers are indicated:

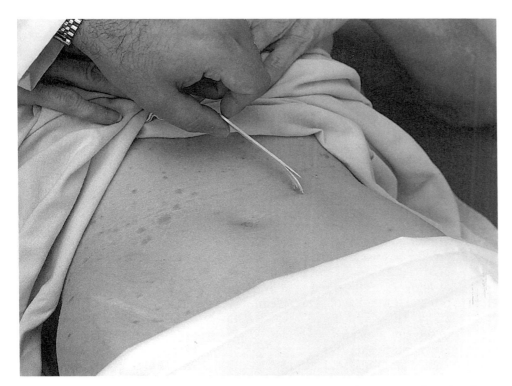

Figure 11.17   Superficial abdominal reflexes. Reflex of the left upper quadrant has been stimulated.

1. **Light touch:** To delineate the affected area, move the stimulus from the area of hypesthesia to each of its margins, drawing with a skin pencil the boundaries of the loss.
2. **Superficial pain:** Usually, the complaint is either that of **loss of sensation** or **paresthesia (numbness, tingling, or crawling sensation)** in the abnormal area. Delineate the margins of the affected area by moving the stimulus from areas of normal sensation to the impaired area, marking the margins with a skin pencil. Repeat the test to confirm its consistency. If there is demonstrable and reproducible loss (anesthesia or hypesthesia) or increase in skin sensitivity (hyperalgesia), assessment of deep pain and temperature perception can be tested.
    a. **Deep pain:** Squeezing of the Achilles tendon, the gastrocnemius or quadriceps muscles, or the biceps tendon may demonstrate a loss of deep pain responsiveness. Pressure on the sternum of an obtunded or comatose patient can be used for the same purpose.
    b. **Temperature:** If superficial pain is absent in a limb or if the patient complains about loss of perception of temperature extremes, the loss may be demonstrated by asking the patient to discriminate, with eyes closed, between two test tubes of water: one hot and one iced or frozen. Work from normal skin to the area of apparent abnormality, marking limits with a skin pencil. Be wary of perfect responses. For example, the patient may be feeling the "dew" on the iced tube rather than perceiving temperature. Most patients try not to fail their examinations and thus may not reveal that they are "cheating."
3. **Joint position sense:** Expand the previously described tests of joint position sense proximally when
    a. Distal (toe) sense is impaired.

    b. Balance (Romberg) is abnormal **only with eyes closed.**

    c. Gait is unsteady **only with eyes closed.**

4. **Vibratory sense:** Expand the previously described tests of vibration proximally when

    a. Distal (foot) perception is impaired.

    b. Joint position sense, closed-eye balance, or gait is impaired. Proximal testing of vibration should move from the periphery, i.e., from the ankle to the shin to the femoral condyle to the iliac crest and from the wrist to the humeral epicondyle to the clavicle; the test is discontinued after normal vibratory sense has been found and localization of the lesion has thus been permitted.

5. **Cortical sensory perception:** These subtle modes are tested when there is mental status abnormality, tactile agnosia, a positive cortical release sign, or an ignoring of body parts (**neglect**) or of the presence of disease (anosognosia).

    a. **Simultaneous double stimulation:** Two equal stimuli are applied simultaneously to symmetrical body areas, as demonstrated on the patient in Figure 11.18, and the patient is asked (eyes closed) to indicate where she feels the stimulus. First, you must demonstrate that the patient can perceive and localize the single stimulus accurately at each site (Fig. 11.18*A* and *B*). If so and if she only loses the perception when both sides are tested simultaneously (Fig. 11.18*C*), the test—also called **bilateral simultaneous stimulation**—is positive. Consistent failure to recognize the double stimulus on one side of the body is called **extinction** and is characteristic of integrative sensory failure, i.e., contralateral parietal lobe disease at or near the cortical representation of the areas in question.

    b. **Stereognosis and graphesthesia:** These are discussed earlier under tests for recognition of sense stimuli.

    c. **Two-point discrimination:** The area in question is examined with the patient's eyes closed. Two equivalent sharp points are applied near one

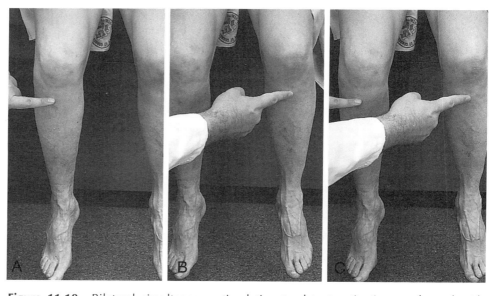

Figure 11.18 Bilateral simultaneous stimulation to detect extinction, performed with patient's eyes closed. **A.** On right leg touching, patient correctly identifies site. **B.** On left leg touching, patient correctly identifies site. **C.** With bilateral leg touching, patient identifies only the right-sided stimulus.

another on the skin surface in question. The points are moved apart until the patient can discriminate both. Normally, two separate points applied simultaneously can first be appreciated at 3–4 mm from one another, although there is some normal variation in sensitivity from one skin site to another. Since it is quantitatively reproducible, this test can be used for side-to-side comparison as well as day-to-day comparison.

Rapid Alternating Movement and Balance

Rapid alternating movement and balance maneuvers require integrity of many nervous system functions: motor, cerebellar, proprioceptive, and the cortical ability to understand and perform as instructed. They work, therefore, as described under the screening examination. Incoordination of movement, poor balance, and abnormal gait must be assessed by the expanded examinations of each of the nervous system functional components potentially involved.

Additional Maneuvers Indicated in Highly Specific Situations

A few clusters of maneuvers are indicated when the clinician is seeking a specific nervous system abnormality, usually in the emergency or urgent situation. Because of the potential hazard in not adequately evaluating for these findings, the useful physical examination maneuvers are explicated or, if previously described in this text, are referenced.

1. **Possible meningeal irritation:** meningitis or subarachnoid bleeding.
   a. **Brudzinski's** test for **nuchal rigidity (the nape of the neck sign):** With the patient supine, the neck is passively flexed toward the chest by the examiner's hands cradling the occiput. A complaint of neck pain, resistance to flexion, or involuntary flexion of the hips and knees are all considered characteristic of meningeal irritation. This test is positive in 80% of cases of meningitis (Fig. 11.19).
   b. **Brudzinski's contralateral reflex (hip) signs:** When the hip and knee on one side are passively flexed by the examiner (Fig. 11.20*A*), the contralateral leg begins to flex (Fig. 11.20*B*) (**identical contralateral reflex sign**). If the leg that has flexed in response to passive flexion of the other leg begins to extend spontaneously, the **reciprocal contralateral reflex** has occurred. A contralateral reflex was present in 66% of the cases of meningitis reported by Brudzinski a century ago.
   c. **Straight-leg-raising (Lasègue) test:** With the patient supine, the examiner flexes the thigh by lifting the leg by the heel, thus keeping the knee in full extension (Fig. 11.21). A positive sign consists of limitation of hip flexion by pain, involuntary hamstring muscle spasm, or both. In contrast to the positive unilateral straight-leg raising found in localized lumbosacral nerve root irritation, *the meningeal irritation response is bilateral.*
   d. **Kernig's sign:** The examiner seeks this sign in the supine patient by flexing the hip and then sharply extending the knee by raising the patient's heel and knee together (Fig. 11.22*A* and *B*). Reduction in the ability of the knee to fully extend because of pain or hamstring spasm is considered a positive test for meningeal irritation.
2. **Possible increased intracranial pressure (IIP).**
   a. **Funduscopic examination** (see Chapter 4): The examiner looks for loss of venous pulsations, which occurs within minutes of the rise in pressure. Blurring of optic disc margins, elevation of the disc, and edema of the macula—later ophthalmoscopic signs of papilledema—may be delayed

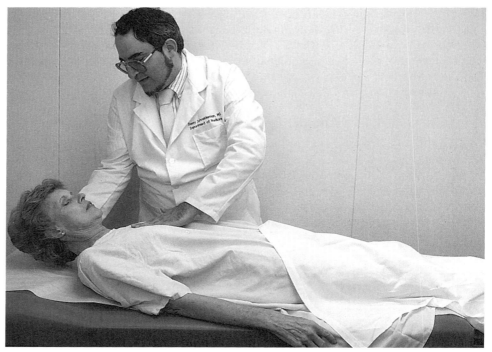

Figure 11.19   Testing for Brudzinski's nape-of-the-neck sign.

24 hours after the pressure rises and may persist 24 hours after it falls, giving rise to misleading information.

b.   Unilateral or bilateral **pupillary dilation,** with decreased or absent light responsiveness.

c.   **Lateral rectus muscle weakness** (see the discussion of "Cranial Nerve VI" in Chapter 4): Bilateral weakness of lateral gaze may be a relatively early sign of IIP.

d.   **Nuchal rigidity** (see Brudzinski's sign above): nonspecific.

e.   **Increasing blood pressure with decreasing pulse rate.**

f.   **Cheyne-Stokes respiratory pattern** (see the Extended Examination section of Chapter 7).

3.   **Abnormal level of consciousness:** For purposes of standardized communication, five levels of consciousness are described:

a.   **Hypervigilant:** This patient is abnormally intensely responsive to even the lightest activity in the environment. This is characteristic of delirium and psychiatric disease.

b.   **Alert:** This patient is normally awake and attentive.

c.   **Lethargic:** This term implies drowsiness, a mild blunting of consciousness, and/or slowed reactions. The lethargic patient is not spontaneous and may show cognitive impairment in other spheres resembling that of one who is demented.

d.   **Stuporous (obtunded):** Severely drowsy and difficult to arouse except with aggressive stimuli, the stuporous patient responds slowly if at all to verbal commands and seems nearly oblivious to the world around him.

e.   **Comatose:** The patient in coma does not respond, except reflexly, to any stimulus. In profound coma, the patient does not even withdraw from

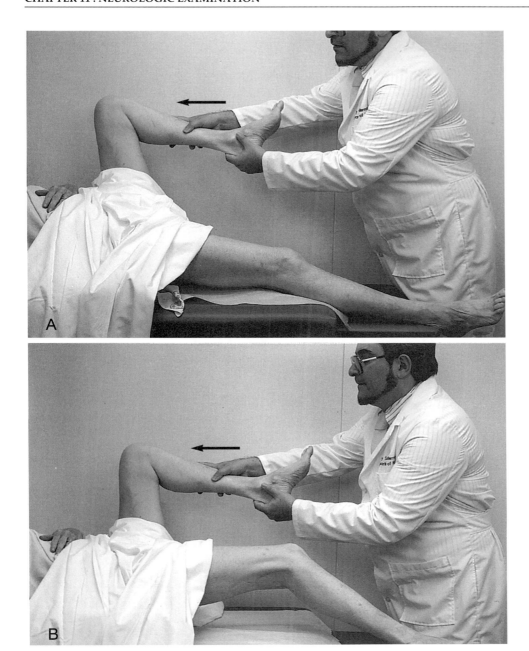

Figure 11.20   Brudzinski's hip signs. **A.** Testing for contralateral reflex. **B.** Involuntary flex-ion of the opposite hip and knee have occurred, a positive sign.

pain. The specific characteristics of coma are determined by its etiology as well as its depth. The reader is referred to textbooks of neurology for features that discriminate one type from another.

INTERPRETING THE FINDINGS

A preliminary analysis of the information gained from an expanded neurologic examination can be made from some basic principles of regional nervous system function.

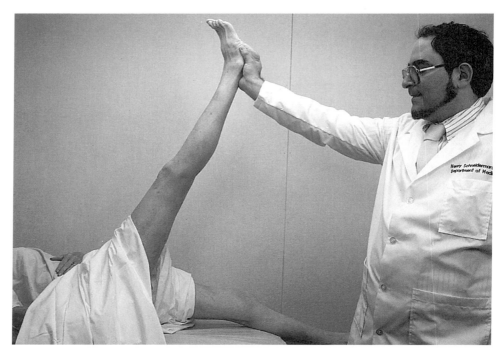

Figure 11.21   Straight-leg-raising (Lasègue) test.

Principles of Regional Nervous System Function

CEREBRAL HEMISPHERES

Symptoms and signs of *cortical disease* concern higher-level integration and inter-pretation of language, memory, intellect, personality, and sensorimotor function. In the majority of persons the **left hemisphere** is **dominant** and therefore controls both written and spoken language and complex motor tasks. Note that 97% of right-handed persons are left-hemisphere dominant, as are some 50% of left-handed persons. Impaired consciousness, intellectual or behavioral aberrations, and impairment of motor and sensory function on both sides of the body suggest **bilateral (or diffuse) hemispheric involvement.**

Certain cortical (and subcortical) functions are lobe specific. **Anterior frontal lobe** disease may impair intellectual function and personality without other neu-rologic signs. **Posterior frontal lobe** lesions involving the motor area result in contralateral monoparesis or hemiparesis. Alter has described a subtle sign of very mild hemiparesis (**digiti quinti sign**) in which the fifth digit of the hand of the affected limb is abducted from its fellows when the patient's arms are extended with palms down and fingers pressed initially into adduction by the examiner, while the digit of the normal side remains adducted.

Cortical sensory defects (i.e., stereognosis, graphesthesia, extinction) and/or failure to recognize one-half of the body (disturbance in body imagery) suggests a contralateral **parietal lobe** lesion. Nonpsychogenic denial of deficit—**anosog-nosia**—usually localizes the lesion to the nondominant parietal lobe.

Most of the visual radiations lie in the **temporal lobes,** such that loss of vision (homonymous hemianopia or quadrantanopsia) indicates a defect contralateral to the defect, e.g., left temporal lobe with right homonymous hemianopia. A domi-nant temporal lobe lesion may also result in receptive aphasia and auditory agnosia.

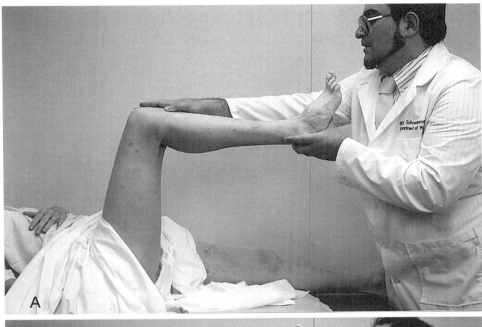

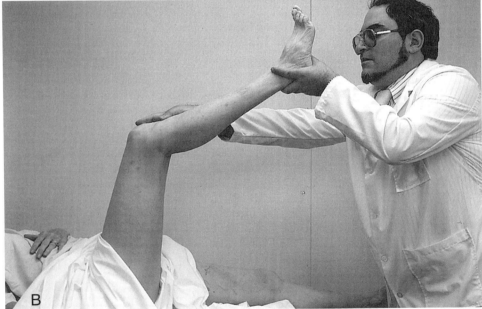

Figure 11.22   Kernig's sign. **A.** Test is begun with both hip and knee flexed to 90°. **B.** Test is completed by assessing whether the knee can then be extended beyond 135°.

Occipital lobe disease is suggested by contralateral homonymous hemianopsia, visual agnosia, and loss of reading comprehension. When bilateral, it can produce the extreme of visual agnosia, cortical blindness.

BASAL NUCLEI AND EXTRAPYRAMIDAL SYSTEM

Most of the movement disorders occur as a result of disease of the extrapyramidal system, with the limb movements occurring contralateral to the brain lesion. Other signs arising in this system are muscle rigidity and slowness of movement (bradykinesia) associated with Parkinson's disease. If the lesions are unilateral, the clinical manifestations are contralateral; more commonly they become bilateral, resulting in widespread dysfunction of all limb and trunk muscles.

DIENCEPHALON

Since disease occurring in the diencephalon results in specific visual symptoms and signs or leads to neuroendocrine and/or metabolic dysfunction, the reader is referred to Chapter 4 and to standard textbooks of medicine for systemic manifestations of disease of the hypothalamus and the pituitary gland.

CEREBELLUM

Three general cerebellar dysfunction patterns correlate with its anatomy:

1. **Cerebellar hemispheres** modulate motor activity, and each is related to the opposite motor cortex; therefore, a unilateral cerebellar hemispheric lesion will result in dysfunction on the **ipsilateral** side of the body, since the cortical fibers have already crossed the midline when they reach the cerebellum. Muscle hypotonia, loss of coordination, and ataxia with falling toward the abnormal side are all signs indicative of cerebellar hemisphere disease.
2. Wide-based gait ataxia, falling to both sides, and *truncal ataxia* characterize lesions of the midline **vermis.**
3. **Diffuse cerebellar disease,** i.e., involvement of all portions by toxins or encephalitis, leads to generalized ataxia (limb and trunk), speech ataxia, and bilateral nystagmus, often vertical or rotatory. In the specific instance of alcoholic cerebellar dysfunction, testing of rapid-alternating movements in the hands gives normal results, but the patient cannot perform the heel-to-shin maneuver normally.

PONS AND MEDULLA

Because of the dense packing of sensory and motor tracts that traverse this region, even small lesions can produce multiple functional deficits. Cranial nerve nuclei V–XII also cluster here. For the vast array of clinical syndromes related to tiny lesions in the pons and medulla, the reader is referred to neurology texts.

SPINAL CORD

Regardless of its axial location, a lesion of the spinal cord, either intrinsic or externally compressing it, will eventually result in (*a*) segmental signs (lower motor

Table 11.5
Signs of Upper versus Lower Motor Neuron Disease

	Upper Motor Neuron	Lower Motor Neuron
Tone	Spastic,[a] greater in flexors of arms, extensors of legs	Flaccid
Reflexes	Accentuated stretch reflexes[a]	Normal, decreased, or absent
Babinski	Present	Absent
Clonus	Frequently present	Absent
Muscle bulk	Slight atrophy of disuse only, late	Atrophy, often marked
Fasciculations	No	Yes

[a]Note that very shortly after an injury to the brain or spinal cord, upper motor neuron signs may be lacking, and there may even be falsely localizing lower motor neuron signs. This transient state is known as **cerebral shock** or **spinal shock,** respectively, notwithstanding that it produces no hypotension.

neuron signs, see Table 11.5), dermatomal sensory loss (Fig. 11.4), and reflex depression or loss and (*b*) long tract signs, both sensory and motor.

Lesions of the **conus medullaris,** which is the inferior termination of the "solid" part of the cord as it "breaks up" into the cauda equina, can give rise to bilateral lower motor neuron signs in the legs (particularly below the knee), impairment of bowel and bladder sphincter function, and sensory loss in the "saddle area" of the perineum.

The **cauda equina** consists of anterior and posterior roots from the lower levels of the cord. Lesions involving the cauda also often involve the conus, so the clinical picture may be mixed. Lower motor neuron paralysis involving both the thigh and leg, often asymmetrical in severity, associated with reduction of patellar and Achilles reflexes, dermatomal sensory loss below the upper lumbar segments, and bladder and rectal dysfunction characterize the cauda equina syndrome. Pain is usually a prominent symptom, and positive straight-leg-raising response may be bilateral.

NERVE ROOTS

See Chapter 12 for a complete discussion of lower (L1–S1) nerve roots.

PERIPHERAL NERVES

Disease of the peripheral nerves is usually spoken of as falling into one of three categories:

1. Polyneuropathy: Many peripheral nerves are involved. Systemic in etiology, it is usually symmetrical and worse in the lower limbs. Motor signs are those of the lower neurons with muscle weakness, atrophy, and often fasciculations. The skin may be abnormally sensitive with spontaneous paresthesias. Involvement of autonomic fibers in the nerve may result in trophic skin changes, loss of hair, and edema and erythema resulting from vasodilatation.
2. Mononeuritis multiplex: Single nerves at various (unpredictable) sites are damaged. This condition is systemic in etiology, **spotty** in distribution, and widely variable in magnitude of involvement.
3. Mononeuropathy: A single nerve, usually a large nerve, is involved. Most often, mononeuropathy is secondary to local mechanical compression, e.g. entrapment neuropathy.

SELECTED SAMPLES OF NEUROLOGIC SYNDROMES

As you proceed with each segment of the extended examination, you may come up with certain constellations of symptoms and signs that can be categorized for problem solving. We make no (false) attempt to be comprehensive here; rather, we suggest a selection of useful clusters. For the next steps, those of constructing a differential etiologic diagnosis, the reader is referred to textbooks of neurology.

Cortical Function

Loss of higher cortical functions such as intellect, memory, rational behavior, reasoning ability, or orientation with disproportionately less impairment in other neurologic function is generically referred to as **dementia.** The causes of "pure" dementia are many, with primary degenerative dementia (Alzheimer disease, i.e., "senile dementia of the Alzheimer type") being the commonest in the United States. Functional loss of cortex may be part of a host of metabolic and neurologic disorders also. Psychiatric disease may initially mimic dementia, e.g., the **pseudodementia** of depression. On the other hand, isolated loss of speech or impairment in the language spheres is most commonly due to focal disease such as vascular occlusion or neoplasia and is usually accompanied by evidence of anatomically consistent motor or sensory loss. Sudden *global aphasia* without motor loss is seen in a few embolic strokes and other multifocal processes (e.g., cerebral metastases of carcinoma). In contrast, gradual-onset loss of speech and comprehension without motor loss, in the context of cognitive loss, is typical of dementing illness.

Motor Function

Interpretation of motor loss begins with an understanding of the anatomical level of the lesion. The **upper motor neuron (UMN)** lesion may lie in the cerebral cortex, the corticobulbar tracts, or the corticospinal tracts; the **lower motor neuron (LMN)** lesion involves the anterior horn cells of the spinal cord or their axons. UMN lesions typically cause muscle weakness with increased tone (spasticity), accentuated muscle stretch reflexes, and a Babinski sign, whereas the LMN lesion results in weakness with hypotonia, muscle wasting, and fasciculations, reduced or absent reflexes, and no Babinski sign. See Table 11.5 for the features differentiating upper from lower motor neuron disease.

The differentiation of motor lesions of the brain and cord from those of peripheral nerves is generally straightforward. By contrast, clinical distinction between forms of flaccid weakness—caused by anterior horn cell, nerve root, plexus, peripheral nerve, myoneural junction, and, to a lesser extent, primary muscle disorders—is not always possible. Some "rules of thumb" are useful, as long as the clinician recognizes that there are variants and exceptions:

1. Classic *nerve root* problems cause weakness, pain, sensory loss, and reflex depression exclusively in the distribution of the affected nerve(s).
2. *Plexus* or multiple nerve root lesions produce parallel symptoms and signs that extend over multiple nerve root distributions, both sensory and motor.
3. Weakness, decreased stretch reflexes, and decreased sensation over a distinct peripheral nerve course or in a stocking-glove pattern point at *peripheral neuropathy,* although they do not pinpoint the site of disease, e.g., cell body, axon, or sheath.
4. Muscle weakness without sensory loss may be *either neuronal or myopathic.* Atrophy may occur in either but is usually more marked with neural disease. Muscle stretch reflexes are diminished or lost when the nerve is involved, but they tend to be preserved if the problem arises in the muscle. In the setting of profound myogenic weakness, however, reflexes may become undetectable. Muscle fasciculation strongly suggests a neural rather than a primary muscular disorder.

Sensory Loss

The pattern of sensory losses in an alert, cooperative, and articulate patient is an excellent key to lesion localization. Table 11.6 summarizes the most common patterns. Careful physical examination to map the borders of deficient areas can provide rather precise anatomical placement. You can also find yourself on a wild goose chase if the patient is a fabricator, malingerer, or psychiatrically disturbed.

Coordination, Balance, and Gait

Since coordination, balance, and gait are integrative functions, the examiner must find intact motor, sensory, and muscular function before assuming an integrative or cerebellar abnormality is responsible for a deficit. The following clusters of dysfunction are suggestive of regional disease:

Table 11.6
Common Sensory Loss Patterns

Site of Lesion	Distribution of Sensory Loss
Cerebral hemispheres	Contralateral face and body: loss of discrimination and/or integration
Brainstem	Ipsilateral face/contralateral body: loss of pain and temperature
Transverse section of spinal cord, complete	Below level of lesion: bilateral loss all sensory modalities
Hemitransection of spinal cord (Brown-Séquard syndrome)	Below level of lesion: ipsilateral loss of position sense and vibration, contralateral loss of pain and temperature
Posterior columns, spinal cord	Below level of lesion: bilateral loss or attenuation of position sense (proprioception) and vibration
Spinal nerve roots	Variable, may have none at all (see also Fig. 11.4)
Polyneuropathy	Varying degrees of loss in stocking-glove distribution, gradually improving from distal to proximal
Major peripheral nerves	See Fig. 11.5

1. Hypotonia, difficulty in performing tests of coordination, and imbalance of stance or a wide-based gait even with **eyes open** implies cerebellar disease.
2. Lack of coordination and impaired accuracy of gait and stance with **eyes closed** that correct when the patient **watches his movements** suggests proprioceptive dysfunction, although cerebellar dysfunction with visual compensation is an alternative explanation.
3. Cogwheel rigidity, a shuffling gait with knees and arms slightly flexed, armswing diminution or loss, and **festination** (progressive increase in rate of tiny steps such that the patient's legs seem to be trying to catch up with the trunk) are typical of the common basal nucleus disorder known as parkinsonism. This occurs spontaneously, as well as after exposure to neuroleptic drugs such as haloperidol.

RECORDING THE FINDINGS

Following is the neurologic examination of a 72-year-old right-handed man whose chief complaint is "I'm slowing down."

Mental status: Appears slightly depressed; slow to respond to questions, although responses are accurate. Oriented × 3. Language and speech functions all normal; Folstein score 26/30 points, with loss on concentration items.

Cranial nerves: II–XII within normal limits.

Motor: Facies symmetric, not mask-like. Strength normal. Cogwheel rigidity in elbow flexors, left. Otherwise, muscle tone and bulk normal. "Pill-rolling" tremor, left hand at rest, 4 cycles/second, disappears on intention. No arm drift.

Reflexes: Muscle stretch reflexes 2+ and symmetrical throughout. Plantar responses downgoing.

Sensory: Light touch, pain, and proprioception all normal. Diminution of vibratory sense both ankles; vibration normal at knees and hands.

Cerebellar: Rapid alternating movement slowed but accurate both upper limbs; finger-to-nose, heel-to-shin slow but accurate. Romberg intact.

Cortex: No cortical release signs. Two-point discrimination normal.

Gait: Slow, mildly shuffling, not festinating. Right arm swing normal; left arm held slightly flexed with very little swing. Can accomplish only two steps of tandem walking, complaining of feeling unsteady, but walks on heels and toes. Takes three small steps to turn.

Impressions: Left basal ganglia disease, early parkinsonism; overlay of depression.

BEYOND THE PHYSICAL EXAMINATION

The past two decades have seen a revolution in the special studies available for refined neurologic diagnoses. New imaging techniques have rendered many older radiographic studies, such as pneumoencephalography, obsolete. Accuracy and precision of definition of small lesions in the central nervous system by means of costly, high-technology procedures provide exciting new possibilities for extending the findings of careful neurologic history and physical assessment. As with any innovative technology, the temptation to bypass the sometimes tedious physical examination and leap directly to computed tomography (CT) or magnetic resonance imaging (MRI) can become overwhelming. The skilled clinician will continue to use primary physical assessment skills to narrow the differential diagnosis as far as possible before ordering these tests. Why? Not merely to honor tradition, but to benefit patients. When imaging studies are needed, they prove most useful. When substituted for thorough history and neurologic examination, they have the potential for becoming unacceptably expensive and diagnostically confusing or even misleading (at times with fatal consequences for patients). First, interview and examine carefully; then, with a cogent differential diagnosis in hand, consider the need for one or more of the procedures discussed below.

Brain Dysfunction

1. Selected **radiographic views of the skull,** including tomography, are of help in assessing for depressed or basilar skull fracture.
2. **Bloodwork** may help discover *treatable* systemic metabolic or endocrine bases for dementia or delirium. While a full discussion calls for a textbook of neurology, the commonest "treatable dementia panel" studies include electrolytes, with calcium, glucose, BUN, arterial blood gases, thyroid function tests, B_{12} and folate levels, VDRL and FTA-Abs, HIV antibodies, and lead and fasting ammonia levels.
3. **Lumbar puncture (LP)** with Gram staining, culture, counterimmunoelectrophoresis, and acid-fast studies of the cerebrospinal fluid (CSF) remain the mainstay of specific diagnosis of central nervous system infection, particularly when meningitis is suspected. Testing is also done for cryptococcosis, especially in AIDS patients. CSF cytology is a major means of discovering carcinomatosis, while CSF VDRL and Lyme titers are used to diagnose neurosyphilis and borreliosis, respectively. Oligoclonal protein analysis assists in the diagnosis of multiple sclerosis.
4. **Electroencephalography (EEG)** is essential in the study of seizure disorders and is useful in following the course of metabolic or toxic cortical dysfunction.
5. **CT and MRI** are indicated when it is important to (*a*) assess brain or ventricular volumes, (*b*) search for mass lesions, (*c*) define the size and nature of suspected strokes, and (*d*) study the dynamics of CSF flow.
6. **Cerebral angiography** is essential for planning possible surgical interventions for vascular lesions and some tumors and occasionally for confirming thrombosis, hemorrhage, or vasculitis.
7. **Brain biopsy** may be required to confirm infection with herpes simplex virus (HSV) or, in the patient with AIDS, to differentiate between toxoplasmosis and lymphoma.

8. **Auditory evoked potential (AEP) and visual evoked potential (VEP)** are useful in the workup of the patient suspected of having multiple sclerosis and in sensory testing of patients with severe mental retardation who cannot cooperate at the bedside.
9. **Neuropsychologic testing** is sometimes necessary when neurologic signs and symptoms raise the possibility of psychiatric or dementing disorder.

Spinal Cord or Nerve Root Disease

1. **Radiography** of the spine is still vital in assessing for bone disease, fracture, loss of alignment, and structural anomalies. For bone density bearing on neurologic symptoms, bone densitometry appears to be preferable.
2. **Radioisotope scanning** of the spine is sometimes useful in localizing and differentiating infectious from neoplastic and metabolic bone lesions.
3. **CT and MRI** have refined the ability to localize cord tumors and extruded disc material.
4. **Electromyography** and nerve conduction velocity testing are sometimes useful in confirmation and localization of nerve function loss.
5. **Myelography,** alone or combined with CT or MRI, retains a selected role in localizing and defining the extent of nerve root compression, especially when surgical intervention is being considered.

Peripheral Nerve and Muscle Disorders

1. **Electromyography and nerve conduction studies** are indicated when there is confusion about the site of the process causing muscle weakness and/or sensory loss, e.g., neural versus primary muscle disease.
2. **Bloodwork** carefully tailored to the differential diagnoses is very helpful in confirming or ruling out certain metabolic, endocrine, toxic, genetic, and immune myopathies and neuropathies. Blood creatine phosphokinase and aldolase levels can rise with muscle damage from any cause.
3. **Muscle** and, less commonly, **nerve biopsies** may be required for definitive diagnosis.
4. Blood **Lyme titers** are now routine in facial (Bell's) palsy, since borreliosis is a common cause of this disorder.

RECOMMENDED READINGS

Adams RD, Victor M. Principles of neurology. 5th ed. New York: McGraw-Hill, 1992.

Alter M. The digiti quinti sign of mild hemiparesis. Neurology 1973;23:503–505.

Chimowitz MI, Logigian EL, Caplan LR. The accuracy of bedside neurological diagnoses. Ann Neurol 1990;28:78–85.

DeMyer W. Technique of the neurologic examination: a programmed text. 3rd ed. New York: McGraw-Hill, 1980.

Editor. Forgotten symptoms and primitive signs. Lancet 1987;1:841–842.

Folstein MF, Folstein S, McHugh PR. Mini-mental state: a practical method for grading the cognitive state of patients for the clinician. J Psychiatr Res 1975;12:189–198.

Gray CS, Walker A. The plantar response: caution in the elderly. Br J Hosp Med 1989;42:105–106.

Jacobs JW, Bernhard MR, Delgado A, Strain JJ. Screening for organic mental syndromes in the medically ill. Ann Intern Med 1977;86:40–46.

Jacoby R. Loss of memory and concentration. Br J Hosp Med 1985;33:32–44.

Keane JR. Neuro-ophthalmic signs and symptoms of hysteria. Neurology 1982;32:757–762.

Kiernan RJ, Mueller J, Langston JW, Van Dyke C. The neurobehavioral cognitive status examination: a brief but differentiated approach to cognitive assessment. Ann Intern Med 1987;107:481–485.

Landau WM. Training of the neurologist for the 21st century. Arch Neurol 1989;46:21–22.

Landau WM. Strategy, tactics, and accuracy in neurological evaluation. Ann Neurol 1990;28:86–87.

Levin BE. The clinical significance of spontaneous pulsations of the retinal vein. Arch Neurol 1978;35:37–40.

Mackinnon SE, Dellon AL. Two-point discrimination tester. J Hand Surg 1985;10A:906–907.

Massey EW, Scherokman B. Soft neurologic signs. Postgrad Med 1981;70:66–70.

Molloy DW, Alemayehu E, Roberts R. Reliability of a standardized mini-mental state examination compared with the traditional mini-mental state examination. Am J Psychiatry 1991;148:102–105.

Munetz MR, Benjamin S. How to examine patients using the abnormal involuntary movement scale. Hosp Community Psychiatry 1988;39:1172–1177.

Nelson KR. Use new pins for each neurologic examination. N Engl J Med 1986;314:581.

Schneiderman H. Mental status examination. In: Willms JW, Lewis J, eds. Introduction to clinical medicine. Media, Pennsylvania: Harwal, 1990:112–115.

Schwartz RS, Morris JGL, Crimmins D, Wilson A, Fahey P, Reid S, Joffe R. A comparison of two methods of eliciting the ankle jerk. Aust N Z J Med 1990;20:116–119.

Van Horn G, Hawes A. Global aphasia without hemiparesis: a sign of embolic encephalopathy. Neurology 1982;32:403–406.

Verghese A, Gallemore G. Kernig's and Brudzinski's signs revisited. Rev Infect Dis 1987;9:1187–1192.

Walshe TM. Neurologic examination of the elderly patient: signs of normal aging. Postgrad Med 1987;81:375–378.

Wartenberg R. The Babinski reflex after fifty years. JAMA 1947;135:763–767.

Ziegler DK. Is the neurologic examination becoming obsolete? Neurology 1985;35:559.

12

Lower Back

SCREENING EXAMINATION OF THE LOWER BACK

APPROACH AND ANATOMICAL REVIEW

Examination of the back is begun as a part of the examination of the neck (Chapter 5) and is continued during the assessment of the thorax (Chapter 7). It is completed, with the patient standing, with the inspection, palpation, and assessment of range of motion of the lower back and the pelvic girdle.

Below the twelve thoracic vertebrae and in alignment with them are (a) the larger **lumbar vertebrae** (five), (b) the usually fused **sacral vertebrae** (five), and (c) the tapering fused **coccygeal vertebrae** (four). This chapter concerns the spine from L1 down and its associated structures. Each **ilium** articulates with the sacrum (Fig. 12.1A). Between each vertebral body and the next lies a fibrocartilaginous **intervertebral disc.** Each disc contains a fibrogelatinous core called the **nucleus pulposus.** See Figure 12.1B for a lateral view of the relationships of these components of the lumbosacral spine. The spinal column and pelvis are supported and moved by the major **muscles** of the back and of the buttocks.

Important surface landmarks of the back include the previously noted protuberant **spinous process** of the **seventh cervical vertebra** and the lesser prominences of the other vertebral spinous processes, the longitudinal paramedian depression created by the long erector muscles along both sides of the **spinal column,** the tips of the **scapulae,** the **crests of each ilium,** the **gluteal cleft,** bilateral dimples over the **sacroiliac (SI) joints,** and the **gluteal folds** (Fig. 12.2A). Viewed laterally, the spine has three visible **curves.** The minimal concave **cervical curve** begins at C2 and ends at T2 (physiologic cervical lordosis), the **thoracic curve** is convex from T2 through T12 (physiologic dorsal kyphosis), and the concave **lumbar curve** involves the lumbar vertebrae (physiologic lumbar lordosis). The **pelvic curve** of the sacrococcyx forms a convexity that is not visible or directly palpable on physical examination (Fig. 12.2B) except per rectum.

TECHNIQUE

This lower back examination is done with the patient standing. Full exposure of the posterior trunk and legs is accomplished by having the patient wear an examination gown with the opening of the gown in the back, such that it covers the anterior body but can be separated to allow full view of the back. Preferably, the feet are bare to permit optimal assessment of gait. See Table 12.1 for the sequence of the examination.

Inspection

Facing the patient's back, after having done a careful inspection of the skin of the buttocks, thighs, and legs, observe the **alignment** of the spine, the scapulae, the iliac crests, and the gluteal folds. Assess the **curves** of the spine from the patient's side. Ask the patient to walk away from you, so that ordinary **gait** may be observed.

Palpation

Palpate the **lumbar** and the **sacral spine** for tenderness and the long **paraspinal** muscles for tenderness or spasm. With your palms placed on the posterior iliac

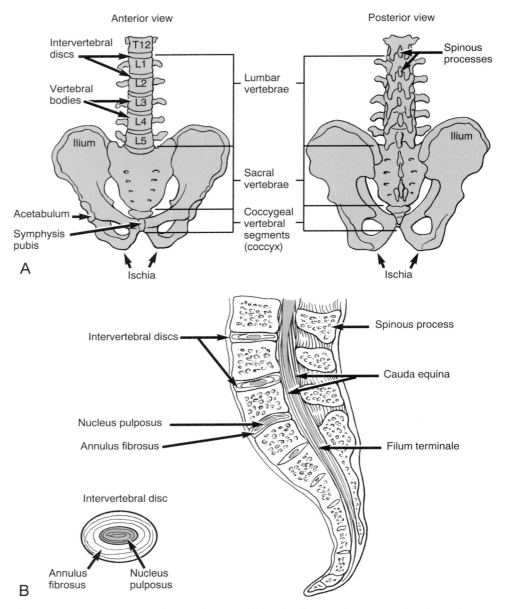

Figure 12.1   A. Bones and articulations of the lumbosacral spine and pelvis, shown schematically in anterior and posterior views. **B.** Sagittal section of the lumbosacral vertebrae illustrates the relationship of the vertebral bodies, the spinous processes, and the nucleus pulposus (intervertebral disc) lying between the vertebral bodies.

crests on each side of the patient's spine, put your thumbs over the dimples that mark the sites of the **sacroiliac joints.** Assess the joints for tenderness or swelling by pressing them firmly (Fig. 12.3). (See also Patrick's test in the Extended Examination section of Chapter 10).

Range of Motion

HIP EXTENSION

Note that **extension of the hip joint** is assessed at this time by asking the patient to hyperextend each leg posteriorly while supporting himself at the end of the

Table 12.1
Sequence of the Screening Back Examination[a]

Inspection	Percussion
Skin of buttocks, posterior thighs and legs	Spinous processes
Spinal alignment (examiner facing patient's back)	
Spinal curves (examiner at patient's side, right or left)	Range of motion
Gait	Hip joint extension
	Back
Palpation	Flexion
Dorsal processes of spine (spinous processes)	Extension
Paraspinal muscles	Lateral motion
Sacroiliac articulations	Rotation

[a]All maneuvers of the screening examination are done with the patient standing.

examining table. Alternatively, if the patient feels insecure standing on only one leg, he may bend over the end of the examining table and raise each leg backward as far as it will extend (Fig. 12.4*A* and *B*).

Flexion of the spine. Ask the patient to bend forward as far as possible, keeping the knees straight. Standing behind the patient, observe the movement of the spine, the symmetry of the scapular wings, and the curvature of the flexed spine.

Extension of the spine. Ask the patient to bend backward at the waist; note the degree of extension achieved.

Lateral motion of the spine. Ask the patient, standing with his feet slightly separated, to bend at the waist (but not to rotate) to each side. Assess the lateral flexion movement for degree and symmetry.

Rotation of the spine. Place your hands on the patient's iliac crests to fix the pelvis, and ask the patient to *rotate* the upper body first to one side and then to the other. Note the degree of rotation.

For illustration of the techniques of the back motion assessment and the expected normal ranges, see Figure 12.5.

NORMAL AND COMMON VARIANTS

Inspection

On inspection from behind the patient the spine appears straight. An imaginary line dropped from the crown of the head should overlie all the spinous processes of the vertebrae and meet the gluteal cleft. Parallel horizontal planes are formed by the two shoulders, inferior tips of the scapulae, posterior iliac crests, and infragluteal folds. The angles between each of these planes and the vertical midline should be 90° (Fig. 12.2*A*).

Occasionally, a lateral midspinal curve (**scoliosis**) is entirely **postural** and will disappear with maximal spinal flexion. If there is a slight **inequality in leg length** (see the Extended Examination section of Chapter 10), a compensatory pelvic tilt may lead to a **functional scoliosis.** When difference in leg length is suspected as the basis for spinal curvature or asymmetry of level of the iliac crests, the leg length is measured for confirmation in the following way: With the patient lying supine and legs spread very slightly, a cloth tape measure is stretched from just beneath the anterior superior iliac crest along the length of the leg, crossing medially near the knee, and brought to the inferior margin of the **medial** malleolus. Each leg is thus measured for length. Any difference greater than 1 cm may account for or contribute to a pelvic tilt and subsequent scoliosis. Once the inequality in leg length is determined, the difference is made up and the patient is equilibrated by having the patient stand and then place the sole of

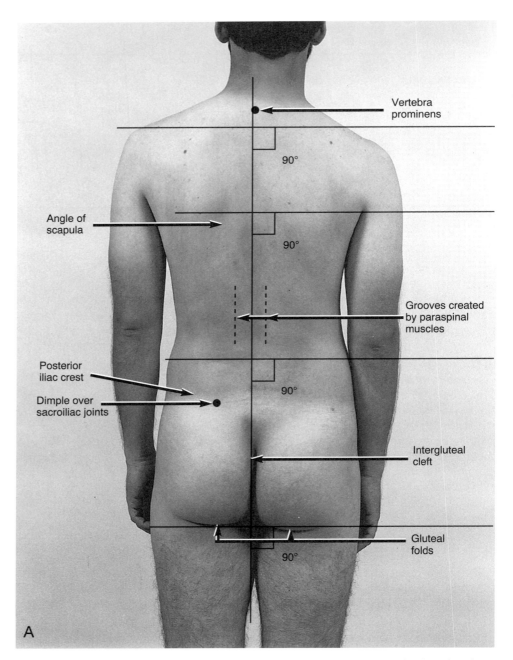

Figure 12.2   A. Posterior skin landmarks are superimposed on the normal back with indication of the *perpendicular (right) angles* that should coincide with the alignment of the spine in relationship to the shoulders, the tips of the scapulae, the posterior iliac crests, and the gluteal folds. **B.** Lateral view of the back showing the expected curvatures of each portion of the normal vertebral column, with the invisible sacrococcygeal curve superimposed.

the foot of the shorter leg on a measured lift (pad of paper, block of Styrofoam, etc.). The spine is reassessed for curvature with the inequality in leg length thus compensated.

Normal anteroposterior spinal curves are variable. Dorsal kyphosis is discussed in Chapter 7. The concavity of the **lumbar curve** (**lordosis**) is exaggerated

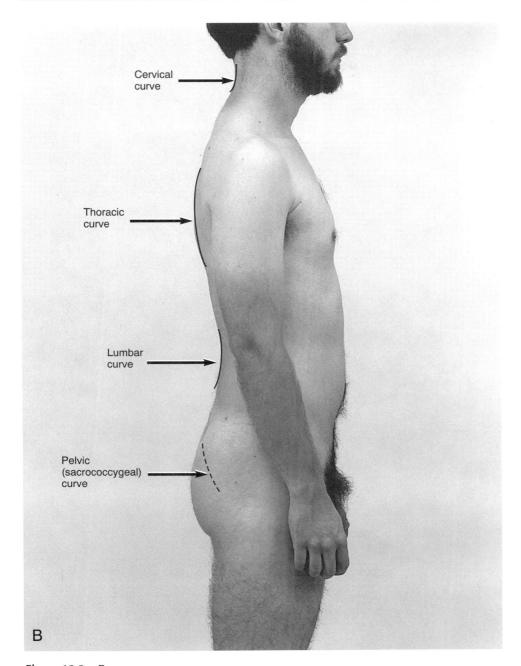

Figure 12.2   B.

in **obesity** and **pregnancy** as compensation for protuberance of the abdomen. There is also some normal individual and racial variability in the degree of lumbar curve. A **flattening** of the lumbar curve suggests paraspinal muscle spasm or disease of the vertebral articulations. This is rarely seen as a normal (or an asymptomatic) variant.

Palpation

On **palpation** there is no tenderness to finger pressure or light percussion with fist or percussion hammer over the **spinous processes.** When palpated bilater-

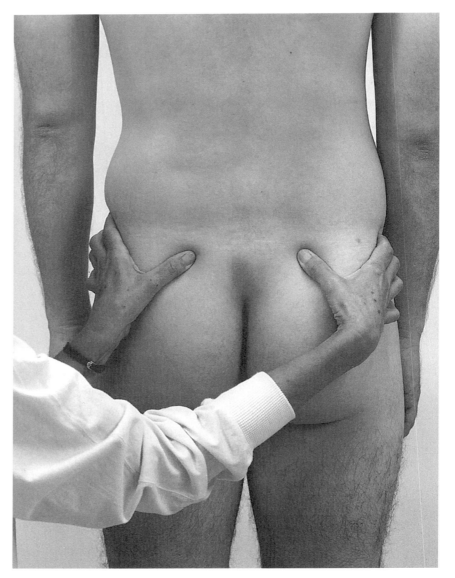

Figure 12.3 Technique for palpation of sacroiliac joints. Note position of examiner's thumbs pressing over both joints in search of swelling or local tenderness.

ally, the mass and tension of the **back muscles** are symmetrical. These muscles should be nontender. The **sacroiliac** joints are equally flat, firm, and nontender to deep pressure.

Range of Motion

Assessment of **range of motion** should meet the criteria shown in Figure 12.5. With aging, some loss of spinal flexibility is to be expected; however, any pain on movement or a greater than 20% reduction of expected motion in any plane suggests neuromuscular, articular, or bone disease and requires more detailed assessment (see the Extended Examination section).

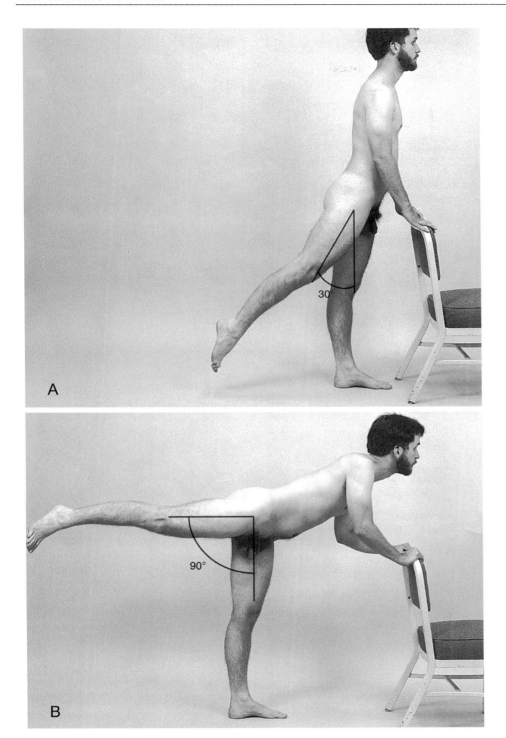

Figure 12.4 Range of hip extension. **A.** Lateral inspection with patient standing on one leg and extending hip as far as possible. Expect 30° from the vertical. **B.** Patient supporting himself with back of chair (or bent over examining table) to achieve maximal hyperextension of the hip to 90° to the vertical.

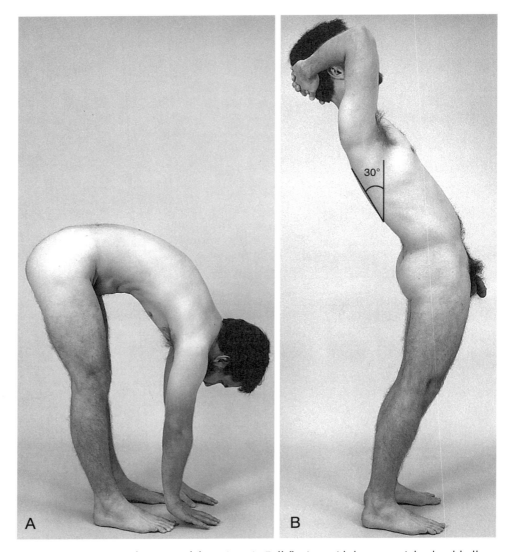

Figure 12.5   Range of motion of the spine. **A.** Full flexion with knees straight should allow the patient to place the fingertips or, in the case of a healthy young adult, the palms nearly flat on the floor. **B.** Extension in standing position is expected to approximate 30° to the vertical. **C.** Lateral bending (right and left) normally reaches 35° to the vertical. **D.** Rotation (with examiner's hands fixing the pelvis) to right and left at 35–40°.

RECORDING THE FINDINGS

The findings on the back examination are conventionally recorded with or immediately after those of the MUSCULOSKELETAL system. A sample recording of the back examination follows:

Lower back: Slight C-shaped scoliosis, convex to left, disappears completely with flexion. Otherwise alignment normal, as is standard gait. Lumbar lordosis normal. Spinous processes, paraspinal muscles, and SI joints normal to palpation. Flexion, extension, lateral bending, and rotation of lumbar spine all normal.

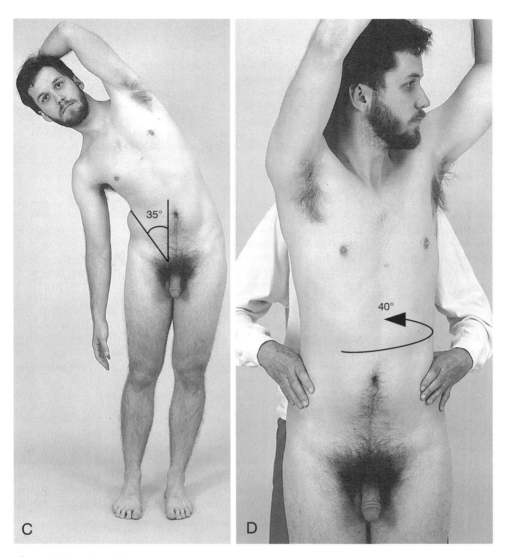

Figure 12.5   C and D.

EXTENDED EXAMINATION OF THE LOWER BACK

In the literature, there are large numbers of special physical examination maneuvers available for assessment of the back. In the presence of specific indications from the history or of unexpected abnormalities detected on the screening examination, the clinician undertakes to choose among these in order to do a more detailed evaluation. We present some of the more common and/or reliable special maneuvers utilized by the primary care provider in the extended assessment of a patient with back complaints or abnormalities on the screening examination. The results of the findings on the extended back examination will dictate any necessary radiographic or laboratory investigations.

INDICATIONS

Far and away the most common indication for special physical examination maneuvers related to the back is the complaint of **pain in the back and/or radiating down one leg.** Rarely will the examiner find on screening examination a previously unknown or unexpected abnormality of any import that has not been anticipated by a history of pain. The indications for special maneuvers are discussed in relationship to their potential differential diagnoses and are summarized in Table 12.2.

Indications Derived from the History
Pain in the Back

Pain in the back may be either chronic or acute and either related to trauma or without apparent antecedent. The considerations for possible diagnoses are categorized accordingly in the following discussion.

Chronic or recurrent back pain. The chronology and details of the parameters of the pain are key to approaching an explanation. The age and sex of the patient are important in formulating hypotheses. For example, a clinician would not strongly consider osteoporosis and its complications in a young man nor ankylosing spondylitis in an elderly woman. Prior therapy and its efficacy provide critical insights, as do aggravating and alleviating factors. Several common and significant causes of chronic back pain are briefly considered below. For more detail on each entity, the reader is referred to textbooks of medicine, rheumatology, and orthopedics.

The most common basis for chronic low back pain is **lumbosacral strain,** an entity found in both sexes and all ages. The complaint is that of daily aching or recurrent bouts of moderately disabling pain in the low back without clear-cut traumatic antecedent. This musculotendinous-skeletal problem must always be differentiated from the symptoms of a progressively deteriorating and protruding **intervertebral disc** and, in the older patient, from **osteoarthrosis.** The inflammatory articular disease known as **ankylosing spondylitis** occurs predominantly in young adults, most often men, whereas the discomfort of progressive bone loss and anterior compression of vertebral bodies (compression fractures) seen in **osteoporosis** is age-related and much more common in women. **Spondylolisthesis** presents as a complication of a congenital weakness or a fracture in the lower lumbosacral area and is much less common than the other diseases discussed. **Primary bone or marrow cancer** including **multiple myeloma** and **metastatic cancer** in the spine may present as chronic back pain, typically progressive.

Acute back pain with a history of trauma. A clear temporal relationship between direct trauma to the back—such as from a fall in which the spine takes the brunt of the stress or from total-body trauma in which the back may be one of many structures involved—and the onset of sudden pain directs the clinician to specific sites in the back and to a consideration of *fracture.* The **fracture of a vertebral body** may occur with minor trauma or even spontaneously in the predisposed osteoporotic spine or with major trauma to a healthy spinal column. Direct blows may lead to the less common **fractures** of a **transverse process** or of **lamina(e)** of one or more vertebrae. **Metastatic malignancy** involving any portion of the vertebrae predisposes to *pathologic fracture* and must be considered in the differential diagnosis of acute localized back pain related to what appears to be disproportionately mild trauma. The integrity of supporting ligaments plays a major role in the stability of any spinal fracture and thus in the potential for spinal cord damage.

Acute back pain without a history of trauma. Both **lumbosacral strain** and **herniated intervertebral disc** may occur without a history of specific trauma. The

Table 12.2
Common Back Problems Emerging in History or Screening Examination[a, b]

From the medical history
  Pain in the back
    Chronic or recurrent pain
      Lumbosacral strain
      Protruding intervertebral disc material (HNP)
      Osteoarthrosis
      Ankylosing spondylitis
      Other spondylitides, e.g., Reiter's syndrome
      Osteoporosis or osteomalacia with vertebral body collapse
      Spondylolisthesis
    Acute pain with history of trauma
      Compression fracture of vertebral body
      Fracture of transverse process of vertebra(e)
      Fracture of lamina(e) of vertebra(e)
      Malignancy of vertebra(e), metastatic or primary
    Acute pain without history of trauma
      Lumbosacral strain
      Herniated intervertebral disc or disc fragments (HNP)
      Osteoporosis with spontaneous collapse of vertebrae
      Neoplasm
  Pain radiating down one leg
    Herniated intervertebral disc (HNP)
    Dorsal root irritation from malignant disease of spine
    Involvement of dorsal root or column with neoplasm of the spinal cord
    Sciatic nerve irritation due to inflammation or entrapment at the sciatic notch of pelvis
  Paresthesias in nerve root distribution of an extremity
    Herniated intervertebral disc (HNP)
    Nerve root irritation from malignant disease of spine
    Entrapment in intervertebral foramen due to osteoarthrosis
    Involvement of nerve root or spinal column with neoplasm of the spinal cord
  Localized tenderness or pain over vertebra(e)
    Neoplastic involvement of spine
    Inflammatory disease of spine, e.g., osteomyelitis, tuberculosis
  Loss of bowel or bladder function (see Chapter 11)
    Neoplastic lesions of spinal cord or spinal column
    Spinal stenosis
    Spondylosis
    (HNP)
  Leg weakness (see Chapters 10 and 11)
  Gait disturbance (see Chapters 10 and 11)

From the screening examination
  Loss of postural height with dorsal kyphosis
    Osteoporosis with anterior vertebral body compression
  Localized tenderness over a dorsal spinous process
    Neoplasm of bone
    Infection of bone
  Marked "C" lateral scoliosis or "S" scoliosis
    Developmental (see Chapter 15)
    Secondary to disc disease, lumbosacral strain, etc.
  Limitation of motion in any plane of spinal movement
    Any disease of spine, spinal articulations, or muscles

[a]Any of the above symptoms and many of the signs can potentially be manifestations of lack of patient cooperation resulting from malingering (desire for secondary gain) or emotional overlay. See text for methods of separating organic from nonorganic disease.
[b]**Boldface** indicates most commonly seen; HNP, herniated nucleus pulposus.

vulnerable **osteoporotic vertebral body** may collapse—typically anterior compression fracture, usually in the thoracic spine—without trauma. **Cancerous bone** also may undergo spontaneous fracture.

Pain Radiating down One Leg

A primary spinal problem may present without clear-cut back symptoms, but with a history of pain in the lateral or posterior thigh, knee, leg, or, less commonly, the foot. The location of the pain depends on the spinal root(s) involved (see Chapter 11), and the etiology could be any of the problems that are known to cause back pain and in which nerve root encroachment occurs. **Sciatica** is the term commonly given to compression or irritation of the sciatic nerve at the sciatic notch through which it leaves the pelvis to enter the posterior thigh.

Paresthesias in a Limb with or without Pain

If a primary spinal problem leads to compression or irritation of the sensory nerve root, such as a posterolateral disc protrusion, the patient's complaint may be numbness and tingling in a specific spinal nerve root distribution (see Chapters 10 and 11).

Localized Tenderness or Pain over the Spine

Malignant or inflammatory disease of any portion of the vertebral column or associated structures may give rise to a complaint of very discrete pain or, more commonly, tenderness to pressure. Fracture can also do this, but *uncomplicated* metabolic bone disease (osteoporosis, osteomalacia, or Paget's disease of bone) should not.

Loss of Normal Bowel or Bladder Function

Neoplastic lesions or compression of the cauda equina or lower sacral cord segments may cause urinary retention, producing a huge bladder, loss of sensation of need to void, and overflow incontinence. Anal sphincter tone impairment with fecal incontinence can also accompany compression syndromes such as spinal stenosis, spondylosis, or herniated nucleus pulposus. These will prompt extended evaluation of both the lower back and the neural structures.

Leg Weakness

Weakness of one or both lower limbs demands careful low back and neurologic examination (see the Extended Examination section of Chapter 11).

Gait Disturbance

An isolated complaint of gait disturbance is rarely attributable to a pure low back syndrome and is discussed in detail in the Extended Examination section of Chapter 11.

Indications Derived from the Screening Examination

Occasionally, without a specific history related to the back or limbs, the clinician discovers an abnormality on the basic back assessment. If any one of the following abnormalities is noted, more extensive maneuvers are indicated.

Loss of Height with Kyphosis

Progressive painless anterior compression of vertebral bodies, especially in the thoracic spine, may lead to increasing kyphosis and overall loss of height. The patient who measured 160 cm in height 10 years ago and who now measures 150 cm offers no other rational differential diagnosis (barring errors of measurement, recording, or transcription).

Unexpected Localized Tenderness over a Spinous Process

Unexpected localized tenderness over a spinous process is rare but, when found, requires confirmation (see the discussion of spinal or paraspinal tenderness under the subheading *Palpation with the Patient Standing*) and further workup.

C-Shaped (Single) or S-Shaped (Double) Scoliosis

Marked C-shaped (single-curvature) scoliosis that does not disappear with flexion and cannot be accounted for by unequal leg length or S-shaped (double-curvature) scoliosis needs further assessment. Scoliosis may be secondary to degenerative disc disease with fragment protrusion and related paraspinal muscle spasm or may be caused by lumbosacral muscle strain. Special maneuvers to evaluate the congenital or progressive developmental scoliosis of children are discussed in Chapter 15.

Limitation of Motion in Any Plane, with or without Pain on Movement

The discovery of unexpected restriction of spinal movement requires assessment by means of the extended examination described below.

CONDUCTING THE EXTENDED EXAMINATION

A set of standard special maneuvers are carried out if any of the indications for extended examination are present. Some maneuvers are relatively specific to confirm a particular hypothesis; however, the clinician needs to know and be prepared to perform all of them during the patient encounter, to utilize the information gained to narrow (or alter) the diagnostic possibilities and to select any necessary special investigations. The extent and detail of the extended examination will, of course, be modified if the patient's physical condition precludes some of the maneuvers.

In the setting of trauma, protection of the spinal cord is paramount and may obviate all manipulation until **after** radiographs are obtained and studied, to exclude any lesion that would threaten cord integrity with the manipulation required for examination. See Table 12.3 for a summary of the special maneuvers in an extended and focused back examination.

Inspection with Patient Standing

Lateral curvature (listing). Look again for subtle lateral curvature (listing). A list or leaning of the body to one side or the other is a reflection of paraspinal muscle spasm or involuntary guarding, usually because of pain. The list, when observed, is characteristically toward the affected side.

Transverse crease. Observe carefully for a transverse crease in the skin of the lower flanks at or above the posterior superior iliac spines.

Schober's flexion test. To perform this test, mark the skin over the vertebral column at the level of the posterior iliac spines and make a second mark 10 cm above the first (Fig. 12.6A). As the patient bends forward in an attempt to touch the floor, measure the new distance between the two marks (Fig. 12.6B). In young adults, an increase of less than 4 cm in this distance indicates impaired flexion characteristically based on inflammatory disease of the articulations of the spine, usually ankylosing spondylitis, and/or inflammation of paraspinous tissue.

Table 12.3
Summary of Extended Maneuvers

Patient standing
  Inspection
    For lateral curvature
    For list
    For transverse crease
    For gap in spinous processes
    Schober's flexion test
  Palpation
    For gap in dorsal spinous
      processes
    For localized spinal tenderness
    For localized paraspinal muscle
      tenderness
    For tenderness or leg pain
      reproduction at sciatic notch

Patient supine
  Observe for position of maximal
    comfort
  Straight-leg-raising test
  Crossed straight-leg-raising test
  Foot dorsiflexion test
  Sensory examination of anterior
    aspects of legs and thighs

Patient prone
  Reverse straight-leg-raising test
  Sensory examination of posterior aspect of
    legs and thighs

Patient sitting
  Muscle stretch, patellar (knee), and Achilles
    (ankle) reflexes
  Muscle group strength

Other special maneuvers when indicated
  Measurement of chest expansion
  Measurement of leg length
  Stoop test
  Tests when lack of cooperation is suspected
    Aird's test
    Bench test

Palpation with Patient Standing

Gap. Palpate the spinous processes for a gap.

Spinal or paraspinal tenderness. Palpate for localized spinal or paraspinal tenderness. If the patient has complained of a painful or a tender area, ask him to point to it, and then mark it with a skin pencil. Return to it at a later point in the examination and ask the patient to show its site by pointing, unprompted by a second touch, to the tender area in question.

Sciatic notch. Palpate the sciatic notch (Fig. 12.6C). With palpation at the **sciatic notch** on the affected side, a complaint of (*a*) pain radiating down one leg or the other, (*b*) an increase in preexisting pain, or (*c*) a reproduction of pain in the radiation previously described by the patient suggests nerve root irritation.

Examination with Patient Supine

Ask the patient to arrange his trunk and legs in the supine position that feels most comfortable to him. Note whether he voluntarily flexes his knees or hips or objects to lying flat on his back because of pain.

Straight-leg raising. This maneuver is carried out by passively lifting each of the patient's extended legs in turn from the examining table and then noting any degree less than 90 at which he begins to complain of pain in the back or down the lifted leg.

Crossed straight-leg raising. Ask the patient to raise the leg *on the pain-free side* to 90° from the table. Note any complaint of exacerbated pain in the affected limb or of pain in the previously unaffected limb (either response is considered a positive crossed straight-leg-raising test).

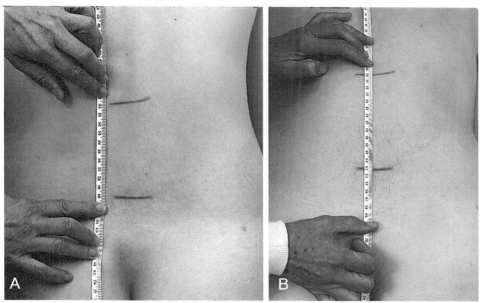

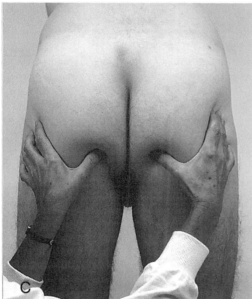

Figure 12.6 Special maneuvers. **A** and **B.** Schober's test for impaired spinal flexion. With the patient standing, a distance of 10 cm is marked off with a skin pencil (**A**). On maximal spinal flexion, the increase in distance between the skin marks should reach or exceed 14 cm (**B**). **C.** Palpation of the sciatic notch. The examiner's thumbs press deeply through the gluteus to the bony notch where the sciatic nerve exits from the pelvis, seeking direct tenderness or reproduction of pain in the thigh or leg.

   Foot dorsiflexion. This test is considered complementary to or a slightly inferior substitute for the straight-leg-raising test. With the patient's legs on the examination table, sharply passively dorsiflex each ankle in turn. A complaint of back pain or a complaint of pain radiating down the leg on the affected side is considered a positive test for nerve root or sciatic nerve irritation.
   Sensory examination. See Chapter 11.

Examination with Patient Prone

Reverse straight-leg raising. Ask the patient to flex the knee maximally against the thigh. A positive test is the complaint of pain in the back or in the sciatic nerve distribution on the affected side.

Sensory examination. See Chapter 11 and Table 12.4.

Examination with the Patient Sitting

Patellar and Achilles reflexes. See Chapters 10 and 11.
Muscle group strength. See Chapters 10 and 11.

Other Special Maneuvers

Measurement of chest expansion. If ankylosing spondylitis is suspected, the expansion range of the chest is measured. This is done with a cloth or paper tape placed at the nipple level around the chest wall. The patient is asked to maximally exhale, and the circumference is noted; then he is asked to maximally inhale, and the circumference is again noted. A chest excursion of less than 2 cm is considered suspicious of thoracic cage disease, likely including the thoracic spine, except in the setting of primary pulmonary restrictive disease or active obstructive airway disease.

Measurement of leg lengths. A significant (greater than 1 cm) difference in leg lengths may account for lateral spinal curvature and low back pain. See the Screening Examination section of this chapter under the subhead Normal and Common Variants and the Extended Examination section of Chapter 10.

Stoop test for entrapment radiculopathy. The patient who complains of intermittent, exercise-related back, gluteal, or posterior thigh pain but has no demonstrable abnormality on the maneuvers outlined above may demonstrate a positive stoop test associated with lumbar degenerative disease. Ask the patient to walk briskly down a long corridor; a positive test consists of a progressive assumption of stooped posture as the patient continues to walk and the appearance of symptoms when the patient is asked to stop walking and to stand upright. (Note that in some instances, especially with spinal stenosis, a patient may adaptively assume a simian posture when walking—stooped, with flexion of the hips and knees—to prevent radicular pain or neurologic symptoms.)

Tests to assess the potentially noncooperative or malingering patient. The complaint of back pain is notorious for its secondary-gain potential. The clinician who evaluates patients with back problems needs to know a few maneuvers for differentiating the "real" from the feigned.

- **Aird's test:** Ask the patient who could not touch his toes in a standing position to do so while sitting with his supported legs extended in front of him. The ability to complete this second maneuver, after the first was impossible, suggests a cooperation problem.
- **Bench test:** Ask the patient to kneel on a bench with his hips and knees flexed and then to place his hands on the floor. The patient with true organic low back pain will be able to carry out this maneuver, since it relieves nerve traction; complaint of the inability (because of pain) to do so suggests a nonorganic basis for the complaint of back pain. However, no single test is perfect, and widespread inflammation might produce a nonsimulated positive bench test.

INTERPRETING THE FINDINGS

Once the clinician has obtained the history of back complaints and completed the extended examination, she organizes the data obtained to construct a differential diagnostic list and to make decisions about subsequent diagnostic tests. Exam-

Table 12.4
Possible Neurologic Abnormalities[a, b]

Muscle stretch reflexes (MSR), lower limb

Reflex	Segmental Level Involved if Reflex Absent or Diminished
Patellar (knee jerk)	L2, L3, **L4**
Achilles (ankle jerk)	L5, **S1**, or S2

Muscles of joint motion

Joint	Motion	Nerve Root Involved if Impaired
Knee	Extension	L2–L4
	Flexion	L4–S3
Ankle	Dorsiflexion	L4–S1
	Plantar flexion	L5–S2
Foot	Supination and pronation	L4–S1
Toes	Plantar flexion	L5–S2
	Dorsiflexion	L4–S1

Loss of cutaneous sensitivity to pain (see also Chapter 11)

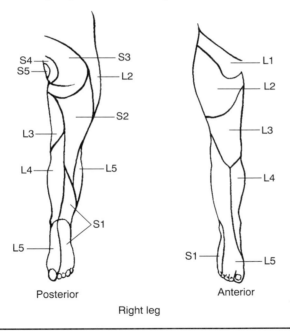

Posterior   Anterior

Right leg

[a]Lesions of single roots may produce *no* sensory deficit as a result of overlap of innervation.
[b]**Boldface** indicates most commonly seen.

ples of constellations of findings suggestive of the more common and/or clinically significant diagnoses are outlined below.

Herniated Intervertebral Disc or Disc Fragments

The onset of symptoms and their specific local and neurologic manifestations depend on the position(s) of the extruded fragment(s) in relationship to the nerve root(s) and on the disc space(s) involved. With careful and thorough physical examination, the clinician is often able to arrive at the probable diagnosis of disc protrusion and to determine its anatomical location. On basic examination, the following abnormalities may be found.

With the patient standing, look for

- **Lateral deviation** toward the affected side, which persists even with the spine flexed
- **Limitation of flexion and extension,** with lateral and rotational motion relatively normal
- **Paraspinal tenderness** and **muscle spasm** lateral to the spine, especially on the affected side

With the patient supine, look for

- Pain on **straight-leg raising** at less than 50° on the affected side
- Increased pain in the back and/or sciatic region with **crossed straight-leg raising** on the affected side and complaint of sciatic pain in the opposite leg
- Increased pain in the back and/or sciatic nerve distribution with sharp **dorsiflexion** of the foot on the affected side

With the patient prone, look for

- Pain in the back and/or sciatic nerve distribution on the affected side during **reverse straight-leg raising**

Focused neurologic testing is imperative in the assessment for possible disc protrusion. Sensory and motor abnormalities consistent with specific nerve root involvement are tabulated in Table 12.4. At the **most common site, the L5-S1 disc,** the key neurologic finding is unilateral loss of the Achilles (ankle) reflex.

Lumbosacral Strain

With the patient standing, observe for

- Accentuation of pain with spinal **flexion**
- Accentuation of **lumbar lordosis**
- **Spasm of paraspinal muscles** on affected side

With patient supine,

- Ask patient to assume the position most comfortable for him; with lumbosacral strain, he will usually prefer to **flex hips and knees** and sometimes to curl (flex) the spine also.
- **Straight-leg raising, crossed straight-leg raising, and foot dorsiflexion** typically will not accentuate pain.

As there is no spinal root involvement, the **neurologic** examination is entirely normal.

Ankylosing Spondylitis

Ankylosing spondylitis is a generalized inflammatory disease of the articulations of the spinal column that most commonly presents in young men from their teenage years onward. The elements of the history suggesting ankylosing spondylitis are discussed by Calin et al., and the systemic manifestations are discussed in Luthra's paper. In early disease there may be only **flattening of the lumbar curve,** but later the entire spine becomes fused and rod-like with a progressive compensatory anterior thrusting of the head. On **palpation,** there is **tenderness** over any involved joint, and the **sacroiliac** joints are often exquisitely tender (sacroiliitis). **All ranges of spinal motion** are impaired. Often, **chest expansion** is reduced to less than 2 cm as a result of spinal fixation. There is often a positive Patrick's test (see the Extended Examination section of Chapter 10).

Spondylolisthesis

This anterior slippage of one vertebral body on another can occur as the result of fracture or degeneration of a segment of the neural arch or may be an adult manifestation of a congenitally incomplete lamina. Most commonly, the fifth lumbar vertebra slips forward relative to the sacrum. The low **back pain is referred to the lateral leg** or, on occasion, to the **coccyx.** Inspection may reveal a **transverse crease** of the skin surface at or above the iliac crests, and palpation may show a **gap between spinous processes** where the involved vertebra has slipped so far anteriorly that its spinous process is no longer palpable. Spinal **flexion** is impaired.

Osteoarthrosis of the Lower Spine

Osteoarthrosis of the lower spine, a very common change of aging, is often asymptomatic (in contrast to the common age-related cervical osteoarthrosis, which is often symptomatic). When back pain is present, it is usually low-grade and remitting. The findings on extended examination are nonspecific, although there may be limitation of movement of the spine in any plane. Very occasionally, a calcified protrusion may encroach on a nerve root; however, symptoms and signs of nerve root irritation should not be attributed to osteoarthrosis until other potential causes have been ruled out.

Osteoporosis of the Spine

Elderly women are the usual victims of osteoporosis of the spine, a common disorder secondary to loss of bone mass in the axial skeleton and long bones. Osteoporosis is often asymptomatic until the increasingly fragile thoracic vertebral bodies develop microfractures from ordinary weight-bearing; their anterior portions begin to collapse ("wedging", the radiographic appearance of anterior compression fractures). Chronic **middorsal back pain, progressive loss of stature,** and **increasing kyphosis** make up the constellation of symptoms and signs. In some instances, particularly after a fall onto the buttocks, **acute severe pain** may herald a **major vertebral collapse,** the diagnosis of which is confirmed by radiographs of the painful portion of the spine. Osteomalacia tends to produce the same symptoms, signs, and complications.

Traumatic Fractures of the Spine

Fractures of the spine may involve the vertebral body, the transverse process, the spinous process, or the lamina. If the fracture is **undisplaced, pain** and **local tenderness** may be the only signs; however, when ligamentous tears accompany the fracture, it may become unstable. A palpable **gap** between **spinous processes in the setting of trauma** to the back suggests **unstable fracture** and a potential hazard to spinal cord structures. Radiographic evaluation is then mandatory.

Lumbar Spinal Stenosis

A congenital narrowing of the spinal canal usually remains asymptomatic until foraminal osteophytes or spondylitic spurs add to the anatomical encroachment on nerve tissue. A characteristic, albeit uncommon, complaint is that of heaviness or numbness of the legs after modest physical activity. The symptoms subside with rest, thus the term **intermittent claudication of the cauda equina** (or pseudoclaudication, or neurogenic claudication). Neurologic signs, e.g., muscle weakness or decreased muscle stretch reflexes, may be present only immediately after exercise and may abate (normalize) after a short rest period.

RECORDING THE FINDINGS

An example of recording the findings of an examination of the back follows:

Lower back: Slight list to the left in standing position, accompanied by lateral deviation of the spine to the left, accentuated by attempts at spinal flexion. Resistance to flexion beyond 15°; extension limited to 5°. Lumbar curve absent. Paraspinal muscles from T12 downward in spasm and tender. No direct tenderness to percussion over spinous processes. Straight-leg raising positive at 30°, left. Crossed straight-leg raising positive. Foot dorsiflexion and reverse straight-leg raising confirmatory.

Neurologic: Loss of toe and foot dorsiflexor strength, left; absent left ankle jerk, right normal; both knee jerks normal. Hypalgesia to pinprick left lateral leg and foot.

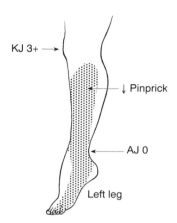

Assessment: Probable herniated intervertebral disc, L5–S1, left, with motor and sensory compromise, chiefly implicating L5 root.

Plan: Lumbosacral spine radiographs and neurosurgical consultation; complete bed rest pending results.

BEYOND THE PHYSICAL EXAMINATION

The radiologist holds the key to many definitive diagnostic procedures related to the back. Radiographs of the spine, directed by the examining physician to the suspicious area, will confirm most fractures, spondylolisthesis, and the sacroiliitis and later spinal fusions of ankylosing spondylitis. Narrowing of disc space(s) on radiographs is highly suggestive of degeneration and/or extrusion of disc material. Osteoarthrosis and significant osteoporosis of the spine are confirmed by radiographs, although early osteoporosis may require bone density studies.

Metastatic cancer in the spine may be visible as abnormally hypermineralized or hypomineralized zones known respectively as osteoblastic or osteolytic lesions; however, *a negative plain film of the spine does not rule out neoplasm*. Radionuclide bone scanning, computed tomography (CT), or magnetic resonance imaging (MRI) may be vital for further study. Contrast medium injected directly into the subarachnoid space (myelography) is still sometimes necessary to define precise disc space and position of fragments before surgery for disc disease. Nerve conduction studies such as nerve conduction velocity (NCV) and electromyography (EMG) may be indicated to define the extent, severity, and precise anatomic location of nerve root dysfunction or to determine any contribution of primary muscle dysfunction unrelated to nerve root encroachment.

Adjunct or confirmatory laboratory tests are sometimes useful in defining the precise etiology of inflammatory articular disease, such as the (nonspecific) elevation of erythrocyte sedimentation rate (ESR) in several disorders. The lymphocyte histocompatibility antigen HLA-B27 is usually present in persons with ankylosing spondylitis, but the test is less specific than sensitive and is costly. The decision to order such ancillary tests should await the collection and interpretation of "harder" and more useful data.

With osteoporosis, the ionized serum calcium and the levels of phosphorus and alkaline phosphatase are normal. With osteomalacia, the calcium may be reduced. In Paget's disease, the alkaline phosphatase is usually elevated. Tumors and hyperparathyroidism can elevate the calcium and sometimes the alkaline phosphatase. Immobility in the setting of Paget's disease of bone also causes hypercalcemia.

RECOMMENDED READINGS

Calin MA, Porta J, Fries JR, Schurman DJ. Clinical history as a screening test for ankylosing spondylitis. JAMA 1977;237:2613–2614.

Dyck P. The stoop-test in lumbar entrapment radiculopathy. Spine 1979;4:89–92.

Hall H. Examination of the patient with low back pain. Bull Rheum Dis 1983;33(4):1–8.

Hoppenfeld S. Physical examination of the spine and extremities. 1st ed. Norwalk, Connecticut: Appleton-Century-Crofts, 1976:276.

Hudgins WR. The crossed-straight-leg-raising test. N Engl J Med 1977;297:1127.

Luthra HB. Extra-articular manifestations of ankylosing spondylitis. Mayo Clin Proc 1977;52:655–656.

Murphy M, Ogden JA, Southwick WO. Spinal stabilization in acute spinal injuries. Surg Clin North Am 1980;60:1035–1047.

Nelson MA, Allen P, Clamp SE, de Dombal FT. Reliability and reproducibility of clinical findings in low-back pain. Spine 1979;4:97–101.

Polley HF, Hunder GG. Rheumatologic interviewing and physical examination of the joints. 2nd ed. Philadelphia: WB Saunders, 1978:286.

Simkin PA. Simian stance: a sign of spinal stenosis. Lancet 1982;2:652–653.

Waddell G, Main CJ, Morris EW, Venner RM, Rae PS, Sharmy SH, Galloway H. Normality and reliability in the clinical assessment of backache. Br Med J 1982;284:1519–1523.

Waddell G, McCulloch JA, Kummel E, Venner RM. Nonorganic physical signs in low-back pain. Spine 1980;5:117–125.

13

Male Genitalia and Rectum

APPROACH AND ANATOMICAL REVIEW

The examinations of the genitalia, of the groin for hernia, and of the rectum and prostate constitute the final steps in the physical examination of the adult man. Except when disability prevents standing, the genital and groin inspection and palpation are best done with the patient upright, and the rectal and prostatic palpation is best done with the patient bending over the end of the examination table. Alternative positions for the disabled patient are described below.

The anatomical structures to be examined include the penis, the scrotum and its contents, the inguinal canal, the perineum, the anus and rectum, and the prostate gland. The anatomy of the area is reviewed below (Fig. 13.1).

Penis

The dorsal shaft of the penis is made up of bilateral columns of erectile tissue, the **corpora cavernosa.** The ventral **corpus spongiosum,** also erectile, contains the urethra, the urine conduit from the bladder to the **urethral meatus.** The **glans penis** is the smooth terminal structure of the shaft. It is separated from the shaft by a circumferential corona (sulcus) from which the foreskin (**prepuce**) of the uncircumcised male arises and covers, in hood fashion, the glans. The meatus pierces the most distal extremity of the glans as a small round to vertical orifice.

Scrotum

The scrotal sac is a pouch of skin, smooth muscle, and fascia that lies posteroinferior to the base of the penile shaft. It is asymmetric in that the left side hangs lower than the right in many men and higher than the right in some others. It is divided in the midline by a **median raphe** or furrow that extends from the ventral surface of the penis to the perineal body. Each half of this divided sac contains a **testis, epididymis,** and the group of structures collectively known as the **spermatic cord;** these structures include the **vas deferens, arteries and veins, lymphatics, and nerve supply.**

The **testis** is elongated and ovoid, oriented vertically, and suspended in the hemiscrotum by the spermatic cord and other proximal attachments. The posterior surface of the upper pole of the testicle is capped by the head of the **epididymis.** The epididymis courses along the posterolateral surface of the testicle toward its inferior pole. Proximally, it becomes continuous with the **vas deferens,** which joins blood vessels and lymphatic channels (Fig. 13.1*B*) at the spermatic cord.

The **spermatic cord** constituents (vas deferens and associated structures) pass upward from the scrotal sac into the inguinal canal and, thence, through the **abdominal inguinal ring** into the pelvis. In this extraperitoneal space, the vas deferens continues behind the bladder to join the ipsilateral **seminal vesicle.** Semen generated in the testis travels this route, then traverses the ipsilateral **ejaculatory duct** that emerges from the prostate gland to enter the urethra adjacent to its contralateral counterpart.

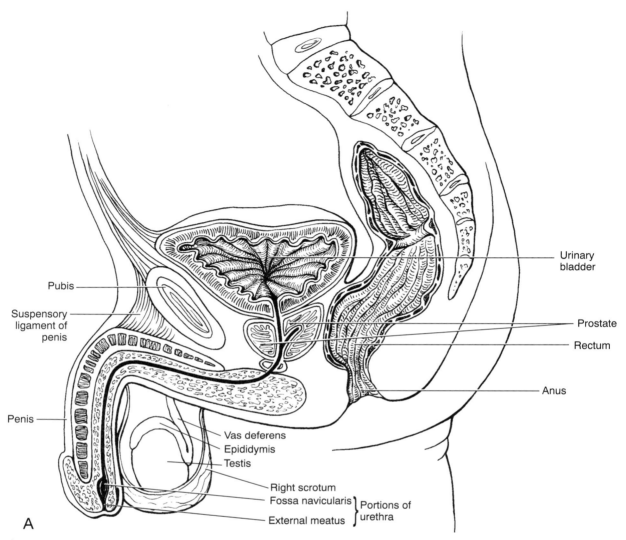

Figure 13.1   Male pelvic anatomy. **A.** Sagittal section of male pelvis showing the major internal structures. **B.** Frontal view of scrotal and suprascrotal contents of a normal adult man (penis retracted ventrally).

Anus and Rectum

See Chapter 14, under Approach and Anatomical Review, for description of the anus and rectum.

Prostate Gland

The prostate is a glandular structure lying in the pelvis, approximately 2 cm dorsal to the symphysis pubis. The posterior surface is contiguous with part of the anterior rectal wall and is therefore accessible to digital examination via the rectum. The two lateral lobes and the posterior lobe of the prostate may be assessed through the rectal wall. The remainder of the gland is nonpalpable. A critical issue to comprehend is the nonpalpability of the portion of the prostate that immediately encircles the urethra. If the patient has symptoms of urethral obstruction but the prostate feels normal, the problem is likely that the median

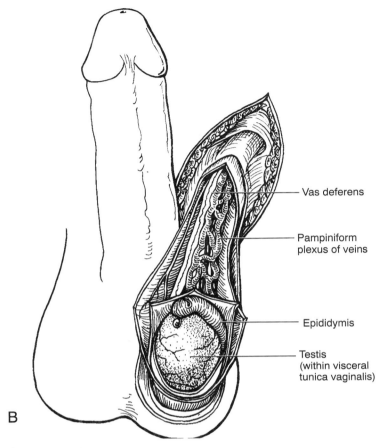

Vas deferens

Pampiniform
plexus of veins

Epididymis

Testis
(within visceral
tunica vaginalis)

B

Figure 13.1   B.

bar—an inaccessible anterior part of the prostate abutting the urethra but not the rectum—has undergone a comparatively selective enlargement.

TECHNIQUE

It is important that the clinician keep in mind that this examination may be culturally and personally anxiety-provoking for the patient. Concerns about the "normality" of his genitalia, nervousness about having this very private part of his body invaded by a stranger, and fear of an involuntary erection are all potentially present. The clinician must be alert to the possibility of an erection in response to genital manipulation and address it directly with the patient if it occurs: "This is a common physical reaction to this examination, so please do not worry about it" is a nonjudgmental and appropriate response. Provide the patient with as much time and space, as well as verbal understanding, as is necessary for his comfort.

Gravity facilitates the male genital examination, particularly the assessment for inguinal hernia. The patient is asked to stand, and the examiner sits facing him. *The clinician always gloves both hands for the conduct of the examination.* The inguinal area and genitalia are fully exposed, either by asking the patient to lift and hold up his gown, or to lower his underpants to the ankles. The required supplies and the steps of the examination are summarized in Table 13.1 and illustrated in Figures 13.2–13.4.

Table 13.1
Male Genital Examination: Supplies and Sequence[a]

Supplies
    Disposable gloves (nonsterile)
    Lubricant
    Supplies for stool occult-blood testing (test cards, developer)
    [Light source for scrotal transillumination]

Sequence of examination

Patient standing	External genitalia
	Inspection
	Penis
	Shaft and prepuce
	Glans
	Corona and sulcus
	Urethral meatus
	Scrotum
	Palpation
	Each hemiscrotum
	Testis
	Epididymis
	Vas deferens and associated structures
	[Transillumination]
	Inguinal canal
	Inspection
	Inguinal bulge (with cough)
	Palpation
	External ring (with cough)
	Canal
	Internal ring (with cough)
	Femoral triangle (with cough)
Patient bent over end of table	Anorectal and prostate gland
	Inspection
	Perianal area
	Anus
	Palpation
	Anal sphincter
	Anal verge
	Rectal ampulla
	Prostate gland
	Test stool for occult blood

[a][. . .] means when indicated by an intrascrotal mass.

External Genital Examination

INSPECTION

Begin the inspection of the genital area with its general contours and the distribution of hair, which is diamond-shaped in the fully developed adult, although the escutcheon often shrinks in old age. Assess each organ as follows (see Fig. 13.2):

- Inspect the **penis** first. The skin of the **shaft** and the **prepuce** is noted for general pigmentation and any visible lesions, of both dorsal and ventral aspects (Fig. 13.2*A* and *B*).

- In the uncircumcised male, retract or have the patient retract the **prepuce (foreskin)** in order to inspect all surfaces of the **glans.** The glans is noted for its hygiene and for the presence of any skin lesions or breaks (Fig. 13.2*C*).

- Examine the **urethral meatus** for its position relative to the center of the glans, for any signs of inflammation, or for discharge. *Gentle* ventral-dorsal pressure on the sides of the glans will promote some gaping of the urethral meatus to better inspect its most anterior 1–2 mm (Fig. 13.2*D*). Do not touch the meatus itself unless cultures are indicated because of a history or visible presence of secretion. After inspection of the glans, the corona, and the urethral meatus, replace the foreskin.
- Note the position of each half of the **scrotal sac,** its general appearance, and normal variation in position.
- Elevate each hemiscrotum to inspect the rugated surfaces for evidence of skin lesions, e.g., nodules, ulcerations, or discoloration. Every surface of the scrotum should be systematically inspected, including the dorsal median furrow as it courses toward the anus (Fig. 13.2*E*).

PALPATION OF SCROTAL CONTENTS

Palpate each side of the scrotal sac separately, with attention paid to any asymmetry in its contents (Fig. 13.3). With your hands, cradle the hemiscrotum being palpated, with palmar surfaces toward the organs. The patient is instructed to indicate if any area proves tender.

- Palpate the **testis** between your posteriorly (ventrally) placed palm or surfaces of the index through ring fingers and your anteriorly (dorsally) placed thenar eminence and thumb. From upper to lower pole, assess the gland for contour, for lumps or bumps, and for areas of tenderness (Fig. 13.3*A*).
- The **head of the epididymis** is usually easily located at the superoposterior pole of the testis, and from there is followed caudad along the posterior surface. It is distinctly tubular, multiply knobby (bosselated), and separated from the body of the testis by connective tissue (Fig. 13.3*B*). At the lower pole of the testis, the epididymis turns to course cephalad as the **vas deferens,** one of the components of the spermatic cord. As you examine each epididymis, compare it with the other regarding size, position, and tenderness.
- Palpate the **spermatic cord** in each hemiscrotum in like fashion. From the testis or termination of the epididymis, the **vas deferens** and accompanying vascular structures course cephalad into the inguinal canal (Fig. 13.3*C*). Again, compare the two sides in terms of size, position, and tenderness of cord contents.

Inguinal Hernia Examination

There are two possible sites of presentation for an inguinal hernia, with one being a congenital defect near the pubic tubercle (**direct hernia**) and the second, and much more common, a weakness in the integrity of the abdominal ring through which the contents of the spermatic cord exit from the pelvic cavity (**indirect hernia**). For anatomic discrimination between these hernia presentations, see Figure 13.4.

INSPECTION

Observe the inguinal area for evidence of bulging or asymmetric prominence of one or the other proximal scrotal sac. A cough, a laugh, or the Valsalva maneuver may bring out bulging.

PALPATION

Palpation for inguinal hernia should follow these steps:

- Locate the **pubic tubercle(s)** (Fig. 13.5). Place the palmar surface of the index or middle finger directly over the area immediately lateral to each pubic

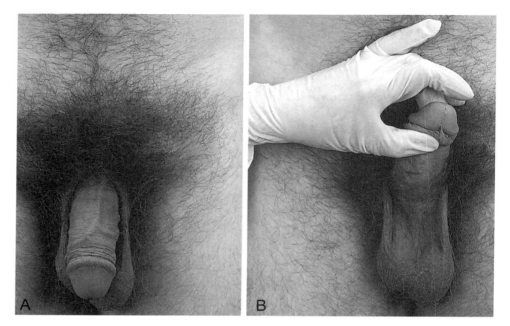

Figure 13.2 Inspection of external genitalia. **A.** General inspection of genitalia. Note the typical male hair distribution and the asymmetry of the hemiscrotal sacs with the left lower than the right. The corona of the glans penis is clearly visible in this circumcised man. The dominant dorsal veins are normal in the flaccid, dependent penis. **B.** The penis is elevated to show its undersurface. Prepuce is surgically absent. The underside of the glans and shaft is normal. **C.** The corona and glans are inspected circumferentially for evidence of skin lesions. In the uncircumcised male, this is accomplished by retraction of the prepuce until the corona becomes visible. **D.** Note the lateral retraction of the periurethral part of the glans penis to expose the outermost 2 mm of urethra. **E.** Penis and scrotum are retracted cephalad to permit inspection of the undersurface of the scrotal sac.

tubercle, and ask the patient to cough or bear down (Fig. 13.5*A*). Observe for a single forceful pulsation against the finger, which suggests a defect in the fascia, permitting egress of a **direct inguinal hernia.**

• Beginning well down on the lateral scrotal sac or at its most dependent point, gently insert the index or middle finger alongside the spermatic cord, invaginating (indenting) the rugate, redundant scrotal skin as the finger is moved up the inguinal canal (Fig. 13.5*B* and *C*). With the palmar surface of the finger against the abdominal wall, the **internal inguinal ring** may be felt as a depression above the inguinal ligament and 2–4 cm lateral to the pubic tubercle. Ask the patient to cough or bear down, with your finger in this position; a soft bulge descending along the canal suggests an **indirect hernia.** It takes experience to decide whether a very minor sensation without a bulge is a true hernia or merely transmission of transient physiologic elevation of intraperitoneal pressure. Repeat the procedure on the opposite side.

• To evaluate for the occasional **femoral hernia** presenting in the male patient, locate the femoral arterial pulse immediately below the juncture of the medial and middle thirds of the inguinal ligament. With the palmar surfaces of the index and middle fingers pressed into the femoral triangle just medial to the arterial pulsation, ask the patient to cough or bear down. The occurrence of a soft bulge against your fingers during such increase in intra-abdominal pressure suggests a femoral hernia. Repeat the examination on the opposite side, or palpate the two femoral triangles simultaneously.

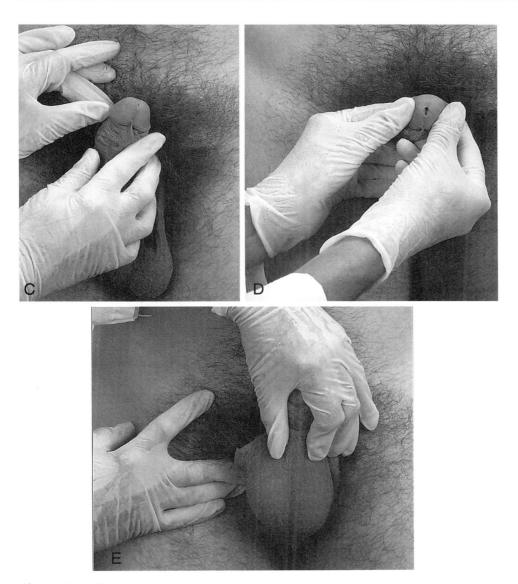

Figure 13.2   C–E.

If the patient is unable to stand for the genital examination, the steps may be conducted from the bedside, with the patient lying supine, hips slightly abducted and externally rotated if possible, and genitalia dependent between the thighs. Subtle or small inguinal hernias cannot be excluded if the hernia examination conducted in this position is negative for bulging.

Anorectal Examination

See Chapter 14 for more detail on inspection and palpation of the anus and rectum. There are several patient positions that suffice for this examination. If able to stand, the patient is, after completion of the genital and inguinal palpation, asked to bend forward over the end of the examining table with legs slightly spread and elbows resting on the table. The anorectal and prostatic examination may also be accomplished with the patient in the Sims position (left lateral decubitus, with right knee flexed toward his chest), knee-chest position on bed or examining

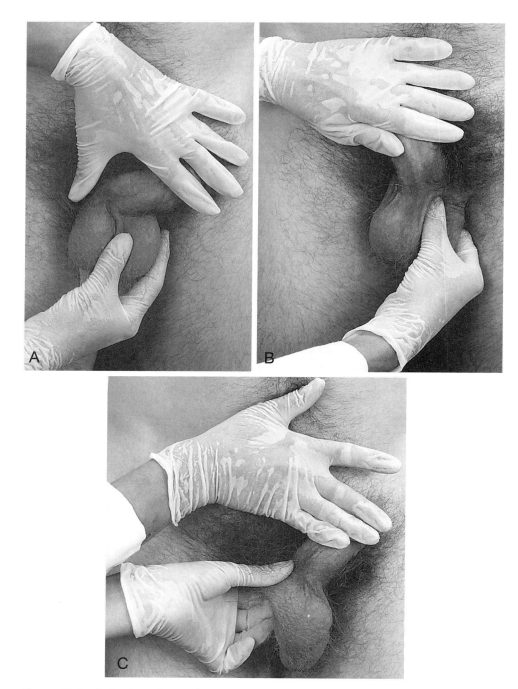

Figure 13.3   Palpation of scrotal contents. **A.** Each testis is palpated between thumb and fingers in the manner illustrated. **B.** Each epididymis is isolated between the thumb and index finger and palpated throughout its posterolateral course along the surface of the testis. **C.** Each spermatic cord is palpated from the superior pole of the testis to its retreat into the inguinal canal.

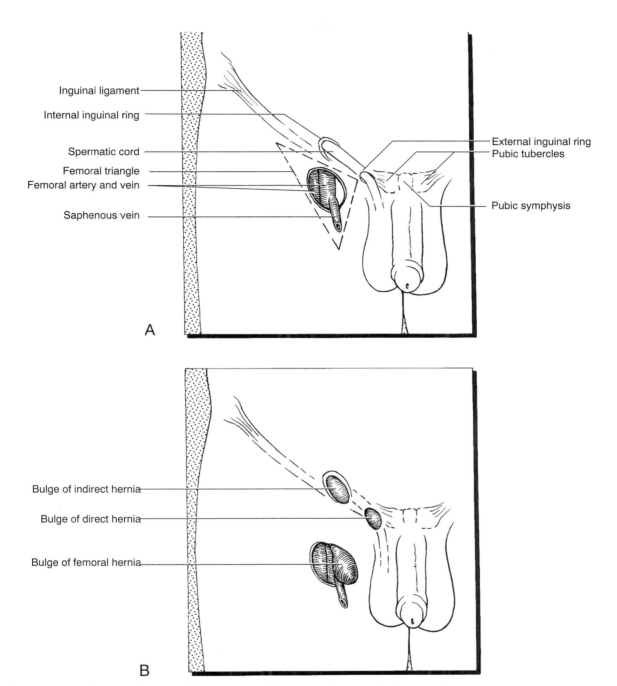

Figure 13.4 Schematic drawing of the anatomy of the inguinal area as it relates to the presentation of hernias. **A.** Anatomical relationships of the inguinal structures. **B.** Sites of presentation of indirect and direct inguinal hernias and of the infrequent male femoral hernia.

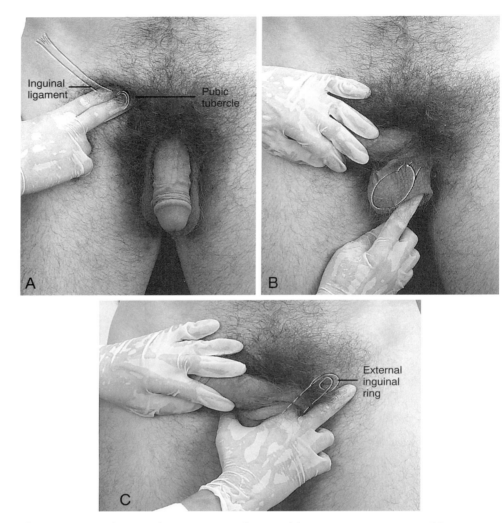

Figure 13.5   Techniques for assessment of inguinal hernias. **A.** Direct inguinal hernia presents through a potential fascial defect just lateral to the pubic tubercle. Increase in intra-abdominal pressure by cough or Valsalva maneuver, which results in pulsation against the examiner's fingerpads, suggests the presence of this *direct* hernial defect. **B.** You must begin inverting the scrotum from well down on the scrotal sac to achieve effective invagination of scrotal tissue to the level of the inguinal ring. **C.** Note the extent to which the invaginating finger can carry scrotal tissue along the course of the spermatic cord without creating discomfort for the patient.

table, or, least satisfactorily, lithotomy position (patient supine with hips abducted and externally rotated, both knees flexed). See Figure 13.6 for illustration of the preferred first two of these positions.

Prostatic Examination

Palpation of the prostate gland is included in the digital examination of the rectal vault (Fig. 13.7). The gland abuts the anterior part of the rectal ampulla. Its most cephalad extremity is reached by deep penetration of the gloved and lubricated middle finger. Rarely, the seminal vesicles that emerge at the upper lateral poles of the gland are palpable. The prostate is characterized by its relative elasticity and its bilobar configuration. After identifying the median raphe, which

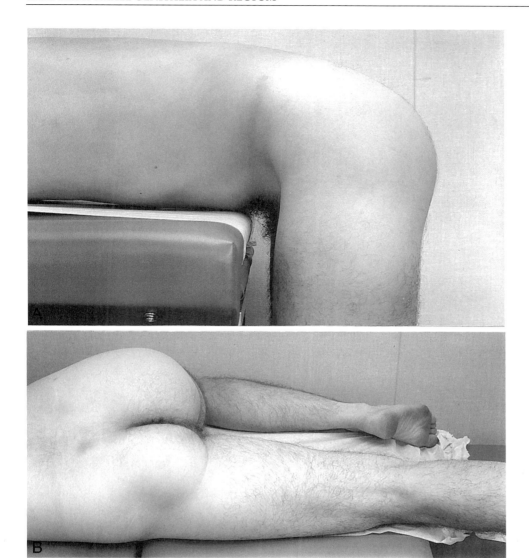

Figure 13.6 Positioning the patient for anorectal and prostate examination. **A.** For the patient who is able to stand and bend over the end of the examining table, this position works well. The perianal structures may be easily inspected by separating the buttocks (or asking the patient to use his hands to do this), the anus is clearly visualized, and the rectum and prostate gland are readily palpated. **B.** For the patient who is less mobile, a completely satisfactory anorectal and prostatic examination can be done in the left lateral decubitus position as illustrated. The right buttock is elevated by the examiner's left hand in order to expose the anal area. The palpating finger of the right hand is inserted into the anal orifice with its palmar surface toward the ventral prostate gland.

feels like a definite central sinking inward without clear-cut borders, palpate the rectal surfaces of each lobe, noting size, consistency, any irregularities, or areas of tenderness. The two lobes are normally symmetrical in all of their characteristics, and the rectal mucosa slides freely over them. At the upper extremity of the gland, the median furrow widens, and a flattened area may sometimes be appreciated.

Transfer stool on the withdrawn examining finger to a card for direct inspection and occult blood testing.

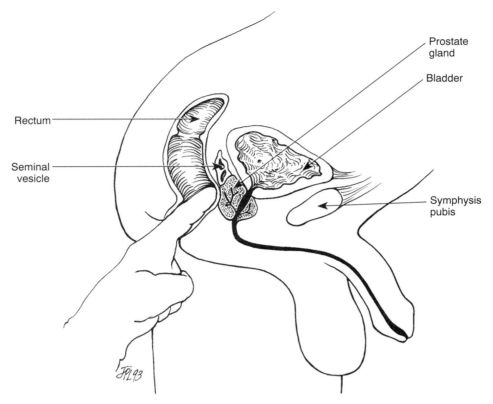

Figure 13.7 Schematic representation of prostatic palpation. Note the position of the examiner's finger relative to the median sulcus and lateral lobes of the gland. The depth of penetration of the examiner's index finger is dependent on the degree of flexion of the examiner's middle finger.

After completion of the anorectal and prostatic examinations, the patient is provided with tissue to clean residual lubricant from his perianal area. The physical examination is now finished.

NORMAL AND COMMON VARIANTS

Inspection of External Genitalia

INGUINAL HAIR DISTRIBUTION

Inguinal hair distribution is subject to wide variation. It is heavy in the pubic area and extends pyramidally upward toward the umbilicus. There is variable hair on the scrotum and lateral thighs, usually reaching in the midline to the perianal area. Inguinal area hair is characteristically darker, more coiled, and stiffer than scalp (capital) hair. The thickness and extent of pubic hair is individually variable and tends to thin with aging, although the male escutcheon pattern may be maintained.

PENIS

The **penis** varies widely in nonerect size among normal men. The foreskin should retract easily, and it is not unusual to discover a small amount of white secretion and debris, **smegma,** under the skin and in the sulcus of the corona. The slit-like **urethral meatus** is located at or a few millimeters ventral to the tip of the glans. It is glistening and pink-gray when gently compressed to slightly gape. Its skin is usually darker than that elsewhere.

URETHRAL MEATUS PLACEMENT

There may be congenital displacements of the urethral orifice, with the most common being **hypospadias,** in which the orifice appears on the ventral surface of the glans or the penile shaft. Less common is **epispadias,** in which the orifice is located on the dorsum of the penis. These anomalies, especially when they are positioned on the glans itself rather than more proximally, are often inconsequential.

The skin of the penis is slack to allow for the expansion of erection. On palpation, the shaft of the penis feels uniformly flaccid and rubbery and should be nontender. The skin of the glans is pinkish, very finely grainy in texture, and uniform in appearance.

SCROTAL SAC

The skin of the **scrotal sac** is usually more deeply pigmented than elsewhere, thick, and heavily rugated. The left hemiscrotum usually is slightly longer than the right as a result of the longer left spermatic cord, giving the scrotum the appearance of asymmetry. The scrotal sac responds to external stimuli and, for example, may be seen to contract and thicken if the room or the examiner's hands are cold or the patient is apprehensive. **Sebaceous cysts** (epidermoid cysts) are relatively common in the skin of the scrotal sac, as they are on the trunk, neck, and scalp.

Palpation of Contents of Scrotal Sac

TESTIS

The normal adult **testis** is approximately 5 cm long and 2–3 cm thick, being oval in shape. The two testes should be of the same size, and appreciable size difference in any given patient indicates abnormality. The consistency of the gland is moderately firm, and its palpation may elicit a visceral sensation, often experienced as diffuse pain. The surfaces of the testis are smooth (apart from where the epididymis covers it) and very regular, and any lump or other irregularity requires further assessment once one is confident that it is not merely epididymis under the examining fingers.

The most common variant associated with the testis is the **hydrocele,** a fluid accumulation in the cavity of the **tunica vaginalis.** It presents as a progressive painless swelling in the scrotal sac and is usually noted first by the patient as he sees the sac enlarge. Palpation reveals a smooth and resilient mass with its larger dimensions toward the lower pole of the testis. It almost always lies in front of the testis, and the gland can usually be palpated as a separate structure. **Transillumination** (Fig. 13.8) will verify that the mass is filled with a transparent fluid. See Figure 13.9*A* for the anatomical definition of a hydrocele.

EPIDIDYMIS

The **epididymis** is a soft, elongated structure that usually lies on the posterior lateral surface of each testis, growing progressively smaller as it courses from its head, on the superior pole of the gland, to its tail in transition to the vas deferens near the inferior pole. In 7–10% of normal adult men, the testicle is rotated congenitally such that the epididymis lies anterior to the gland. It is tubular to corrugated and nontender. Epididymal structures should be symmetrical bilaterally.

Two common variants should be considered while palpating the epididymis: spermatocele and epididymal cyst. **Spermatocele** (Fig. 13.9*B*) is a retention cyst of the epididymis, usually located near its head, and appreciated as a soft, compressible sac not distinctly free of the epididymis itself. It is generally asymptomatic, although it may have been discovered by the patient on his own self-examination.

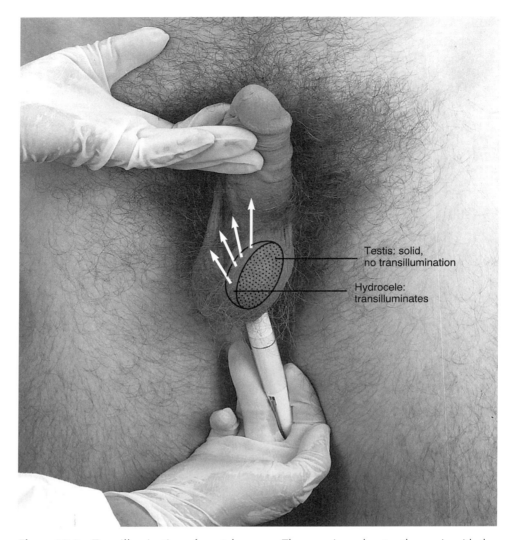

Figure 13.8	Transillumination of scrotal masses. The examiner elevates the penis with the nondominant hand in order to expose the scrotum to full view. With the room darkened, a concentrated beam (as from penlight or sinus transillumination light) is held behind the palpated mass and is directed anteriorly. Failure of the mass to transmit light suggests solid tissue; transmission of the beam through the mass is suggestive of a fluid-containing cyst, either a hydrocele or a spermatocele.

This variant rarely becomes large enough to create cosmetic changes. It contains milky spermatic fluid that is sometimes appreciated with transillumination. The more common **epididymal cyst** (Fig. 13.9C) may be found anywhere along the course of the epididymis, and it is often multiple and bilateral. As with the spermatocele, these fluid-filled cysts are not important in themselves but must be distinguished from solid or inflammatory masses (Fig. 13.9B and C).

SPERMATIC CORD

The *vas deferens* and associated vessels and nerve supplies to the testis are normally bilaterally symmetrical structures palpable near the apex of the upper scrotal sac as it courses toward the inguinal canal and thus into the pelvic cavity. The vas deferens is usually distinguishable by its firm, cord-like consistency. It is

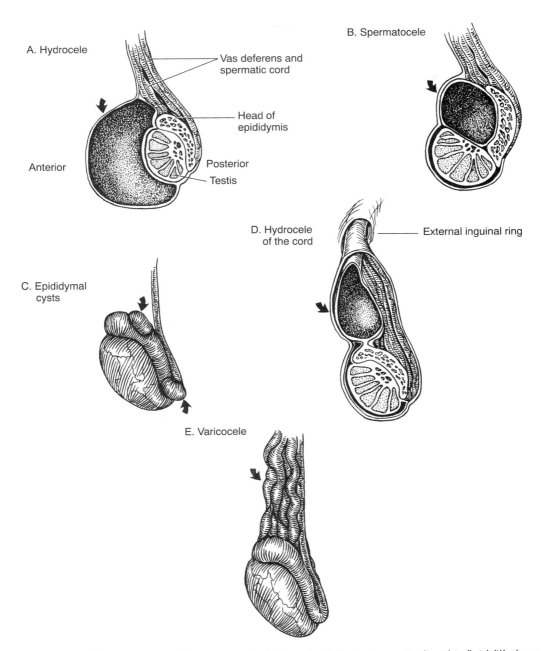

Figure 13.9   Common benign masses of the scrotum. **A.** Hydrocele of the tunica vaginalis. This fluid-filled sac anterior and adjacent to the testis but palpably separate from it should transilluminate. **B.** Spermatocele is palpated as an enlargement of the epididymis, often not distinctly separable from it. If large enough, it may transilluminate. **C.** Epididymal cysts. These small nodules, often multiple, are compressible and located along the course of the epididymis. **D.** Hydrocele of the cord usually lies high in the scrotum and is sometimes difficult to distinguish from a varicocele because the position may be the same. **E.** Varicocele of the spermatic cord is usually distinguishable by its worm-like consistency; it is often bilateral.

smooth, regular, and nontender. Absence of a palpable vas is an important sign (see the Extended Examination section). The other cord structures are not usually distinguishable from one another but make up a clump of soft strands accompanying the vas.

Hydrocele of the cord (Fig. 13.9D) may form in the congenitally persistent cavity in the tunica vaginalis surrounding the cord structures. Like the hydrocele of the testis, this presents as a soft and compressible mass but lies above the testicle along the course of the cord. It also transilluminates and is clinically unimportant unless it becomes very large. Hydrocele of the cord must occasionally be distinguished from inguinal hernia because of its position relative to the spermatic cord and its soft consistency.

Varicocele of the pampiniform plexus is a common variant whose only suspected adverse effect is reducing fertility, particularly if bilateral. It is made up of a convoluted mass of dilated veins in the venous plexus of the cord. Its consistency has led to its being described as feeling like a "bag of worms" (Fig. 13.9E). Because the varicocele is made up of blood-filled veins, it does *not* transmit light. It may become a surgical consideration if it enlarges sufficiently to be mechanically uncomfortable or cosmetically objectionable or when infertility is a problem.

Anus and Rectum

The common variants found during the **perianal** inspection and **anal** and **rectal** palpation are discussed in Chapter 14.

Palpation of Prostate Gland

There is some normal variation in prostatic size after puberty, but the gland should be less than 4 cm in diameter and protrude less than 1 cm into the rectum. The lateral lobes should be symmetrical in size, shape, and consistency and nontender to palpation. Any unilateral variation or bilateral enlargement requires further assessment (see the Extended Examination section).

Normal and common variants of the male genitalia are summarized in Table 13.2.

Table 13.2
Normal and Common Variants[a]

Inspection: external genitalia	Palpation: inguinal canal and femoral triangle
Inguinal hair distribution	**[Indirect inguinal hernia]**
Wide individual variations in	[Direct inguinal hernia]
pattern and thickness	[Femoral hernia]
Thinning with age	
Penis	Inspection: perianal area and anus
Wide normal variation in size	(see Chapter 14)
Urethral meatus placement	
[Hypospadias]	Palpation: rectum (see Chapter 14)
[Epispadias]	
Scrotal sac	Palpation: prostate gland
Individual variation in symmetry	**Variation in size with age**
Palpation: external genitalia	
Scrotal contents	
Hydrocele	
Spermatocele	
[Varicocele]	

[a]**Boldface** indicates very common, and [. . .] indicate potentially clinically significant.

RECORDING THE FINDINGS

This portion of the examination is often recorded as the final entry in the patient's physical examination database.

Sample Write-up

Genitalia: Pubic hair normal with adult male distribution. Penis circumcised; normal glans and corona. Urethral meatus in usual location; no irritation or discharge. Penile shaft unremarkable. Left hemiscrotum slightly lower than right. A 1 × 1.5-cm, freely mobile, subcutaneous soft mass felt lateral side of right scrotal sac. Both testes present in the scrotum, normal in consistency, equal in size, without mass or tenderness. Epididymis palpable in usual position bilaterally, without mass, enlargement, or tenderness. At root of left scrotal sac, 2 × 3-cm mass of soft, compressible structures associated with the spermatic cord. It does not transilluminate. Vas deferens palpable and normal bilaterally.

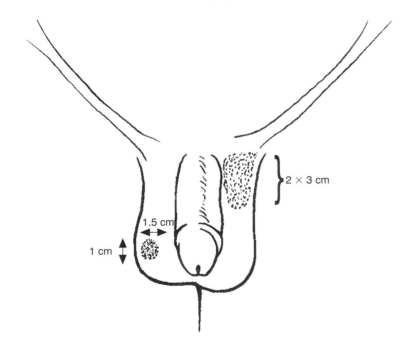

Inguinal: Both inguinal rings felt, and no bulge with cough.
Rectal: Perianal area normal to inspection. Finger easily inserted, no anal tenderness. Rectal vault free of mass, small amount of stool in ampulla. Brown stool on examining glove negative for occult blood.
Prostate: Easily palpable; lateral lobes smooth, of normal size, and nontender.
Impression: Subcutaneous mass, right scrotum. Varicocele, left scrotum.

EXTENDED EXAMINATION OF THE MALE GENITALIA AND RECTUM

INDICATIONS

Although anatomic proximity links the structures discussed in this chapter, they are sufficiently functionally distinct that any indication tends to lead toward extended examination of just one or two of the areas. The following subheadings are indications for the extended examination. Any local pain or discharge also calls for extended genital evaluation, as does impotence and any known or suspected sexually transmitted disease.

Infertility

Infertility calls for close scrutiny of the male genitalia whether or not his partner has a problem that contributes to the condition. Male infertility may coexist with female infertility. Thus the status of *both* partners always requires assessment at the outset.

Venereal Symptoms

Penile discharge requires smear and culture, as described at the end of this chapter, and extended examination of the genitalia, including prostatic palpation. The discovery of any sexually transmitted disease will lead to the same extended examination. Of course, the clinician will want to examine both or all sexual partners, whether the index case is male or female.

Continence Issues

The second step in workup of urinary incontinence or retention, after the history, is careful examination of the genitalia. This also includes examination of the rectum, since fecal impaction can cause partial urethral obstruction with overflow incontinence, as can an enlarged prostate. The same rationale for rectal examination also applies to the other symptoms lumped as prostatism. Fecal incontinence or retention requires meticulous anorectal and perianal examination.

Anemia or Positive Fecal Occult Blood Test

Any patient with unexplained anemia will need rectal examination, both for palpation of the potentially cancerous prostate or rectum and to secure a fecal sample for occult blood testing. A patient who has defecated a stool sample that has tested positive for fecal occult blood but who has not had a rectal examination, should have a rectal examination, partly for restudy of stool but more vitally to palpate for the responsible pathology.

Diarrhea

Patients with diarrhea often experience perianal erosions with discomfort on examination, but they too ought to have a careful rectal examination—not so much to secure stool, which is expelled spontaneously, but to check for responsible pathology, e.g., a villous adenoma of the rectum.

Bowel Obstruction

The patient with small bowel obstruction needs a careful search for hernias: direct inguinal, indirect inguinal, femoral, and, outside the scope of this chapter, ventral. An entrapped hernia can present as small bowel obstruction, with nausea, vomiting, and the absence of flatus or stool. Incarcerated hernia is surgically correctable. Operative technique is simpler and outcome is better if the diagnosis is made promptly, i.e., before the incarcerated segment becomes strangulated and necrotic.

Cancer

A scrotal mass requires extended examination. Men who present with metastatic cancer and no known primary site need extended examination of the rectum and genitalia, as either may reveal the source of the metastasis. Such a discovery sub-serves diagnosis and affects the selection of therapy.

CONDUCTING THE EXTENDED EXAMINATION
Scrotal Contents

If the scrotal contents are so retracted that palpation is difficult or impossible, give the patient time and physical warmth, both of which will help reduce the involuntary muscle contraction that is responsible.

PALPATION

The **vas deferens** is best found by gently bringing the palpating thumb and forefinger together at the top of the testis (Fig. 13.3C). The vas has the size and consistency of a pipe cleaner, although not its texture. The vas will usually be found posteriorly, above the **epididymis.** When the epididymis is hard to find, you can locate the vas as described, then move inferiorly until a more irregular structure than the smooth globe of the testis is encountered. That will be the epididymis.

TRANSILLUMINATION

A major technique in assessment of **scrotal masses** is transillumination. This is done in a darkened room, with a strong, narrow light source such as a penlight. The light is held to the skin to minimize light leakage, which will otherwise render interpretation difficult or impossible. If the room cannot be blacked out, a low-intensity ambient light can be used, such as an x-ray viewing box. Transilluminate the normal side first, to have a sense of the particular patient's baseline, and then repeat the test across the pathology. The light is held behind the hemiscrotum and directed forward. Observe from the front (Fig. 13.8): Cystic masses transmit light; solid masses do not.

In the study of an apparent testicular mass, three principles apply:

1. The patient should be warm enough and comfortable, so that the testes hang freely to permit optimal palpation.
2. Try to feel a superior pole of the mass. If you can, you have excluded inguinal hernia, a great mimic of primary testicular masses.
3. If this maneuver fails, auscultate the mass. The presence of bowel sounds suggests hernia, with small bowel present in the hernia sac (although no data are extant on transmission of bowel sounds to bowel-free scrota). If there are no sounds, no safe conclusion can be drawn.

SELF-EXAMINATION

Testicular self-examination by palpation has been advocated to reduce mortality from testicular cancer. Data proving its efficacy are lacking.

Penis

To see more of the **urethral meatus, very gently** retract from a point 1 cm posterolaterally on either side of it, looking for erythema of the exposed distal mucosa. In addition, gently sliding the finger on the underside of the shaft and glans from the inferoposteriormost point of the root of the penis to the tip (Fig. 13.10) may demonstrate urethral tenderness and can occasionally "milk" forth a drop of exudate that was not leaked spontaneously.

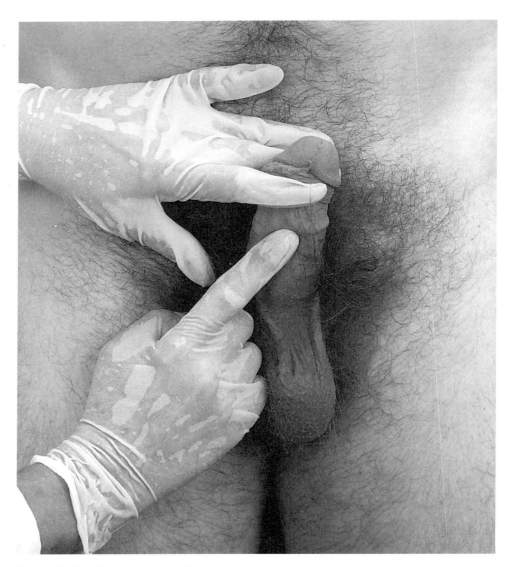

Figure 13.10   Palpation for urethral tenderness.

Anorectum and Prostate

Visualization of the perianal skin is best accomplished by placing the patient in a modified Sims position rather than standing bent over. The patient is asked to extend the left hip and knee that are in contact with the examination table, then to flex the right hip and knee, and finally to turn the trunk and pelvis toward the table (Fig. 13.6*B*). Once the patient is in this position, you put gloves on *both* hands, and then warning the patient in advance of each action, touch each buttock with your ipsilateral fingers, and retract the buttocks as widely as needed to see the anus and surrounding skin. This technique also results in the best lighting. If rectal prolapse needs to be sought because of a compatible history (e.g., fecal soilage), the patient is asked to bear down as though moving his bowels, while buttock retraction is sustained.

Although the technique of rectal examination was described earlier, several fine points that reduce patient discomfort are reiterated:

1. Do not stint on lubricant, and do not use water in place of a jelly for this purpose.
2. Reassure the patient, and make sure that each action *follows* your words, rather than accompanying or preceding them.
3. When you place your fingertip on the anal skin, leave it there a moment, and then insinuate it gently and slowly. Every person's anal sphincter tightens when the finger first touches, and relaxes to one degree or another with a bit of time.
4. Position the finger so that the sensitive pad is directed forward to the prostate to maximize the diagnostic accuracy of palpating this structure. You may later rotate your hand 180° in each direction from this point, about the fulcrum of the intrarectal finger, to palpate the lateral walls of the rectum and the presacral zone.

In the extended rectal examination, ask the patient to bear down once again while you reach for any high rectal lesion to bring it within range of the palpating finger. Bearing down does not seem to move the prostate. It is seldom possible to reach above it to the seminal vesicles or even all the way to the posterolateral margin of an enlarged prostate. To reach higher on the prostate,

1. Use the middle rather than the index finger for rectal palpation, since this is the longest digit.
2. Don't hesitate to press the whole hand inward, i.e., up toward the navel, while tightly flexing the knuckles and interphalangeal joints of all fingers except the middle (Fig. 13.11). This will produce pressure on the patient's perianal skin but no pain unless the pressure is sudden or excessive. The effect will be to compress the elastic subcutaneous fat and allow an extra centimeter or so of prostate to be reached.

When **prostatitis** or **prostatic abscess** is being sought, feel for fluctuance and localized prostatic tenderness, and massage the prostatic fossa with the palpating

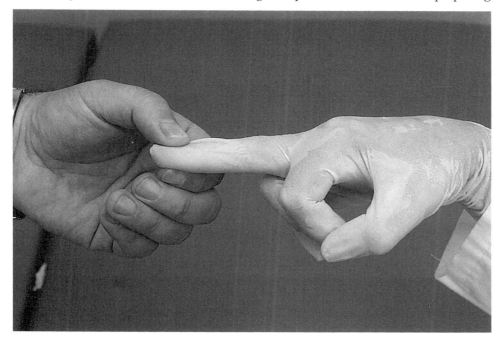

Figure 13.11   Flexion of other fingers to extend reach of palpating middle finger in rectal examination (ungloved hand stretches the gloved finger for demonstration only).

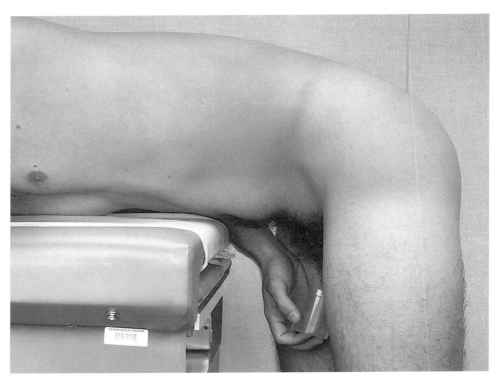

Figure 13.12   Patient holds cup to catch any prostatic exudate expelled during prostatic massage.

finger several times. Have the patient hold a sterile cup just beneath his penis (Fig. 13.12) in case the maneuver expels intraprostatic exudate. If it does not do so, a postmassage voided urine specimen will contain material for culture that was expelled from prostatic glands or ejaculatory ducts by the maneuver.

Hernia

A suspected *inguinal hernia* can be rendered more visible by a variety of means. Gravity assists diagnosis in the upright posture compared with the supine position. The most pleasant augmentation technique for the examiner, patient, and, in pediatrics, the parent is to have the patient laugh out loud several times. This can reveal a visible bulge before it is detectable with other means.

INTERPRETING THE FINDINGS

Scrotum and Its Contents

VAS DEFERENS

If the vas deferens cannot be found by careful physical examination—if necessary repeated by a urologist—the patient is likely to have agenesis or dysplasia of the vas. This condition has a high association with ipsilateral renal agenesis. If normal vasa can be felt, an otherwise tenable diagnosis of cystic fibrosis can be confidently discarded or at least questioned.

Men who have had vasectomy—resection of a short superficial segment of each vas—often develop a variably symptomatic enlargement and firmness of one of the cut ends of the vas. This condition, called **vasitis nodosum,** may produce a palpable nodule high in the scrotum distinctly above and separate from the testis but not always palpably in continuity with the rest of the vas remnants.

EPIDIDYMIS

A very tender epididymis—sometimes palpably enlarged but more often not detectably so—is most characteristic of **acute epididymitis,** which is usually a venereal infection often caused by gonococci or coliforms. Sometimes there is an associated urethritis, but not always. In the child with very localized point tenderness over a spot on the testis or epididymis, consider a diagnosis of **torsion** of the minute testicular adnexum called the appendix testis.

An indurated epididymis, especially if nontender, may represent **tuberculosis. Primary epididymal tumors** are very rare.

TESTES

Normal testes in adults measure over 3 cm and usually over 4 cm in longest dimension, which is usually the vertical. Smaller testes are called **atrophic.** Unilateral atrophy reflects remote injury, the nature of which will be indeterminate from examination, although the history may offer clues. *Symmetric small firm testes*—palpated when the upper pole as well as the lower is accessible—suggest a relatively short differential diagnosis. In the young man with tall, thin habitus and a small penis, **Klinefelter's syndrome** is likely. In the alcoholic, **cirrhosis-associated atrophy** may be inferred, which is endocrinopathic and due to unclear mechanisms. In the intravenous drug abuser, **HIV-associated testicular atrophy** will lead the list. **Remote trauma, orchitis, or pressure atrophy** are also possibilities. Small soft testes suggest **hypogonadotrophic hypogonadism.**

Orchitis produces a tender testis with or without enlargement. One of many conditions may be responsible. Mumps is a prototype of systemic disease that involves the testes. Transient orchitis has also been produced by *excessive testicular self-examination,* with symmetric testicular tenderness as the only physical finding.

Enlarged firm testes with minor tenderness, nontender enlarged testes, or testicular nodules suggest **testicular neoplasm.** Soft, "wormy," or yielding intrascrotal masses may represent various processes including **hydrocele, varicocele, hernia, and epididymal cyst.** In young men, **germ cell tumors** are likely to be the cause of neoplastic enlargement or nodules. In older men, **lymphoma of the testis** leads the list. Although both offer excellent prospects for combined-modality cure, even with disseminated disease, the necessity of prompt diagnosis and early therapy remains evident. Perhaps the most crucial issue for the clinician is *not to dismiss testicular enlargement as inflammatory (nonneoplastic) because of some tenderness.* If there is not rapid, complete resolution of both enlargement and pain with antimicrobial therapy, reconsideration of underlying neoplasia will be most helpful. In the further assessment of a testicular mass, the *absence of inguinal lymphadenopathy* offers no reassurance about nodal spread. The lymphatic drainage of the testes recalls their embryonic descent from an intra-abdominal position: the para-aortic lymph nodes will be affected first. Inguinal lymphadenopathy, if found, most likely results from another cause, such as irritation of the skin of the feet. More ominously, in advanced lesions, inguinal lymphadenopathy may result from drainage from a scrotum involved by fixation and extension of the tumor.

SCROTUM

The scrotum and penis can swell if the iliac veins or lymph nodes are obstructed by tumor in the pelvis. In this setting there will be severe leg and thigh swelling, along with scrotal and penile swelling. The absence of penoscrotal edema, in the case of bilateral swelling up through the topmost parts of the thighs, implies the preservation of at least some flow in the iliac veins and lymph vessels, whereas their presence mandates investigation of the pelvis and, if there is edema of the lower abdominal wall also, of the inferior vena cava.

Transient, bright pink *acute idiopathic scrotal edema* in boys, usually under the age of 10, has been described.

An *empty scrotum* signifies undescended or retracted testes. The latter are common. If all methods fail to bring testes within reach, the clinician should consider **nondescent** and **cryptorchidism,** unilateral or bilateral, in the differential diagnosis. The importance of undescended testes lies in the frequency of dysplasia and the potential for malignancy developing in these gonads. Surgery to relocate the testes does not prevent this complication.

Primary squamous cancer of the scrotum was the first recognized occupational malignancy, described by Sir Percival Pott in chimney sweeps over two centuries ago. Their scrota remained in protracted contact with carcinogenic smoke residues on their clothing.

Besides the usual skin conditions that can occur in any intertriginous zone, the commonest scrotal findings are minute bright-red to dark-red smooth-domed papules representing **cutaneous hemangiomas,** called Fordyce spots. In men over 40, they are normal. In children they are associated with Fabry's disease, a rare inborn metabolic error with prominent renal and cerebral manifestations.

The most ominous penoscrotal finding is **Fournier's gangrene,** a mixed anaerobic and Gram-negative aerobic infection whose hallmarks are extensive black necrosis of penile, scrotal, perineal, or perianal skin with typically prominent symptoms and pronounced ulceration.

MISCELLANEOUS

Most **varicoceles** occur on the left. An old pearl, unproved by quantitative studies, claims that *sudden* appearance of a left varicocele should prompt consideration of a left renal cell carcinoma with extension into the left renal vein and consequent obstruction of the left testicular vein that empties into the long left renal vein. Others have advocated seeking underlying problems with any *right-sided* varicocele!

Penis
POSITION OF MEATUS, PENILE COLOR, AND PENILE SHAPE

The skin of the penis is often darker than skin elsewhere, regardless of the general pigmentation of the patient. Sometimes the glans has irregular darker mottling. Thus you needn't seek an abnormal pituitary-adrenal axis based on darkening in this area.

A foreskin that cannot be retracted constitutes **phimosis,** whether the glans is edematous or not. A retracted foreskin that cannot be brought forward to recover the glans is a **paraphimosis.** Both call for referral for elective circumcision to prevent hygienic, infectious, or vascular complications.

Penile edema can be part of anasarca as well as a manifestation of iliac venous or lymphatic obstruction. Penile edema can also result from sexual trauma. Transient isolated penile edema in both adults and children sometimes defies explanation.

An *apparently bent penis* usually indicates **Peyronie's disease,** a fibromatosis of the corpus cavernosum, although the deformity may represent a soft-tissue fracture of the penile shaft. Lesser degrees of Peyronie's disease present as deep palpable plaques or nondeforming areas of induration deep within the penile shaft. Whatever the degree, the patient may complain that the deformity increases with penile erection. Any of several sexual difficulties may follow, ranging from psychologic difficulty for either patient or partner, to dyspareunia, to inability to achieve erection, intromission, or orgasm.

Hypospadias can be innocent or can be associated with reduced fertility. It serves as an external marker for internal disease in that there is an increased incidence of other genitourinary malformations in afflicted men.

SEXUALLY TRANSMITTED DISEASES, ULCERS, AND SEXUALLY ASSOCIATED PROBLEMS

The classic nontender, painless solitary penile ulcer—which may occur anywhere on the organ—is the **chancre of primary syphilis.** After a long decline, the incidence of syphilis has risen sharply. Thus, this lesion is now again likely to be seen by the reader.

In **gonorrhea,** local physical findings may be absent or may be limited to an erythematous urethral meatus with or without diffuse urethral tenderness or expressible purulent urethral discharge. Asymptomatic gonococcal urethritis has now become common in men as well as women. Associated epididymal tenderness suggests that the same pathogen has ascended to the epididymis.

A red anterior urethra can occur in **anterior urethritis** from any cause. **Excessive sexual intercourse** is a mechanical noninfective cause of this inflammation.

Genital herpes simplex virus produces pain or tingling paresthesia a day or so before the first classic sign, namely, multiple minute vesicles, typically on erythematous bases, appears. Any part of the penis may be affected. In recurrent genital herpes, the lesions may or may not reoccupy the same spots as originally.

Typical **condylomata acuminata** result from infection with human papilloma virus (HPV). They produce genital warts that favor the moistest areas, e.g., the corona and sulcus; however, they may occur anywhere, including the base of the penile shaft. The lesions range from under 1 mm to about 1 cm in size. Their fronds are randomly oriented and usually consist of an intact epithelium over a very scant core.

Atypical (flat) condylomata acuminata consist of flat lesions that may or may not be discolored. Two special physical examination techniques for visualizing HPV lesions deserve mention:

1. A 5-minute application of a 5% solution of acetic acid, i.e., white vinegar, to the penis and scrotum, with soaked gauze sponges. Although false-positive results may occur, the development of whitening of the epithelium upon this maneuver, particularly in a patient with known HPV lesions, provides strong evidence of flat condyloma.
2. Colposcopy, a form of in vivo microscopy much more commonly done on women.

Penile ulcers are seen in diverse conditions but are often infective in origin. Use of the dorsal veins of the penis for intravenous drug abuse, with extravasation and infection, is one striking cause.

Sexual trauma can follow sexual activity incorporating undue force, poor lubrication, or an inadequately distensible orifice. It is seen in the most extreme forms among cocaine users. Lesions include diffuse erythema, bite-marks from incautious fellatio, ecchymoses, and hard, thrombosed, very tender superficial penile veins. Users of certain sexual aid devices, notably penile rings—which are legitimately prescribed for impotence as well as used indiscriminately by others—may also suffer penile injury.

Priapism is the term applied to persistent, uncontrollable penile erection. It is usually painful. It is seen as an adverse drug reaction (e.g., in some men receiving trazodone), with thrombotic diatheses (e.g., sickle cell anemia), and in other settings including after the use of prescribed penile rings and corpus cavernosum injections for impotence.

SKIN DISEASES

Psoriasis commonly affects the penis. The characteristics of penile psoriasis resemble psoriasis found elsewhere on the body. A related finding apparently limited to the penis and soles is seen in **Reiter's syndrome.** The penile lesions include a noninfectious urethritis and a marked inflammation of the skin of the glans, corona, and sulcus called **circinate balanitis.**

A line of minute papules or fronds, arrayed in parallel around the coronal sulcus, is the hallmark of a condition called **pearly penile papules,** whose import lies in distinguishing it from venereal lesions, especially condylomata acuminata.

INFECTIONS AND CANCER

Poor hygiene, particularly in uncircumcised men, predisposes to **balanopos-thitis,** an infective or mechanical inflammation of the glans penis and overlying foreskin that is often pruritic. Cases due to candidal infection tend to be the most intensely erythematous. A balanoposthitis in which the scrotum is also involved or that includes small satellite nodules or papulopustules suggests *Candida* as the most likely cause. Dermatophytes may cause browner lesions, sometimes with central clearing. *Gardnerella vaginalis*—the agent of nonspecific vaginitis— can produce balanitis whose distinguishing characteristic is said to be a fishy odor, although such an odor is also common with poor hygiene.

Persistent penile erythema after appropriate therapy for balanoposthitis raises the question of **carcinoma in situ,** also known as erythroplasia of Queyrat. Such redness may occur in a small patch or in a larger area. Uncircumcised men are most subject to both conditions, which cannot always be distinguished reliably by physical examination.

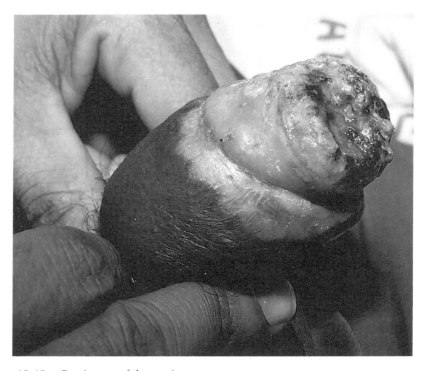

Figure 13.13 Carcinoma of the penis.

Adverse medication effects can also cause a red zone or patch anywhere on the skin that tends to recur with each exposure to (or course of) the medicine. The penis is a surprisingly common site of such **fixed drug eruptions.**

An ulcerated, exophytic mass that appears stuck onto the penis or that replaces all of it (Fig. 13.13) is likely to be **invasive squamous cell carcinoma.** The dictum that neonatal circumcision confers lifetime immunity to penile cancer no longer obtains in the era of HPV oncogenesis.

PENILE DISCHARGE

Naked-eye examination of any available body fluid is a vital part of physical examination. A frankly purulent discharge is likely to represent gonorrhea. Chlamydial and mycoplasmal urethritis are alternative explanations, but the discharge may be thinner (more mucoid). Mucoid discharge is, however, most typical of Reiter's syndrome. Epidemiology plays a role in weighing diagnostic choices: Gonorrhea is commonest in men of lower socioeconomic status, whereas chlamydial infection is more prevalent in middle-class men. Always follow up with microscopy (see below).

RELATIONS TO ABDOMEN AND TO TRAUMA

With **tense ascites,** intraperitoneal ascitic fluid may spread along tissue planes to cause prominent scrotal and/or penile swelling, so that a separate cause need not be sought when this combination is present.

Retroperitoneal hemorrhage can also track to the penis and scrotum, producing **nontraumatic penoscrotal ecchymosis,** which carries the eponym of *blue genital sign of Bryant.* Classically, this is considered to represent ruptured abdominal aortic aneurysm with inferoanterior tracking of blood, but a similar sign has appeared after aorto-bifemoral bypass surgery.

In the setting of blunt trauma, typically in a motor vehicle accident, a butterfly-shaped hematoma over penis and scrotum is considered evidence of urethral rupture.

Prostate

DIFFUSE ENLARGEMENT

Diffuse enlargement of the prostate is common in men above age 60 and is sometimes found earlier. It is usually due to hormonally mediated benign glandular and stromal prostatic hyperplasia. The clinician palpates as much of the posterior surface of the gland transrectally as possible, without skipping areas. Usually, diffuse enlargement will occur without obscuring the midline vertical depression known as the median raphe of the prostate. As mentioned above, prostatic hyperplasia can occur without enlargement of the portion of the gland accessible to palpation, so that an anterior median bar compromises urethral flow despite posterolateral lobes that feel normal. Thus, you have to be realistic about the limited specificity of normal findings on prostatic palpation with regard to excluding prostatism.

PROSTATIC NODULES

Nodules may occur in isolation or with generalized prostatic enlargement. Among the less common but important noncancerous causes of prostatic nodules are (*a*) **benign hyperplasia,** which is often a bit soft but sometimes quite hard, (*b*) **calcinosis,** especially with hard nodules, (*c*) a **prostatic infarct** complicating benign hyperplasia, and (*d*) **granulomatous prostatitis.**

Many **prostatic cancers** begin in the posterior lobe, where they are often palpable as hard nodules. The sensitivity of palpation is imperfect because other cancers may arise out of reach or may have a less distinctive texture. Part of the physical examination of any prostate with a nodule is to try to feel whether the induration extends to and beyond the edge of the prostate and whether the prostate retains normal mobility with respect to adjacent structures such as the pelvic wall. Extraprostatic extension and fixation elevate the clinical stage of a prostate cancer and render surgery with curative intent unlikely. They lead to a combined-modality team approach.

TENDERNESS

Marked and localized or diffuse prostatic tenderness is a hallmark of **prostatitis** and **prostatic abscess,** diagnoses that may coexist with nodularity and enlargement. If pus drains from the urethra upon prostatic palpation or massage, the pathologic diagnosis is clear, although the microbiologic etiology remains to be determined.

PERITONEAL SHELF

If a peritoneal shelf is palpable at the upper edge of the prostate, there is likely to be **intraperitoneal carcinomatosis** with settling of cells at the most dependent portion of the peritoneal cavity. The eponym **Blumer's shelf** is frequently used.

Anorectum

TRAUMA

Both gay and straight men can have sexual practices that include anal penetration. Depending on violence and frequency, there may be perianal ecchymoses, lacerations, abrasions, loss of sphincter tone, or normal physical findings.

Nontraumatic perianal ecchymosis has the same significance as the parallel penile finding, i.e., retroperitoneal hemorrhage. One group described such a "black-bottom sign" after rupture of an abdominal aortic aneurysm.

INFLAMMATION AND INFECTION

Many of the lesions of sexually transmitted diseases described with the penis can be found in the anus or perianal skin. Chancres, herpetic vesicles, and condylomata (both typical and flat) resemble their penile counterparts. **Progressive necrotizing herpetic infection** can cause large ragged ulcers and eschars that begin at the anus and spread outward. This striking finding was among the first published manifestations of AIDS, even before the syndrome was named or the retrovirus incriminated.

Perirectal abscesses, identified by visibility and palpable swelling, are always accompanied by severe pain and tenderness and usually by erythema or purulent drainage. Even if the infection begins in an anal crypt, i.e., internally, the resultant bulge usually distorts perianal skin and contours, *without* prolapse having occurred.

HEMORRHOIDS, FISSURES, FISTULAS, AND PROLAPSE

Hemorrhoids in men resemble those in women. *External hemorrhoids* are usually smooth blue domes that are painful or tender when inflamed or thrombosed. They often have surface erosions or ulcers. Generally, their contour and surface are far more regular than those of neoplasms. **Internal hemorrhoids,** above the anal verge, are rounded or elongated structures under a mucosa that feels intact. Characteristically, the pain of hemorrhoids is continuous, whereas pain on defecation is more characteristic of anal fissure.

Anal fissures are minute linear breaks in epithelial integrity, often shallow and frequently free of erythema, visible blood, or pus. They are painful, and the clinician may be puzzled if she fails to locate them or if she finds them and considers the pain disproportionate to the lesion.

Perianal fistulas represent pathologic connection between the skin surface and the anal canal or rectum. They may be seen with any tissue-destroying process, including neoplasia, and are most commonly seen in the setting of Crohn's disease.

Rectal prolapse is extrusion of otherwise normal-appearing anal or rectal mucosa out of the anal orifice. The process is common during and after severe diarrhea, resulting from local irritation, and is often accompanied by severe erythema, erosion, and maceration of the anal skin. Almost all rectal prolapse can be readily reduced by simply pushing the tissue back in. If the tissue comes out often enough to bother the patient and persists apart from acute diarrhea, specialty referral is indicated.

RECORDING THE FINDINGS

Sample Write-up

HPI: Patient seen because of diffuse penile soreness after protracted intercourse with three male partners. Active partner with each act, and had no receptive intercourse. Used condoms at all times, and claims not to be excessively concerned with sexually transmitted infection. No drug use during the episode or ever. No other symptoms.

Genitalia: Penis circumcised, with mild diffuse erythema around the glans and sulcus. No deep penile tenderness, deformity, or Peyronie's plaques. Mild urethral tenderness with direct pressure but no expressible exudate. No ulcers, vesicles, condylomata or other masses, or thrombosed vessels. Testes nontender, free of nodules. Epididymides minimally tender bilaterally, vasa normal. Prostate normal size, nontender, and free of nodules; no secretion expressed with palpation or massage.

Anorectum: Perianal skin normal, anal sphincter tone normal, no rectal mass. Scant stool in ampulla, formed, brown, and negative for occult blood.

Hernia: No hernial bulges including with coughing and laughing.

Impression:
   1. Mechanical balanodermatitis.
   2. Minimal epididymitis (?), doubt infective cause.

BEYOND THE PHYSICAL EXAMINATION

The urologist is almost always the consultant of choice. Occasionally, a dermatologist, an infectious disease specialist, or a colorectal surgeon is indicated.

Testicular Problems

Imaging modalities are limited. **Ultrasound** has been used to define scrotal masses, and a nuclear medicine technique can be used for torsion.

Fertility Issues

Analysis of semen is one of the methods available for further workup. **Culture of semen** for *Chlamydia* and other pathogens is another.

Penile Problems

Microscopic examination of a **Gram stain of discharge** will help if Gram-negative intracellular diplococci—the hallmark of gonorrhea in men—are present. This is usually combined with **culture.** If there is no spontaneous discharge, a minute urethral swab can obtain specimens for culture for *Neisseria, Chlamydia,* and *Mycoplasma.*

Dark-field microscopic examination of material from a penile ulcer can make the diagnosis of syphilis. A modified Tzanck smear can be used to delineate herpetic infection here as anywhere on the skin surface (see complete instructions in the Extended Examination section of Chapter 3). Viral culture may be necessary. Colposcopy in men is usually combined with biopsy in delineation of HPV lesions and in the issue of related carcinogenesis.

Empiric circumcision may be followed after 1 month by reinspection of a persistently red area of penile skin that has not cleared with antimicrobial therapy for balanoposthitis. If the discoloration disappears, carcinoma in situ has been excluded. If not, biopsy is indicated.

Prostatic Disease

There is a vigorous debate about the indications for transrectal ultrasonic screening for prostatic nodules in asymptomatic men. By contrast, the technique of transrectal ultrasound has an established role in the workup, assessment, and directed-needle biopsy of such nodules once they have been discovered by physical examination. Neither ultrasound nor MRI helps with staging (determining presence and extent of spread) of prostate cancer. Most practitioners will employ bloodwork including measurements of calcium, alkaline phosphatase, acid phosphatase, and prostate-specific antigen (PSA) for any patient with a prostatic nodule that feels cancerous. Most clinicians would perform radiographs of the pelvis and a total-body bone scan in the search for extraprostatic spread. Some persons have advocated PSA measurements for screening patients with no symptoms and no prostatic nodules. This does not appear to be justified by diagnostic yield or enhanced prognosis, and false-positive results cause great anguish and wasteful investigations.

In the realm of suspected prostatic infection, culture of exudate or of *postmassage urine* may be of help.

Anorectal Difficulties

Staining of fecal specimens for occult blood is a laboratory procedure, but one performed at the bedside by most clinicians. All practitioners are encouraged to think of this as part of the physical examination and a part that can be repeated by the laboratory on defecated stool if suspicion persists when the first test is negative. Staining for fecal leukocytes, which is best done on a part of a diarrheal stool that is rich in mucus, helps define the cause of diarrhea. Any of several stains can be used; *methylene blue* is the simplest. *Gram's stain* has the further utility of staining the fecal flora. The latter becomes important when a dominant bacterial or fungal morphology is sought in the setting of fecal neutrophils. Stool can be studied for a host of other problems, including parasitic infection, by various morphologic and cultural techniques. Visualization of the distal colorectal and anal mucosa can be accomplished with anoscopy and proctosigmoidoscopy.

RECOMMENDED READINGS

Screening Examination of Male Genitalia and Rectum

Amelar RD, Dubin L. Importance of careful palpation of vas deferens. Urology 1974;4:495.

Amerson JR. Inguinal canal and hernia examination. In: Walker HK, Hall WD, Hurst JW, ed. Clinical methods: the history, physical, and laboratory examinations. 3rd ed. Boston: Butterworths, 1990:484–485.

Blumer G. The rectal shelf: a neglected rectal sign of value in the diagnosis and prognosis of obscure malignant and inflammatory disease within the abdomen. Albany Med Ann 1909;30:361–366.

Kulbaski MJ, Goold SD, Tecce MA, Friedenheim RA, Palarski JD, Brancati FL. Oral iron and the hem-occult test: a controversy on the teaching wards [letter]. N Engl J Med 1989;320:1500.

Pedersen KV, Carlsson P, Varenhorst E, Lofman O, Berglund K. Screening for carcinoma of the prostate by digital rectal examination in a randomly selected population. BMJ 1990;300: 1041–1044.

Schneiderman H. Carcinoma in situ of the penis. Consultant 1990;30:49–52.

Wallis LA, Tardiff K, Deane K, Frings J. Teaching associates and the male genitorectal exam. J Am Med Wom Assoc 1984;39:57–58, 62.

Zornow DH, Landes RR. Scrotal palpation. Am Fam Physician 1981;23:150–154.

Extended Examination of Male Genitalia and Rectum

Ackerman AB, Kornberg R. Pearly penile papules: acral angiofibromas. Arch Dermatol 1973;108: 673–675.

Barrasso R, Brux JD, Croissant O, Orth G. High prevalence of *Papillomavirus*-associated penile intraep-ithelial neoplasia in sexual partners of women with cervical intraepithelial neoplasia. N Engl J Med 1987;317:916–923.

Donohue RE, Fauver HE. Unilateral absence of the vas deferens: a useful clinical sign. JAMA 1989; 261:1180–1182.

Najmaldin A, Burge DM. Acute idiopathic scrotal oedema: incidence, manifestations and aetiology. Br J Surg 1987;74:634–635.

Rosemberg SK. Sexually transmitted papillomaviral infections: IV. The white scrotum. Urology 1989;33:462–464.

Roy CR, Wilson T, Raife M, Horne D. Varicocele as the presenting sign of an abdominal mass. J Urol 1989;141:597–599.

Wheeler RA, Atwell JD. Horizontal testis with a varicocele: a new physical sign. Br J Surg 1991;78:225.

White WB, Barrett S. Penile ulcer in heroin abuse: a case report. Cutis 1982;29:62–64.

14

Female Genitalia and Rectum

APPROACH AND ANATOMICAL REVIEW

Approach

The pelvic and rectal examinations frequently constitute the last portion of the physical examination of the woman. The examination of the pelvic organs may be appropriately deferred or deleted in the asymptomatic patient under only very few circumstances:

1. Documentation of a complete assessment within the preceding calendar year, including a normal (class I) Papanicolaou (Pap) smear in any woman who has ever been sexually active
2. Active menstrual bleeding, which makes interpretation of the Papanicolaou smear unreliable and may necessitate a second visit when active flow has ceased
3. Known current pregnancy unless specific indications for the examination exist
4. Certain special circumstances in the setting of adolescence or the very elderly

The decision to delete the pelvic examination from any comprehensive physical assessment requires that the clinician have a sound reason for not including it.

PREPARATION

Preparation for the pelvic examination includes awareness of the date of the last menstrual period and an assessment of the patient's prior experiences and current concerns about the examination itself. A brief but thoughtful dialogue including any necessary explanation about the procedure before it is begun will reduce time expenditure and possibly discomfort for both parties during the examination. The decision to have a third party (chaperone) present for this portion of the examination depends on the clinical setting, the preference of the patient, and the needs of the examiner. An extra pair of hands to pass equipment and supplies may shorten the procedure; on the other hand, the privacy preferences of the patient should be considered in making the decision about third party presence. In some circumstances, it is prudent to have a chaperone present for the legal protection of the examiner.

INSTRUMENTS AND SUPPLIES

The instruments and supplies required for the pelvic and rectal examinations are listed in Table 14.1. When possible, the examination is conducted with the patient in the lithotomy position on a standard examining table with retractable foot extensions and stirrups. A movable light source, either a goose-neck lamp or a flexible gynecologic light, illuminates the external genitalia for effective inspection; in the absence of a light attachment for a transparent speculum, a movable light source permits inspection of the vaginal wall and cervix, including visually directed acquisition of the Papanicolaou smear. The pelvic examination begins with evaluation of the external genitalia, proceeds to inspection of the cervix and vagina with use of the speculum, is followed by bimanual palpation of the pelvic organs and, lastly, the anal and rectovaginal examinations.

Anatomical Review

EXTERNAL GENITALIA

The **external genitalia** (Fig. 14.1) include those structures visible on inspection of the **vulva.** They are described and defined as they appear when the patient is in a lithotomy position (on her back with knees and hips flexed, hips externally rotated, and thighs separated). The **mons pubis** is the fleshy mound padding the symphysis pubis and, in the fully developed adult woman, is covered with dark, coarse hair in the distribution of an inverted triangle with the flat base extending onto the abdomen and the apex at or near the perineal body.

The **labia majora** are the folds of skin, fat, and connective tissue that surround and protect the deeper surface structures. They extend from the mons to a bit behind the posterior commissure. At the ventral bifurcation of the labia majora lies the **clitoris** encased in its hood. Immediately posterior (inferior, as the structures appear to the examiner who faces the patient's perineum as described above) to the clitoral structures, the **labia minora** bifurcate and follow the general contour of the labia majora. The labia minora are thinner and are covered with squamous mucous membrane. The posterior reapproximation of the labia minora is known as the **posterior fourchette.** Within the **vestibule** medial to the two labia minora lie the remaining surface structures of the external genitalia.

The **urethral meatus,** or opening of the urethra, appears as a slightly vertical elongated dimple or orifice approximately 2 cm posterior (inferior) to the clitoris.

The **vaginal orifice** is a long vertical slit extending from just posterior to the urethral meatus to the posterior fourchette (**hymenal ring at the introitus**), its most posterior extremity.

The 2–3-cm expanse of skin between the posterior commissure and the anal orifice is technically known as the **perineum,** although the term perineum is also used more loosely for the whole external genital–anal complex.

Table 14.1
Instruments and Supplies

Examining table with	For cervical/vaginal cultures and other
Retractable stirrups	studies for infection
Padding for stirrups	Glass slides
Retractable foot tray	KOH solution
Flexible light source	Saline solution
Examiner's stool or chair	Thayer-Martin medium (for gonococci)
Cloth drapes (sheets)	Chlamydia transport medium
Running warm water	Culturette tubes
Examination gloves, disposable (nonsterile)	
Assortment of speculum sizes	For fecal occult blood testing
Hand mirror (for patient education)	Smear cards (guaiac-impregnated)
Water-based lubricant	Developing fluid
For Papanicolaou smears	
Bifid spatula	
Cotton swabs or endocervical brushes	
Glass slides/pencil	
Spray fixative	

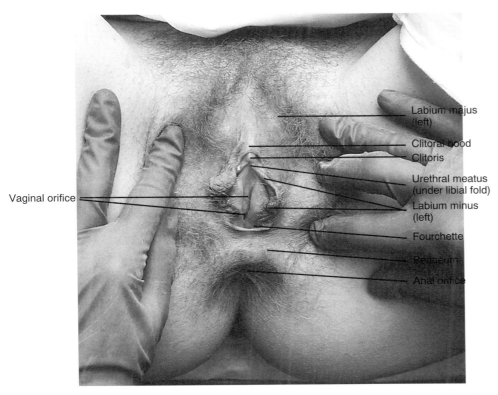

Figure 14.1 External female genitalia. In this view the urethral meatus, lying between the clitoris and the anterior part of the vaginal orifice (anterior fourchette), is hidden in a labial fold. Note the redundant tissue of the right labium minus; this type of labial asymmetry is a very common normal variant.

The openings to the **greater vestibular glands (Bartholin's glands)** lie in the cleft between the labia minora and the vaginal orifice. The glands themselves are located in the labia majora. The openings to the **periurethral glands (Skene's glands)** lie on either side of and posterior to the urethra.

The **anal orifice,** the puckered exit of the gastrointestinal tract, is located at the juncture of the gluteal folds.

INTERNAL GENITALIA

The representation of the internal organs of the female pelvis and their relationship to the rectum are presented in a schematic sagittal view with the subject upright (Fig. 14.2*A*) and in a coronal view constructed to depict the anatomical structures as they might be mentally perceived by the clinician conducting an examination with the patient in the lithotomy position (Fig. 14.2*B*). The pelvic organs of the woman include the vagina, the uterus with its two components, the cervix and the corpus, the bilateral Fallopian tubes, and the two ovaries with their ligamentous attachments. The relationship of the sigmoid colon and rectum to the pelvic organs becomes clear with study of the figures indicated.

From the **introitus,** the **vagina** extends superoposteriorly to end in a blind pouch encasing the uterine cervix. The vaginal wall is rugated during reproductive years but flat-walled in childhood and long after menopause. It is an expansile tube composed of muscular fibers lined with squamous mucosa and separated from the bladder anteriorly and the rectum posteriorly by thin connec-

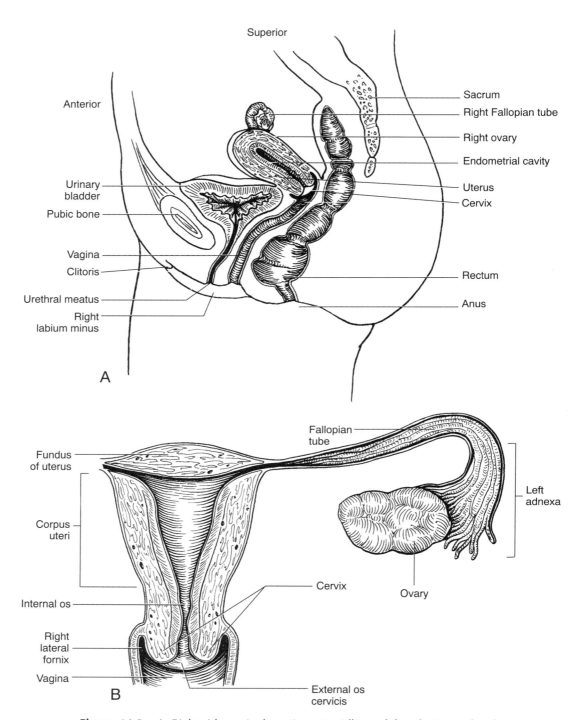

Figure 14.2   **A.** Right-side sagittal section at midline of female internal pelvic organs. **B.** Schematic coronal section of uterus and adnexal structures, with adnexa greatly magnified.

tive tissue layers. The **cervix** protrudes into the apex of the vagina. The pocket of the folded vaginal wall surrounding the cervix is divided for descriptive surfaces into four **fornices** (recesses), anterior and posterior and left and right lateral.

The roughly pear-shaped **uterus** is a muscular organ that is flattened in its anteroposterior dimension and may be inclined slightly forward or folded on itself anteriorly or posteriorly. The normal sexually mature but nulliparous uterus is 5–8 cm long and 3–4 cm wide, relatively mobile, and covered by peritoneum, the posterior reflection of which separates it from the rectosigmoid. The cul-de-sac (recess) of peritoneal space between the posterior surface of the uterus and the anterior surface of the rectum is referred to as the **pouch of Douglas.** The body of the uterus is a hollow organ lined with specialized mucosa called **endometrium;** the uterus tapers to terminate in the **cervix.** The external, or distal, end of the cervix contains an opening visible on speculum examination of the vagina, referred to as the **cervical (external) os.** The dome, or broadest upper portion of the uterine corpus, is often palpable on bimanual examination as the **uterine fundus.**

Inserted into the upper lateral angles of the uterus are the two **Fallopian tubes** (also called salpinges (singular: salpinx) or oviducts). Each salpinx is several centimeters long and terminates in fimbriated ends that capture an ovum expelled from the ovary at ovulation. Each tube is suspended by its **mesosalpinx,** a fold of the broad ligament.

The **ovaries,** suspended from the Fallopian tubes and the uterus by ligamentous attachments (mesovaria), are small, pecan-shaped glands resting approximately at the level of the anterosuperior iliac spine near the lateral pelvic wall. The internal pelvic organs are supported by ligamentous attachments to the bony pelvis, the four pairs of which are called the **round, broad, cardinal, and uterosacral ligaments.**

The **anus** is the distal communication of the **rectum,** which is separated from the posterior surface of the vagina by the thin **rectovaginal septum.** The anal canal is surrounded by a series of striated muscles (e.g., levator ani) that provide its voluntary **sphincter** control. At the level of the internal sphincter, the **anal verge** opens into the pouch of the distal rectum.

TECHNIQUE

The examination of the female pelvis and rectum is usually conducted at the end of the physical examination for practical reasons and for comfort. It requires major repositioning of the patient and the examiner, a well-organized and well-arranged set of instruments and supplies (see Table 14.1), and some detailed explanation of procedure. Because the patient is required to be in a relatively blinded and uncomfortable position throughout this portion of the physical examination, it should be conducted as quickly and efficiently as possible, short of compromising efficacy or accuracy. The following advance preparations must be completed by the examiner and, if indicated, an assistant:

1. Before positioning the patient, briefly explain the steps of the examination, answering any questions she may have.
2. **Give the patient the opportunity to empty her bladder.** A full bladder compromises the bimanual examination and creates discomfort for the woman being examined.
3. Arrange all supplies near at hand, such that they can be reached without confusion or interruption of the examination.
4. Determine that privacy is ensured.

5. Proper positioning of the woman is essential to conducting the examination. Elevation of the head of a breakable examining table to 45° permits eye contact and enables observation of the patient's facial expression throughout the examination.

6. The metal stirrups on the standard examining table should be padded with fabric, or the woman should be allowed to put on shoes, slippers, or socks.

7. The length of the stirrup supports is adjusted to allow the greatest comfort in terms of hip flexion. This will vary depending on the height, weight, and joint mobility of the patient.

8. Draping for this examination provides warmth for the thighs and abdominal wall and a modicum of privacy, but it must not obstruct eye contact between patient and clinician (Fig. 14.3) or the visibility of all perineal structures.

Evaluation of External Genitalia

Ask the patient to slide her buttocks toward the end of the table until she feels your bilaterally gloved hands. The buttocks should be flush with the end of table, with the foot-support extension retracted. Ask her to externally rotate her hips as far as is comfortable. The drape is adjusted to cover the thighs. You should be seated comfortably and have available an adjustable light source that permits a well-illuminated view of the external structures. **Always notify the patient**

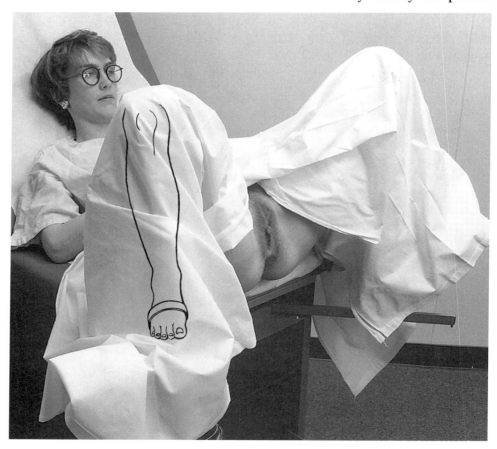

Figure 14.3   Patient is positioned and draped for the pelvic examination. The head of the examining table is elevated 45° to permit visual contact between seated examiner and patient. The drape is arranged to cover the patient's thighs and legs without imposing visual barrier.

before touching. She is unable to see your hand movements from her position. It is useful and reassuring to the woman if you explain what is being observed as the external genitalia are sequentially inspected and palpated. The examination proceeds as indicated below (Table 14.2).

INSPECTION

Inspect the external structures from anterior to posterior. Distribution of pubic hair is noted for the female pattern. Gently retract the labia major laterally to expose the hood of the clitoris, which is inspected for skin lesions. With the index finger, retract the hood anteriorly to allow visualization of the clitoris itself, also inspected for irritation or skin lesions. Now, with index fingers and thumbs, spread the labia minora laterally in order to view the urethral orifice, which is examined for redness or discharge. *Do not touch the urethral meatus.* Posterior (inferior) to the urethra, the vaginal orifice comes into view. Examine it for patency and the normal, glistening pink mucosal surface (Fig. 14.4).

Then, inspect the perineum and the anal orifice. Note the normal puckering of the gray-pink to brown mucosa of the anus, with attention paid to the presence of skin tags or venous prominences.

PALPATION

Palpation of the external genitalia includes assessment for possible enlargement of the Bartholin's or Skene's glands; the former are palpable within the substance of the labia majora, while the latter are palpable in the periurethral area. This is accomplished by palpating each labium between thumb and index finger and by observing for swelling or tenderness.

Table 14.2
Sequence of the Pelvic Examination

Preliminaries	Bimanual examination of internal organs
Preliminary discussion	Inspection: none
Assembly of equipment	Palpation
Positioning and draping of patient	Cervix
Donning of gloves	Fundus
External genitalia	Adnexal structures
Inspection	Changing of gloves
Pubic hair	
Skin of perineum	Rectovaginal examination
Clitoris and hood	Inspection
Urethral meatus	Perianal area
Vaginal introitus	Anal mucosa
Anal orifice	Palpation
Palpation	Anal verge
Labia majora and nearby glands	Rectovaginal septum
Labia minora	Uterine fundus and cervix
	Rectal vault
Vagina and cervix: the speculum examination	
Inspection	Fecal occult blood testing
Cervical surface and os	
Vaginal mucosa	
Obtaining specimens	
Pap smear(s), if indicated	
Culture(s), if indicated	

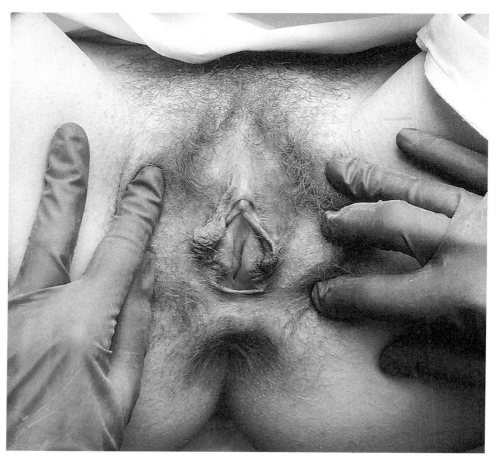

Figure 14.4   Labia are gently retracted laterally to expose more tissue of the external genitalia for inspection. The urethral slit is brought into view by shifting fingers to retract labia minora superolaterally.

Examination of Vagina and Cervix

EQUIPMENT

The next step in the pelvic examination is the inspection of the vagina and uterine cervix, which requires insertion of the vaginal **speculum**. The choice of speculum size and style is dependent on the anatomy of the patient and the preference of the examiner. After having inspected the external genitalia the clinician should have a sense of the best speculum to use. The nulliparous patient, especially one who has no history of vaginal penetration may require a smaller speculum or one with very narrow blades. The presence of an intact hymen or a hymenal membrane that is still evident may also require modification of speculum choice. If you are in doubt about the appropriate speculum, insert a finger that has been *lubricated with tap water* into the vaginal introitus to assess for relaxation and dimensions of the orifice. The options of speculum sizes and styles are depicted in Figure 14.5.

The choice between the transparent plastic speculum and the metal speculum is a matter of examiner preference. The plastic speculum has the advantages of (*a*) disposability, (*b*) transparency, allowing better visualization of the vaginal mucosa, and (*c*) adaptation for an attached light source. Its disadvantages include

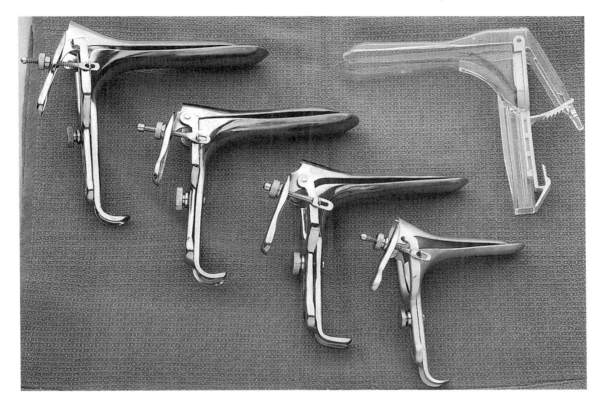

Figure 14.5 Variations on the vaginal speculum. Pictured from left to right are a large Graves speculum with blades 13 cm long × 3½ cm wide, a standard Graves speculum (11 × 3 cm), the narrow and flatter Pedersen speculum (11½ × 2½), and a pediatric speculum, which is 8½ × 2 cm. The plastic speculum is seen in *right upper corner.*

(*a*) a higher frequency of dysfunction, (*b*) lack of size and length options, and (*c*) a disturbing ratcheting noise when it is being opened.

INSERTION OF SPECULUM AND INSPECTION

The speculum is warmed and lubricated with **warm tap water. Do not lubricate with gel** if a Papanicolaou smear is to be done, as the gel renders the specimen unusable for the cytologist. Before inserting the speculum, gently exert downward (posterior) pressure with a finger at the posterior fourchette in the introitus, thus relaxing the perineal muscles at the posterior vaginal orifice. Introduce the speculum, with blades closed, at an angle 45° to the vertical, maintaining downward pressure against the perineal muscles in order to avoid traumatizing the anterior urethra. Direct the speculum toward the sacrum as you pass it slowly into the vaginal canal. When the full length of the speculum blades has entered the vagina, rotate the instrument so the blades are at right angles to the introitus and the handle is posterior (Figs. 14.6 and 14.7).

Now open the speculum blades, adjust the light source, and look for the uterine cervix. The latter should slide into view at the distal end of the opened speculum blades—unless the patient has had a hysterectomy. If slight manipulation of the position of the blades does not bring the cervical os into full central view, close and retract the blades slightly, and reposition. When the cervix lies between the blades, the latter are fixed in the open position by the thumbscrew at the han-

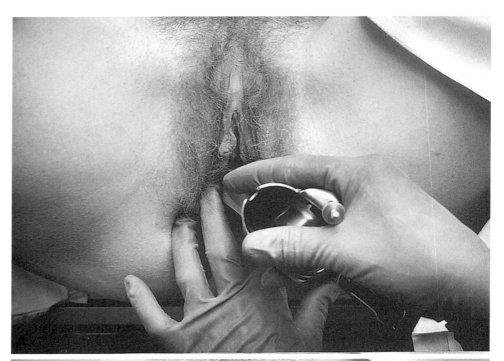

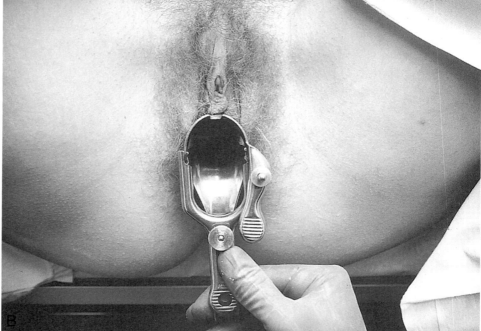

Figure 14.6   A. Insertion of vaginal speculum. The tip of the examiner's left index finger is inserted slightly into the posterior vagina while exerting gentle downward traction. The examiner's right index finger rests on the superior blade of the speculum, which is angled at 45° to the horizontal plane. **B.** After insertion of the speculum blade tips, the instrument is rotated to the horizontal plane before opening the blades. The insertion is completed under direct visualization. (Note the normal redundant fold of labium minus resting on the superior blade.)

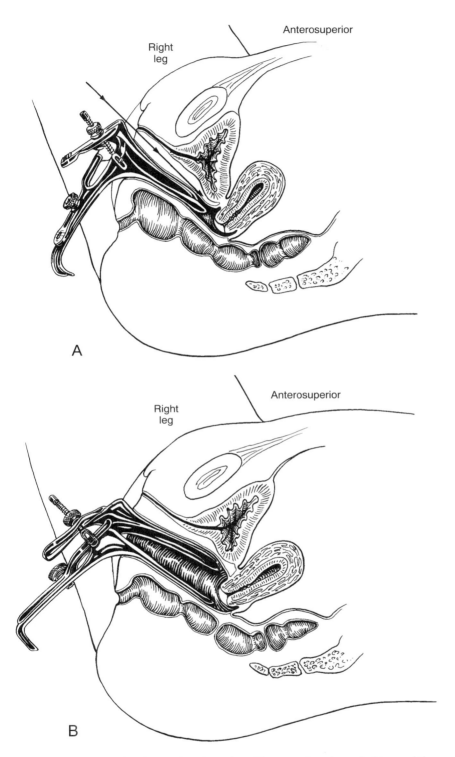

Figure 14.7   **A.** Angle of speculum insertion. The speculum is angled toward the sacrum as it is advanced along the vaginal canal toward the cervix. **B.** Once the speculum is inserted to its full length, the blades are slowly opened to expose the cervix to view.

dle. The speculum, if properly placed and fixed, should remain in position such that your hands are both freed to obtain the cervical samples.

The cervix and its os are inspected for color, shape, and the presence of friability or bleeding. Any surface irregularities or discoloration are noted as to location and physical characteristics.

OBTAINING CYTOLOGIC SAMPLES

Cell samples are obtained from two sites: the endocervix and the (exo)cervical surface. **Endocervical cells** may be gathered by inserting a saline moistened swab 0.5–1 cm into the cervical os (roughly to the hilt of its cotton tip) and twirling 360° in this position or by the use of a specially designed brush. The cells are transferred immediately to a clean and labeled glass slide and **fixed at once** with spray (Spray-cyte, etc.). If a commercial fixative is unavailable, a jar filled with 95% ethanol works well. Immediacy is critical; even a few extra seconds of air-drying can render the cells uninterpretable. **Cervical cells** are obtained by inserting the elongated end of a bifid spatula into the cervical os and scraping the surface of the cervix by rotating the spatula. Again, the sample is transferred to a glass slide and fixed immediately. Some clinicians obtain a third sample from the posterior fornix, where cells have been shed into the pooled secretions. This **vaginal pool** sample is picked up by a cotton swab and transferred to a slide (Fig. 14.8). Cervical cell sampling should induce no pain; at most, it may create a slight sensation of pressure; however, some patients may have **slight** vaginal spotting for a few hours.

WITHDRAWING THE SPECULUM

Once the specimens have been obtained and fixed, the speculum blades are "unfixed" by releasing the thumbscrew and are slowly withdrawn and simultaneously rotated gently so the vaginal mucosa may be inspected for inflammation, lesions, or adherent discharge. After the cervix has fallen from the blades and the deep two-thirds of the vaginal canal has been inspected, the blades are fully closed to facilitate withdrawal from the introitus. If disposable, the speculum is placed with the discarded cellular sampling devices, into the appropriate container for disposal. A reusable metal speculum is transferred to a transport container for cleaning; it is *not* placed in the sink where hand washing takes place.

Bimanual Palpation of Internal Organs

The third step in the sequential examination of the female pelvis is palpation of the uterus and adnexal structures. If you intend to use one hand for all internal

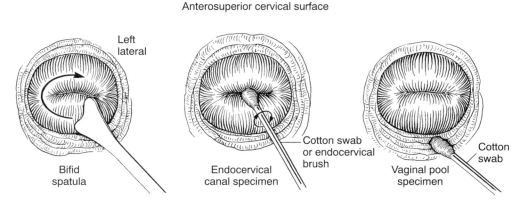

Figure 14.8 Obtaining cervical samples.

manipulation, the glove on the other hand may be removed for better tactile appreciation through the abdominal wall. This examination is done standing, so that you may continue to watch the patient's face for any expression of discomfort and to allow effective positioning of the hands.

Introduce the index and middle fingers of the dominant hand into the introitus, palmar surface upward, and pass them along the vaginal canal to the posterior fornix. Palpate the cervix for variations in consistency; each fornix is entered by the fingertips in search of tenderness or irregularities. Then, grasp the cervix between the fingertips and move it side to side, seeking its range of mobility and any tenderness elicited by motion. Next, position the fingers in the posterior fornix and elevate the uterine cervix anteriorly to bring the fundus toward the anterior abdominal wall. Then, with the outer ("upper") hand on the abdominal wall, palpate the elevated uterus through the abdominal wall just above the symphysis pubis. In this position, the commonly anteverted anteflexed fundus may be assessed between the internal fingers and the abdominal hand. If the fundus does not become palpable with cervical elevation, it is likely retroverted or retroflexed and will be better assessed on rectovaginal palpation (see Fig. 14.9 for variations of normal uterine position).

The fundus of the uterus, thus captured between the examining hands, is assessed for size, smoothness of contour, mobility, and tenderness. The normal uterus moves freely from side to side and anteroposteriorly without motion tenderness. It is smooth, firm, and nontender (Fig. 14.10A).

Next, palpate the adnexal structures. The fingers are placed in one lateral fornix, palmar surfaces anterior (upward), and projected along the inguinal ligament toward the anterosuperior iliac spine. Simultaneously, the hand on the abdomen, beginning at the level of the anterosuperior iliac spine, is drawn, palmar surface against the skin, toward the symphysis. The motion of the fingers is that of a continuous stroke, attempting to trap the ovary between the fingers on the abdomen and those in the vagina. The freely mobile ovary is elusive and will slip between the two hands quickly, but with a distinct visceral sensation experienced by the patient. If you fail to encounter the ovary on the first "sweep," you may repeat the motion until the patient is certain that the ovary has or has not been felt. The ovary is noted for its mobility, size, and consistency (Fig. 14.10B).

Only in exceptionally thin and relaxed patients can normal Fallopian tubes be appreciated as separate structures. The failure to feel the Fallopian tubes has no significance, therefore, even in "easy to examine" patients.

The above procedure is repeated on the opposite side for the adnexal structures.

Anal and Rectovaginal Examination

The final segment of the pelvic examination is the assessment of the uterus and abdomen via the rectum and of the anus and rectum themselves. For this portion of the examination, the clinician should be seated in order to directly visualize the anal orifice. Fresh gloves are donned to avoid any microscopic blood or microbial contamination from the vagina.

Inspect the skin surrounding the anus. Place a finger on either side of the anus and spread the tissue laterally, separating the puckers of the anus to allow better visualization of its surface.

After describing the procedure to the patient, ask her to bear down slightly against your well-lubricated *middle* fingertip placed at the anal orifice. This relaxes the anal sphincter and facilitates the painless introduction of the middle finger into the rectum. Now stand. Next, introduce the *index* finger into the posterior (inferior) aspect of the vagina at the posterior fourchette, and the two fin-

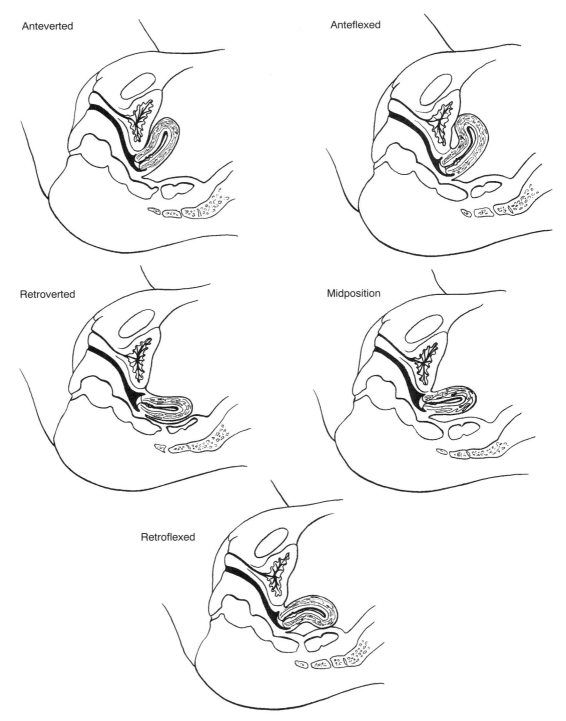

Figure 14.9   Range of normal uterine positions.

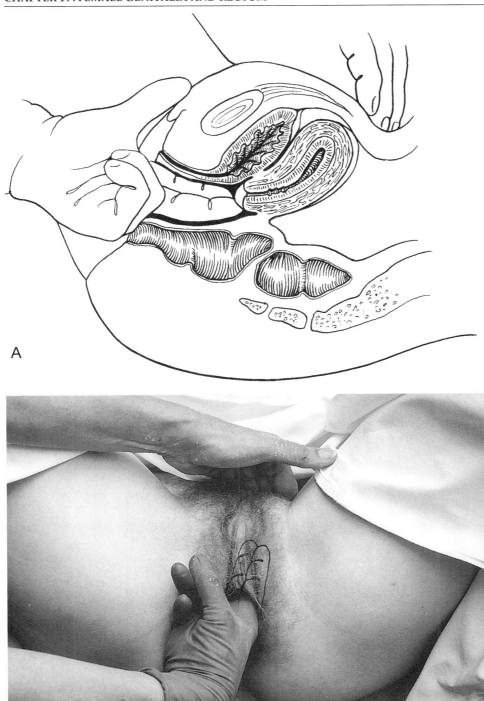

Figure 14.10 **A.** Uterine palpation. The two vaginal fingers find and elevate the cervix anteriorly, while the abdominal hand palpates the uterine fundus as it is pushed up from behind the pubic bone. **B.** Adnexal palpation. The intravaginal fingers press superolaterally into each adnexal region, while the abdominal fingers sweep parallel to the corresponding inguinal ligament, attempting to trap the ovary between the fingers of the two hands.

gers are approximated across the thin rectovaginal septum and swept side to side, assessing for tenderness or mass in the septum (Fig. 14.11). You may then remove the vaginal finger. Use the remaining rectal finger to palpate the posterior surface of the uterine fundus if it is retroverted and thus has not been clearly palpable on bimanual vaginal examination. Again, assess the fundus for its texture, for tenderness, and for the presence of irregularities or masses. When the uterine examination is completed, palpate the rectum through 360°, feeling for rectal masses or tenderness. When you are satisfied that the rectal vault, anal verge, and surrounding abdominopelvic contents have been completely palpated, remove the rectal finger and transfer adherent stool to a specimen card for occult blood testing.

At the completion of the pelvic and rectal examination, the patient is helped into the sitting position, given a box of tissues to cleanse herself of the lubricant, and allowed privacy to dress before the discussion of findings and plans from the encounter are conducted.

NORMAL AND COMMON VARIANTS

The normal female pelvic structures and some common variants are discussed in the order in which the examination proceeds: from inspection of the external genitalia and the cervix and vagina, to palpation of the pelvic organs, to inspection and palpation of the anus and rectovaginal area.

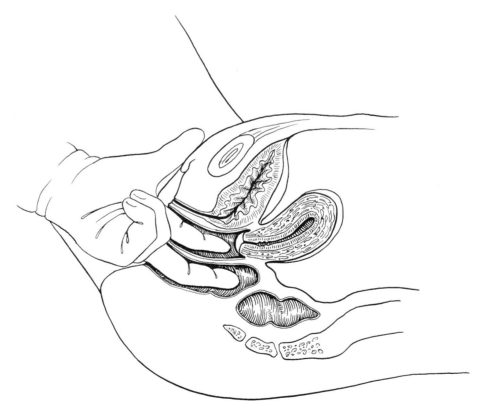

Figure 14.11   Rectovaginal examination. The rectovaginal septum is palpable between the two fingers as shown. The posterior surface of the uterus and cervix is palpated through the thin rectal wall. The fundus of a retroflexed uterus may be palpable only via the rectum.

Inspection of External Genitalia

The thickness and the distribution of pubic hair vary widely. Some normal women have sparse pubic hair, and hair thinning and loss are common in the years after menopause and usual in old age. Although hair distribution is most commonly that of the inverted triangle described earlier, many women will have extension of pubic hair in the midline of the abdomen toward the umbilicus, to produce a diamond-shaped escutcheon, and laterally along the groins and the upper medial thighs. Only if there has been a *change* in hair distribution after full development of secondary sex characteristics should such a widened distribution be a cause for concern.

The color of the vulvar skin is usually uniformly dark pink to brown, although there may be genetically determined variations in pigment. Several years after cessation of estrogenic stimulation, the tissue will lighten in color and become slightly atrophic and dry.

During pregnancy (and rarely in the woman with proximal venous obstruction), prominent veins may be seen on the vulva. These are rarely symptomatic or cause for concern, although a unilateral engorgement may indicate compression of the pelvic venous system.

The posterior introitus may reveal evidence of an intact hymen, skin tags as remnants of a perforate hymen, or, on palpation, a distinct band of hymenal ring tissue. Occasionally, the hymen is sufficiently well developed to prevent introduction of more than one finger or of the speculum blades. When vaginal and cervical inspection are required in this setting, the narrow Pedersen speculum or the small pediatric speculum should be considered, although even these are not inevitably successful.

Inspection of Cervix and Vagina

The angle of the cervix relative to the plane of the vaginal canal is a function of the position of the uterus (see Fig. 14.9 for normal variants of uterine position). The cervical surface is mucosal, pink, and moist in appearance, and has been compared to that of another nonkeratinized squamous mucosa, the buccal mucosa. A bluish discoloration is normally present in pregnancy. It is common to see small mucus-filled (retention) cysts, **Nabothian follicles,** on the surface of the cervix. Occasional enlargement of the cervix, causing symmetrical elongation of the lips, is noted and has no clinical significance.

The cervical os varies in appearance with parity. The nulliparous os is usually tightly closed, a small pore in the center of the cervical surface. Vaginal delivery permanently changes the configuration of the os, giving it a slit-like appearance or, if cervical lacerations occurred during childbirth, irregularity (see Sample Write-up in the Extended Examination section). Some eversion of a patulous os may bring into view the redder, pebbly-appearing tissue of the endocervix at the rim of the os. It is not uncommon to discover a soft pink mass at the os, an **endocervical polyp.** Only if it is symptomatic (postcoital bleeding) or diagnostically questionable on inspection is biopsy or removal of this common variant necessary.

The mucosa of the vagina in the adult woman during her reproductive years is pink, heavily rugated, and moist with normal glandular secretions. A small amount of clear to white mucus is often but not inevitably seen, distributed along the walls of the vagina and pooled in the posterior fornix. With physiologic loss of estrogen production, the postmenopausal vagina eventually thins, flattens, and becomes less fully lubricated. In the very aged woman, the mucosa may become gray-white with punctate friability and cicatrix (scar) formation leading, respectively, to petechiae and to adhesions (synechiae) between opposite walls.

Palpation of Internal Genitalia

The cervix may be deviated in any direction as a function of uterine position and is sometimes directed somewhat laterally. However, the cervix should always be freely mobile without pain on manipulation. Pregnancy softens the surface of the cervix, which in the nonpregnant state has a palpable consistency similar to that of the tip of the nose. Occasionally, the Nabothian follicles or a cervical polyp may be palpable with the intravaginal examining fingers.

Parity increases nonpregnant uterine size by at least as much as 25% over nulliparous size; the enlargement gradually diminishes after the cessation of estrogen stimulation. The wide range of uterine positions is noted in Figure 14.9. Appreciation of such normal variability is important in selecting a method for optimal palpation. For example, the fundus of a sharply retroflexed uterus may be palpable only via the rectum.

The Fallopian tubes are rarely palpable when they are normal. During reproductive years, the adult ovaries are $3 \times 2 \times 1$-cm soft ovoids that slip between the abdominal and intravaginal fingers. A slightly tender unilateral enlargement may be present during the luteal phase (postovulation) of the menstrual cycle. In this situation, it is prudent to ask the patient to return for reexamination during or just after her next menses; the ovary should have returned to normal size and become nontender by then.

After menopause, the ovary decreases progressively in size as its cyclic functions cease. A palpable ovary 3 years or more beyond menopause is considered abnormal until proven otherwise.

Anal Inspection and Palpation

Visible anal mucosa is grayish-pink to brown-pink and tucked inward in multiple folds. Distended veins (**hemorrhoids**) may be seen at the skin-mucosa interface and disappearing into the anal canal. Soft and nontender veins are commonly present and require no attention unless they are accompanied by pruritus or thrombosis or are contributing to chronic fissure formation. Skin tags are evidence of previous surgery or irritation.

Muscle tone of the anal sphincter should resist but not prevent admission of a finger into the canal. The most common cause of a very tight sphincter is apprehension with involuntary tightening of the sphincter muscles. This resistance is overcome by asking the patient to bear down as if she were going to have a bowel movement, which relaxes the muscles of the sphincter. Lax sphincter tone is most often a result of perineal trauma during childbirth, although it is also seen in various neurologic disorders, in local problems, and nonspecifically with critical illness.

Rectovaginal and Rectal Palpation

The membrane separating the rectum from the vagina is thin and flexible between the examining fingers. As the rectal finger is advanced, it encounters anteriorly—sequentially and readily palpable through the septum—the cervix, the fundus or posterior corpus of the uterus, and the rectouterine pouch. Posteriorly, the finger drops over the anal verge into the soft, distensible rectal pouch, which is relatively rugate and should be free of mass. Each lateral rectal wall is normally also soft and mobile under the examining finger. Soft stool may or may not be felt in the rectal pouch, but there is usually enough stool or mucus on the glove when it is withdrawn to permit a smear for occult blood testing.

RECORDING THE FINDINGS

By convention, the pelvic and rectal examinations are recorded after the abdominal but before the musculoskeletal and neurologic examinations or, alternatively, at the end of the physical examination in the write-up. The routine examination of a normal woman in her reproductive years might read as follows:

Pelvic and rectal: Normal pubic hair distribution. External genitalia normal to inspection and palpation. Introitus easily entered with speculum, vaginal mucosa pink and moist with small amount of mucus. Cervical surface dotted with Nabothian follicles; color normal. Os parous with small degree of eversion at posterior lip. No bleeding induced by obtaining Papanicolaou specimen. Cervix anteverted, freely mobile, and nontender. Fundus anteflexed, freely mobile, smooth, firm. Size consistent with parity. Rectovaginal examination confirms vaginal findings; posterior aspect of uterus normal. Rectovaginal septum thin and free of nodularity.

Anal orifice looks normal apart from external skin tags. Sphincter tone normal, as is rectal pouch. No masses felt. Scant soft brown stool in ampulla, negative for occult blood.

EXTENDED EXAMINATION OF THE FEMALE GENITALIA AND RECTUM

INDICATIONS

With a few exceptions, the sequence and maneuvers of the pelvic examination are the same for the extended examination (symptomatic patient) as for the screening examination. The extensions beyond the routine are described as they are indicated by patient history, new symptoms, or unexpected abnormalities detected on examination.

- Patient's medical history, with or without symptoms
  1. Maternal diethylstilbestrol (DES) exposure
  2. Multiple (simultaneous or serial) sexual partners
  3. Unexplained infertility
- New or recurrent pelvic symptoms
  1. Change in character, frequency, regularity, or duration of menstrual bleeding
  2. Midcycle, postcoital, or postmenopausal vaginal bleeding
  3. Lower abdominal pain or swelling, especially unilateral
  4. Painful sexual intercourse (dyspareunia)
  5. Vulvar or vaginal pruritus
  6. Change in quantity or character of vaginal discharge
  7. Urinary incontinence
  8. Burning or pain on urination (dysuria), with or without diagnosed urinary tract infection
  9. Lower back pain or any other symptoms that bear consistent relationship to menstrual cycle
  10. Unexpected onset of menarche or menopause
- New or recurrent rectal symptoms
  1. Blood in or on stool or on toilet paper, or bleeding following defecation
  2. Pain in anorectum, either constantly or on defecation
  3. New constipation or change in configuration of stool
  4. Perianal itching
  5. Melena

- Abnormalities detected on screening examination (any of the following signs noted on screening examination call for further maneuvers or procedures even in the absence of symptoms)
    1. On inspection of the external genitalia—skin lesions, swelling, or erythema
    2. On speculum inspection—erythema, irritation, or mass of vaginal wall; erosion, friability, or mass on the cervical surface
    3. On bimanual palpation of uterus and ovaries—enlargement, tenderness, immobility, or mass of uterus, ovary, salpinx, parametrium (tissue surrounding pelvic organs), or rectovaginal septum
    4. On rectal examination—perianal skin lesions or bleeding, tenderness, or mass of anus or rectum

CONDUCTING THE EXTENDED EXAMINATION

Symptoms Referable to Pelvic Organs

Any of the complaints noted below require full inquiry regarding the parameters of the symptom itself and baseline information about menstrual history, pregnancy history, use and type of contraceptives, sexual activity, and prior pelvic symptoms or treatment for disease or dysfunction.

Change in menstrual pattern. Obtain full details of the change. The examination is conducted the same as the routine screening. Additional maneuvers are dictated by any abnormalities that are noted.

Postcoital bleeding. In conducting the examination, special attention is paid to the vaginal wall and cervix. Are bleeding points visible? Is the cervix friable? Does the spatula used to obtain smears induce bleeding? Is an endocervical polyp visible? Does it have a spotted appearance suggesting the *colpitis maculata* appearance of vaginal trichomoniasis?

Lower abdominal pain. In this instance, the screening pelvic examination should be preceded by a full abdominal examination and followed by additional procedures determined by the findings (see the Extended Examination section of Chapter 9).

Painful sexual intercourse. Local pathology may account for this symptom. On inspection of the external genitalia, observe for erythema or local skin disease and for discomfort induced by palpating the labia. Is the hymen sufficiently perforate to allow admission of two fingers without discomfort? Is there muscular spasm or pain with introduction of the speculum (vaginismus)? If so, does the speculum reproduce the type of pain experienced on intromission? The vaginal wall is inspected for evidence of inflammation or atrophy; the cervix, for visible pathology. On bimanual palpation, is pain produced by movement of the cervix, compression of the uterine fundus, or palpation of the adnexa? Are all organs of normal size, position, and shape? Is there edema of the labia?

Vulvar or vaginal pruritus. Inquire about local irritants, such as soaps, douche products, synthetic fabrics in underclothing, spermicides. Ask about genital symptoms of the patient's partner(s) if she is sexually active. Consider risk factors for vulvovaginal candidiasis, such as antibiotic therapy or use of oral contraceptives or systemic corticosteroids. Observe the vulva for evidence of atrophy or local skin disease and secondary excoriation, and examine the vaginal canal for inflammation or discharge.

Vaginal discharge. A history of increased or foul-smelling discharge indicates possible infection. Samples of the discharge are obtained for microscopic examination and/or culture. See Table 14.3 for a summary of smear and culture techniques based on the character of the discharge noted on examination.

Urinary incontinence. In the multiparous, postmenopausal, or posthysterectomy patient, the complaint of *urge or stress incontinence*—leaking or dribbling of

Table 14.3
Vaginal and Cervical Specimens for Smear and Culture[a]

Purulent cervical discharge in sexually active patient
Consider: *Neisseria gonorrhoeae*
Procedure: With cotton swab, obtain cervical and vaginal secretions. To prepare culture,
    spread specimen in "Z" pattern on Thayer-Martin (chocolate agar) plate or insert swab
    into culture tube. Follow local instructions for labeling, prompt transporting, and storage.

Cheesy white discharge with vulvar pruritus
Consider: *Candida albicans* (monilia) infection
Procedure: Obtain generous sample of discharge with swab, smear broadly on glass slide,
    mix with a drop of potassium hydroxide, add coverslip, examine immediately under
    microscope for budding hyphae or fungal branches, or after brief gentle warming of slide.
    Cultures for *C. albicans* are seldom clinically indicated; if needed, consult local labora-
    tory for proper medium and handling.

Watery, foul-smelling, copious discharge
Consider: *Trichomonas vaginalis* or *Gardnerella vaginalis*
Procedure: For trichomoniasis, collect vaginal pool specimen on spatula and transfer to
    glass slide; add 2 drops of saline solution, cover with glass coverslip, and examine
    promptly under microscope for motile flagellates. For *G. vaginalis,* obtain specimen in
    same fashion but apply to dry slide and examine immediately under microscope for
    "Clew cells," the intracellular inclusions suggestive of infection with this organism.

**Cervical erosion with surface purulence, urethritris with discharge, or history of exposure
    to infected male**
Consider: *Chlamydia trachomatis*
Procedure: A number of methods are currently available for obtaining and handling speci-
    mens for culture of this organism of increasing clinical significance. Consult local labora-
    tory for latest methods.

[a]The indications for obtaining material for culture or smear are history and physical examination dependent. Some common considerations are listed.

urine with increased intra-abdominal pressure (such as cough or laugh) or after
prolonged voluntary retention of urine—raises the question of reduced muscular
efficacy of the pelvic support structures. To assess for this possibility, ask the
patient to bear down while you observe the introitus. If the anterior or posterior
vaginal wall bulges with this maneuver, a **cystocele or a rectocele** respectively,
may be present. Then ask the patient to do a Valsalva maneuver, using the
demonstration technique described previously in the Extended Examination section of Chapters 2 and 8. The supporting structures of the bladder, urethra, and
anterior vaginal wall are thus evaluated. If the bladder and/or urethra bulges
outward, it is likely that muscular support is deficient, which may account for
impaired bladder control. Make an analogous observation of the rectovaginal
region, seeking bulging of the rectum into the posterior vaginal canal with
increased intra-abdominal pressure. During these maneuvers, look for leaking of
urine from the urethra or of stool from the anus.

   Painful urination. When the patient complains of burning during the passing of urine, of frequency or urgency of urination, or of postvoiding suprapubic
pain, there may be visible clues as to cause. Carefully inspect the urethral
meatus for atrophy, local erythema, and edema signalling inflammation, local
hypertrophy, or purulent discharge. Downward abdominal pressure immediately above the symphysis pubis is sometimes helpful in evaluating for bladder
tenderness secondary to cystitis. Upward pressure with a single digit placed

superiorly in the vagina may reveal midline urethral tenderness if *urethritis* is present.

Rectal bleeding. A history of bleeding from the rectum demands (*a*) a local inspection of the perianal area for venous distension or breaks in the integrity of the anal mucosa and (*b*) digital palpation of the anal verge and rectum for masses or tenderness. Analysis of the stool for gross and occult blood should be carried out on any specimen obtained. If the explanation of a history of bleeding from the rectum is not readily apparent on this examination—and some would say even if it is—more sophisticated assessment is required (see Beyond the Physical Examination).

Painful defecation. Inspection and palpation of the perianal area, anal canal, rectum, and rectovaginal septum are carried out as described for the screening examination.

Abnormalities Discovered on Screening Examination

Most asymptomatic abnormalities discovered on the screening examination are either inconsequential or will require diagnostic procedures beyond the scope of the physical examination. Any abnormality noted should prompt a review of the history to explore for overlooked or subtle, unvolunteered symptoms. Note the abnormality, assess its characteristics, and refer to the last two sections of this chapter for interpretation and further diagnostic steps.

Pelvic Examination in Suspected Pregnancy

If the history indicates possible pregnancy (i.e., delayed menses, unexplained vaginal spotting, nausea, breast changes), the pelvic examination may be of help in confirming this diagnosis. Prior to the fourth to sixth week of gestation, false-negative examinations are common, but some of the following pelvic signs have been noted to be associated with pregnancy:

1. Bluish discoloration of the cervix (Chadwick's sign)
2. Soft generalized uterine enlargement
3. Focal uterine softening (Dickinson's sign)
4. Uterine pulsation

The monitoring of the progress of pregnancy by means of pelvic examination is beyond the scope of this work but may be studied in any standard textbook of obstetrics.

Pelvic examination in the setting of suspected pregnancy, especially after 24 weeks of gestation, must be conducted with caution and only if specifically indicated by abdominal or pelvic symptoms or under the supervision of an experienced obstetrician. The introduction of infection and the induction of bleeding (as in the presence of a placenta previa) are possible complications of vaginal examination in advanced pregnancy.

Examination of the Rape Victim

Detailed discussion of this painful but very important issue clearly lies outside the scope of this textbook, and the interested reader is referred to reviews of the topic. The most basic principles to be borne in mind are

1. Pelvic examination is emotionally charged and difficult for patients in general, and it is all the more so for a victim of violence. Rape is a crime of violence. Thus it is absolutely essential that you be physically gentle and explicitly emotionally supportive for the examination not to compound the psychic and physical trauma that the patient has already experienced.

2. The purposes of the examination include not only the traditional one, establishing diagnoses with an eye to treatment, but also the collection of evidence that may help convict a criminal. Both purposes are well served by examining the patient before she has washed or douched and, ideally, with at least an initial interview and examination before voiding.

3. Look for evidence of trauma, not only in the genital area but also about the mouth, the anus, the face, the trunk, and the limbs. Although body orifices are the usual sites at which the rapist intromits either the penis, digit(s), fist, or a foreign body, any area may be struck with intent to harm. It may be worthwhile to take *photographs for documentation*, with patient permission.

4. Semen is important evidence and can be collected from the vagina, the anorectum, or the skin; dried semen, which appears yellow-white and flaky, is usable as evidence.

5. *Do not assume that the history is complete.* Fear and shame are powerful silencers, and the victim may tell only part of the story. It is wise to presume that vaginal, rectal, *and* oral penetration may have occurred.

6. Once the diagnostic and legal data collections are complete, reassurance is given, follow-up is arranged including companionship for the immediate present—often from a rape counseling service—and the patient is given an opportunity to wash and to change clothing in private, if desired. Remember that clothing, particularly if damaged and stained, constitutes evidence as well and should be collected, labeled, and bagged directly from the patient's hands.

7. The desire to be medically complete is tempered with mercy and perspective. For example, it is of greater import to inspect the vagina for lacerations than to be absolutely positive that the ovary is impalpable. Routine assessment can wait.

INTERPRETING THE FINDINGS

As a general rule, the role of the nonspecialist in the diagnosis of pelvic and rectal pathology is that of locating abnormalities, recognizing their significance, ordering the primary additional special procedures, and deciding whether referral for further diagnostic or therapeutic consultation and management is indicated. Interpretation of common abnormalities is broadly reviewed as a guide to decisions about further procedure. Suggestions for further studies and referral for pelvic pathology are incorporated into the final section of this chapter.

Common Abnormalities of Female Pelvis

A host of abnormalities are frequent in the organs under discussion (Table 14.4).

VULVA

Skin Lesions

The basic principles of interpretation of skin abnormalities apply to the vulva (see Chapter 3); however, there are some guidelines specific to this region. **Ulcers** of the vulva may be seen in venereal infection (such as the chancre of primary syphilis), granulomatous disease, neoplasm, and, less commonly, drug eruptions and treatable vasculitides, characteristically Behçet's syndrome. Each of the possibilities demands specific diagnosis in order to direct appropriate treatment, and the details are beyond the scope of a physical diagnosis text. **Melanoma** of the vulva has the significance of melanoma elsewhere, and when it is suspected, the patient should be referred for wide excisional diagnostic biopsy. Because of the relative invisibility of the vulva to patient self-examination (except with mirrors

Table 14.4
Common Abnormalities on Pelvic Examination

Vulva	Uterus
Skin lesions	Prolapse
Erythema	Tenderness
Atrophic vulvovaginitis	Enlargement
Laceration	Irregularity or mass
Hematoma	Fixation to surrounding structures
Edema	Adnexa
Melanoma	Tenderness
Ulcers	Enlargement
Masses	Irregularity or mass
Retention cyst	Rectovaginal septum
Condyloma acuminatum	Tenderness
Bartholin's gland cyst	Irregularity or mass
Urethral meatal signs	Anus and rectum
Edema	Engorged veins and hemorrhoids
Erythema	Fissures
Discharge	Fistulae
Atrophic urethritis	Hypertrophied anal papilla
Urethrocele/cystocele	Rectal mass or thickening
Vagina	Rectocele
Mucosal lesions	Dermatitis
Ulcer	
Erythema	
Laceration	
Masses	
Atrophy	
Cervix	
Mucosal lesions	
Erythema	
Friability	
Erosion or ulcer	
Cyst (Nabothian follicle)	

and persistence), particular care must be taken in determining the significance of any skin peculiarity noted by the clinician.

Generalized erythema of the vulva is most commonly secondary to candidal vulvitis, which can be established as noted in Table 14.3.

The most common benign **mass** of the vulva is the **retention cyst,** which is a mucosa-covered mucoid pocket found at the posterior introitus. Unless this cyst causes cosmetic or functional problems for the patient, it requires no further consideration. **Condyloma acuminatum** is the fleshy, frond-like, usually clustered collection of papules caused by the **human papilloma virus.** Because of its propensity for spread to the cervix and the association of some strains with neoplasia both there and in the vulva itself, the presence of condyloma on the vulva requires both local treatment and referral for colposcopic examination of the cervix. **Bartholin's gland cyst and/or abscess** presents as a unilateral swelling in one labium majus. When tender and inflamed, this abscess requires surgical drainage and/or excision.

Urethral Meatal Abnormalities

Redness and swelling at the urethral opening may be the result of local *trauma, urethral infection, or urethral caruncle,* which looks and feels more like a mass.

Specifics of the history of symptoms, culture of any discharge, and careful inspection will usually serve to define the etiology of periurethral inflammation.

VAGINA

Evaluation of **prolapse** of vaginal folds with other pelvic organs is discussed below. If **cystocele, urethrocele, or rectocele** is *symptomatic*—usually in the form of urinary incontinence—referral to a specialist may be indicated.

Ulcers of the vagina have the same etiologic spectrum as ulcers of the vulva, and *violent sexual intercourse* is a recent addition to the differential diagnosis. Vaginal **inflammation** is most commonly a result of local *trauma*, of *irritation* (e.g., contact "dermatitis") caused by the use of external products such as deodorant sprays or by douches, or of infection, e.g., candidal infection, trichomoniasis, and the "nonspecific vaginitis" of *Gardnerella* infection. Evaluation for infection as the source of an inflammatory reaction is outlined in Table 14.3.

Neoplasia of the vagina is uncommon except in women whose mothers received DES during pregnancy, but the presence of localized mucosal changes or masses must be evaluated for this potential. This is best done as a special procedure by an experienced gynecologist.

CERVIX

Friability, ulcer, erosion, or color irregularity of the cervical surface should be carefully sampled for Papanicolaou smears and cultured for *Chlamydia trachomatis* (see Table 14.3). If any doubt exists about the cause of cervical abnormality, the patient must be referred for colposcopy and biopsy. Irregular exophytic masses with surface necrosis occur late in cervical cancer, and the absence of visible abnormality does not guarantee the absence of serious disease.

UTERUS

Prolapse of the uterus along the vaginal canal or into or beyond the introitus is most commonly the result of damage from previous childbirth(s). The severity of symptoms and the degree of prolapse dictate whether and when referral is indicated. A minor, vaginally contained prolapse apparent only on increased intra-abdominal pressure may often be left alone; by contrast, a uterine cervix that extrudes from the vagina (grade 3–4 prolapse) should usually be referred for a pessary or for surgical correction.

Tenderness on manipulation indicates inflammation from infection or endometriosis. Neoplastic involvement of the organ or its suspensory tissue can cause fixation of the uterus. **Enlargement** of the uterus is most commonly due to **pregnancy** in the childbearing years and to **fibroid tumor** (benign leiomyoma) in midlife or later. Discrete **tumors** of the serosal surface of the uterine body are usually leiomyomas and, if asymptomatic, can be followed by observation only or at most with an ultrasonogram.

ADNEXA

Symptoms pointing to, or palpable abnormalities of, the adnexal structures are usually of concern. Enlargement and/or tenderness of the **salpinx** is indicative of either infection or ectopic pregnancy until proven otherwise. This condition is a relative medical emergency requiring immediate attention, usually including hospitalization and laparoscopy or laparotomy. **Ovarian** enlargement in the woman of childbearing age may be the result of a benign cyst, of polycystic ovary disease, or of ovarian neoplasia. Any unilateral enlargement of an ovary in this age group demands, at a minimum, careful reexamination at the end of the next menstrual period and, preferably, ultrasonic assessment sooner. Ovarian enlargement in the perimenopausal woman must be considered a potential malignancy, as must a distinctly palpable ovary in the woman who is more than 3 years past menopause.

RECTOVAGINAL SEPTUM

Scar tissue, nodules of **endometriosis,** or, more rarely, infiltrative carcinoma can create a rigid or lumpy rectovaginal septum. Any abnormality of this tissue requires expert assessment.

ANUS AND RECTUM

Hemorrhoids (venous distension with engorgement) of the anal veins and **fissures** (tissue breakdown) of the mucosa of the anus are common abnormalities of this region. A **thrombosed hemorrhoid** is a painful distension caused by coagulum in an obstructed vein. It often requires local surgical relief. **Fissures** cause

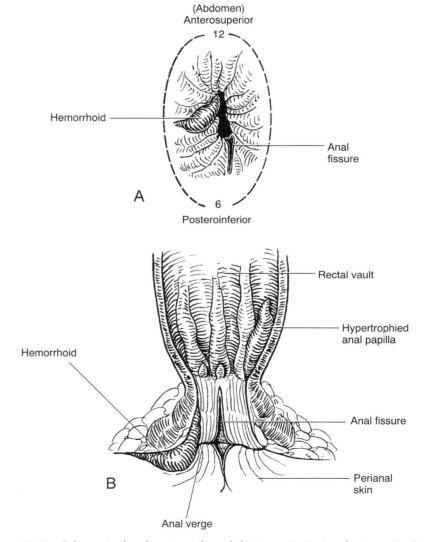

Figure 14.12 Schematic localization of anal lesions. **A.** Perineal view. **B.** Coronal schematic.

painful defecation and may result in streaking of blood on the stool or spotting of blood on the toilet tissue after defecation. They are superficial breaks in the mucosal or skin integrity, usually barely visible to inspection with the anal tissue spread. **Anal or anorectal fistulae** are much more serious. They present as sites of drainage of fecal material, with or without purulent matter, onto the perianal skin. They may be the result of old trauma, including iatrogenic injury, or represent necrosis from neoplasm or chronic inflammatory bowel disease, classically Crohn's disease. The presence of a fistula requires surgical assessment for diagnosis and definitive therapy. (See Figure 14.12 for representation of the positions of common anal pathology.)

At the anal verge, a mass may be indicative of either an internal hemorrhoid or a **hypertrophied anal papilla.** The distinction between the two usually requires visualization with an anoscope. Any palpable anorectal mass or area of thickening or rigidity also demands visual inspection via instrumentation to exclude *carcinoma of the anus.*

RECORDING THE FINDINGS

The findings on female pelvic and rectal examinations are recorded by narrative as noted previously, with liberal use of sketches when they are useful in delineating position or dimensions of a finding. An illustrative record of an abnormal pelvic examination follows.

Sample Write-up

External genitalia: Normal except for 1 × 1-cm mucoid cyst at 5 o'clock.

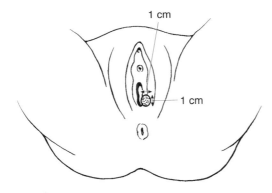

Vaginal vault: Moist, pink, and free of lesions. Cervical os parous. Small erosion, anterior lip, which bleeds easily with spatula contact.

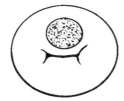

Bimanual examination: Mobile cervix, sharply anteflexed uterus, normal size and contour. Left adnexal structures normal. Right adnexal mass: soft, freely movable, 4 × 6 cm in dimension and nontender; not fluctuant and not clearly cystic. No ovary or tube distinct from this mass palpable on right side. Percussion note unchanged over this area.

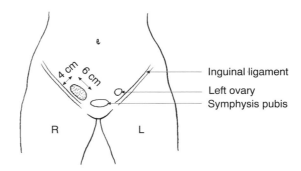

Inspection of anus: Cluster of small, fleshy papules, up to 3 mm across, gray to pink to right (9 o'clock) of orifice; remainder of rectal and rectovaginal examination normal. Right adnexal mass not appreciated by rectal palpation.

Impressions:
1. Right ovarian mass, ?teratoma.
2. Anterior cervical erosion, ?etiology.
3. Mucoid cyst, vulva.
4. Skin tags, anus.

BEYOND THE PHYSICAL EXAMINATION

Because of their routine nature or common occurrence, techniques for obtaining **Papanicolaou smears** and cervical, vaginal, and urethral smears and **cultures** have been outlined in the earlier part of this chapter. **Biopsies,** acquired by experienced personnel either with a punch curette or by blade excision, are required for lesions of the skin and mucosa that demand microscopic study. Uterine or adnexal enlargement or mass is, at the present time, best initially studied for its characteristics by pelvic **ultrasonography.** Palpable anorectal abnormalities usually require **anoscopy** or **proctoscopy.**

Rectal bleeding or change in bowel habits not clearly explained by inspection, palpation, and/or proctoscopic examination may require **colonoscopy** or **double-contrast (air-barium)** radiographic visualization of the lower tract. Lower urinary tract symptoms or cystourethral abnormalities not attributable to acute infection will sometimes call for **cystourethral visualization by endoscopy** (cystoscopy) and, in selected cases, for **contrast radiography,** i.e., excretory or retrograde urography. The majority of these procedures are best chosen, conducted, and interpreted by a specialist in the appropriate field.

Infertility evaluation is complex and outside the scope of this text.

RECOMMENDED READINGS

Barber HRK, Graber EA. The PMPO syndrome (postmenopausal palpable ovary syndrome). Obstet Gynecol 1971;38:921–923.

Broadmore J, Carr-Gregg M, Hutton JD. Vaginal examinations: women's experiences and preferences. N Z Med J 1986;99:8–10.

Buchwald J. The first pelvic examination: helping students cope with their emotional reactions. J Med Ed 1979;54:31–34.

Clyman SG. Why do we chaperone the female pelvic exam? Del Med J 1982;54(2):105–108.

Deneke M, Wheeler L, Wagner G, Ling FW, Buxton BH. An approach to relearning the pelvic examination. J Fam Pract 1982;14:782–783.

Editorial. Vulvovaginal candidiasis—what we do and do not know. Ann Intern Med 1984;101:390–392.

Jones RH. The use of chaperones by general practitioners. J R Coll Gen Pract 1983;33:25–27.

Lamphier TA. Rape. Md State Med J 1982;April:37–43.

Magee J. The pelvic examination: a view from the other end of the table. Ann Intern Med 1975;83:563–565.

Munsick RA. Dickinson's sign: focal uterine softening in early pregnancy and its correlation with the placental site. Am J Obstet Gynecol 1985;152:799–802.

Phillips S, Friedman SB, Seidenberg M, Heald FP. Teenagers' preferences regarding the presence of family members, peers, and chaperones during examination of genitalia. Pediatrics 1981;68: 665–669.

Primrose RB. Taking the tension out of pelvic exams. Am J Nurs 1984;84(1):72–74.

Rosen L. Physical examination of the anorectum: a systematic technique. Dis Colon Rectum 1990;33:439–440.

Sargentis V. Uterine pulsation as sign of early pregnancy. Lancet 1974;2:900.

Scherger JE. Changing gloves between vaginal and rectal examination: an additional reason. JAMA 1987;257:191.

Waradzin M, Pinto MM. Efficacy of combined spatula/Cytobrush smear for cervical sampling. Conn Med 1990;54:433.

Wertheimer AJ. Examination of the rape victim. Postgrad Med 1982;71:173–180.

Wilbanks GD. Changing gloves between vaginal and rectal examination: reinstitution of old practices for new diseases. JAMA 1986;256:1893.

Wolner-Hanssen P, et al. Clinical manifestations of vaginal trichomoniasis. JAMA 1989;261:571–576.

15

Pediatric Examination

Editor's Note: This chapter was adapted from Algranati PS. *The Pediatric Patient: An Approach to History and Physical Examination.* Baltimore: Williams & Wilkins, 1992.

Because there are so many unique considerations involved in examining younger patients, this chapter departs in format from the previous chapters. In recognition of those differences related to developmental stage, most of the information in this chapter has been organized in relation to the patient's age group rather than by body region.

PEDIATRIC HISTORY

OVERVIEW

Pediatric history is obtained in a variety of circumstances. Regardless of the setting or the reason for the contact, common features characterize most pediatric interviews.

The history is usually recited by someone other than the patient (e.g., a parent). Therefore, the content of the history may be profoundly affected (both in accuracy and flavor) by the parent's innate observational abilities and by the parent's interpretations of the child's signs or symptoms. Longstanding patterns of parent-child interaction influence what "story" is told. The clinician who explores beyond the factual data to uncover factors influencing each parent's perspective (e.g., parent's perceptions of their child's vulnerability to illness, parent's hidden agendas) will be more successful at achieving accuracy, honesty and, ultimately, compliance.

Children can contribute to history telling far more than is usually appreciated. Information about a child's developmental stage (e.g., abilities and fears) can be used to structure the interview in order to minimize fears and maximize participation. Both physical and verbal techniques are useful. **Physical techniques include involving the child in age-appropriate play, encouraging the child to physically explore the immediate environment, and allowing the child to remain as close to a parent as desired. Verbal techniques include tailoring statements and questions to the developmental level of the child (e.g., the 5-year-old can supply information in response to "What did you eat for lunch?" or can respond to a request to "Point to the ear that hurts"), using humor cautiously to put the child at ease (e.g., joking not teasing, friendliness without intrusiveness), addressing developmentally predictable fears with honesty, and giving reassurance when possible (e.g., offering reassurance such as "no needles today").**

Looking at a problem from the child's vantage point may be quite useful in both clarifying the nature of the problem and designing a solution. Probably even more important is the unspoken message conveyed to the child by a request for information or an offer of explanation. The child whose participation is acknowledged as valuable experiences an enhancement of self-esteem. This, in turn, may improve cooperation during the examination. It may also contribute to future efforts to empower the child with responsibility for his own health care.

Information about the child's day-to-day functioning is vitally important. These data include the child's usual patterns in activities of daily living (e.g., eating, sleeping, elimination, activity level), as well as the child's usual functioning in the affective, cognitive, and physical spheres (e.g., temperament, mood, verbal abilities, motor skills). One technique for obtaining this information is to ask the parent or older patient to "describe a typical day." During health supervision this information is vital for the assessment of the child's overall state of well-being and progress in each major area of development. During an investigation of a problem or an illness, the child's usual or baseline level of functioning is compared and contrasted with his current level of functioning. The comparison not only helps to clarify the nature and severity of a problem but also provides guidance when planning therapy.

TYPES OF PEDIATRIC HISTORY: CONTENT AND INDICATIONS

The content of the pediatric history is tailored to fit the patient's needs and the setting in which the encounter occurs.

Comprehensive Pediatric History

The comprehensive pediatric history is the most complete type of pediatric history database. The patient's entire past medical and psychosocial history and family history are explored. Current affective, cognitive, and physical functioning is also explored. A comprehensive pediatric history is obtained when a child is admitted to the hospital. In the outpatient setting, it is obtained for any new patient seeking health supervision, a "second opinion," or an evaluation of a complicated, vague, or potentially serious problem. The attention that each area receives is determined by the patient's age and problems.

COMPREHENSIVE PEDIATRIC HISTORY[a]

Identifying Information: Name of patient, date of birth, sex, date of interview. Record name of historian.

  I **Chief Complaint (CC):** Direct quotation from patient or parent, if possible

  II **History of Present Illness (HPI):** Narrative description of the events involving present illness or illnesses, including the relevant past medical history, review of systems, family health, and psychosocial history

  III **Past Medical History (PMH)**
    A. **Prenatal, natal, neonatal history**
      1. **Prenatal**
        a. Maternal
          i. Age
          ii. G (gravida status—no. of pregnancies)
          iii. P (para status—no. of potentially viable infants delivered)
          iv. Ab (abortus status—no. of miscarriages or abortions)
          v. EDC (estimated date of confinement or due date)
        b. Pregnancy
          i. Planned
          ii. Prenatal care
          iii. Complications and therapies

[a]Adapted with permission from Algranati PS. Pediatric clinical encounter. In: Willms JL, Lewis J, eds. Introduction to clinical medicine. Media, Pennsylvania: Harwal, 1991:121–158.

          iv.   Medications

          v.   Substance abuse (timing, extent of exposure)

  2. **Labor and delivery**

     a. Labor onset, spontaneous or induced (reason for induction)

     b. Duration of labor

     c. Duration of ruptured membranes, meconium staining

     d. Medications during labor and delivery

     e. Presentation: vertex, breech, other

     f. Delivery vaginal or cesarean section (reason for cesarean section)

     g. Maternal reaction to experience of labor and delivery

  3. **Neonatal**

     a. Birth date, birth weight, estimated gestational age

     b. Apgar scores, condition of newborn in delivery room

     c. Resuscitation or intervention required

     d. Problems in nursery (e.g., jaundice, poor feeding, Rx)

     e. Hospital discharge of mother and infant, including reasons for prolongation of hospitalization of either

     f. Circumcision done; results, complications

B. **Childhood illnesses and exposures**

  1. **Childhood illnesses** (e.g., varicella)

  2. **Recent exposures to contagious diseases**

  3. **Travel, pets** (potential exposures via travel, animals)

C. **Immunizations and reactions:** dates, specific nature of reaction

D. **Medications:** include over-the-counter medicines

E. **Allergies**

  1. **Medication allergies:** describe reaction

  2. **Other allergies** (e.g., seasonal rhinitis): symptoms and remedies

F. **Injuries** (include ingestions, burns): circumstances of event

G. **Hospitalizations, surgery, and transfusions**

H. **Prior screening results** (e.g., vision, anemia, tuberculosis)

I. **Nutrition**

  1. **Infant feeding history:** breast/formula feeding, solids (timing, problems, satisfaction)

  2. **Childhood eating history:** preferences, diet, weight concerns

J. **Growth and development:** Present age and level of functioning should determine extent of questioning. Examples of general introductory questions include, "Overall, what do you think about your child's growth and development up until now?" and "Do you have any concerns about any area of your child's growth or development?"

  1. **Growth and physical development**—infant and child growth patterns: concerns about growth rate or pattern, comparisons to other family members or peers. Actual measurements may be recorded when available.

  2. **Development and developmental milestones:** Query about the patient's progress along each line of development (e.g., motor, affective, cognitive) and elicit concerns. List age at which major milestones achieved (e.g., lifted head off bed, rolled over, sat alone, pulled to stand, held cup or spoon, smiled, babbled, said first word, said two-word phrases, dressed self, tied shoelaces, skipped).

IV **Review of Systems:** Review of systems is tailored to the purpose of the visit. Ask a few global questions in each system; pursue areas of concern in further detail. Below are some representative areas to explore.

A. **General:** weight concerns, activity and energy level, sleep patterns, fever, drinking habits, mood, missed school, growth concerns
B. **Skin:** rash, birthmark, acquired lesions; hair or nail problems
C. **Head:** abnormal size or shape, headache, dizziness, trauma
D. **Eyes:** vision problem, crossed eyes
E. **Ears:** hearing problem, infections
F. **Nose:** drainage, irritation, bleeding
G. **Mouth and throat:** sore throats, dental problems, speech, snoring
H. **Lymphatics:** enlarged or painful lymph nodes
I. **Neck:** thyroid problem, neck mass, wryneck
J. **Breasts:** mass, asymmetry, pain, nipple discharge
K. **Respiratory:** frequent infections, cough, asthma, exercise tolerance
L. **Cardiovascular:** heart murmur or abnormality, high blood pressure, chest pain, palpitations
M. **Gastrointestinal:** abdominal pain, constipation, encopresis, vomiting, food intolerance, diarrhea, jaundice, colic
N. **Urinary:** infection, enuresis, hematuria, dysuria
O. **Genital**
    1. **Male:** congenital abnormality (e.g., hypospadias, undescended testicle), testicular pain, hernia; puberty: age at onset, sexually transmitted diseases (STDs), sexual activity and contraception, concerns
    2. **Female:** vaginal discharge or irritation; puberty: age at onset of puberty, menarche—nature of cycle, concerns, last menstrual period; STDs, sexual activity and contraception, pregnancies, concerns
P. **Musculoskeletal:** bone, joint, or muscle pain; injuries, congenital abnormalities, scoliosis
Q. **Neurodevelopmental:** seizure, fainting, abnormal movements or vocalizations (e.g., tics, tremors); problems with handwriting, balance, coordination; weakness or paralysis; CNS infection; school functioning, delayed development
R. **Psychiatric:** mood, memory, behavior, hallucinations

V **Psychosocial History:** This history seeks information about the child's behavioral, emotional, and cognitive functioning and about the home environment. Questions are tailored to the patient's age and circumstances. Parental concerns are elicited. Potential areas to explore include:
A. **Affective functioning and development:** child's mood; behavior; relationships with peers, family, and others. (For example, topics may include temperament—"easy baby" or "difficult baby"; reaction to rules and discipline; leisure pursuits; strengths and weaknesses; risk taking behaviors—substance abuse, disregard for obvious danger.)
B. **Cognitive functioning and development:** intellectual functioning, including language and speech development, school readiness, school progress and functioning, plans for future education or employment
C. **Habitual behaviors:** habits and attitudes toward them (e.g., thumbsucking)
D. **Household:** List and describe household members (e.g., names, ages, occupations) and the relationships between members. Inquire about parent or siblings absent from household and about childcare arrangements, financial resources, recent changes or problems in household. Is the child worried about a family member?

VI Family Health History
   A. **Parents, siblings, grandparents:** ages, medical problems
   B. **Family history of:** inherited diseases or diseases that "run" in the family, infant or childhood deaths, congenital anomalies, early cardiovascular deaths, lipid problems, hypertension, cancer, diabetes, kidney disease, mental illness, alcohol or drug abuse, AIDS, consanguinity, TB, anemia, arthritis

Prenatal and Perinatal History

The prenatal and perinatal history is indispensable to the clinicians who are responsible for the care of a newborn. It includes prenatal, natal, neonatal history; family health and social histories; and home preparations for the new baby. During the interview, the clinician observes the baby's mother (or parents) and attempts to answer the following questions: What is the mother's overall mood and interest in hearing about the baby? Does she ask questions about the baby? If the baby is present, how does she interact with the baby: Does she touch him? hold and cuddle him closely? look at him? speak endearingly to him? If the answers to these questions are affirmative, there is evidence that the parent is beginning to form a strong attachment or bond to the baby. Assuming the mother is not experiencing a lot of pain or under the influence of narcotics or sedatives, if the answers to the above questions are negative, concern about her psychologic state or bonding should be raised. Similar observations are made about the baby's father.

Health Supervision History

The health supervision history seeks information that is necessary to evaluate the patient's current functioning. It is an interval update of the child's comprehensive history. It includes information about the child's current day-to-day functioning, recent developmental progress (in affective, cognitive, and physical areas), recent health status, and relevant family health and psychosocial issues. This is the history obtained at health supervision encounters. Selected parts of this history are useful during problem encounters. Suggestions for age-related topics are supplied. Actual content should be determined by clinician and parent together.

INFANT: HEALTH SUPERVISION TOPICS

1. **Daily functioning:** Topics may include feeding, sleep, bowel and bladder control, measures taken by parents for baby's safety and play.
2. **Developmental progress:** Parents are queried for their impression of the baby's progress and for any concerns about growth, physical development, or other areas of development.
   a. **Affective development:** Parents are encouraged to describe the infant's temperament (e.g., easy versus difficult). Appearance of stranger anxiety (12 months) and separation anxiety (6–9 months) is discussed.
   b. **Cognitive development:** Baby's emerging interest in searching for hidden objects (object permanence) and interest in wind-up toys (causality) (9–12 months) are noted.
   c. **Developmental milestones:** Inquiry is made about the infant's latest accomplishments in the areas of motor skills, social interaction, language, vision, and hearing (see Fig. 15.8)
3. **Recent health:** Areas of concern may include crying, teething, colds, thumbsucking, immunization reactions, vision, or hearing.

4. **Relevant family health and psychosocial issues:** Adjustments of family to baby, changes in routine, and employment are discussed.

TODDLER: HEALTH SUPERVISION TOPICS

The older toddler can supply information in some of these areas.

1. **Daily functioning:** Topics may include diet, sleep, toilet training, tooth care, child safety, and play preference.
2. **Developmental progress:** At this age, parents are frequently concerned about a deceleration in the child's growth rate, high activity level, or appearance of the limbs. History addresses overall impressions and elicits specific concerns.
    a. **Affective development:** Parents are encouraged to discuss the toddler's struggles with autonomy and independence, including negative behaviors, lack of impulse control. Other topics include the child's interactions with peers and play (e.g., pretend play, parallel play).
    b. **Cognitive development:** Major topic is the emergence of language, including its content, complexity, and intelligibility. Other questions may include evidence that the child is beginning to understand things or individuals not actually present (representation) and is demonstrating curiosity by asking questions such as "What's this?" For the older preschooler (4–5), school readiness is a major issue.
    c. **Developmental milestones:** Inquiry is made about toddler's latest accomplishments in the areas of fine and gross motor skills, social and personal skills, and language (see Fig. 15.8).
3. **Recent health:** Areas of concern may include recent illnesses, habits (e.g., masturbation), vision, hearing, or speech concerns.
4. **Relevant family health and psychosocial issues:** Toddler's effect on household, including sibling rivalry and "goodness-of-fit" between toddler's behaviors and abilities versus parent's expectations, is discussed.

SCHOOL-AGE CHILD: HEALTH SUPERVISION TOPICS

The clinician involves the school-age child as an active participant while obtaining the health maintenance history. For the older school-age child, or preadolescent, the style of the upcoming adolescent visit may be previewed by conducting part of the interview with the parent outside of the room.

1. **Daily functioning:** Topics may include diet, body image, sleep habits, independence in elimination, exercise and sports participation, safety habits, and leisure preferences.
2. **Developmental progress:** Parents and patient may report impressions or concerns about growth, body changes, or other areas of development.
    a. **Affective development:** Major issue is child's increasing involvement with peers. Topics of discussion may include same- and opposite-sex friends, parent-child communication, and risk-taking behaviors. The preadolescent may be asked to provide a verbal "weather report" for an overall assessment of current functioning.
    b. **Cognitive development:** Major topic is school adjustment and school functioning.
    c. **Developmental milestones:** For the school-age child over 6, data about school performance, athletic pursuits, and peer interactions are appropriate for developmental monitoring.
3. **Recent health:** Inquiry is made about illnesses, aches and pains of childhood, habits, vision, and hearing, concerns and knowledge about puberty.

4. **Relevant family health and psychosocial issues:** Effect of child's school entry on household is sought. For older child, inquiry focuses on evidence of the preadolescent's "declaration of independence" and its ramifications.

ADOLESCENT: HEALTH SUPERVISION TOPICS

The adolescent is the primary historian. If the parent has special concerns, time is allotted to obtain history from the parent also. The main body of the adolescent interview should be conducted without the parent in the room. The subject of confidentiality should be introduced at the start of the interview so that ground rules are understood by both patient and parent.

This history seeks information to assess how well the adolescent is currently functioning in the physical, emotional, and cognitive spheres. Much attention is focused on the patient's progress through puberty and adolescence. These subjects may be difficult for both patient and inexperienced interviewer to discuss. It is helpful to plan a tentative sequence of topics ahead of time. Begin with topics that the adolescent is most likely to feel comfortable with (e.g., discussing a "typical day," home life, school, or recent health). Discussion of the most sensitive issues (e.g., risk-taking behaviors, sexual activity) is best left until rapport is established. Sensitive topics should be introduced in an open and matter-of-fact manner. Asking the adolescent if friends experiment with _____ (substances of abuse, e.g., smoking, drinking, drugs, or other risk-taking behaviors) is a non-threatening way to introduce these topics. This may be followed by the question, "Do you ever _____, too?" The same technique may be used to inquire about sexual activity. "Are any of your friends involved in a sexual relationship?" may be followed by "Have you ever been involved in a sexual relationship?" Most adolescents, when assured of confidentiality, will acknowledge their activities when approached in this manner. The clinician should acknowledge the difficulty in discussing sexuality while emphasizing its necessity because of the impact on the patient's health.

1. **Daily functioning:** Topics may include usual diet, body image, sleep habits, exercise and sports pursuits, safety habits, and dental care.
2. **Developmental progress:** Self-impression of progress and concerns about puberty, growth, strength, sexual identity, and intimacy. Presumptions about sexual preference are avoided.
    a. **Affective development:** Major issues are progress toward achieving autonomy and independence from one's parents and texture of peer relationships. Topics include relationships with parents and other significant adults and with same- and opposite-sex peers. Participation in risk-taking behaviors is explored. The patient may be requested to provide a "weather report" or overall summary "on a scale of 1–10" of current functioning.
    b. **Cognitive development:** School progress and current functioning are main topics. The older adolescent may discuss future plans for higher education or employment.
    c. **Developmental milestones:** For the adolescent, data about school performance, athletic pursuits, and Tanner staging are appropriate for developmental monitoring.
3. **Recent health:** Inquiry is made about general concerns and, specifically, about any related to skin, musculoskeletal system, and genitourinary system (puberty and sexual activity).
4. **Relevant family health and psychosocial issues:** Prior discussion is summarized, and further concerns are elicited. Family cardiovascular history is

reviewed. The clinician closes this section of the interview by inquiring as to whether there is anyone in the family or household the patient is worried about.

MEASUREMENTS IN CHILDREN

Many physical findings can be measured objectively. Norms for these measurements have been established, and data for an individual child can be evaluated in comparison to those of other children of the same gender and chronologic age at one point in time or over a period of time. Data for an individual child can also be evaluated in comparison to other data for that same child. The importance of using proper technique to obtain accurate measurements in children cannot be overstated. Clinicians responsible for child health care rely heavily on data obtained through measurement. Errors in measurement may produce unnecessary anxiety or, conversely, may be falsely reassuring.

VITAL STATISTICS

Length/Height

Supine length is measured in children up to age 2–3 years. Beyond age 3 years, standing height is measured. When **length** is obtained, results are recorded on the chart labeled **"Birth to 36 months."** When **height** is obtained, results are recorded on the chart labeled **"2 to 18 years." This is especially important to remember when a toddler is measured, because values for children ages 2–3 years can be recorded on either type of chart. Inadvertent recording of supine measurement on a "height" chart rather than a "length" chart will falsely lower the child's stature percentile.**

LENGTH

The infant is placed supine on a flat hard surface as shown on the baby in Figure 15.1. The distance between the vertex (top of the head) and soles of the feet is measured. The best way to do this is to place either vertex or feet against a hard nonmovable board (i.e., at a 90° angle to the table surface). A second board at the other end of the child is moved toward him with his legs extended until resistance is encountered. The distance between the two boards is the supine length. Two people are required to measure a squirming infant. This is an imprecise measurement in the full-term newborn and very young infant in the first weeks of life. Term newborns are born with flexion contractures at the elbows, hips, and knees. Attempting to "stretch out" the legs in order to obtain an accurate length is an exercise in frustration for examiner and infant alike; it is unnecessary to force the issue with a healthy baby.

HEIGHT

For standing height, the child without shoes is directed to stand up straight ("stand tall") with eyes looking straight ahead and feet together. The top of the child's head should be positioned so that the crown is approximately parallel to the floor. A ruler or another flat-surfaced object is placed across the top of the head, and at the point at which the ruler makes contact with the adjacent wall or scale, a measurement from the floor or bottom of the scale is obtained.

Plot length or height on the age- and gender-appropriate growth chart at the child's exact age. The diagonal lines across each chart correspond to the reference-group percentiles. Length or height is obtained and plotted at each health super-

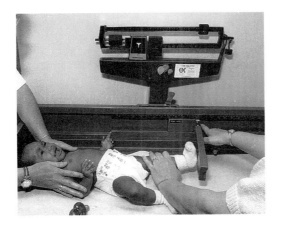

Figure 15.1   Measurement of supine length.

vision visit and may also be obtained at other visits when there are concerns about growth or health.

Weight

The infant is placed on the scale wearing no more than a diaper. The older infant may sit up during this measurement. Children who are able to cooperate are weighed (in their underwear or gown) on a standard upright scale. Weight is plotted on the age- and gender-appropriate charts. Children are weighed at all health supervision visits. Weight is also measured in sick children, especially if their intake has been poor or when medication dosages need to be calculated (Figs. 15.2*A* and *B* and 15.3*A* and *B*).

Head Circumference

Head circumference is measured by using a paper or cloth tape measure. The head is surrounded to obtain the maximal occipital-frontal circumference (OFC). Younger children often have to be restrained for this procedure. The measurement may need to be repeated to ensure accuracy. The results are plotted on the gender-relevant chart. Head circumference is measured at every health supervision visit for the first year (the period of maximal brain growth), at every initial visit, or whenever there are concerns about growth or neurologic status (Figs. 15.4*A* and *B* and 15.5).

VITAL SIGNS

Heart Rate

Heart rate is determined either while listening directly over the precordium with a stethoscope or by palpating a convenient peripheral pulse. In an infant whose anterior fontanelle is patent, the heart rate may be determined by counting the pulsations visible through the anterior fontanelle (Table 15.1).

Respiratory Rate

Respiratory rate is optimally determined when the child is calm. The rate is counted either during auscultation of the chest or by observing the rise and fall of the chest. As with heart rate, there is wide variation, depending on activity level (Table 15.2).

BOYS: BIRTH TO 36 MONTHS
PHYSICAL GROWTH
NCHS PERCENTILES*

NAME _____ RECORD # _____

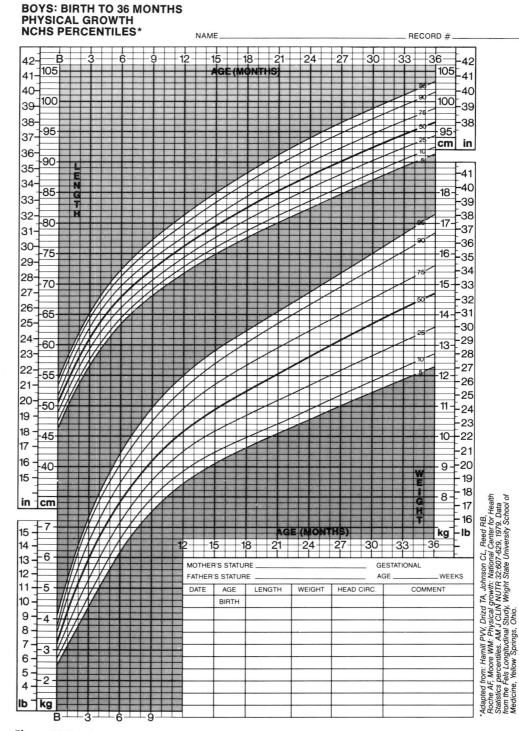

Figure 15.2   A.

GIRLS: BIRTH TO 36 MONTHS
PHYSICAL GROWTH
NCHS PERCENTILES*

NAME _____ RECORD # _____

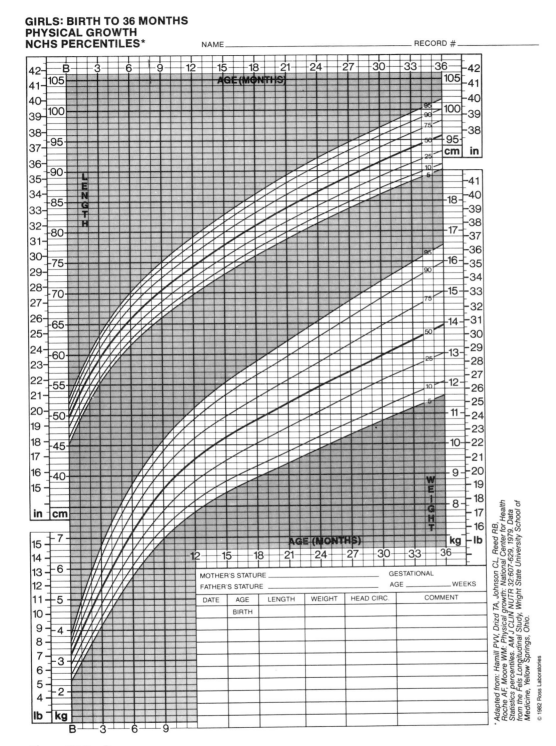

* Adapted from: Hamill PVV, Drizd TA, Johnson CL, Reed RB,
Roche AF, Moore WM: Physical growth: National Center for Health
Statistics percentiles. AM J CLIN NUTR 32:607-629, 1979. Data
from the Fels Longitudinal Study, Wright State University School of
Medicine, Yellow Springs, Ohio.

© 1982 Ross Laboratories

Figure 15.2   B.

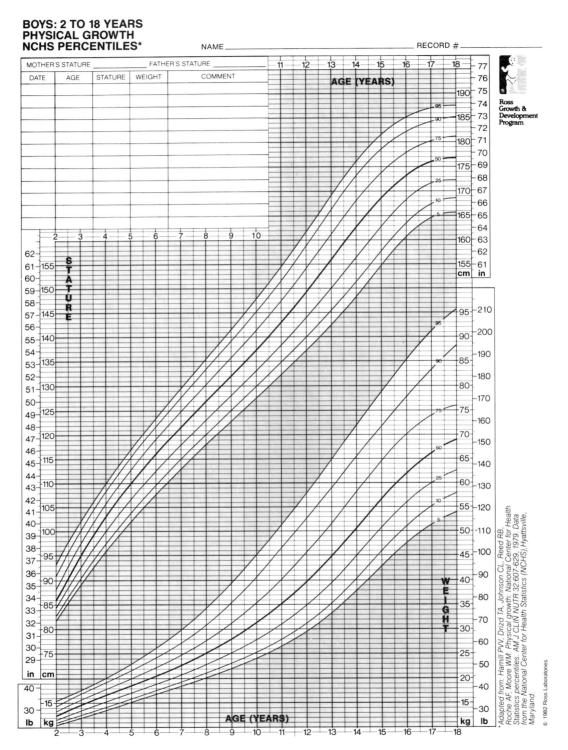

Figure 15.3   A.

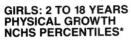

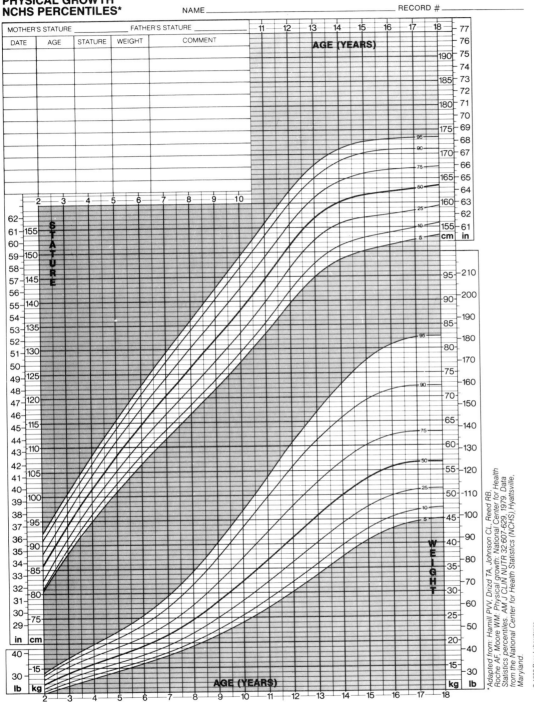

Figure 15.3   B.

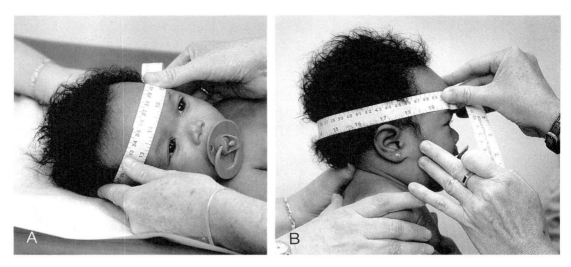

Figure 15.4 **A** and **B.** Measurement of head circumference. Anteriorly, the tape is positioned over the smooth area on the frontal bone, just above the eyebrows. Posteriorly, it is positioned at the level of the occipital protuberance.

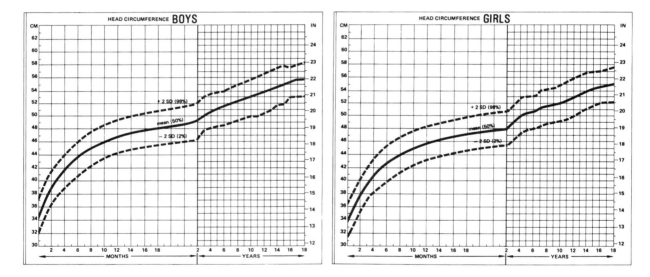

Figure 15.5 Head circumference from birth to 18 years.

Temperature

Normal body temperature varies with age, activity, and time of day. Newborns have a slightly higher normal temperature than young children, who in turn have a slightly higher normal temperature than adolescents. The variation by age approximates 1°F in total. More important is the diurnal variation in an individual child: Body temperature rises to its highest level by early evening and falls to its lowest point at midnight. The average diurnal variation in temperature is usually at least 1°F and may be as much as 2°F or 3°F. In young children in particular, heavy clothing may significantly influence body temperature. In the young infant (under 2 months of age), subnormal temperature is sometimes a more ominous sign of illness than an elevated temperature.

Table 15.1
Average Heart Rates in Children at Rest

Age	Average Rate	2 SDs
Birth	140	50
First month	130	45
1–6 months	130	45
6–12 months	115	40
1–2 years	110	40
2–4 years	105	35
6–10 years	95	30
10–14 years	85	30
14–18 years	82	25

Table 15.2
Normal Respiratory Rates in Children

Age	Respirations/min
Newborn	30–75
6–12 months	22–31
1–2 years	17–23
2–4 years	16–25
4–10 years	13–23
10–14 years	13–19

Rectal temperatures are generally about 1°F higher than oral temperatures. Forehead temperature strips are inaccurate. Axillary temperatures are said to be about 2°F lower than rectal temperatures. Many pediatricians believe that axillary temperatures are also inaccurate.

Rectal temperature is the best method to use until children are able to safely hold a mercury thermometer under their tongue. The age at which this occurs is around 4 or 5 years. To obtain a rectal temperature, the child is placed prone in the parent's lap or on the examining table or bed. Approximately ¾ inch of the lubricated metal bulb end (the rectal thermometer has the short metal bulb) is inserted into the rectum at an angle of approximately 25° to the floor and held in place for 1–2 minutes. Gently squeezing the patient's buttocks together will facilitate holding the thermometer in place. Oral temperature is obtained by having the patient place the long metal bulb under the tongue for 2 minutes.

Electronic thermometers are especially useful because they work quickly. Some facilities use a device inserted into the ear canal that measures infrared energy emitted from the eardrum. At this time, the accuracy of this device in children is under investigation.

Rectal Fahrenheit temperatures from approximately 97.5° to 100.4° are generally considered in the normal range. Temperatures are routinely obtained in newborns and hospitalized children. In the outpatient setting, they are generally reserved for ill children.

Blood Pressure

Blood pressure readings are performed at routine health supervision visits, starting at the age of 3. Prior to age 3, special circumstances or concerns may initiate a blood pressure measurement (e.g., heart or renal disease, a very ill infant, or when there is difficulty palpating the femoral pulse). A mercury-gravity sphygmomanometer is most commonly used in children beyond infancy.

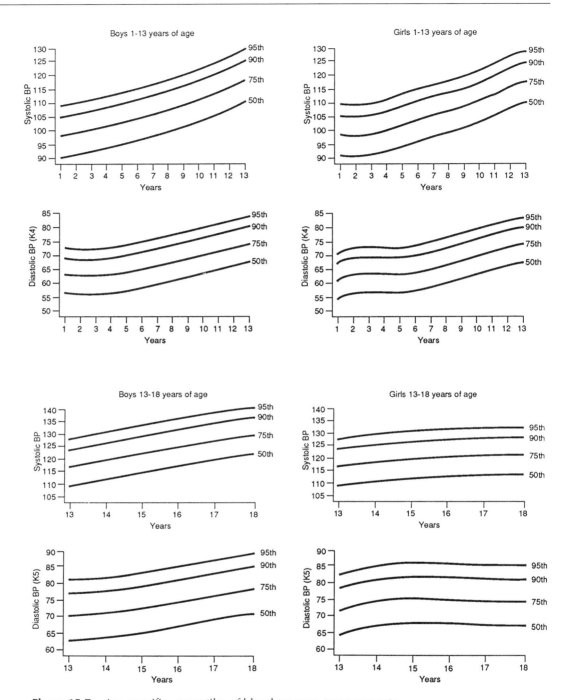

Figure 15.7   Age-specific percentiles of blood pressure measurements.

added up to a possible total of 10. Most babies do not "get a 10," because a point has been taken off for color. A score of 8–10 is excellent; 4–7 is worrisome; and 0–3 is critical. The score, particularly at 1 and 5 minutes, should not be equated with long-term significance. A mnemonic to remember APGAR is: **A** for appearance (skin color); **P** for pulse; **G** for grimace (reflex irritability); **A** for activity; and **R** for respiration.

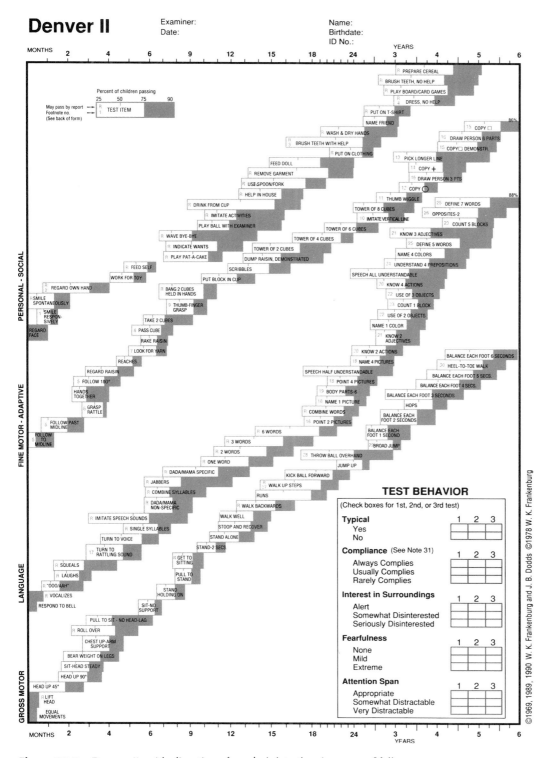

Figure 15.8 Denver II, with directions for administration (see page 614).

DIRECTIONS FOR ADMINISTRATION

1. Try to get child to smile by smiling, talking or waving. Do not touch him/her.
2. Child must stare at hand several seconds.
3. Parent may help guide toothbrush and put toothpaste on brush.
4. Child does not have to be able to tie shoes or button/zip in the back.
5. Move yarn slowly in an arc from one side to the other, about 8" above child's face.
6. Pass if child grasps rattle when it is touched to the backs or tips of fingers.
7. Pass if child tries to see where yarn went. Yarn should be dropped quickly from sight from tester's hand without arm movement.
8. Child must transfer cube from hand to hand without help of body, mouth, or table.
9. Pass if child picks up raisin with any part of thumb and finger.
10. Line can vary only 30 degrees or less from tester's line. |/
11. Make a fist with thumb pointing upward and wiggle only the thumb. Pass if child imitates and does not move any fingers other than the thumb.

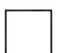

12. Pass any enclosed form. Fail continuous round motions.

13. Which line is longer? (Not bigger.) Turn paper upside down and repeat. (pass 3 of 3 or 5 of 6)

14. Pass any lines crossing near midpoint.

15. Have child copy first. If failed, demonstrate.

When giving items 12, 14, and 15, do not name the forms. Do not demonstrate 12 and 14.

16. When scoring, each pair (2 arms, 2 legs, etc.) counts as one part.
17. Place one cube in cup and shake gently near child's ear, but out of sight. Repeat for other ear.
18. Point to picture and have child name it. (No credit is given for sounds only.)
    If less than 4 pictures are named correctly, have child point to picture as each is named by tester.

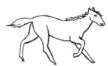

19. Using doll, tell child: Show me the nose, eyes, ears, mouth, hands, feet, tummy, hair. Pass 6 of 8.
20. Using pictures, ask child: Which one flies?... says meow?... talks?... barks?... gallops? Pass 2 of 5, 4 of 5.
21. Ask child: What do you do when you are cold?... tired?... hungry? Pass 2 of 3, 3 of 3.
22. Ask child: What do you do with a cup? What is a chair used for? What is a pencil used for?
    Action words must be included in answers.
23. Pass if child correctly places and says how many blocks are on paper. (1, 5).
24. Tell child: Put block **on** table; **under** table; **in front of** me, **behind** me. Pass 4 of 4.
    (Do not help child by pointing, moving head or eyes.)
25. Ask child: What is a ball?... lake?... desk?... house?... banana?... curtain?... fence?... ceiling? Pass if defined in terms of use, shape, what it is made of, or general category (such as banana is fruit, not just yellow). Pass 5 of 8, 7 of 8.
26. Ask child: If a horse is big, a mouse is __? If fire is hot, ice is __? If the sun shines during the day, the moon shines during the __? Pass 2 of 3.
27. Child may use wall or rail only, not person. May not crawl.
28. Child must throw ball overhand 3 feet to within arm's reach of tester.
29. Child must perform standing broad jump over width of test sheet (8 1/2 inches).
30. Tell child to walk forward, ∞∞∞∞∞► heel within 1 inch of toe. Tester may demonstrate.
    Child must walk 4 consecutive steps.
31. In the second year, half of normal children are non-compliant.

OBSERVATIONS:

Reproduced with permission from Frankenburg WK, Dodds J, Archer P, Shapiro H, Bresnick B. The Denver II: a major revision and restandardization of the Denver developmental screening test. Pediatrics 1992;89:91–97.

Figure 15.8 Continued.

PEDIATRIC PHYSICAL EXAMINATION

Organization of the Pediatric Physical Examination Sections

The sections on pediatric examination are presented in chronologic order: **Newborn, Infant, Toddler, School-Age Child, Adolescent.** Each age group, in turn, is divided into two major subsections: **Techniques of Examination** and **Normal** and Common Variants and *Clues to Abnormalities.* Several age groups contain an additional subsection called **Special Maneuvers.** The reason for the overall arrangement of the text into age groups rather than into body regions is to demonstrate the enormous influence of developmental stage on the approach to, and on the content of, pediatric physical examination. **The patient's stage of development determines, at minimum, how the child is verbally and physically approached, how the examination is sequenced, what areas of the body are emphasized, what findings are expected, which equipment is used, and how the child is likely to respond to the clinician.**

This chapter is written with the assumption that the reader has a working knowledge of the content and sequence of a comprehensive physical examination in the adult. In the Techniques of Examination section under Newborn, the text is actually presented in the sequence in which the examination might be performed, with a comprehensive discussion of the examination. The reason for this is that the newborn examination is the most unique and different of pediatric examinations, compared with a standard adult-type "head-to-toe" sequence.

Beyond the Newborn section, each component of a complete examination is not discussed. The material is presented with the assumption that a relatively complete examination will be performed. What the other sections contain are (a) techniques that are unique to a particular age group or are introduced beginning at a particular age, (b) parts of the examination that are particularly important for a certain age group, and (c) findings that are uniquely, logically, or significantly age-related. For simplicity, the sections beyond the Newborn section follow a "head-to-toe" order. Suggestions for modifying the actual examination sequence in age groups beyond the neonatal period are clearly noted.

The text emphasizes basic techniques and normal and common findings. The beginner may start by reading the Techniques of Examination sections and, with increased clinical exposure, continue to the Normal and Common Variants and *Clues to Abnormalities* sections. Clues and signs of a more pathologic nature, which may require further investigation or intervention, are set off from the regular text in special italic type. The Special Maneuvers sections contain maneuvers that, though not part of the basic screening examination, may easily be incorporated if clinically indicated.

NEWBORN

Techniques of Examination

AREAS OF EMPHASIS

The newborn examination screens for (1) congenital anomalies, major and minor, (2) consequences of birth trauma associated with labor or delivery, (3) neonatal medical problems, and (4) the infant's gestational age and appropriateness of size for that gestational age.

GENERAL STRATEGIES

In the newborn, as in older children, there are a great many findings that are variations of normal or fall within the spectrum of normal and, therefore, are without pathologic significance. Strategies to use during the examination, which may assist in making these determinations, include the following:

1. **Compare sides (right versus left) as the examination proceeds down the body** (e.g., if there is uncertainty about the normal color of the red reflex, compare the finding on one side to the finding on the other). Caution is advised, as some abnormalities are bilateral.

2. **Compare the baby's features to those of his parents and siblings.** What may appear unusual and questionably abnormal may be a family trait. Caution is advised here too, as some family traits have pathologic significance.

3. **When concerned, make repeated observations of a behavior or finding during the examination.** State-to-state transitions in the newborn are predictably unpredictable. There is tremendous variation in state and behavior from day to day and hour to hour. This instability in behavior may confound observations during the examination.

4. **View deviations from normal in the context of the whole child. When one abnormality is found, look for others.** One minor structural feature that departs from normal may have no significance if found in an otherwise healthy child. If, on the other hand, the child has multiple, even subtly abnormal features that depart from the expected, these features may be linked together as a syndrome.

5. Some asymmetries and deformities result from forces within the intrauterine environment. **When external deformities are noted, attempt to simulate the infant's intrauterine positioning by "folding" the infant (e.g., flexing the limbs) into a position that offers the least resistance (e.g., a position of comfort).** This maneuver may contribute to understanding the origin of an external deformity (e.g., curvature of the foot or asymmetry of the head or neck).

6. **Some structural features may be evaluated by using objective measurements and findings compared with established norms** (e.g., when eyes appear to be widely spaced, the interpupillary distance may be measured).

7. **Some structural features must be evaluated subjectively.** Findings should be compared with those of the population at large, as well as with family members (e.g., an upturned nose, a flattened nasal bridge).

ORIENTING TO THE NORMAL NEWBORN NURSERY AND EQUIPMENT

Prior to entering the newborn nursery, scrub hands and forearms and put on an overgown. Leave personal equipment behind and use the nursery's equipment. **Equipment that is routinely necessary includes stethoscope, ophthalmoscope, flashlight, tongue blade, tape measure, clock, gestational age assessment worksheet, newborn growth charts, and pacifier.** Additional equipment that may be required under special circumstances includes rubber gloves, sphygmomanometer, otoscope, and flexible feeding tube for passage through posterior nares. The newborn may be examined either in the nursery or at the mother's bedside. The bedside provides an opportunity for parents and clinicians to discuss findings and features as the examination proceeds.

OVERALL SEQUENCE

Be flexible and prepared to vary the sequence, depending on the infant's state. After initial observation, if the newborn is quiet, begin with three maneuvers: cardiac auscultation, abdominal palpation, and inguinal-femoral palpation. Turn to the head and continue head-to-toe anteriorly, then head-to-toe posteriorly, and end with any remaining neurologic/developmental maneuvers. In addition, keep the ophthalmoscope close by. Whenever the infant is alert with eyes open, take advantage of the opportunity by interrupting the examination and inspecting the eyes both with and without the ophthalmoscope.

Crying during the Examination

The clinician's hands should be warm, as should the equipment that makes contact with the baby (e.g., stethoscope diaphragm). If the infant's fussing interferes with the examination or is prolonged and disturbing, a variety of maneuvers may be attempted in order to console. These include offering something to suck on (e.g., nipple or gloved finger), rocking, feeding a small amount of water, burping, changing diaper, and talking to the baby in a soothing voice.

THE EXAMINATION
General Appearance and Initial Observations

Observe the infant at rest. Form impressions about overall maturity (premature, full term), appearance of wellness (well or sick), and state and level of activity (e.g., awake, alert, irritable, calm). Note gross asymmetries or abnormalities in body size or configuration and observe the infant's positioning (e.g., limbs extended or flexed). Inspect visible skin surfaces for overall color (e.g., pink, ruddy, jaundiced, pale, cyanotic) and any visible bruises, swellings, or other lesions.

If the infant is quiet, count respirations per minute and listen for respiratory sounds. Review the chart and note length and weight.

Observations throughout the Course of the Examination

While proceeding through the examination, note how easily (or suddenly) the infant makes transitions from waking to sleeping or fussing to calming. Some infants do this handily and calmly while others react suddenly and uneasily. Excess or extremes of activity (e.g., unconsolability, unresponsiveness) are abnormal. When the baby fusses, observe movements for symmetry, fluidity, and limitations. Before consoling, do not neglect to note the quality of the cry. When the infant is awake and active, pay attention to the sounds accompanying breathing. Excess nasal sounds, stridor, or hoarseness may not be audible when the infant is sleeping, only to become apparent with increased respiratory rate or effort.

If the infant is quiet, begin with auscultation of the heart and anterior lung fields. This should be accomplished with a minimum of disruption to the infant.

Heart and Anterior Lung Fields

The baby may be swaddled. Attempt to avoid disturbing the infant by gingerly opening the blanket and placing the warmed diaphragm of the stethoscope under the T-shirt onto the precordium. Auscultate the heart. This deviates from the usual order of the cardiac examination when inspection and palpation are performed prior to auscultation. Inspection and palpation of the precordium are performed later in the examination when the infant is undressed. Determine that the heart sounds are loudest in the left chest in order to screen for a congenital abnormality in cardiac position. Count heart rate, evaluate rhythm, identify first (S_1) and second (S_2) heart sounds, and listen for murmurs or extra sounds.

Auscultate the anterior lung fields. Note regularity of breathing, quality of aeration, and adventitious sounds. Because the chest wall is so thin and small, sounds from within are easily transmitted and may be difficult to localize.

Continue with minimal disturbance to the infant. If the infant is not yet in the supine position, roll the baby onto his back. Open the front of the diaper to expose the abdomen. After the abdomen is examined, continue caudad and examine the femoral pulses, inguinal region, and genitalia. As you proceed, open the diaper only as much as is necessary for optimal exposure.

Abdomen

Expose the entire abdomen and inspect overall contour and symmetry. After inspection, cover the penis with the diaper. Inspect the umbilicus and note the placement of its insertion into the abdominal wall. If the umbilical stump is moist, identify two smaller-caliber, thick-walled arteries and a single, thin-walled vein. Bowel sounds will be audible within a few hours after birth.

Initiate palpation very gently and superficially. Most infants grimace in reaction to the initial touch of the examiner. Proceed slowly, allowing the infant to adjust to you as you move from quadrant to quadrant and increase depth of pressure. Abdominal musculature is most relaxed when the infant is calm and sucking. Assess overall muscle tone and integrity. The infant may grimace if there is tenderness. Palpate for the lower margins of the liver and spleen and estimate the extent to which the liver edge is palpable below the anterior costal margin in the midclavicular line. Follow superficial palpation with deep palpation, searching for masses in all quadrants. Unless there are concerns about intra-abdominal pathology, percussion is not routinely performed in the newborn.

Palpation of the kidneys is especially important in the newborn, as the most common abdominal masses in this age group are associated with the genitourinary tract. The bimanual technique is described as follows.

Place your fingers (palm side up) under the baby's back on the side you wish to examine (e.g., right fingers for the infant's left side) at a level just above the iliac crest. With your free hand on the abdomen beginning medially and working laterally, palpate down toward your posterior hand until you feel a firm but soft mass approximately 2 cm wide (and as much as 4 cm in length) between the fingers of your two hands. You may be able to ballotte (gently move) the kidney between your two hands. Perform this maneuver on both sides, remembering to change hands. This requires a great deal of practice. Sometimes, even an experienced examiner will be unable to palpate the kidneys, even though they are both present and in a normal position. The right kidney is easier to feel because its position is lower (Fig. 15.9).

Palpation with Crying. When the infant is crying and you are unable to successfully console him, but must examine the abdomen, what should you do? Palpate at the end of expiration: Your hands should be in place on the body, ready to palpate. At the completion of a "wail," as the baby prepares to take a deep inspiration, quickly palpate inward. With the next expiratory wail, resistance will be encountered again. Do not remove your hands; wait for the cry to end and palpate inward once again. Continue to work with this cycle until the region has been examined.

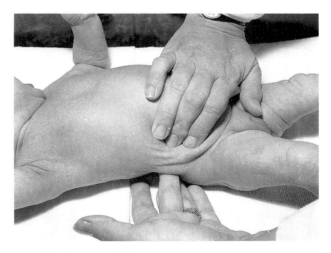

Figure 15.9   Bimanual palpation of kidney.

Inguinal Region

After palpating for masses and enlarged lymph nodes, femoral pulses are palpated bilaterally. In a squirming infant, it is not always easy to locate the femoral pulse. In this instance, an acceptable alternative is to palpate the dorsalis pedis pulse. After confirming strong lower limb pulses, simultaneously palpate the right brachial pulse and the femoral pulse. There should be no delay when comparing the lower artery pulse with the right brachial pulse. The purpose of these maneuvers is to screen for **coarctation of the aorta.**

Open the diaper completely.

Genitalia

Female genitalia. Inspect the labia majora.

Flex, externally rotate, and abduct the thighs. Apply gentle lateral traction on the labia majora in order to fully visualize the genitalia (Fig. 15.10).

Inspect, from superior to inferior, the clitoris (appearance and size), urethra, vagina, and anus. Be certain that there is a vaginal opening. The anus is inspected for patency and for adequate separation between the anus and vagina.

Male genitalia. Inspect the penis for adequacy of size, absence of curvature, and location of urethral opening. *Do not attempt to forcefully retract the foreskin.* In the uncircumcised newborn, at most, the tip of the glans and the urethral opening will be visible.

Inspect scrotal color and appearance of rugae and median raphe. Inspect the anus for patency. Palpate the scrotum for masses and fluid. Locate the testicles and palpate for size and consistency.

If both testicles are not palpable in the scrotum, carefully palpate the lower abdomen for masses, then continue to palpate while progressing caudally along the entire length of each inguinal canal. If the testicle is located in the canal, attempt to bring it down in to the scrotum by using a milking or stroking action with your fingers. If the testicle can be brought into the scrotum, the testicle is referred to as **retractile** and is normal.

If the male infant voids during genital manipulation, observe whether the stream is straight and forceful.

Replace the diaper temporarily. Return to the head region. Proceed from head to toe anteriorly.

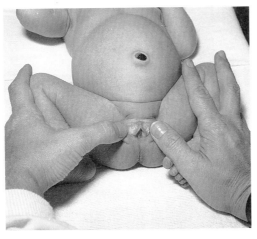

Figure 15.10   Position to inspect newborn female genitalia.

Head: Hair, Face, Eyes, Ears, Nose, and Mouth

Whenever the infant is quiet and alert with eyes open, perform the ophthalmoscopic examination.

Hair. Inspect hair on the head and face (including eyebrows) for quantity, color, and distribution. Rub the hair between your fingers to determine texture.

Head. Inspect and palpate the skull. Measure and record the head circumference. Assess the overall contour, noting asymmetries, swellings, and bulges. Palpate along the suture lines, noting separation or overriding of the sutures; estimate the extent of either. Outline the margins of the anterior and posterior fontanelles and estimate the approximate dimensions of both (Fig. 15.11).

Assess for bulging of the fontanelle by palpating the scalp within the fontanelle margins. If bulging is noted when the infant is lying down, repeat the assessment while holding the infant upright when he is not crying or struggling. True bulging of the fontanelle can only be assessed when the effects of gravity have been eliminated.

Face. Inspect overall appearance and color. Note any unusual aspects and asymmetries, remembering to compare paired structures. Many syndromes are associated with abnormalities in appearance or size of structures on the face. Actual measurements of individual features are reserved for situations in which there is suspicion of significant abnormality.

Eyes. Inspect the eyes for overall size (large or small), symmetry, and shape. Estimate whether or not the eyes are positioned correctly (not too close together or too far apart) and determine in which direction the palpebral fissures are slanted.

The **palpebral fissure slant** is determined by drawing an imaginary line through the medial and lateral canthus of each eye. If this line slants upward as it moves from medial to lateral, then the palpebral fissure has a so-called Mongoloid slant. If it slants downward as it moves laterally, then it has a so-called anti-Mongoloid slant (Fig. 15.12).

If objective measurements are required, the **width of the palpebral fissure** (distance from the medial canthus to the lateral canthus of the eye) can be measured to determine whether the eye is of normal width. The **interpupillary distance** may be measured to determine whether the eyes are too close (hypotelorism) or too far apart (hypertelorism).

The baby may open his eyes spontaneously. If not, speak to the baby. Even at this young age, the newborn will respond to the sound of the human voice by

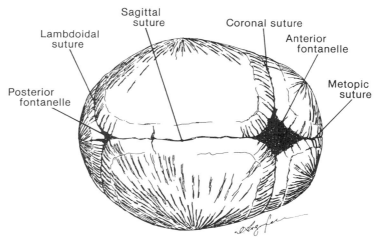

Figure 15.11 Cranial sutures and fontanelles, viewed from above. Baby's face is to viewer's right.

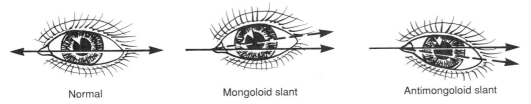

Normal   Mongoloid slant   Antimongoloid slant

Figure 15.12   Determining the angle of the palpebral fissure in three left eyes.

opening eyes. Dimming the lights in the nursery may encourage the baby to open the eyes wider. It is important to perform the eye examination without forcing the lids open. When the lids are forced open, most babies will respond with crying and resistance.

If the baby still does not have his eyes open, lift the baby's head off the mattress by cradling the occiput in your hand. The usual response is a reflex opening of eyes. Some of the time it is necessary to lower the head back down and raise it again multiple times in sequence in order to encourage the infant to open or keep the eyes open. When cradling the occiput in one hand, the ophthalmoscope may be held in the other hand.

When the baby's eyes are open, inspect the individual structures within each eye. Look for gaps in structures, called colobomas. Inspect the globes for symmetry of size and absence of bulging. Inspect the irides for completeness and symmetry of color, the sclerae for color (e.g., jaundice, hemorrhage), and the corneas for clarity. The lids are inspected for swelling, absence of ptosis or deformity, and presence of **epicanthal folds** (a small vertical skin fold at the medial canthus).

The pupils are inspected for shape, equality of size, and absence of visible opacities. The newborn pupillary response to light may normally be quite sluggish, but it is present. Set the ophthalmoscope at 0 diopters. Assess presence, clarity, and symmetry of the red reflexes. When a light is shined in the infant's eyes, note whether he blinks in response.

Lift the infant into the upright position by supporting the axillae in the crook of your hands while cradling the occiput with your fingertips. The eyes open reflexively (Fig. 15.13).

In this position, it may be possible to engage the infant in visual fixation. At this age, the infant can see shadows and shapes, particularly at a distance of about 1 foot. The infant may or may not subsequently follow the examiner's face. Attempt to assess visual fixing, following, conjugate eye movements, and doll's eye reflex.

To assess **fixation,** hold the infant approximately 12 inches from your face and observe whether he fixes on your face. If the infant appears to look away from you, he is not fixing. If you are not successful, attempt this maneuver again. Do not use a flashlight for this, as the infant will blink and shut his eyes tightly until the light is removed.

To assess the infant's **ability to follow movement,** hold the infant steady and move your head horizontally from side to side and vertically up and down, watching to see if the infant's eyes follow your movements. The infant may be able to follow up to 90° from the midline to either side. Most of the time (but not always), the eyes will move together (conjugately).

To assess the **range of eye movements and conjugate movements,** the doll's eye reflex may be used. While supporting the infant's head, rotate the head from side to side and flex it gently back and forth. During these maneuvers, observe whether the eyes move in all directions and move together. Also observe whether

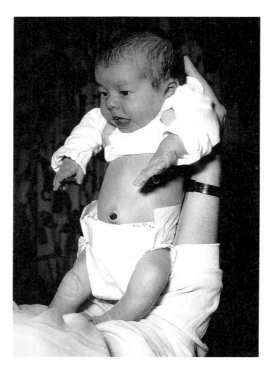

Figure 15.13   When the infant is held upright, he reflexively opens his eyes.

the eyes deviate in the direction opposite to the direction that the infant's head is moving. If rotation of the head is maintained, the eyes will return to midline after a few seconds (**doll's eye reflex**).

Place the infant back on the mattress in the supine position.

Ears. Inspect the ears for placement on the head, appearance, including size and shape of the auricle, and patency of the canal. Placement refers to the vertical location of the ear relative to the rest of the head. To determine whether ears are normally "set" (placed high enough), draw an imaginary horizontal line through the medial canthi (inner corners of the eyes) across to the ears. At least one-tenth to one-fifth of the total ear height should fall above the line. If less than that amount and, definitely, if the entire ear falls below that line, the **ears are low set.** This determination can be made in patients of all ages (Fig. 15.14). *This observation is important because low-set ears are associated with renal and auditory abnormalities.*

The total size of the auricle is estimated by inspection, as is the appearance of the normal contours. Skin tags or pits on or near the ear are noted.

Fold back the top of the helix and release it. Determine the degree of firmness, as well as how readily it springs back into position when released.

During the first days of life the canal is filled with amniotic debris. It is not necessary to assess the tympanic membranes in a healthy newborn whose external ears and canals appear normal otherwise.

Nose. The nose is inspected for overall size and shape, patency of the nares, and any swellings or deformities. The nasal bone is palpated to determine whether it is intact.

Mouth. Observe the lips both at rest and during yawning or crying for symmetry. If there is asymmetry, note which side does not follow the expected con-

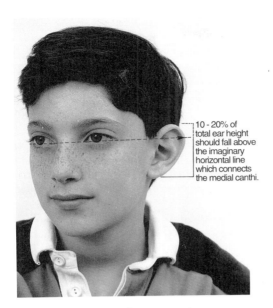

10 - 20% of total ear height should fall above the imaginary horizontal line which connects the medial canthi.

Figure 15.14   Determining whether or not the ears are low-set.

tour. The jaw may quiver intermittently for a few seconds. Note whether this movement, a form of clonus, becomes frequent or sustained.

Inspect the interior oral structures. A light source and tongue depressor may be of help but are not obligatory. A glove is mandatory for universal precautions. Inspect the gingivae, uvula, and pharynx. A bifid uvula is noted. Inspect and palpate the entire length of the palate for a midline hard palate ridge and normal domed shape and for the absence of a cleft. Assess whether the tongue fits easily inside the mouth and whether its tip protrudes to at least the alveolar ridge. Determine that the tongue moves in all directions and lacks sustained quivering or trembling movements. A **gag reflex** is usually provoked during these manipulations. Note its presence and that the infant recovers spontaneously.

Allow the infant to suck on your finger and assess whether the suck creates firm pressure and an adequate seal (**sucking reflex**). Remove your finger from the mouth and lightly stroke the skin to elicit a **rooting reflex;** i.e., stroke horizontally from the corner of the mouth toward the cheek. The infant who is calm and relaxed will turn his head toward the side where your finger stroked and begin to suck.

Remove the infant's upper-body clothing, hyperextend the neck by cradling the occiput in the palm of one hand and slightly elevate the upper back off the mattress in the other hand. Allow the head to *gently* fall backward enough to fully expose the neck.

Neck, Thorax, and Upper Limbs

Because the newborn's neck is so short, it must be hyperextended in order to adequately inspect it. Subtle goiters are not visible otherwise. Inspect for bulges or masses, midline placement of the trachea, and absence of neck webbing (an excess of skin particularly posteriorly and laterally).

Place the head back down on the mattress.

Palpate the neck all around, including palpation for head and neck lymph nodes. Turn the head from side to side, flex, and extend to assess range of motion and flexibility at the neck. Palpate the clavicles along their full length to assess for fractures, feeling for continuity of bone and absence of crepitus.

Observe the unclothed chest for respiratory rate and pattern, symmetry, movement during respirations, and absence of retractions. The thorax is rounded, and the chest wall is thin and pliable. The precordium should not bulge. The point of maximal impulse (PMI) may be visible. The abdomen moves prominently during normal respiration.

Palpate the sternum, breasts, and precordium. In the newborn, chest percussion is not helpful.

Upper limbs are inspected for symmetry, overall appearance, (size, shape, bulk, length), and symmetry of spontaneous movements. Hands are inspected for palmar creases, and fingers are inspected for number, taper, curvatures, and webbing (syndactyly). Nails are inspected for size and configuration. Nailbeds are inspected for color. Bones and muscles are palpated along their full length, and all joints are assessed for range of motion. The brachial pulses are palpated simultaneously. Muscle tone is assessed as the limbs are passively manipulated, and strength is estimated when the infant is actively moving.

Place your little finger in the ulnar side of the infant's palm. The baby's fingers will close around your finger, demonstrating the presence of a **grasp reflex.**

The diaper should be opened during the inspection and manipulation of the hips.

Lower Limbs

Gently extend the limbs as far as they will straighten without using undue pressure. Normal flexion contractures at the hips and knees will prevent the examiner from totally straightening the limbs at these joints. The limbs are inspected for symmetry, overall appearance (size, shape, bulk, length, and angulation), and symmetry of spontaneous movements. The anterior medial thigh creases are inspected for symmetry.

The feet are inspected for appearance and for edema. Look at the plantar surface (the sole) of each foot. Assess whether the forefoot (toes and metatarsals) is straight in line with the hindfoot. Count toes and inspect for webbing, overlapping, and other deformities and for restricted range of motion. Nails are inspected for size and configuration, and nailbeds are inspected for absence of cyanosis.

The bones and muscles are palpated along their full length, and joints at the knees and feet are assessed for range of motion. Muscle tone is assessed as the limbs are passively manipulated, and strength is estimated as the infant actively resists parts of the examination.

Congenital hip dysplasia (CHD) is one of the most difficult but important diagnoses to make in the newborn. Early recognition and treatment significantly influence prognosis. The initial portions of the screening examination for CHD have already been performed: inspection of the lower limbs for symmetry of size, length, placement of medial thigh creases, and degree of flexion of hips and knees. Any or all of these might be asymmetric in unilateral hip dysplasia.

The Ortolani and Barlow maneuvers are the maneuvers utilized to diagnose CHD in the newborn. They may be performed on one hip at a time, as shown on the baby in Figure 15.15, or on both hips simultaneously. While standing at the "feet" end of the baby, use your right hand to examine the left hip and your left hand to examine the right hip. Use your nonexamining hand to stabilize the opposite hip simultaneously. Begin by examining the left hip with your right hand.

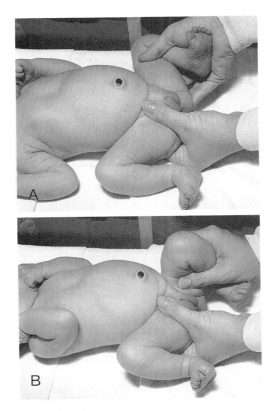

Figure 15.15   The Ortolani and Barlow maneuvers.

1. First, stabilize the baby's right hip. Place your left thumb on the baby's symphysis pubis and the fingers of your left hand under the right buttock.
2. Next, with your right hand, bring the baby's left hip into 90° of flexion and hold the knee fully flexed. The midanterior tibia will rest against the palm of your hand. Place your thumb on the baby's left anteromedial thigh just distal to the inguinal fold and your second and third fingers on the posterolateral thigh (over the greater trochanter).
3. Gently abduct the thigh at the hip joint while lifting toward the ceiling with your second and third fingers. This is called the **Ortolani maneuver.**
    A dislocated hip may "reduce," and you will feel (or hear) either movement or a "clunk." In normals, you will feel nothing, or you may feel a "click" (not a clunk), usually emanating from the knees.
4. The second maneuver is the **Barlow maneuver.** This evaluates dislocatability. With your right hand still wrapped around the left leg and thigh, bring the thigh back toward the midline while pressing toward the floor onto the anteromedial thigh with your thumb. *A hip that is "dislocatable" may slide out and dislocate over the rim of the acetabulum; you may feel or hear a clunk.*
5. Repeat both maneuvers on the opposite hip.

Skin

Before turning the infant, inspect the anterior skin surfaces from head to toe. Turn the baby over to the prone position, extend the lower limbs, and examine the skin. The skin is inspected, front and back, for color, birthmarks, rashes, masses, tags, and pits.

Back

While the baby is prone, look closely at the back and posterior aspects of the lower limbs. Inspect from head to toe the appearance of midline and parallel structures: occiput (birthmarks), posterior neck (webbing), spine along its full length (straightness, lesions, or defects overlying the spine, including soft tissue masses, hair tufts, hemangiomas, and dimples), scapulae, and iliac crests. For complete visualization, separate the buttocks and inspect the sacrum and anus. Evaluate the symmetry of the posterior medial thigh creases and buttocks creases. Palpate the spine along its full length.

Auscultate the posterior and lateral lung fields.

Return the infant to the supine position.

Neurologic System and Development

General observations. Consider the state of arousal and the ease with which the infant changes from state to state and the ease with which the infant is consoled. Consider the fluidity and spontaneity of movements and the posture at rest. How easily does the baby startle, cry, or develop leg or facial movement? How difficult is it to arouse the infant? How much spontaneous activity does the infant demonstrate? When moved about, does the infant startle very easily, cry excessively (or with a high pitch), or develop sustained leg or facial clonus?

Cranial nerves. Mentally review the cranial nerves and fill in the missing maneuvers. Several of the cranial nerves (e.g., cranial nerve I) are nearly impossible to evaluate in the newborn. Most have already been assessed in the course of the general examination by observing the extraocular movements and doll's eyes, response to light, red reflex, sucking, crying, swallowing, gag, and tongue movements. The corneal reflex is reserved for a formal neurologic examination. For a gross assessment of hearing (VIII), introduce a novel sound (e.g., a bell), expecting the infant to "alert" by quieting his movements and opening his eyes. Cranial nerve XI is a little difficult to evaluate in newborns, but in the absence of torticollis, it is unlikely to be abnormal.

Sensation is not routinely formally evaluated in the healthy newborn. If necessary, withdrawal to pinprick may be used.

Reflexes. In the screening newborn examination, the deep tendon reflexes are not routinely included. The Achilles and brachioradialis reflexes are not present until age 6 months. The patellar reflex is present at birth. If a detailed neurologic assessment is required, you may use your fingertip to tap the tendon to assess this reflex. Assessment of the plantar reflex is not part of the routine newborn examination because both flexion and extension of the toes may be seen in normal newborns.

Special newborn reflexes. In contrast to deep tendon reflexes, primitive reflexes are routinely evaluated in the newborn. These provide information about the general integrity of the neurologic system. In the newborn the following primitive reflexes are assessed for presence and symmetry.

- **Moro reflex.** To test for the Moro reflex, the infant should be lying supine, as in Figure 15.16. Cradle the infant's head and upper back in your hands and forearms. Next, allow the infant's head to fall back with your hands as you abruptly (but gently) move your hands back toward the surface of the bassinet. The normal response is a symmetric abduction of the arms with extension of the fingers (and some lesser abduction of the legs), followed by a return to the resting flexed posture. A "complete" Moro tells the examiner that the brain, nerves, and muscles are working together. It also tells the examiner that there is no unilateral paralysis or injury of a limb. The Moro reflex sometimes triggers a few beats of unsustained clonus of the arms or legs, which are normal at this age.

- **Placing and stepping.** To observe placing and stepping, lift the infant upright by supporting him with your hands under the axillae. Next, gently scrape the top of the baby's foot along the underside of a table or bassinet edge. He will respond by flexing, then extending his leg (i.e., placing). When the sole of the baby's foot touches a flat surface, he will "walk" (i.e, stepping).
- **Reflex grasp, suck, root.** These primitive reflexes are routinely assessed and are described earlier.

Motor examination. Much of the required information has been obtained during the course of the examination. Posture at rest (flexed versus extended) provides information about tone and symmetry of limbs. Observation of primitive reflexes provides information about function and symmetry of large muscle groups. The limb examinations also provide the opportunity to assess muscle bulk, strength, and tone.

Head lag. This provides further information about tone. Grasp the infant's hands in yours and pull the infant up gently by the hands from supine to sitting. Observe whether the baby's head remains totally extended as he is pulled to a sitting position or whether it begins to flex slightly as it comes up off the mattress.

Ventral suspension. Hold the infant aloft by supporting him around the thorax and abdomen and assess his ability to maintain a horizontal posture (Fig. 15.17).

Slip through. This is assessed with the infant in the upright position (as used to assess placing and stepping, with your hands in the infant's axillae). The newborn

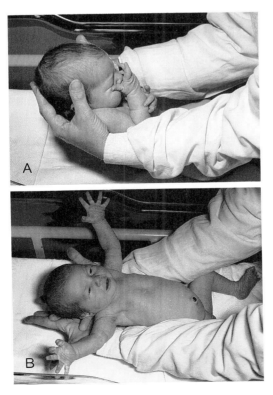

Figure 15.16   The Moro reflex.

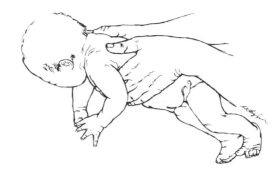

Figure 15.17   Ventral suspension: full-term newborn.

with normal tone and strength will not "slip through" your hands (or be totally supported by you); you should not have to hold the baby upright, just support her.

Determining gestational age. Gestational age is calculated as the number of weeks elapsed from the first day of the mother's last normal menstrual period to the date of the infant's delivery. A reliable estimate of gestational age or degree of fetal maturation is crucial in order to provide appropriate care and an accurate prognosis for the newborn. Unfortunately, maternal dates and prenatal ultrasound estimations of gestational age may be inaccurate or unavailable. In addition, the infant's measurements (e.g., weight, length) do not necessarily correctly correlate with gestational age. It is, therefore, important for the clinician evaluating the newborn to be able to determine gestational age by physical examination.

Infants are categorized into three groups based on their gestational age: (1) **premature,** 37 weeks of gestation or less; (2) **full term,** 38–42 weeks; (3) **post-mature,** more than 42 weeks of gestation.

The principle behind determining gestational age by physical examination is that certain physical and neurologic attributes mature in a progressive and predictable fashion during the latter half of gestation. Rating scales of these physical and neurologic attributes assign numerical values to specific findings (values increase with maturity), which are then summed. Numerical totals are compared with standards that have been correlated to specific gestational ages. There are several versions of this method. Some versions use either physical or neurologic criteria; others use both.

The **New Ballard Score** is a recently refined version of a combined scale (using both physical and neurologic criteria) that may be used to assess gestational age in infants, beginning at 20 weeks of gestation. Physical maturity criteria are external physical findings that are assessed by inspection and palpation. Neuromuscular maturity criteria assess posture, flexibility, and passive flexor tone. For optimal validity, when using the New Ballard Score, the extremely premature infant (26 weeks gestation) must be assessed when less than 12 hours of age. Each of the neurologic and physical criteria is assessed, and a score is assigned for each criterion. The scores are summed and correlated with a maturity rating in weeks according to the table (Fig. 15.18*A* and *B*).

Determining appropriateness of size for gestational age. After determining the gestational age, plot the weight, length, and head circumference on the newborn growth charts under the appropriate gestational age. Measurements will fall in one of three areas: **AGA** (appropriate for gestional age—between the 10th and 90th percentiles), **SGA** (small for gestational age—less than the 10th percentile), **LGA** (large for gestational age—greater than the 90th percentile). As stated previously, the newborn's size does not necessarily correlate with gestational age. Regardless of maturity, the newborn's measurements will be AGA, SGA, or LGA.

The baby whose measurements are absolutely normal will "plot out" as AGA. SGA and LGA babies, whatever the gestational age, have a higher incidence of certain in utero and postnatal problems. SGA babies are also known as growth retarded. Some common examples of SGA babies are those with congenital viral infections, placental insufficiency, and infants of alcoholic mothers. Maternal cigarette smoking is associated with lower weight for gestational age. The LGA baby is often large for either familial or unknown reasons. If there is a pathologic cause, its most common association is with maternal diabetes (Fig. 15.19).

Whether the infant is examined before or after you meet the parents, be sure to speak to them immediately after you have completed the examination. Most of the time the infant will be healthy and normal. When that is the case, make sure that this unspoken question is the first thing you tell them.

Figure 15.20 is an example of one form presently used to record the newborn physical examination. It assumes that the clinician has performed a complete examination. While it does not ask for a description of every finding, there is room to record anything of significance.

Normal and Common Variants and *Clues to Abnormalities*

General Appearance

Many, if not all newborns, demonstrate "battle scars" such as bruises, swellings, or asymmetries acquired during intrauterine life, labor, or delivery. A careful review of the prenatal and perinatal history will assist in determining the logical etiology of a particular finding (e.g., a facial bruise may be explained by a forceps delivery). Most "battle scars" fade or resolve rather quickly but may be alarming or disappointing to new parents.

Another "alarming" but normal group of findings relates to the newborn's relative peripheral vascular instability, thin skin, and limited amount of subcutaneous fat. The infant's skin and superficial vessels manifest remarkable changes in response to changes in ambient temperature. The responses are most visible in the hands, feet, perioral skin, and trunk and include cyanosis and mottling. The clinician must be adept at distinguishing these findings from those that imply underlying pathology (e.g., cyanosis of the lips).

Head: Hair, Face, Eyes, Ears, Nose, and Mouth

Head and hair on head. Irrespective of its appearance at birth, most hair on the head is shed during the first few months of life and will be replaced by hair of a different texture. Various characteristics of hair may be clues to underlying abnormalities. *Some rare systemic disorders and syndromes are associated with abnormalities in color or texture of hair (e.g., fragile hair, twisted hair, very blond hair, hair with a white forelock, and absent hair and eyebrows). Other disorders are associated with abnormal patterns of hair (e.g., more than one hair whorl on the head is considered a dysmorphic feature). The presence of multiple hair whorls should stimulate a search for other craniofacial anomalies.*

Palpation of the head may reveal the following asymmetries and other types of "battle scars" on the head. These resolve gradually during the days and weeks following birth:

Molding. This is from pressure on the presenting part and is therefore more common in vaginal deliveries. The head looks or feels asymmetric or elongated.

Caputsuccedaneum. This is edema of the scalp tissues and is also secondary to intrauterine or vaginal pressure. This swelling is usually found on the top or back of the head; it crosses the midline. The swelling feels somewhat firm but is ill-defined in circumference and pits with pressure applied with a fingertip (Fig. 15.21).

MATURATIONAL ASSESSMENT OF GESTATIONAL AGE (New Ballard Score)

NAME ______ DATE/TIME OF BIRTH ______ SEX ______

HOSPITAL NO. ______ DATE/TIME OF EXAM ______ BIRTH WEIGHT ______

RACE ______ AGE WHEN EXAMINED ______ LENGTH ______

APGAR SCORE: 1 MINUTE ______ 5 MINUTES ______ 10 MINUTES ______ HEAD CIRC. ______

EXAMINER ______

NEUROMUSCULAR MATURITY

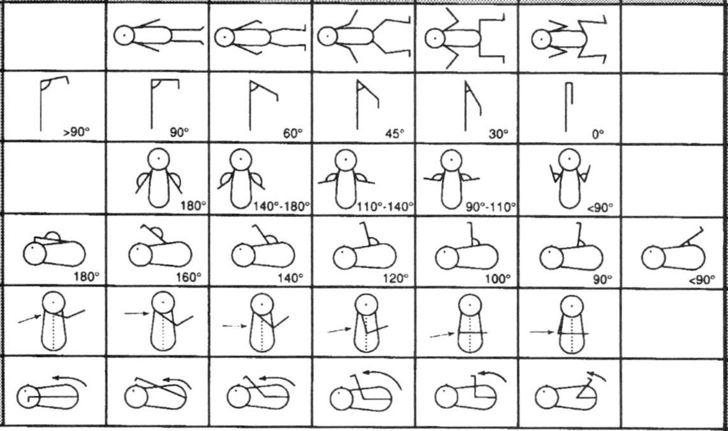

NEUROMUSCULAR MATURITY SIGN	SCORE -1	0	1	2	3	4	5	RECORD SCORE HERE
POSTURE								
SQUARE WINDOW (Wrist)	>90°	90°	60°	45°	30°	0°		
ARM RECOIL		180°	140°-180°	110°-140°	90°-110°	<90°		
POPLITEAL ANGLE	180°	160°	140°	120°	100°	90°	<90°	
SCARF SIGN								
HEEL TO EAR								
							TOTAL NEUROMUSCULAR MATURITY SCORE	

PHYSICAL MATURITY

PHYSICAL MATURITY SIGN	SCORE -1	0	1	2	3	4	5	RECORD SCORE HERE
SKIN	sticky friable transparent	gelatinous red translucent	smooth pink visible veins	superficial peeling &/or rash, few veins	cracking pale areas rare veins	parchment deep cracking no vessels	leathery cracked wrinkled	
LANUGO	none	sparse	abundant	thinning	bald areas	mostly bald		
PLANTAR SURFACE	heel-toe 40-50 mm: -1 <40 mm: -2	>50 mm no crease	faint red marks	anterior transverse crease only	creases ant. 2/3	creases over entire sole		
BREAST	imperceptible	barely perceptible	flat areola no bud	stippled areola 1-2 mm bud	raised areola 3-4 mm bud	full areola 5-10 mm bud		
EYE/EAR	lids fused loosely: -1 tightly: -2	lids open pinna flat stays folded	sl. curved pinna; soft; slow recoil	well-curved pinna; soft but ready recoil	formed & firm instant recoil	thick cartilage ear stiff		
GENITALS (Male)	scrotum flat, smooth	scrotum empty faint rugae	testes in upper canal rare rugae	testes descending few rugae	testes down good rugae	testes pendulous deep rugae		
GENITALS (Female)	clitoris prominent & labia flat	prominent clitoris & small labia minora	prominent clitoris & enlarging minora	majora & minora equally prominent	majora large minora small	majora cover clitoris & minora		
							TOTAL PHYSICAL MATURITY SCORE	

SCORE

Neuromuscular

Physical

Total

MATURITY RATING

score	weeks
-10	20
-5	22
0	24
5	26
10	28
15	30
20	32
25	34
30	36
35	38
40	40
45	42
50	44

GESTATIONAL AGE (weeks)

By dates ______

By ultrasound ______

By exam ______

Reference
Ballard JL, Khoury JC, Wedig K, et al: New Ballard Score, expanded to include extremely premature infants. *J Pediatr* 1991; 119:417-423. Reprinted by permission of Dr Ballard and Mosby-Year Book, Inc.

A

Figure 15.18 **A.** Maturational assessment of gestational age (New Ballard Score). **B.** Notes on techniques of assessment of physical and neurologic criteria.

NOTES ON TECHNIQUES OF ASSESSMENT OF PHYSICAL CRITERIA

Plantar surface foot length	Foot length is measured from the tip of the great toe to the back of the heel. (This is measured in the premature infant in whom no plantar creases are present.)
Eye/Ear	Loosely fused eyelids are defined as closed but able, in the case of one or both lids, to be partly separated by gentle traction. Tightly fused eyelids are defined as bilaterally inseparable by gentle traction. (This is useful in evaluating the very premature infant. In the more mature premie, the ear pinnae are evaluated for this category.)

NOTES ON TECHNIQUES OF ASSESSMENT OF NEUROLOGIC CRITERIA

Posture	Observed with infant quiet and in supine position. Score 0: arms and legs extended; 1: beginning of flexion of hips and knees, arms extended; 2: stronger flexion of legs, arms extended; 3: arms slightly flexed, legs flexed and abducted; 4: full flexion of arms and legs.
Square window (wrist)	The hand is flexed on the forearm between the thumb and index finger of the examiner. Enough pressure is applied to get as full a flexion as possible, and the angle between the hypothenar eminence and the ventral aspect of the forearm is measured and graded according to the diagram. (Care is taken not to rotate the infant's wrist while doing this maneuver.)
Arm recoil	With the infant in the supine position the forearms are first flexed for 5 seconds, then fully extended by pulling on the hands, and then released. The sign is fully positive if the arms return briskly to full flexion (Score 2). If the arms return to incomplete flexion or the response is sluggish, it is graded as Score 1. If they remain extended or are only followed by random movements the score is 0.
Popliteal angle	With the infant supine and his pelvis flat on the examining couch, the thigh is held in the knee-chest position by the examiner's left index finger and thumb supporting the knee. The leg is then extended by gentle pressure from the examiner's right index finger behind the ankle, and the popliteal angle is measured.
Scarf sign	With the baby supine, take the infant's hand and try to put it around the neck as far posteriorly as possible around the opposite shoulder. Assist this maneuver by lifting the elbow across the body. See how far the elbow will go across, and grade according to illustrations. Score 0: elbow reaches opposite axillary line; 1: elbow between midline and opposite axillary line; 2: elbow just reaches midline; 3: elbow will not reach midline.
Heel to ear maneuver	With the baby supine, draw the baby's foot as near to the head as it will go without forcing it. Observe the distance between the foot and the head as well as the degree of extension at the knee. Grade according to diagram. Note that the knee is left free and may draw down alongside the abdomen.

B

CLASSIFICATION OF NEWBORNS (BOTH SEXES)
BY INTRAUTERINE GROWTH AND GESTATIONAL AGE [1,2]

NAME _____ DATE OF EXAM _____ LENGTH_____

HOSPITAL NO. _____ SEX _____ HEAD CIRC. _____

RACE _____ BIRTH WEIGHT _____ GESTATIONAL AGE _____

DATE OF BIRTH_____

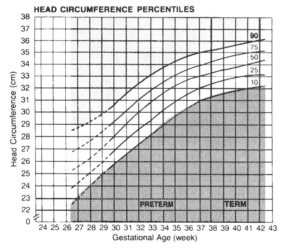

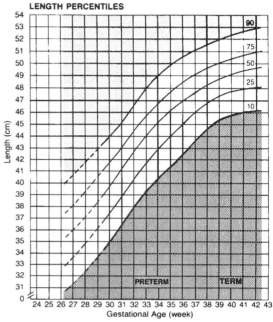

CLASSIFICATION OF INFANT*	Weight	Length	Head Circ.
Large for Gestational Age (LGA) (>90th percentile)			
Appropriate for Gestational Age (AGA) (10th to 90th percentile)			
Small for Gestational Age (AGA) (<10th percentile)			

*Place an "X" in the appropriate box (LGA, AGA or SGA) for weight, for length and for head circumference.

References
1. Battaglia FC, Lubchenco LO: A practical classification of newborn infants by weight and gestational age. J Pediatr 1967; 71:159-163.
2. Lubchenco LO, Hansman C, Boyd E: Intrauterine growth in length and head circumference as estimated from live births at gestational ages from 26 to 42 weeks. Pediatrics 1966; 37:403-408.

Reprinted by permission from Dr Battaglia, Dr Lubchenco, Journal of Pediatrics and Pediatrics.

A service of **SIMILAC®** Infant Formulas

The Ross Hospital Formula System

A5860(0.05) / OCTOBER 1991

ROSS LABORATORIES COLUMBUS, OHIO 43216 Division of Abbott Laboratories, USA

LITHO IN USA

Figure 15.19

Admission Examination

Wt: (lbs.)	Lgt: (in.)	HC: (cm)

	WNL	(If abnormal, describe)
Skin Clear?	☐	_____
(Note jaundice/cyanosis/rash)		_____
Head		
Fontanelles palpable/normal?	☐	_____
Sutures OK?	☐	_____
(note significant molding/caput)		_____
Eyes		
Red Reflex present?	☐	_____
Conjunctiva clear?	☐	_____
Ears		
Position & shape normal?	☐	_____
Cartilage present?	☐	_____
Nose patent?	☐	_____
Mouth		
Palate intact?	☐	_____
Neck		
Clavicles intact?	☐	_____
Chest		
Breast tissue palpable?	☐	_____
Lungs		
Clear?	☐	_____
Heart		
Rate/Rhythm normal?	☐	_____
Murmur absent?	☐	_____
Pulses adequate?	☐	_____
Abdomen		
Organomegaly/masses absent?	☐	_____
Anus patent?	☐	_____
Cord vessels normal?	☐	_____
Genitalia		
Normal ♂ or ♀?	☐	_____
Testicles↓↓?	☐	_____
Hernia/Hydrocele absent?	☐	_____
Musculoskeletal		
Hips in place?	☐	_____
Digits all present?	☐	_____
Neurological		
Strong moro/suck/root?	☐	_____
Good grasp/tone?	☐	_____

Term: ☐   Preterm: ☐   Post Term: ☐   AGA: SGA: LGA:
Plan:

_____ M.D.
Date   Physician

Figure 15.20   Newborn physical examination.

Cephalohematoma. This is a subperiosteal hematoma. This type of swelling does not cross the midline (limited by suture lines). It feels firm and more circumscribed than a caput. The center of the swelling may have a "mushy" or tense consistency, depending on the amount of blood contained within it. A cephalohematoma may be associated with a linear skull fracture; this is usually clinically inapparent. The clinician should palpate for a depression in the skull contour, which may indicate the less common, but more serious, association of a depressed skull fracture. The cephalohematoma may leave behind small, hard nodules of no significance (Fig. 15.22).

The key to the "benign" swellings is to distinguish them from more important swellings such as **encephaloceles** and **meningoceles.** Make sure that there is bone underneath the "usual swellings." That tells you that there is probably no brain communication with the scalp (as with an encephalocele).

Cranial sutures are not fused at birth. Pressure on the head during labor and delivery may push cranial bones together so that suture lines feel ridged. **Ridging** when secondary to molding resolves during a period of weeks to several months. *Ridging that is very marked and bony asymmetries of the skull are abnormal.* Conversely, there may be a small palpable separation between sutures. This is also normal as long as the head circumference is normal and there are no signs of increased intracranial pressure. *Extremely wide separation of sutures (significantly wider than the width of your fingertip) may indicate increased intracranial pressure, especially when accompanied by an abnormally large head circumference.*

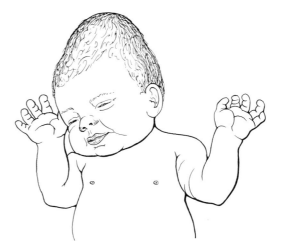

Figure 15.21   Newborn with molding of the head and a caput.

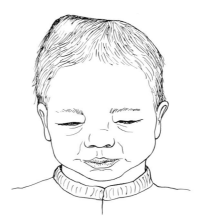

Figure 15.22   Cephalohematoma.

The anterior fontanelle is diamond-shaped and averages 2 × 2 cm in size but may be as much as 3 × 4 cm; the posterior fontanelle is usually about a fingertip open. Small and large fontanelles may be normal variants. Abnormally large fontanelles may be seen with hydrocephalus (and some skeletal, chromosomal, congenital, and metabolic disorders); small fontanelles may be seen in such conditions as microcephaly and hyperparathyroidism.

A small scab will be visible on the scalp at the site where an intrauterine fetal monitor was placed. It will heal over a week's time.

Head circumference. **Macrocephaly** is a large head circumference or a head that measures more than 2 SDs above the norm for age. A large head may be a normal and/or familial variant. It may also result from a pathologic process (e.g., hydrocephalus). A macrocephalic head may contain a small, normal, or large brain inside. **Microcephaly** is defined as a head circumference that is more than 2 SDs below the norm for age. A small head reflects a small brain.

Face. Depending on the age of the infant and the innate skin tone, the face may appear pink, reddish, or pale. In the healthy baby, "pale" appearance usually reflects fair skin tone rather than significant anemia or impending shock. Absence of true pallor is confirmed by everting the lower eyelid and noting that the blood vessels of the palpebral conjunctivae are dark pink or red.

Clusters of small yellow-white papules found on the bridge of the nose, chin, or cheeks are called **milia.** They result from retained keratin, sebum, and sweat, and are transient.

Forceps deliveries are associated with several facial findings. Bruising or **forceps marks** are linear purple marks that heal in the same manner as bruises in older children. The facial nerve may be damaged during a forceps delivery. *A **facial nerve palsy** will manifest as palpebral fissure asymmetry (taller fissure on the paralyzed side) and a flattening of the nasolabial fold with the face deviating to the nonparalyzed side. This injury may be heralded by forceps marks found medial to the infant's ear.*

Eyes. When silver nitrate eyedrops are instilled when the infant is in the delivery room, he may manifest a transient (up to 48 hours) chemical conjunctivitis with swelling of the lids and slight eye drainage. In the newborn, infectious conjunctivitis may manifest the same signs, but this usually begins after the first 2 days of life.

The conjunctivae are often dotted with focal hemorrhages, a result of labor and delivery. These are harmless and resolve spontaneously.

Epicanthal folds may be noted. An **epicanthal fold** is a small fold of skin that covers the medial canthus. This may be a normal variant. It is only significant if it is found in association with other abnormal features (e.g., as in Down syndrome).

The palpebral fissure may manifest a so-called **Mongoloid or anti-Mongoloid slant.** This may be related to the patient's family or ethnic origin; it may be an isolated finding; or like an epicanthal fold, it may be part of a syndrome. For example, patients with Down syndrome have palpebral fissures with so-called Mongoloid slants. *Many syndromes are associated with abnormal interpupillary distances or palpebral fissure widths. For example, narrow palpebral fissures are seen in fetal alcohol syndrome.*

The corneas should be clear, not cloudy. Cloudiness may indicate the presence of congenital glaucoma or a cataract. *Early recognition and treatment of congenital glaucoma and large cataracts are extremely important in order to optimize visual function. Absent red reflexes or white pupillary reflexes imply the presence of an abnormality either anterior to the fundus or within the fundus itself (e.g., retinoblastoma). These findings require immediate ophthalmologic referral.*

The newborn and young infant's eyes will periodically appear crossed. This intermittent misalignment disappears by age 3 months. *A fixed limitation of extraocular movement in one or more directions or a **fixed** misalignment is always abnormal and requires further investigation.*

Ears. Pits or tags on or near the ears are found in normal children but are also occasionally a sign of a more extensive branchial cleft abnormality.

Nose. The nose may appear mildly swollen and asymmetric secondary to the birth process. A marked abnormality in nasal shape (e.g., a markedly beaked nose) may be an isolated finding or may be part of a syndrome.

Mild nasal congestion and sneezing may be seen during the first few days of life, secondary to nasal retention of amniotic fluid. Nasal sounds may be particularly apparent in this age group because most newborns breathe through their noses rather than their mouths. *Marked nasal congestion is seen in infants with congenital syphilis beginning at the end of the first week of life, and very frequent sneezing is seen in infants with narcotic withdrawal.*

*If the nasal passages are blocked (i.e., **choanal atresia,** a congenital membranous or bony obstruction of the posterior nasal air passage), the baby is forced to breathe through the mouth. When the mouth is closed or occluded, as in feeding, the infant with bilateral nasal blockage will display severe respiratory distress, usually with apnea and cyanosis. A unilateral choanal atresia may be asymptomatic in* *the newborn period. If choanal atresia is suspected, passage of a flexible catheter through the nares down past the nasopharynx is attempted bilaterally.*

Mouth. The lips and tongue should be pink. In contrast, the skin surrounding the lips, the perioral skin, may be slightly cyanotic. This is called **perioral cyanosis.** This is normal and is associated with the newborn's peripheral vascular instability. *True cyanosis, signifying capillary oxygen desaturation, is manifested by a blue-purple coloration of the lips and tongue.*

*If only one side of the mouth turns down when the infant cries (and the rest of the face is symmetric), the infant may have an **absence of the depressor anguli oris muscle,** a defect that may be isolated or may be part of the **asymmetric crying facies syndrome,** which has associated cardiac and other defects.*

A cleft of the lip or hard palate will be obvious. A soft palate cleft will not necessarily be visible and may only be appreciated with careful palpation. A bifid uvula may be a marker for a submucous cleft of the soft palate.

Whitish papules may be found near the junction of the hard and soft palates or on the gum lines. The papules on the palate (located on either side of the median raphe) are known as **Epstein's pearls.** The papules on the gum lines are called **epithelial pearls.** Both types of "pearls" are shed spontaneously within weeks to months; neither has clinical significance.

Occasionally, a **natal tooth** will have erupted. If it is loose, it will require extraction because of the risk of aspiration to the neonate.

It may appear that the tongue does not reach out of the mouth very far because of a tight or shortened frenulum. A **tight frenulum** rarely produces problems for speaking or eating. Most commonly, as the tongue grows, the frenulum stretches out. *If the tongue does not fit easily inside the mouth, then either the tongue is too large (e.g., Beckwith syndrome), or the jaw is too small (e.g., Pierre Robin syndrome).*

Neck, Thorax, and Upper Limbs

Neck. The newborn neck is quite supple. There should be no limitation to passive motion in any direction. The head should not tilt toward one shoulder or the other. *Congenital neck masses include thyroglossal duct cyst, goiter, and cystic hygroma.*

A webbed neck is found in association with a variety of syndromes. The most common of these is Turner's syndrome (a chromosomal disorder in females in which there is only one X, or one normal X, chromosome).

Thorax. When compared to that of an older child or adult, the normal xiphoid may appear prominent and feel distinct from the rest of the sternum.

Clavicle fractures secondary to the birth process are common. Palpation of the involved clavicle reveals discontinuity with or without crepitance. There may or may not be a visible asymmetry between the two clavicles.

In the term infant there will be approximately 1 cm (in diameter) of palpable breast tissue. Toward the end of the first week of life, breasts may swell, redden, and discharge a milky substance. This phenomenon that occurs in both males and females is known as **physiologic galactorrhea.** This is secondary to the influence of maternal hormone and resolves within several weeks.

Upper limbs. In the normal-term newborn, there are small **flexion contractures** at the **elbows** that resolve within several weeks. *Birth trauma to the upper limbs may result in fractures and/or nerve damage, both of which are manifested by diminished and asymmetric upper limb movements. Damage to the C5 and C6 nerve roots causes **Erb's palsy** (resulting in paralysis of the shoulder girdle and upper arm muscles). Damage to the C7, C8, and T1 roots results in **Klumpke's paralysis** (involving the muscles that control forearm, wrist, and hand movements).*

Hands, fingers, feet, and toes may appear quite blue or purple, particularly in response to decreasing ambient temperature. In the normal child, the nailbeds remain pink. This **acrocyanosis,** like perioral cyanosis, is usually a reflection of the newborn's normal peripheral vascular instability and resolves during the first weeks and months of life. *Hypoplastic or underdeveloped nails are found in several disorders, including fetal hydantoin syndrome secondary to maternal phenytoin exposure during pregnancy. A single palmar crease is seen in Down syndrome and some other syndromes. It may also be present in isolation in normal individuals.*

Cardiorespiratory System

The usual heart rate in the newborn is approximately 140 beats/min (approximate normal range; 90–160/min). It will be on the lower end when the infant is sleeping.

Several innocent murmurs may be audible in the neonate, especially during the first 24–48 hours of life. The etiologies of most of these are uncertain but are thought to be related to either blood flow turbulence produced by a closing ductus arteriosus or to falling pulmonary vascular resistance. These are soft (usually not louder than grade 2/6), blowing, and occupy the ejection period of systole (beginning after S_1); most are heard best along the upper left sternal border. Most of these murmurs disappear within the first 2 days of life.

A common specific innocent neonatal murmur is known as **peripheral pulmonic stenosis (PPS).** This is a short, midsystolic blowing murmur not louder than grade 2/6 and is best heard along the distribution of the peripheral pulmonary arteries. Thus it may be heard in the front of the chest, the axillae, and back. The key to identifying this murmur is that if it is heard in the right chest as clearly as in the left, then one can be fairly certain that it originates from both sides of the chest. This diagnosis is confirmed retrospectively when the murmur disappears by approximately age 3 months.

The newborn with any of the following may have congenital heart disease; pathologic or persistent murmur (not deemed to be PPS), pallor, true central cyanosis, poor pulses, respiratory distress, or poor feeding.

The normal respiratory pattern in the newborn, when compared to that in children and adults, is more irregular. In addition, the normal respiratory rate is substantially faster (30–75/min). Brief pauses in the respiratory cycle, unaccompanied by bradycardia or changes in color or tone, are normal. The pattern in which the infant takes a series of relatively quick breaths and then pauses for even as long as 10 or 15 seconds is known as **periodic breathing.** Periodic breathing is more common in prematures and tends to be less common as gestational age increases, but it is still normal in term newborns. *If breathing ceases for more than 20 seconds or if pauses of any length are accompanied by pallor, limpness, cyanosis, or bradycardia and require vigorous stimulation, this is pathologic and is known as **apnea of infancy.***

During the first few hours of life, scattered long crackles may be auscultated in an otherwise healthy infant. The crackles should disappear within several hours and should be unaccompanied by any other signs of respiratory distress. Thereafter, auscultation reveals clear or bronchovesicular breath sounds.

*The newborn with **respiratory distress** may be observed to breathe very quickly or, alternatively, may manifest apnea. In addition, retractions (intercostal, subcostal, or supraclavicular) and nasal flaring (widening of the alae on inspiration) may be observed. Audible expiratory grunting (sounds like a grunt) may be appreciated. On auscultation, findings will, in part, reflect the etiology of the respiratory distress. For example, crackles may be appreciated in pneumonia or congestive heart failure; alternatively, an infant with overwhelming sepsis may demonstrate poor respiratory effort, poor air entry, and no specific adventitious sounds. As pulmonary failure worsens, cyanosis of the mucous membranes is observed.*

Coughing in the newborn is distinctly uncommon and requires investigation. Hoarseness and stridor are also abnormal in the newborn. Causes for these include anomalies in or around the larynx (e.g., paralyzed vocal cord, congenital subglottic stenosis, tracheomalacia, or a vascular ring pressing onto the airway). One transient type of hoarseness or stridor is not related to an anomaly: The history will reveal that a diagnostic laryngoscopy was performed in the delivery room. The infant may demonstrate mild and transient (1–2 days) hoarseness with crying or stridor, without any other signs of respiratory distress.

Abdomen

The abdomen is rounded convexly and moves prominently with normal respirations. A **diastasis recti** is a separation of the medial rectus sheath. It is palpable and visible as a midline longitudinal outpouching when the baby cries. It is a normal variant and usually disappears when the child is older. If there is skin laxity surrounding the umbilicus, the child may have an **umbilical hernia.** It will be easier to decide this when the infant is a few weeks old, after the umbilical stump has separated.

Marked concavity or marked distension of the abdomen are both abnormal and usually reflect underlying abdominal pathology (e.g., marked distension may reflect bowel obstruction and marked concavity may reflect a diaphragmatic hernia).

Umbilical cord insertion abnormalities that involve underlying abdominal contents are much more ominous than umbilical hernias. If there is herniated bowel through the abdominal wall at a site away from the umbilicus, the defect is called a gastroschisis. If bowel contents herniate through the umbilicus, it is called an omphalocele.

Variations from the normal number of umbilical vessels (e.g., a single umbilical artery) are associated with a high incidence of congenital anomalies, especially skeletal, gastrointestinal, and renal anomalies.

The liver edge is palpable approximately 1–2 cm down from the anterior costal margin in the midclavicular line and is firm. The spleen tip is normally either not palpable or just barely palpable. *An infant with a congenital viral infection (e.g., congenital rubella) may demonstrate hepatosplenomegaly.*

Inguinal Region

If the femoral pulses are very weak or absent or are delayed when compared with the right brachial pulse (and a dorsalis pedis pulse is not palpable either), suspect an obstruction in the aorta (i.e., coarctation of the aorta).

Genitalia

When inspection reveals genitalia that are either abnormal in size (e.g., a large clitoris or a small penis) or abnormal in appearance (e.g., labia majora that are fused) or contents (e.g., undescended testes or labial mass in what is thought to be a female), the diagnosis of ambiguous genitalia is suggested. This situation usually leads to further investigation (e.g., chromosome analysis, hormonal levels) of the infant's actual genetic and gonadal makeup.

Female genitalia. In the term infant, the labia majora cover the labia minora. As with breast tissue, there may be some swelling and erythema of the labia minora (toward the end of the first week) secondary to maternal hormone. There may be a mucoid or bloody vaginal discharge also. The vulva may also be swollen because of intrauterine pressure effects. One must differentiate a diffusely swollen vulva from a unilateral labial mass (e.g., a hernia).

In a full-term baby, the clitoris is covered by the labia when the legs are in the adducted position. *If the clitoris protrudes out from the labia (and the baby is not extremely thin or undergrown), the infant will require further investigation for other signs of virilization.*

Male genitalia. The normal size of the penis in the term infant is 3–4 cm in gently stretched length. *If the penis has a ventral curve, this is called a **chordee**. If the urethral opening is situated on the dorsal (top) surface of the penis, this is called an **epispadias**, and if it is on the ventral (underside), it is called a **hypospadias**.*

The scrotum may be edematous and bruised from intrauterine pressure effects. This is particularly common in breech presentations. *If a testicle is not descended or retractile but is located somewhere along the normal path of descent, this is an undescended testicle or **cryptorchidism.***

A fullness within the scrotum on either one side or both may be visible and/or palpable. Palpate for an underlying, normal-sized (approximately 0.6 cm in length) testicle. Then transilluminate (using the otoscope head) the scrotum on each side. If the scrotum transilluminates clearly except for the small testicular shadow, then the infant probably has a **hydrocele.** This is a fluid remnant. Most hydroceles resorb, although they are sometimes associated with an inguinal hernia.

If a mass is visible in the groin area, the most likely explanation is a hernia. Most inguinal hernias in childhood are indirect in type. An inguinal hernia looks like a bulge in the groin and extends above and lateral to the pubis; it may also extend into the scrotum. A hernia generally increases in size with crying or straining and decreases in size with relaxation. Scrotal transillumination may also be positive when the hernia contains bowel, thus making differentiation from a hydrocele difficult. It is helpful to remember that hydroceles are generally placed more distally, beyond the external inguinal ring. Inguinal hernias are far more common in males.

Lower Limbs

The term newborn has **flexion contractures at the hips and knees** from intrauterine positioning. Like those at the elbows, these resolve within the first few weeks of age.

Asymmetry of thigh or gluteal folds should raise suspicion of a hip abnormality (congenital hip dysplasia), although as many as one-third of normal infants demonstrate this isolated finding.

As the legs are extended, the clinician frequently notes that the newborn's **tibiae are mildly bowed** laterally at their midsection. Like flexion contractures, this is also secondary to fetal positioning.

The feet may be slightly edematous for a period of several days.

When the plantar surfaces of the feet are inspected, the clinician may discover that the forefoot (toes and metatarsals) curve toward the midline rather than remain vertically in line with the hindfoot. If so, the child has **metatarsus adductus** (Fig. 15.23). If the forefoot curves inward, the next maneuver is performed to determine the severity of the problem. Stabilize the heel between the thumb and index finger of your hand. Attempt to straighten out the forefoot using the fingers of your other hand by pushing laterally against the medial curved edge. If you are able to straighten it out using moderate pressure, this deformity may correct spontaneously or with passive stretching exercises during the first 2 months of life. Mild degrees of metatarsus adductus are very common (Fig. 15.24).

*If the entire foot points downward (like the appearance of the foot of a horse) and the lateral border of the foot is more distally placed than the medial border, the child may have a **clubfoot (talipes equinovarus).** This requires early orthopedic attention (Fig. 15.25).*

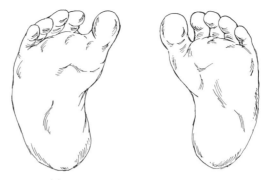

Figure 15.23   Metatarsus adductus.

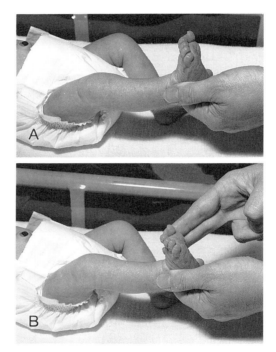

Figure 15.24   **A** and **B.** To assess the severity of metatarsus adductus, stabilize the heel, then apply pressure to the forefoot.

Back

Lesions (e.g., soft tissue masses, hair tufts, hemangiomas, skin defects) located directly over the spine require particular attention. Any of these lesions can be: (1) a marker for an underlying neural tube defect or (2) the most superficial aspect of a connection to the spinal canal. A dimple overlying the lower spine is very common. If it is possible to spread the skin apart to see that the skin under the dimple is intact, then there is not a high probability of an underlying problem. *All lesions overlying the spine, especially masses, require consideration, and possibly evaluation, for an underlying abnormality of neural tube development.*

A black-and-blue macule or patch, which is also commonly found over the lower spine and buttocks and over the posterior aspects of the shoulders is called

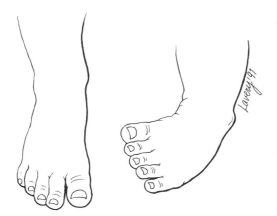

Figure 15.25   Clubfoot.

a **nevus of Ota.** It is a normal variant with absolutely no clinical significance. It is much more common in dark-skinned children. It fades as the child grows older.

Skin

During the first hours of life, some infants appear very ruddy. This intense coloring often resolves to a lighter, less intense pink. If it does not, the ruddiness may reflect underlying polycythemia. At birth, the skin (except for nailbeds and the scrotum) of dark-skinned infants often appears much lighter than it will appear ultimately. The skin deepens in color during the first few months of life.

Another transient finding secondary to the normal peripheral vascular instability of the newborn is **skin mottling.** A superficial lacy pattern of vessels becomes visible over the trunk and limbs, especially in response to decreases in ambient temperature. Another manifestation of this same phenomenon is called a **harlequin color change.** This appears as a sharp vertical demarcation down the center of the body with one side of the body appearing redder than the other.

Lanugo is a fine downy hair that covers the skin, particularly the shoulders and back, of the fetus. Lanugo is not present in the extremely premature infant. Some of this hair is shed prior to term, and the rest is shed within several weeks of life. Aside from lanugo, the variation in the body hair texture and quantity is enormous from baby to baby. In normal infants much of this variation is familial.

Cracking or desquamation in the term infant is normal. The postmature infant demonstrates increased peeling of the superficial skin. The term "newborn rash" is sometimes used.

At birth there may be some residual **vernix caseosa** (vernix means varnish and caseosa means cheesy in Latin), particularly in the skin folds and nailbeds. This fetal covering consists of sebum and desquamated epithelial cells.

Transient puffiness, or slight edema of the limbs and eyelids, may be present during the first few days of life and should resolve thereafter.

Jaundice in the neonate becomes visible on the face first. As the bilirubin rises, jaundice "spreads" caudally to include the rest of the body and the sclerae also. Natural sunlight provides the most accurate illumination in which to inspect for jaundice. It is possible to roughly correlate the extent of hyperbilirubinemia with the extent of the body that is visibly jaundiced. Jaundice in the newborn becomes visible when the bilirubin level exceeds 5–6 mg/dl: this is noticeable on the face. When the jaundice involves the face and upper half of the body (e.g., the umbilicus), the total bilirubin level may be estimated to be approximately 8–12 mg/dl. When the jaundice involves the entire body, including the lower limbs, the total bilirubin level generally exceeds 12 mg/dl.

Common birthmarks. **"Stork bites" or salmon patches** are very superficial, pink to red, flat lesions, which are present at birth mostly over the eyelids, nasal bridge, and nape of neck. These fade during a period of months to years (those on the neck tend to fade less completely).

"Strawberry" hemangiomas are so named because of their bumpy, red surfaces. These may be found anywhere on the body. Although it is a congenital lesion, this type of capillary hemangioma is not usually visible right at birth. However, with very careful inspection, one may find the **forerunner of the "strawberry" hemangioma**—a circumscribed, hypovascularized area with telangiectasias or tiny red threads within it. The characteristic well-demarcated "strawberry" appears within the first weeks after birth and grows rapidly in size and palpability during the first year (Fig. 15.26).

"Port-wine stain" hemangioma are visible at birth. These are flat hemangiomas that are red or pink at birth but eventually darken to a deep red or purple. They grow in proportion to the child. Unlike the "stork bite," these do not fade and, therefore, may be quite disfiguring. Port-wine stains tend to be unilateral; they may be found anywhere on the body but are most common over the face or neck *(Fig. 15.27). If a "port-wine stain" involves the area of the face innervated by the ophthalmic division of the trigeminal nerve, the baby may have **Sturge-Weber syndrome** with cerebral vascular abnormalities and possible mental retardation, seizures, motor, and ophthalmologic problems .*

Rashes. The newborn may manifest one or more of several rashes. The most common newborn rash is called **erythema toxicum.** This has a "flea-bite" appearance with scattered erythematous macules with a predilection for trunk, face, and limbs, not the palms and soles, and sometimes with papulopustular centers. These benign lesions "come and go" during the first 2 weeks of life. This requires no treatment (Fig. 15.28).

Another benign rash, seen much more commonly in dark-skinned neonates, is **transient neonatal pustular melanosis** (TNPM). Vesiculopostules can be present anywhere (including palms and soles) at birth. Within a few days, they rupture. Some of the lesions will leave behind pigmented macules with a fine scale surrounding them. Resolution is ultimately complete (Fig. 15.29).

When pustules are present, particularly with surrounding erythema, the clinician must include Staphylococcus aureus infection in the differential diagnosis. Similarly, when vesicles appear, a spectrum of diagnoses from the benign to the life-threatening will be entertained. The most benign etiology for a vesicle in the newborn is a friction blister; this is usually secondary to in utero minor repetitive trauma, e.g., a blister on the thumb secondary to thumb sucking in utero. These are usually solitary lesions that are not tiny in size; they do not multiply, spread, or enlarge postnatally, as the friction ceases after birth. On the other end of the spectrum, vesicles in the newborn must always raise a suspicion of herpes simplex virus infection.

Neurologic System and Development

General observations. When the infant is moving about, does the baby startle easily, cry excessively or with a high pitch, or develop sustained leg or facial clonus? This behavior would be identified as **jitteriness.** The opposite end of the spectrum for these observations would be the baby who does not react at all when moved about, has no natural flexion of the limbs (if full-term), and feels limp when suspended. Many full-term healthy babies have slight degrees of either types of behavior or transient periods of mild jitteriness. *Significant and, or prolonged jitteriness or limpness are definitely abnormal and usually signify underlying pathology (e.g., hypoglycemia, central nervous system hemorrhage, or sepsis).*

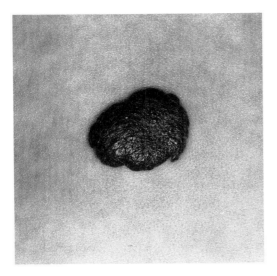

Figure 15.26 "Strawberry" hemangioma.

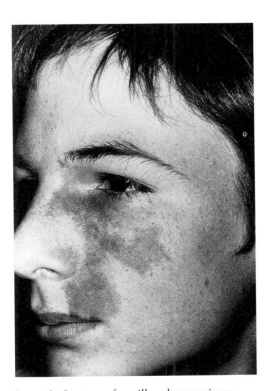

Figure 15.27 "Port-wine stain," a type of capillary hemangioma.

The premature infant is floppy and less spontaneously active than the term infant. Decisions about activity level, spontaneity of movement, and posture at rest should take gestational age into account.

The healthy mature infant has a strong and lusty cry. Weak, faint, or high-pitched cries should be viewed as nonspecific warning signs of other problems.

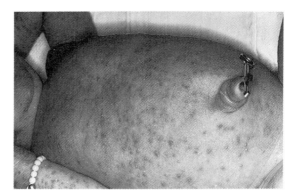

Figure 15.28   Erythema toxicum.

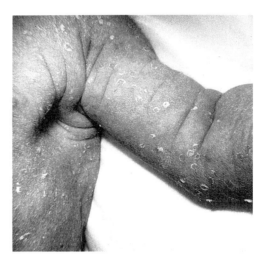

Figure 15.29   Transient neonatal pustular melanosis (TNPM).

Motor. At rest, the full-term infant's limbs are maintained in flexion (Fig. 15.30), while the premature's limbs are maintained in extension.

Head lag. The full-term baby's head will not remain totally extended when he is pulled to sitting from the supine position, so it may begin to flex slightly after the head leaves the mattress. The infant who is hypotonic for whatever reason and the premie will display no ability to flex the neck during this maneuver.

Ventral suspension. In ventral suspension, the full-term infant with normal truncal tone does not roll into a complete circle, but, rather, maintains horizontal positioning. Some newborns can even pick their head up a little from the prone position. The premie almost forms a circle with his head and body when held in ventral suspension (Fig. 15.31).

Slip through. The term newborn with normal tone and strength should not "slip through" the examiner's hands when held upright under the axillae.

Gestational age: Physical maturity. The skin of the **premature infant** is thin, smooth, and red or dark pink, with visible veins. There may be a thick layer of vernix, and except for the extremely premature infant, there is abundant lanugo. There is no palpable breast tissue, the ear pinnae are soft and malleable, there are

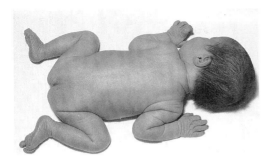

Figure 15.30   Flexed posture of the term newborn.

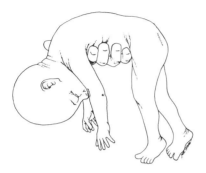

Figure 15.31   Ventral suspension: premature newborn.

no creases on the sole of the foot, and the external genitalia are underdeveloped. The **term infant** has palpable breast tissue, creases over the entire sole, thicker pink skin, and firm pinnae with well-defined folds. The **postmature infant** displays physical characteristics that have progressed further along the continuum: The skin is leathery, cracked, wrinkled, and devoid of lanugo; the nails are long; and the soles have deep creases (see Fig. 15.18).

Neuromuscular maturity. The **premie** is floppy, has limited to no passive flexor tone (at knee, shoulder, and hip), and has limited to no flexibility at the wrist. At rest, the infant lies with limbs in extension. In the more premature infant, when the "heel-to-ear maneuver" is performed, the heel reaches all the way to the ear; in the "scarf-sign maneuver," the elbow reaches the opposite anterior axillary line. At rest, the **term infant's** limbs are held in flexion. The heel-to-ear and scarf-sign maneuvers demonstrate much increased passive flexor tone. That is, the heel may only reach as far as the umbilicus, and the elbow may not even reach the midline of the thorax. The **postmature infant** will demonstrate all of the neurologic criteria on the mature end of the scale, with fewer exceptions than a term infant might demonstrate (see Fig. 15.18).

INFANT

Techniques of Examination

AREAS OF EMPHASIS

The first year of life is characterized by dramatic visible progress along all developmental lines. Consequently, the physical examination for this age group emphasizes (1) progress in physical growth (weight, length, head circumference), (2) progress in motor and verbal development, and (3) quality of infant-parent attachment and interaction. Also important in young infants is continued surveillance for congenital anomalies or conditions not uncovered during the newborn period.

OVERALL SEQUENCE AND STRATEGIES TO MAXIMIZE COOPERATION

In the infant, factors that particularly affect the child's ability to cooperate for the examination include state (awake, asleep), mood, innate temperament, and developmental stage. Alterations in sequence or approach, if specifically adapted to the infant's individual characteristics in these areas, will maximize the clinician's ability to accomplish a complete examination. The infant who is tired, hungry, or ill may resist even the least intrusive parts of the examination. Whenever a reasonably simple solution might dramatically improve the infant's comfort level, take the time to correct the problem (e.g., feeding or changing a diaper). In the end, this extra time is well-spent.

Young Infant

During the first 6 months of life, most infants are relatively easy to examine and do not resist or cry unless physically disturbed. The clinician may request that the infant be weighed, measured, and undressed to the diaper. The examination may be performed on the examining table with the parent standing or seated nearby.

If the infant is quiet, begin with auscultation of the heart and lungs. As in the newborn examination, the clinician may continue with abdominal palpation, inguinal-femoral palpation, and inspection of genitalia. This is followed by turning to the head and proceeding in a head-to-toe sequence (filling in parts not previously examined), deferring intrusive or uncomfortable aspects until the end of the examination, e.g., tympanic membranes, pharynx.

This is an age group that is generally easy to approach. Success is usually achieved when the clinician smiles, uses a gentle gradual touch with warm hands (and stethoscope), and speaks in a soft pleasant voice. Many, but not all infants, will cry during the tympanic membrane, pharynx, and hip examinations. The infant must be adequately restrained (especially if there is resistance) during the tympanic membrane and pharynx examinations in order to avoid injuring the child and to accomplish successful visualization.

Older Infant

During the second half of the first year, the emergence of stranger anxiety and separation anxiety may impact on the clinician's ability to secure cooperation. Prepare to be flexible! By avoiding direct interaction, including eye contact, and maintaining a physical separation from the infant, the clinician should begin data acquisition through observation. The infant is also given the opportunity to observe and begin familiarizing himself with the clinician. During history taking, the infant's mood, state, global developmental level, and parent-child interactions are observed. Based on these observations, the clinician formulates a strategy for proceeding with the examination. The older infant may be sociable, engageable, and playful or terrified, clingy, and crying vociferously. **If the infant does not appear to be afraid, and the parent confirms that the infant is unlikely to resist, the sequence for the younger infant may be followed. For the older infant, particularly for the infant who appears afraid, general guidelines include the following:**

1. **Give the infant who looks afraid time to get used to you.** Approach him gradually. Make your body language as physically and verbally nonthreatening as possible. Sit, talk softly, sit away, and gradually draw your chair

closer. Ignore the baby and look at the parent before looking directly at the child, and begin touching in a to-and-fro manner before sustaining your touching.

2. **Begin with nonintrusive components,** reserving the most intrusive components for last. **Begin actual touching distally, with the outermost parts of the body (e.g., toes, fingers, top of the head) and proceed toward the central parts of the body.**

3. **Maximize each opportunity as it arises** (e.g., auscultate the heart and lungs when the infant is sleeping; check the red reflex and corneal light reflex if the infant is wide-eyed and alert).

4. **Use the infant's developmental stage** (motor and cognitive abilities) **to plan distraction techniques and techniques to familiarize him with the components of the examination.** For the child who can grasp and transfer, give the infant a reflex hammer or pneumatic otoscope bulb to handle and transfer. For the child who has acquired an appreciation of object permanence, play a hiding game with a piece of equipment, then "reward" the infant by allowing him to handle it before using it. Cooperation is enhanced when the infant is occupied and diverted.

5. **When planning strategy, use the information the parent supplies about the baby's temperament to supplement observations in the examining room.**

6. **Do not separate the infant from a parent if the infant looks afraid.** Perform the entire examination in the parent's lap. Specific components of the lap examination (e.g., tympanic membrane examination) are discussed in the text that follows. **A summary of the lap examination sequence is found in the Techniques of Examination section under Toddler.**

The maneuvers for the newborn examination apply to the infant. What is highlighted below are the areas with special significance during the first year of life.

THE EXAMINATION

General Appearance and Initial Observations

Infant and infant-parent interactions are observed. For the infant, focus attention on facial appearance, overall mood, motor activity, and body proportions. Does the infant look well-fed and normally developed? Does the baby seem to see and hear? Does the baby smile or vocalize? When placed on the examining table, does the baby attempt to move or roll over? Is the baby having any difficulty breathing, or is the overall skin color abnormal? The parent-child interaction may be assessed by observing how the parent handles, feeds, and comforts the infant. Consider the following: Does the interaction seem loving and affectionate? Does the baby gaze at and follow the parent? Is handling done gently? During feeding, does the parent look at and interact with the baby? How quickly and appropriately does the parent respond to the infant's cry?

Measurements

When using standard growth charts, the premature infant's measurements may be plotted by using two methods: the chronologic age and the adjusted age. **Adjusted age** is calculated by first subtracting the number of weeks the actual birth date preceded the expected due date (how many weeks early the child was born) and then subtracting that value from the chronologic age (e.g., if a child was born 7 weeks early and is now at a chronologic age of 16 weeks, the adjusted age is 9 weeks). The adjusted age is used to plot weight, length, and head circumference measurements. This method is appropriate when only standard growth charts are available. There are also special growth curves for plotting the postnatal growth of premature infants, using chronologic age. These are more accurate but are not always readily available.

Head: Hair, Face, Eyes, Ears, Nose, and Mouth

Head. Unless there are special concerns, head circumference is monitored routinely during the first year but not thereafter. The examination should seek evidence that the effects of the birth process have successfully regressed and that during this rapid phase of head growth, both size and configuration remain normal. Special attention is paid to the apposition of sutures for separation or overriding and to the progressive closure of the posterior and anterior fontanelles. Percussion of the head in children with open fontanelles does not yield useful information.

Eyes. Vision is assessed grossly by noting the infant's response to bright light; by observing the infant following a light, boldly patterned figure, or the examiner's face; and by observing the older infant reach out for a toy. **The other extremely important point about assessing visual acuity in the infant is to ask the parent whether the child sees. A parent's concern about the infant's vision is usually justified.**

The infant under a few months of age does not usually cry when a light is shined in his eyes. The older infant is less cooperative. Under this circumstance, ask the parent to hold the infant upright over one shoulder (as if to burp the baby). Stand behind the parent and face the infant. In one hand, hold up an attractive object for the baby to fix on; hold the ophthalmoscope with the other hand.

Routine strabismus screening begins when the infant is 3–4 months of age. Parents are queried for evidence of "crossed eyes, lazy eye, or wandering eye" in their infant. Prior to age 3–4 months, the eyes may normally cross periodically. Strabismus or abnormal ocular alignment must be diagnosed early in life in order to prevent permanent visual loss. The **corneal light reflex** is one type of strabismus screen and is appropriate for infants over age 3–4 months. This is performed by observing for symmetric reflection of light shined onto the corneas. The light source can be a flashlight shined at the nose, or it may even be a bright overhead light. When the corneal light reflex is asymmetric, suspect strabismus. Another office screening test for strabismus is the alternate cover test, which is described under Special Maneuvers.

During infancy, the red reflex is inspected, and the rest of the retinal examination attempted. Even the most experienced pediatrician has difficulty with this examination in children too young to cooperate. In experienced hands, pupillary dilation may be of help.

Ears. Confirm that the baby hears by watching for a reaction to a noise that originates out of the line of sight and is made without physical distraction. The infant who is several months old will begin to turn eyes and head toward the source of the sound. Beyond age 6 months, the baby will turn his body to investigate the sound. These are "gross" assessments and somewhat subjective, but they are accurate enough for routine screening. **The same level of attention should be paid to parental concerns about hearing as to those about vision. When parents think their infant does not hear, their concerns should be taken quite seriously.**

Examining the eardrums and the posterior pharynx is the most intrusive part of the infant examination. Adequate visualization of the tympanic membranes is also one of the most difficult skills to acquire in pediatric physical diagnosis. Proper immobilization is the key to success. The very young infant, who is not yet able to sit, is best examined in the supine position on the examination table. The older infant can either sit in the parent's lap or lie on the table.

Ear examination with infant on the table. (The left-handed examiner may follow these directions or reverse hands if it is more comfortable to do so.) Place the infant's arms at his sides. Ask the parent to stand at the baby's feet and lean over him in order to immobilize his knees with her body, while simultaneously restraining the baby's arms down on the table. This frees you up to deal only with the baby's head. You may turn the head to either side and restrain it with your left forearm. Your left hand is free to pull back on the pinna, and the right hand, holding the otoscope, can advance the speculum gently into the ear canal (Fig. 15.32).

Ear examination with infant in the parent's lap. Seat the infant in the parent's lap, facing you (you should also be seated), with his legs restrained between the parent's knees. Have the parent wrap one of her arms around and across the infant's arms and chest tightly. Instruct her to turn the infant's head to one side with her free hand and gently restrain it against her chest. This will enable you to use your left hand to pull on the pinna and your right hand to introduce the otoscope (Fig. 15.33).

Other important guidelines include the following:

1. **Use the largest size speculum that will fit in the canal; in infants, the most convenient size is long and narrow (sizes 2.5 or 3).**
2. The infant's ear canal is directed upward. **Pulling the pinna down and posteriorly as the speculum is advanced into the canal will facilitate visualization of the tympanic membrane.** Note that this angulation differs from the adult's.
3. The shaft of the otoscope should rest in your palm. **The examiner's hand should always rest against the child's head, separating the head from the shaft of the otoscope.** Thus, if the infant moves suddenly, he will push against your hand, which, in turn, controls the depth of penetration of the speculum. This reduces the potential for injury to a struggling infant.
4. **The otoscope should be equipped with a connecting tube and a rubber bulb at the end of it (pneumatic otoscope).** With the otoscope shaft resting in

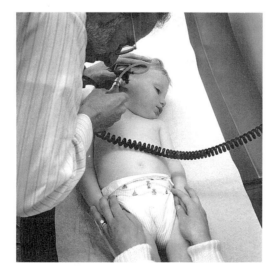

Figure 15.32 Ear examination with child on examination table.

your palm, place the bulb against the outer side of the shaft and hold it in place under your thumb (Fig. 15.34).

5. **Try making whispered noises as you insert and advance the otoscope into the canal.** Some of the time this is sufficient to briefly distract the infant who, as a result, will forget to cry.

6. **You may need to change the angle of the otoscope head in order to visualize the entire tympanic membrane (TM).**

7. **Once you have visualized the TM, push in gently on (insufflate) the rubber bulb and then release it.** The TM should move in as you push against the bulb and then return outward to its initial position as you release it. If you see movement, make sure it's the drum that's moving, not the canal (the external surface of the canal in young infants sometimes moves with bulb insufflation). **It is also important to be sure that there is an adequate seal between the speculum and the canal.** Changing the speculum to a larger size may be required to effect an adequate seal.

Mouth. Whenever the infant cries in a sustained fashion, quickly inspect the mouth and oral pharynx, using a penlight or otoscope. When teeth are present, they are counted and inspected for shape and color. Throughout the examination, do not neglect to note sounds or words the baby utters. If the opportunity to inspect the pharynx does not arise spontaneously, the clinician must decide whether to perform this with the infant on the examining table or in the parent's lap.

Pharynx examination with infant on the table. If the infant is supine on the table, ask the parent to stand at the baby's head. Request that she draw the baby's

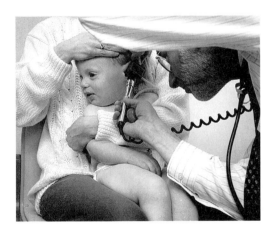

Figure 15.33   Ear examination with child on parent's lap.

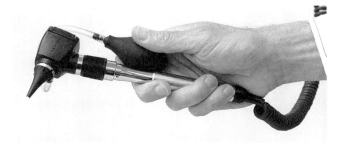

Figure 15.34   Pneumatic otoscope.

arms up over his head and restrain them against his ears. The clinician stands at the baby's feet and leans over him to immobilize his lower body (freeing up both hands for the examination). Hold the light source in one hand and the tongue depressor in the other hand. Attempt to gently tease open the mouth with the tongue depressor; work the depressor gently back into the mouth while pressing down on the tongue (a series of alternating pronation-to-supination wrist movements usually works). Depress the tongue; eventually, a gag reflex is triggered, affording one quick look. In most cases, that is sufficient (Fig. 15.35).

Pharynx examination with infant in the parent's lap. Seat the infant in the parent's lap, facing you (you should also be seated), with his legs restrained between the parent's knees. Request that the parent restrain the baby's arms by wrapping an arm across the baby's chest. Instruct the parent to press the other hand against the baby's forehead in order to restrain his head against the parent's chest (Fig. 15.36).

Whenever the tympanic membrane and pharynx inspections have been completed, move away from the infant and allow the parent to comfort him.

Neck, Thorax, and Upper Limbs

Neck. Inspection of the neck in this age group includes observing for head tilt, for rotational abnormalities, and for degree of head control. The neck and the relationship of the head to the neck are assessed in both the supine and upright positions. To move the infant from the supine to the sitting position, grasp the

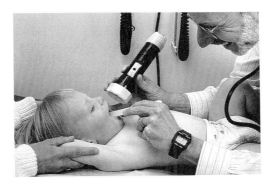

Figure 15.35 Pharynx examination with child on examination table.

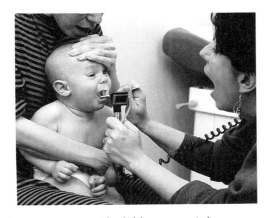

Figure 15.36 Pharynx examination with child on parent's lap.

infant's hands in yours and slowly bring the infant to the sitting position. During this maneuver, observe for head lag. In the sitting position, observe whether the head bobs or remains upright and whether it tilts or rotates asymmetrically.

Until the latter part of the first year, assessment of the neck for nuchal rigidity gives no reliable sign of meningeal irritation.

Thorax and upper limbs. Upper limb symmetry, strength, range of motion, and fine motor manipulation may be assessed in one series of maneuvers. When the infant is able to reach, present an attractive object just outside his range. When he reaches for it, move the object through a variety of directions, observing that the infant is able to reach in all directions. Next, reward the infant by giving him the object to hold and observe for age-appropriate manipulations (e.g., bring it to his mouth, handle it using a pincer grasp, transfer it to the other hand).

Cardiorespiratory System

Begin the cardiac examination with auscultation rather than palpation of the precordium. In young children, especially when cardiac disease is not suspected, auscultation of the heart is much more important than palpating for the PMI. The PMI in infancy is located at the fourth intercostal space just to the left of the midclavicular line. If palpation is performed prior to auscultation, particularly in a wary patient, the clinician risks upsetting the infant and missing the opportunity for a quiet auscultatory examination.

If the infant begins to cry during auscultation, do not remove the stethoscope. Continue to listen to inspiration (inspiration is deep with crying). Next, allow the parent to comfort the child and attempt some distraction techniques. Listen to expiration when the child is calmer.

Infants experience many upper respiratory infections. It is especially important in this age group to distinguish between sounds originating in the nose (called "upper airway noises") and those originating in the lungs. Hold the stethoscope over the nose and compare the sounds that are heard when auscultating the lungs. This maneuver assists the examiner in distinguishing sounds emanating from the upper airway from those emanating from the lungs.

Abdomen

During the first month of life, the umbilical cord insertion site is carefully inspected to determine whether the stump has separated and for evidence of drainage or inflammation. To assess for covert drainage, gentle pressure is applied inward onto the abdomen with fingers placed on either side of the umbilicus.

When proceeding to the groin, remember to palpate the femoral pulses if you have not already done so.

Genitalia

Male genitalia. In an uncircumcised boy, the foreskin is retracted gently, without exerting any excess force. The foreskin of an uncircumcised male will not retract very far in infancy. It should become increasingly easier to do this as the child grows. A circumcised male will have an easily visible meatus and glans.

If a testicle is not palpable, and "milking" the canal does not produce it, attempt either of the following maneuvers next. Place the baby in either a sitting position or a prone position, up on all fours. The increased pressure on the lower abdominal contents may make the testicles more easily palpable or visible.

Parents may report having seen a bulge in the inguinal area or scrotum, thus raising concern about a hernia. When the bulge is not reproducible on physical examination, exploring the external ring with your finger is unlikely to be help-ful. The ring is too small to permit the clinician's finger to enter it. Instead, the spermatic cord may be palpated for a thickening.

Lower Limbs

With the infant supine, inspect the lower limbs in the same manner as in the new-born. Proceed caudally, inspecting symmetry of the hip joint, thigh creases, knee alignment, tibiae, ankle alignment, and feet. The flexion contractures of the hips and knees of the newborn disappear within the first few weeks of life. Examine the feet with special attention to ruling out metatarsus adductus. It is not redun-dant to count toes and inspect for webbing, overlapping, or other deformities. Some minor abnormalities (which may not have been discussed thoroughly dur-ing the newborn period) may become clinically or cosmetically important as the child prepares to ambulate.

Examine the hips. On the younger infant (a few weeks old), perform the Ortolani and Barlow maneuvers. The clinician should continue to examine the hips during the first year, but movement of a dislocated or dislocatable hip in or out of the acetabulum becomes increasingly difficult after the first month or two of life. Thereafter, the most important part of the hip examination consists of externally rotating the hips while they are held in 90° of flexion (Fig. 15.37). The knees should nearly touch the examining table. Differences between the two sides are very significant.

Skin

Special attention is paid to the skin during infancy, as findings related to skin color, birthmarks, and rashes are especially common.

When the infant is ill, clinical determination of *hydration status* is an important component of the examination. This includes: (1) inspecting mucous membrane surfaces for moisture, (2) noting whether tears are present when the infant cries, (3) determining the contour of the anterior fontanelle (if still open)

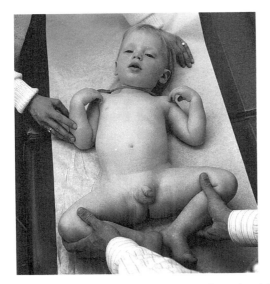

Figure 15.37 Hip abduction examination during infancy; hips should abduct equally, and knees should touch or almost touch the table.

when the baby is upright, (4) assessing abdominal skin turgor, and (5) assessing capillary refill time.

Skin turgor is used as a measure of hydration and nutrition in infants and young children. The examiner gently pinches a small portion of abdominal skin and subcutaneous tissue between the thumb and index finger, pulling up slightly from the plane of the abdominal contour, then quickly releases it. The degree of elasticity of the tissue determines the turgor.

To assess **capillary refill,** briefly squeeze the baby's fingertip between your own thumb and index finger until it blanches. The number of seconds it takes for the color to return to normal is noted.

Neurologic System and Development

The neurologic assessment of the infant includes the traditional neurologic examination (adapted to the young child), assessment of developmental milestones, and assessment of primitive reflexes. Much information about overall neurologic functioning is gained by observing the infant throughout the general physical examination. Components of the general physical examination that may specifically relate to neurologic functioning include growth measurements, head and spine, skin, and the presence of anomalies or asymmetries.

General appearance and mental status. Observations of the child's general appearance and mental status include observations of state, transitions of state, alertness, mood, eye contact, and consolability.

Cranial nerves. Assess the cranial nerves as completely as possible in the manner described for the newborn.

Motor. This is primarily an assessment of tone, strength, and motor milestones. If the history suggests that the patient's motor development is delayed, pay particular attention to tone (floppy or stiff) and strength. **Tone** is the resistance encountered when the infant's limbs are moved passively. Tone is assessed when the infant is not crying and is as relaxed as possible; this is obviously sometimes difficult to accomplish. The clinician must examine many infants to better appreciate what "normal" tone feels like. **Strength** is measured by the amount of active resistance the baby poses against the examiner's manipulations. Information about strength (or weakness) is also supplied by observing the infant's ability to support his own weight against gravity (e.g., supporting himself on his elbows, sitting up and bearing weight).

It is more difficult to assess individual muscles in small children than in adults. Watching infants perform some of their motor "accomplishments" supplies information about muscle groups. Head control, rolling over, sitting, bearing weight, and creeping furnish information about gross motor function; reaching, transferring, and banging toys together furnish information about upper limb muscles and fine motor function.

Head lag and ability to maintain the head without bobbing in the upright position are continuously reassessed during the first year of life. In the sitting position, ability to sit with and without support is observed. Once the infant can sit, the length of time the infant can sit without toppling over is observed. Whether or not the arms are used for support is observed also.

Coordination. A "new" achievement is always performed unsteadily at first. First attempts at sitting independently or walking should not be used to assess balance or coordination. Observation of the infant old enough to reach for or manipulate a small object supplies information about coordination.

Reflexes. During a general screening examination, the clinician may opt to defer evaluation of deep tendon reflexes in the infant whose development and motor examinations are normal. Offering an "extra" hammer to the older infant may serve as a distraction. The plantar reflex may not be of help until after age 1 because of the variability of response.

Primitive reflexes. Primitive reflexes are assessed during the first year. These supply information about the general state of the neuraxis. Primitive reflexes that are present in the newborn disappear at predictable ages. Other primitive reflexes appear at predictable times during the first year of life. *Significant delays in timing of either appearance or disappearance of primitive reflexes are general, nonspecific signs of a brain abnormality. In addition to timing, the symmetry and completeness of the expected response are also important to observe. Asymmetry of response may signify paralysis or fracture.* The primitive reflexes of the newborn period are evaluated for presence or absence (e.g., Moro, grasp, suck). The following primitive reflexes appear later:

- **Tonic neck reflex (also known as the fencing posture).** The infant is placed on his back. Keeping the shoulders level, rotate the head to one side. The limbs on the side the head is facing toward will extend; the opposite limbs will flex (Fig. 15.38). There should not be a striking asymmetry between the tonic neck reflex on one side or the other. During the general physical examination, the baby may assume this posture spontaneously. This reflex emerges at approximately 2–8 weeks (it may be present at birth) and disappears at approximately 6–7 months.
- **Lateral prop.** The infant is placed in a sitting position, supported around the waist if necessary. With the infant's attention directed at something other than the examiner's hands, the clinician gently tilts the child to the side. Beginning at approximately age 4–5 months, the infant will extend his ipsilateral arm to brace the fall in a protective manner.
- **Parachute reflex.** To elicit, hold the infant in ventral suspension and abruptly tilt the baby's head down toward the floor. A normal response is extension of the arms as if to protect himself from hitting the ground in a fall (Fig. 15.39). This reflex emerges at approximately 8–9 months and never disappears.

Sensory system. Formal sensory testing is reserved for children in whom detailed neurologic investigations are required or in whom a true lack of sensation is suspected.

Developmental milestones. Milestones may be assessed during the general physical examination rather than at the end. When the infant is fearful, the entire examination may begin with "games" to assess development and continue with more intrusive components (see Fig. 15.8).

At the conclusion of the examination, the infant should be rewarded with a smile from the clinician and returned to parent's arms.

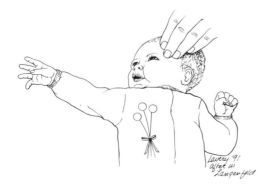

Figure 15.38   Tonic neck reflex.

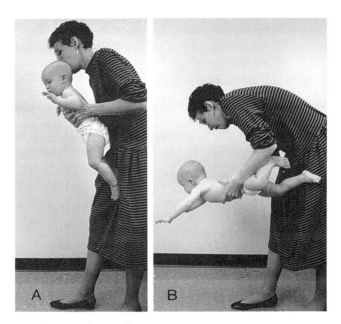

Figure 15.39   **A** and **B.** Parachute reflex.

Normal and Common Variants and *Clues to Abnormalities*

General Appearance

When awake, the healthy infant appears bright-eyed and alert. Breathing is quiet and unlabored. The baby makes eye contact with parent, and vice versa. The infant may be very interested in the surroundings but will respond and react to a parent's interventions. While conversing with the clinician, the attentive parent will continue to cuddle, comfort, interact, or attend in other ways to the infant. The healthy infant will smile, vocalize, and/or move about. The baby's cry is strong and lusty. The responsive parent will attempt to soothe the child, using words, actions, or both.

The infant who is mildly ill will be cranky but consolable and, if sleeping, will arouse easily. Other observations to make when assessing the ill infant are discussed under **Special Maneuvers.**

Measurements

When the infant's weight, length, and head circumference are plotted on the appropriate charts, the clinician looks for evidence that the child is "doing well" with respect to these parameters. Steady progress along any of the curves within a normal range, whether along the 3rd or 95th percentile, is normal. Neither is "better" than the other. *A child who loses weight (except during a brief illness), or consistently fails to gain, or whose rate of gain slows so much that multiple percentiles are crossed in a downward direction is a child who is **failing to thrive.** The etiologies of failure to thrive are numerous and encompass many biologic, psychologic, and social problems. The first step in the evaluation of failure to thrive is to recognize that it exists as early as possible. Even though the individual examination provides only one set of measurements, the clinician is obligated to review these measurements within the context of previous measurements. This is important at any age during childhood but is crucial during periods such as infancy, when rapid growth is of major importance.*

Head: Hair, Face, Eyes, Ears, Nose, and Mouth

Head and hair on head. The premature infant's head appears **long and narrow** with flattening on the sides. During the first months of life, the ex-premie, unable to lift his head up on his own, lies with the head turned to one side or another. The flattening occurs because of the preferential positioning, combined with the softness and malleability of the skull bones at that age.

Another common variation in head contour is the **flattened occiput.** This is particularly common during the first half of the first year among infants who spend a lot of time lying on their backs. It is accentuated in babies with slow development and poor muscle tone.

By age 6 months, palpation of the suture lines should reveal no ridging (overriding). Closure of the fontanelles is a gradual process and, like all other developmental processes, shows normal variations in timing. In general, the posterior fontanelle is closed by age 2 months, and the anterior fontanelle closes between 6 and 18 months (age 2 years at the latest). *Ridging of suture lines beyond expected age, premature closure of the fontanelles or unexpectedly small fontanelles, slow head growth, or abnormal shape must all raise the suspicion of premature fusion of the cranial sutures (craniosynostosis).* **Craniosynostosis** *usually becomes more pronounced over time as the head grows, either with increasingly abnormal head shape and or limitation in size.*

Face. The infant's overall facial appearance may provide clues to hidden problems. *The infant with* **untreated congenital hypothyroidism** *is inactive and coarse-featured. The skin is dry, and the hair is dull and dry. As myxedema involves the face, the infant develops puffy eyelids and the appearance of small, widely spaced eyes with a depressed nasal bridge. The mouth is open, and a thickened tongue protrudes. The cry is hoarse. The neck is thick and short.*

Eyes. Intermittent dysconjugate eye movements are normal up to the age of 3–4 months. *When dysconjugate eye movements are observed beyond that age, the corneal light reflection is asymmetric, or range of motion of either eye is incomplete,* **strabismus** *is suspected. In addition, if the child objects (particularly on one side more than the other) to having his line of vision interfered with, strabismus is suspected.*

One common variation of normal, which may be mistaken for strabismus, is seen in children with epicanthal folds. In these children, the eyes may seem as if they cross without actually doing so, a phenomenon known as **pseudostrabismus.** In a child with pseudostrabismus, the corneal light reflection will be symmetric, and the eyes will move together.

Tears may not be produced in volume until 2–4 months of age. A **congenitally obstructed nasolacrimal duct** ("blocked tear duct") is exceedingly common and becomes symptomatic several weeks after birth, as the amount of eye secretion begins to build and the normal drainage path is blocked. Tearing and/or retention of mucoid or crusted material may be noted in one or both eyes. The conjunctivae are usually only slightly reddened. If the eyes are very reddened and/or produce large amounts of purulent material, the diagnosis is more likely to be infectious conjunctivitis.

The fundus may reveal clues to systemic disease, several examples of which are mentioned. The macula may display areas of pigmentation secondary to congenital toxoplasmosis or a cherry-red spot of Tay-Sachs disease. The optic disc is pale in the anemic child and may be surrounded by gray stippling in lead poisoning. In papilledema, the disc margin is blurred, veins are engorged and without normal pulsations, and there may be retinal hemorrhages. Retinal hemorrhages may also be the only external manifestation of child abuse, although other less common etiologies must also be considered (e.g., coagulopathy, brain tumor, leukemia).

Ears. Infants often cry during the examination of the tympanic membrane. Crying produces vascular engorgement, which may redden the tympanic membranes. The clinician may experience difficulty in determining whether or not the tympanic membranes are actually inflamed. In these instances it is especially important to determine whether landmarks appear normal, whether the response to insufflation is normal, and whether there is a significant difference in intensity of redness between the two sides. The normal tympanic membrane is light gray, semitransparent, and slanted away from the examiner (Fig. 15.40).

*Infection of the middle ear (**acute otitis media**) results in opacity and reddening of the tympanic membrane. Normal landmarks behind the tympanic membrane become progressively more obscured by purulent fluid (either yellow or white). The eardrum itself may appear bright red or patchy red. As fluid accumulates behind the drum, it begins to bulge out toward you. The more fluid that accumulates, the less the drum will move in response to insufflation. Children who appear entirely well may have acute otitis media (Fig. 15.41).*

Mouth. Many young infants have **thrush**. This is a candidal infection manifested by white plaques on the tongue and/or buccal mucosa. To differentiate this

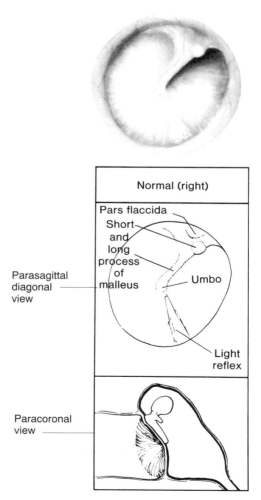

Figure 15.40 Normal right tympanic membrane and adjacent landmarks.

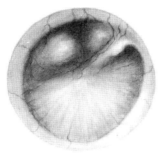

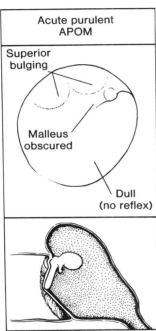

Figure 15.41   Acute purulent otitis media (APOM); orientation same as in Figure 15.40.

from retained milk (which it resembles), attempt to gently scrape a plaque. The lesions of thrush will not scrape off easily and may bleed with this maneuver.

There are several variations of normal in the appearance of the tongue. **Geographic tongue**, in which the surface has the appearance of a relief map, may be normal or signal underlying allergic disease. **Scrotal tongue,** in which there are deep furrows, has no significance. Tremors of the tongue are seen in some neurologic and neuromuscular diseases.

The timing of tooth eruption is somewhat variable. The order of eruption is less so. The first teeth to appear are usually the lower central incisors (one at a time, at 6–8 months), followed shortly thereafter by the upper incisors (at 8–9 months). Less often, the teeth do not begin to erupt until age 1. Further delayed eruption is unusual and may be associated with some disorders of the pituitary axis, rickets, or some syndromes.

Abnormalities in coloring or shape of teeth are not uncommon. Causes of discoloration include the following: iron preparations stain the teeth brown; prenatal tetracycline exposure stains teeth yellow to brown; dentin and enamel dysplasias may result in yellow to brownish teeth; and excessive fluoride ingestion may cause the teeth to acquire chalky white spots. Children with one of the ectodermal dysplasia syndromes may have "tepee"-shaped teeth.

During the latter half of the first year, many infants experience their first upper respiratory infection. Mucus may be visible in the nose and posterior pharynx. The tonsils are small during infancy but, secondary to viral infection, may become reddened, ulcerated, or demonstrate a white or yellow exudate.

Nodes

Beginning in early infancy, small pea-sized, mobile, soft, nontender lymph nodes, known as "shotty" nodes, are palpable in healthy children. **Shotty nodes** are frequently encountered in certain predictable locations, such as the upper portions of the anterior and (less commonly) posterior cervical triangles, occiput, angle of the jaw, axillae, and the inguinal regions. *Anterior cervical lymphadenopathy accompanies upper respiratory infection and inflammation of the anterior portions of the mouth. Posterior cervical lymphadenopathy accompanies otitis media, some viral infections, and scalp irritations. Enlarged lymph nodes can continue to be visible and palpable for many weeks after the inciting cause resolves. It is not uncommon for parents to notice "lumps" in the neck when it is too late to easily discover the etiology. In contrast to the expected distribution of "shotty" nodes, supraclavicular lymphadenopathy is distinctly abnormal. If present, this may reflect lymph system disease or intrathoracic pathology.*

Neck, Thorax, and Upper Limbs

Neck. The head should not be tilted or rotated in one direction or another. If there is a lateral flexion of the head toward one side and rotation of the chin toward the opposite shoulder, this is called **torticollis.** In the young infant, this is usually congenital and represents a shortening (from fibrosis) of one side of the sternomastoid muscle. The head tilts toward the shortened muscle, and the chin rotates away from it *(Fig. 15.42). When torticollis is noted, the cervical spine, scapulae, clavicles, and upper-body neural structures (including the eyes) must be carefully evaluated to exclude other less benign causes of torticollis (e.g., a fourth nerve palsy can produce a head tilt in an older infant as a compensation for strabismus, a posterior fossa tumor, or a fractured cervical vertebra).*

Cardiorespiratory System

Throughout childhood, the rhythm of the heartbeat may vary with respiration. The normal variation is called sinus arrhythmia: The heart rate increases during inspiration and decreases during expiration.

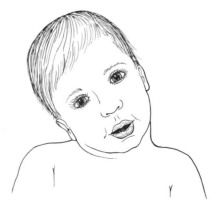

Figure 15.42   Torticollis.

S_1 is loudest over the apex, and S_2 is loudest at the upper left sternal border. S_2 splits during inspiration and narrows during expiration. A normal S_3 may be heard at the lower left sternal border or apex. S_4 is abnormal in children.

The benign murmur of peripheral pulmonic stenosis, first appreciated during the newborn period, may be present for up to approximately 3 months.

A ventricular septal defect (VSD) is the most common congenital heart lesion. The murmur of a VSD may be audible at birth but often is not auscultated until the infant is several weeks old and the pulmonary vascular resistance has significantly diminished. The classic murmur of the VSD is harsh and regurgitant (begins with S_1) and is often holosystolic (ends with S_2). It is heard loudest at the left lower or mid-sternal border. Large defects produce faint murmurs, sometimes accompanied by a middiastolic rumble of relative mitral stenosis from increased blood flow across the mitral valve.

*A complete discussion of signs and symptoms of **congestive heart failure** (CHF) during infancy requires discussion of various individual lesions. In general, heart failure during infancy is characterized by increased heart and respiratory rates, shallow breathing, retractions, and, sometimes, pulmonary crackles or wheezes. With significant pulmonary involvement, there will be pulmonary hyper-inflation with depressed diaphragms and hepatic enlargement. The infant with CHF may be irritable and sweat profusely (involving the total body), especially during feeding and activity. Feeding is poor, and growth is suboptimal. Breathing may be so difficult that grunting is heard, and head bobbing is noted. Unless it is massive, edema may be difficult to appreciate clinically (except as lid puffiness or weight gain); if present, it is usually generalized. Neck vein distension may be impossible to detect in infants because of their short necks. The limbs may be pale, cool to touch, and demonstrate thready pulses. Other findings depend on the specific lesion involved.*

Abdomen

During infancy the abdomen retains a protuberant shape. The umbilical stump dries and usually detaches 1–2 weeks after birth. A slight amount of erythema surrounding a healing umbilical stump may be normal. For a few days following cord detachment, the site may ooze small amounts of serous fluid or blood, especially during cleansing. *If serous fluid continues to drain, an abnormal connection between the abdominal surface and the underlying structures should be considered (e.g., patent urachus). Significant erythema, foul smell, purulent drainage, and edema all suggest omphalitis, a potentially devastating infection.*

By 1 month of age, the site of cord insertion is covered with new skin. Occasionally, after the cord separates, a moist, pinkish, grayish stump of granulation tissue (called an **umbilical granuloma**) is formed. This may heal by itself or may require cauterization with silver nitrate.

Once the umbilicus separates, an **umbilical hernia**, which appears as an outpouching of the abdominal skin around the umbilicus, can become apparent. The outpouching is further exaggerated during Valsalva maneuvers (e.g., during straining at stool or during crying). Umbilical hernias usually reduce easily with gentle pressure. These are usually only of cosmetic, not clinical concern. Most are self-resolving; 60% resolve in the first 2 years of life.

In this age group, the liver edge may be be palpated 1–2 cm below the costal margin. The spleen tip is usually not palpable. In the young infant, the kidneys may still be palpable, even if they are normal-sized. In the older infant, because of decreased cooperation and decreased pliancy of the abdomen, normal kidneys are much less likely to be palpable.

Genitalia

Female genitalia. A **labial adhesion** may be visible. This is a thin layer of tissue stretching across the labia minora, virtually occluding the vaginal orifice but allowing urine to exit the urethra. Labial adhesions form postnatally. These often spontaneously separate from repeated minor trauma with diaper changes. If persistent until adolescence, most shrink in response to endogenous estrogen then.

Male genitalia. The skin at the site of circumcision remains erythematous for several days. This is followed by the appearance of whitish granulation as evidence of further healing.

Scrotal hydroceles are very common during early infancy, and many resorb completely by age 4–6 months.

Over age 6 months, hydroceles are much less likely to resolve. Most children with persistent hydroceles actually have an indirect inguinal hernia.

In the presence of an inguinal hernia, when a finger is rubbed over the lower part of the inguinal area, it may feel as if two pieces of silk are being rubbed together. This is known as the "silk-glove" sign.

Lower Limbs

By age 6 months, most infants begin to bear weight; when held upright by the arms or under the axillae, the infant will begin to participate actively in maintaining an upright posture. Between 9 and 12 months, the infant will pull himself upright while holding on to the crib bars and begin to cruise (walk while holding onto something). The typical stance of the newly upright child has a very wide base with the feet pointing in or out. Parents often want to know if the child will always walk "that way." They will be reassured to know that the wide base provides security for the novice walker. As normal development proceeds, the legs come closer together, and the feet point straight ahead.

Skin

Hydration. When hydration status is normal, mucous membranes are moist, tears are produced with crying, the anterior fontanelle is flat, and the skin is warm and moist. When the abdominal skin is assessed for turgor, it springs back readily to its original contour. Capillary refill time is 1–2 seconds.

With mild dehydration, mucous membranes become dry. As dehydration worsens, tears vanish, the skin may become cold, dry, and mottled, and capillary refill time is prolonged. When dehydration is severe, the surface of the anterior fontanelle becomes sunken or concave, and capillary refill time is more than 3 seconds.

In most instances of significant dehydration, abdominal skin turgor diminishes and demonstrates the phenomenon of tenting; i.e., rather than springing back when released, the skin remains creased in a tent shape beyond the plane of the abdomen. Tissue turgor is also determined by the amount of subcutaneous fat present and by the patient's electrolyte status. Tenting may be absent in an obese infant or in a child with hypernatremic dehydration.

Color. Neonatal **jaundice** may still be visible in a healthy infant during the first 4–6 weeks of age (occasionally up to 3 months). This is most common in breast-feeding infants, and its course is one of gradual resolution. After the second week of life, worsening jaundice is usually of pathologic significance.

Another extremely common and benign skin discoloration, **carotenemia,** may be confused with jaundice. Carotenemia is found in infants who are eating solid foods that include a generous amount of orange and yellow fruits and vegetables. The skin takes on an orange hue that is particularly accentuated on the palms and soles. Carotenemia never involves the conjunctivae. The temporal link to food intake should be established.

Birthmarks. **Strawberry hemangiomas** grow rapidly in size during the first year and then begin a slower period of involution that is completed by middle childhood. No intervention is necessary unless a vital structure is threatened by encroachment (e.g., eye, larynx). This type of hemangioma is often invisible at birth. Almost all "strawberries" resolve completely.

Rashes. The following are common rashes that appear during the first months of life.

Infantile acne. This appears on the face of an infant during the first few months of life and lasts several months. It resembles adolescent acne and consists of papules and pustules with surrounding erythema. Its presence is not predictive of teenage acne.

Seborrhea. This appears during the first few months of life and usually resolves by itself after several months. The greasy, yellow-tinged, scaly rash involving the scalp is called **cradle cap.** The face and eyebrows may also be involved. The skin behind the ears and/or the folds of the neck, axilla, groin, and umbilicus takes on a reddened, scaly appearance. It is not pruritic.

Infantile atopic dermatitis (eczema). This begins slightly later than seborrhea (age 2–6 months). The skin is dry. The rash is red and may be crusted or vesiculated. It is intensely pruritic. Excoriations are common. It involves the face (especially the cheeks), occasionally the scalp, and the limbs in a symmetrical distribution on the extensor surfaces. The infantile form and distribution of atopic dermatitis may last for several years.

Miliaria (heat rash). These lesions may be asymptomatic, clear tiny vesicles without an erythematous base (*miliaria crystallina*). As the eruption intensifies, they become pruritic and papulovesicular with an erythematous halo base (*miliaria rubra*, prickly heat). They are found anywhere on the body but are worse in clothed areas of the body.

Generic or ammonia diaper rash. This is the most common type of diaper rash. It originates from skin "contact" with irritating substances. This rash looks red and dry (almost parchment-like) and usually spares the groin creases (Fig. 15.43).

Candida diaper rash. This is the other most common type of diaper rash. Once a diaper rash has been present for more than a few days, it often becomes secondarily "infected" by the *Candida* organism. When this happens, the rash becomes "beefy" red, and "satellite" papules or pustules develop just beyond the margins (Fig. 15.44).

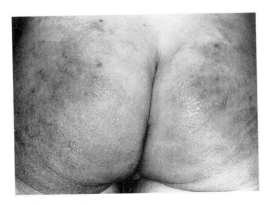

Figure 15.43   "Contact" diaper rash.

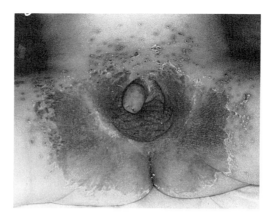

Figure 15.44   *Candida* diaper rash.

Neurologic System and Development

General appearance and mental status. Beyond 2 months of age, the healthy awake infant is expected to display alertness, eye contact, and some manifestation of interest in the examiner, as well as a responsive smile. Some manner of vocalization besides crying (e.g., cooing, bubbling) is often appreciated also.

The child who is lethargic, apathetic, or irritable and not easily consoled mandates further investigation. The child whose cry is high-pitched, coarse, hoarse, or shrill may not be entirely normal. Each of these signs is global and nonspecific. The context in which they occur (e.g., new behavior versus other chronic, associated symptoms, abnormalities on examination) determines the direction of investigation.

Motor. The infant who is calm and relaxed will demonstrate motor achievements when placed on the examining table (e.g., lifting his head when prone, rolling over). Unless the infant is crying and resisting, the clinician should find it relatively easy to move joints through range of motion without encountering either rigidity (hypertonic) or total lack of resistance (hypotonic).

The 2-month-old infant will flex his neck a little when pulled from supine to sitting position; when placed in a seated position, his head will bob. By 4 months of age, the infant will no longer demonstrate significant head lag and, when seated, can hold the head upright and steady. At 6 months of age, the infant when seated will lean forward and support himself on the examining table with his hands (tripoding). A 9-month-old infant can sit erect for prolonged periods (10–15 minutes).

Concern about the motor system is raised when motor milestones are significantly delayed, muscle tone is markedly increased (hypertonic) or markedly decreased (hypotonic), primitive reflexes are globally persistent or globally delayed, and deep tendon reflexes are abnormal. Diagnosis of neuromotor abnormalities is sometimes possible at birth or during early infancy (e.g., spina bifida); conversely, recognition may be delayed until motor developmental delay becomes apparent. Underlying etiologies may relate to the central nervous system (e.g., cerebral palsy) or, less commonly, to the spinal cord, peripheral nervous system, or musculature and may be static or progressive.

*Infants with **cerebral palsy** will demonstrate a variety of abnormalities on examination. If cerebral palsy is severe, its recognition may occur well before the child's first birthday, but if it is extremely mild, its recognition may not occur until school age. One type of cerebral palsy is **spastic diplegia.** An infant with spastic diplegia may demonstrate spasticity in the lower limbs: i.e., increased tone, exaggerated ten-*

don reflexes, tightness of heel cords, and "scissoring" of the legs when the infant is suspended vertically (examiner holds the child upright under the axillae)—the legs are held tightly together and internally rotated, with feet crossed at the ankles.

Other children with cerebral palsy are hypotonic and weak and remain so with advancing age. Other types of cerebral palsy include spastic quadriplegia (involvement of all limbs in spasticity), spastic hemiplegia (asymmetry of motor development may be demonstrated), and choreoathetoid cerebral palsy. Careful attention to developmental milestones, to the results of neurologic examination, and to the status of primitive reflexes will allow the clinician to uncover these problems. Often, repeat examinations in a longitudinal fashion are required to confirm early suspicions.

Reflexes. In young children, the magnitude of a normal response for deep tendon reflexes may be brisker than is normally observed in adults (e.g., a 3 of a possible 4 response). Often, if the clinician has difficulty eliciting a response in a child old enough to have acquired a reflex, the technique may be faulty rather than the reflex abnormal.

Primitive reflexes. Delayed appearance of primitive reflexes or delayed disappearance of primitive reflexes may reflect a problem with neuromaturation. The clinician must keep in mind, however, that abnormalities in appearance or disappearance of primitive reflexes are "gross" signs; they are not specific. Detailed neurologic examination is required to point to more specific areas of dysfunction. It must also be remembered that there is a normal spectrum or range in timing (Table 15.4).

Developmental milestones. For the ex-premature infant, norms for developmental milestones may need to be adjusted downward to account for gestational age rather than chronologic age, in the same way that norms for growth parameters are adjusted (Fig. 15.8).

Special Maneuvers

DIAGNOSIS OF CONGENITAL MUSCULAR TORTICOLLIS

In the congenital variety, when the neck is extended, a hard "mass" (contracted, fibrosed muscle) may be palpated within the sternomastoid muscle on the involved side. This gradually enlarges to a maximum at age 5–6 weeks and may be as large as 2.5 cm long. It gradually regresses over the next several months and may take as long as a half year to completely disappear.

ALTERNATIVE OPHTHALMOSCOPIC EVALUATION IN INFANTS

You have been instructed to examine the adult patient's right eye with your right eye and the patient's left eye with your left eye. If your patient is too young to

Table 15.4
Timing of Primitive Reflexes

Reflex	Present	Disappears
Moro	At birth (term)	6 months
Suck	At birth	6–8 months
Root	At birth	6–8 months
Place and step	At birth	1–2 months
Tonic neck	Birth–2 months	6–7 months
Reflex grasp	At birth	2–3 months
Lateral prop	4–5 months	Does not disappear
Parachute	8–9 months	Does not disappear

actively cooperate, try a switch from the traditional method: Use your right eye to examine the patient's left eye and your left eye to examine the patient's right eye. To distract the patient from looking directly at the light, hold up a toy between you and the child (one hand on the ophthalmoscope, one hand on the toy). The baby will gaze in your direction, but rather than looking directly at you, he will look at the toy.

STRABISMUS SCREENING: ALTERNATE COVER TEST

The alternate cover test is one type of strabismus screen that may uncover a subtle strabismus and should be attempted in older infants. This test assumes that each eye has central vision. This test requires an object that the child will fixate on and an occluder to cover the patient's eyes without touching them. Some examiners prefer to use their thumb for the occluder, which is then moved from eye to eye like a swinging pendulum.

An object for the child to fix on is displayed. Once the child is fixating, cover one eye in as unobtrusive a manner as possible. After several seconds, shift the cover to the opposite eye (allowing no time in between for binocular vision). Observe the recently uncovered eye, as it assumes fixation, for any movement. Shift the occluder repeatedly, from eye to eye, always observing the eye being uncovered for any movement (Fig. 15.45). If there is movement observed, suspect strabismus .

PALPATING FOR THE "OLIVE" WHEN SUSPECTING PYLORIC STENOSIS

The infant with pyloric stenosis usually presents to the clinician after the first week or two of life with progressive forceful projectile vomiting. The diagnosis may be confirmed by physical examination. The findings are best demonstrated when the stomach is empty, either immediately after the infant has vomited or during nasogastric suctioning. Attempt to engage the infant in sucking a pacifier or your finger. Place the infant supine on the examining table or in the parent's lap. While the infant is sucking, observe the upper abdomen for peristaltic waves. Using one hand (the nonpalpating hand), flex the infant's hips. With the other hand, palpate for the olive-sized firm mass (hypertrophied pylorus) in the epigastrium, equidistant between the umbilicus and the costal margin, at the lateral border of the right rectus muscle.

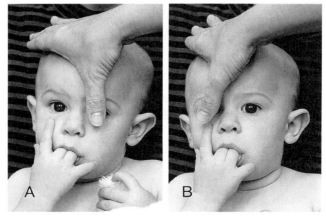

Figure 15.45   Alternate cover test: once the child is fixating, shift the occluder repeatedly from eye to eye while observing the newly uncovered eye for any movement.

An alternative maneuver may uncover the "olive" when the supine examination does not: The infant is placed onto his abdomen. The clinician slides her hand underneath the baby and palpates in the epigastrium as described above.

CLINICAL ASSESSMENT OF THE ILL INFANT: THE ACUTE ILLNESS OBSERVATION SCALES

When evaluating an infant or toddler with a febrile illness, it is important for the clinician to assess "toxicity." Toxicity is an attempt at measuring degree of serious illness or "How sick does this child look?" For years, pediatricians, using their clinical "Gestalt," have recognized that a febrile child who appears "very ill" or "toxic" is more likely to have a serious illness than those who do not have this appearance. This "Gestalt" has now been quantified into observational scales. One of the most widely accepted of these is called the Acute Illness Observation Scales (AIOS). Prior to performing a history and physical examination, this scale may be used by the clinician to assess an infant who is seated in a parent's lap. The result of this evaluation, when combined with a standard clinical evaluation, increases the sensitivity of the clinical assessment of toxicity. The AIOS is most useful in children less than 24 months of age (especially between 6 and 24 months). In very young infants (especially 3 months old and younger), the clinical assessment of toxicity is less accurate because signs of toxicity are less reliable. In this age group, clinicians are more likely to add laboratory investigation to the assessment.

The AIOS is composed of six items to be observed. Each item has a 3-point scale: 1 equals normal; 3 equals moderate impairment; and 5 equals severe impairment. The best possible score on the AIOS is 6 (item) × 1 (normal) = 6. The worst possible score is 30. On the basis of studies performed using the AIOS, a score higher than 10 indicates ill appearance (Table 15.5).

Do not memorize the numbers involved in the AIOS. The observation items and range of findings should serve as a learning tool to help you remember the important clinical signs of "toxicity." See also the Extended Examination section of Chapter 2.

TODDLER

Techniques of Examination

AREAS OF EMPHASIS

The focus of the routine examination in the toddler is different from that in the newborn and young infant. By this age most important congenital anomalies have been uncovered. Attention is directed at (1) assessment of hearing and middle ear function, (2) assessment of speech and language abilities, (3) vision and strabismus screening, (4) assessment of dentition, and (5) observation of gait. The child's behavior and interactions between parent and child are observed. This is an important period for affective development in which autonomy and independence are major issues.

OVERALL STRATEGIES

This age period is characterized by a wide range of behaviors and degrees of cooperation. The 2-year-old child is likely to move continuously throughout the room. Yet, when approached by someone wearing a stethoscope, the child may become very anxious and clingy. Heightened stranger anxiety and separation anxiety are common during the second year of life. The clinician must continue to allow the child to remain close to the parent, if desired, while also allowing the

Table 15.5
Acute Illness Observation Scales

Observation Item	1 Normal	3 Moderate Impairment	5 Severe Impairment
Quality of cry	Strong with normal tone or Content and not crying	Whimpering or Sobbing	Weak or Moaning or High-pitched
Reaction to parent stimulation	Cries briefly then stops or Content and not crying	Cries off and on	Continual cry or Hardly responds
State variation	If awake → stays awake or If asleep and stimulated → wakes up quickly	Eyes close briefly → awake or Awakes with prolonged stimulation	Falls to sleep or Will not rouse
Color	Pink	Pale extremities or Acrocyanosis	Pale or Cyanotic or Mottled or Ashen
Hydration	Skin normal, eyes normal and Mucous membranes moist	Skin, eyes-normal and Mouth slightly dry	Skin doughy or Tented and Dry mucous mem- branes and/or Sunken eyes
Response (talk, smile) to social overtures	Smiles or Alerts (≤2 mo)	Brief smile or Alerts briefly (≤2 mo)	No smile Face anxious, dull, expressionless or No alerting (≤2 mo)

child a certain amount of physical activity and exploration. "Working around" the busy but still very fearful young toddler mandates an examination strategy that emphasizes observation and skillful use of distraction when hands-on examination is required. The young toddler will actively resist rather than actively cooperate.

With progress along verbal, cognitive, affective, and motor areas of development, the toddler's abilities to actively cooperate gradually improve. The clinician must recognize these abilities and capitalize on them. Encouraging a certain amount of physical and verbal activity and autonomy, subtly acquainting the child with the clinician, and demystifying equipment and procedures will maximize success.

One of the secrets to success with the toddler is a toy. **Toys are icebreakers and may be used both for play and for developmental assessment (e.g., small blocks, crayons, little cars, books).** Examination equipment may be placed on a surface accessible to the patient, along with recognizable toys. The child should be allowed free access to these items while the clinician converses with the parent and makes covert observations.

Allow the child who wishes to move around the room and explore time to do so. When you wash your hands, invite the child to wash his hands along with you. Make observations about gait, gross motor movements, strength, skin, facial expression, and speech well before suggesting that his parent bring him closer. When it is time to begin the hands-on part of the examination, request that the parent maneuver the child into her lap while holding on to one or two of the toys that have most intrigued the child.

Do not hesitate to use humor. As long as care is taken to avoid making the child the butt of humor and as long as reality is not distorted permanently, lighthearted levity and fantasy are often effective for making the child feel at ease.

Request that the parent undress the younger or more wary toddler. An older toddler who is fearful may respond well if the examiner begins with the parts of the examination that do not require undressing (e.g., arms, hands, face, development, etc.). Then, either parent or patient can be requested to remove one piece of clothing from the patient at a time (e.g., sometimes it is necessary to start with the shoes). Occasionally, it may be necessary to expose only one part of the body at a time, replacing one item of clothing before removing the next item. Be flexible and patient.

LAP EXAMINATION

All components of a routine examination except for observations of gait may be performed with the child positioned on the parent's lap. The parent should be enlisted to "assist" the examiner by removing the child's clothing as necessary, moving the child into various positions as required for the examination, offering words of comfort, and providing the security of an "anchor" for a feaful child. A maneuver (e.g., auscultation) may be demonstrated either on a parent or by a parent on the clinician or a doll, before attempting it on the patient.

The rule-of-thumb for the sequence of the lap examination is:

Begin with the least invasive and proceed to the most invasive. Observations without touching are first (e.g., inspection of skin, face, and muscles of facial expression, body proportions, speech and language). Developmental milestones may be assessed next.

The clinician may hand the parent (or the child) a few small items intended to intrigue: blocks, balls, crayons and paper. As the child becomes engaged, the clinician may add a few examination tools: a penlight, a reflex hammer, and, for the older toddler, a stethoscope.

The first areas to be touched are the peripheral parts of the limbs and body, e.g., toes, the top of the head and anterior fontanelle, are gently palpated.

If the child resists, stop for a few moments and switch gears to distract and calm him. Disregard the child's reaction, pick out a small interesting item from your "cache," and use that item to begin a new "discussion" with the child. When the situation is defused, and the child again looks comfortable, continue.

Gradually move centrally, completing the limb examinations and head and neck examinations, excluding the tympanic membranes and pharynx.

Penlight and ophthalmoscope are used to assess corneal light and pupillary reflexes (red reflex). A ticking watch may be used to screen hearing in the child too young to cooperate for formal screening.

Continue with assessment of abdomen, inguinal-femoral region, and genitalia. Follow with inspection and palpation of the thorax, axillae, and back.

Final examination components utilize examination equipment. Auscultation of heart and lungs and abdomen, if deemed necessary, is performed. Remaining neurologic examination is completed, including assessment of deep tendon reflexes. The tympanic membranes and pharynx are examined either in the lap position or on the table, if more restraint is necessary.

OLDER TODDLER

Older toddlers are usually much easier to engage than younger ones. They have tremendous language and cognitive abilities. They love being treated as a "big boy or big girl." They also love to pretend. Talk to them in simple, adult language. Show them the medical instruments and demonstrate their use. Ask for help in placing the stethoscope onto the chest. Make a big show of warming up the diaphragm and explain what you are doing. Request that the child touch the diaphragm and decide if it's warm enough to use. When feasible, offer choices. Choices enhance the child's sense of control without diminishing the clinician's effectiveness. For example, ask the child, "Which ear shall I look in first—this one or that one?" This is different from asking for permission to perform a maneuver and is much more effective.

The sequence for the cooperative older toddler resembles the more traditional "head-to-toe" order. In some very cooperative children this may include examination of the tympanic membranes and pharynx in the order traditionally reserved for an older child or adult. An alternative sequence may be head-to-toe, with deferral of only tympanic membranes and pharynx until the end. Highlighted below are the areas with special significance for the toddler years.

THE EXAMINATION

General Appearance and Initial Observations

General appearance and initial observations include observations of both a physical and a behavioral nature. For example, the child who is ambulating is assessed for gait (e.g., intoeing, absence of limp) and for strength, balance, and coordination. The child who speaks is assessed for speech content and clarity. When the child disobeys the parent, both parent and child are observed during the interaction.

Measurements

Blood pressure is measured at routine well-child visits starting at age 3 years. If the child is anxious, defer this measurement until the end of the examination when rapport has been achieved.

Head: Hair, Face, Eyes, Ears, Nose, and Mouth

Head and hair on head. The scalp is palpated, with attention directed toward determining whether the anterior fontanelle is closed; if it is not, its size is estimated.

Eyes. There is wide variation in the age at which a child is able to cooperate for **objective visual screening.** Objective screening should be attempted in all children, beginning at age 3 years. By age 5 years, most children can cooperate for objective screening. One recommended screening instrument is the **Snellen test** of distant visual acuity. This is a chart that is placed at eye level, at a standardized distance (e.g., 10 or 20 feet) from the child. For the preschool-age child, several charts (e.g., the tumbling "E") replace the standard letters on the chart. Each eye should be evaluated separately. While testing one eye, the opposite one should be open but vision occluded. An easy way to accomplish this is to have the child hold an opaque cup over it. In the tumbling "E" test, the child answers by indicating which way the open legs of the "E" are pointing.

Routine screening for strabismus should continue throughout the toddler years. In toddlers this includes (1) a query to parents about the presence of a "squint" or "lazy or crossed eyes," (2) assessment of extraocular muscle function, (3) observation of the corneal light reflex, (4) visual acuity assessment for each eye, and (5) performance of an alternate cover test.

The fundus examination is attempted in the toddler but continues to be hampered by the child's inability to sit still and hold eyes steady, away from the light source. The clarity and equality of the red reflex can easily be assessed, and a fleeting glance at the optic disc, vessels, and background may also be achieved. The clinician should avoid touching the eyes, as it will only disturb the child and decrease the likelihood of success.

Ears. Like vision screening for younger toddlers, hearing screening is performed by using a combination of parent report and observation of the youngster's response to sound outside the line of sight. An older cooperative toddler can answer a question like "What do you hear?" or "Tell me when you hear something" as a ticking watch is brought close to each ear. By age 4 years, most toddlers can cooperate for **objective hearing screening.** This is performed using pure-tone air-conducted stimuli with an audiometer and assesses the child's ability to hear sounds of varying frequencies at varying decibels.

The otoscopic examination is deferred to the end of the examination for the younger child or for the older preschooler who seems frightened or uncooperative. The child under 2 is not only less willing to have his ears examined than the 1-year-old, he is also stronger. The key is to plan immobilization carefully before beginning. This includes giving very specific instructions to the parent. A difficult concept for both novice clinicians and parents to appreciate is that a child who is insufficiently or improperly restrained is at risk for more injury, discomfort, and a lengthy examination than the child who is securely restrained. The ear canal is surprisingly fragile, and contact between a fighting child and an otoscope all too frequently results in a bleeding canal.

Mouth. The anterior regions of the mouth are inspected. Toddlers like to have their teeth "counted," thus affording the clinician the opportunity to inspect some or all of the interior of the mouth. Alternately, the older child may be willing to open and say "ahh," or to "pant like a doggy." Unless the child voluntarily opens his mouth, examination of the tonsils and pharynx is deferred until the end of the examination. General oral hygiene is assessed. Teeth are counted and inspected for stains or decay.

All children should have a dental examination at age 3. The dentist will check for malocclusion, caries, abnormal eruptions, early periodontal disease, and other individual teeth abnormalities.

When the tonsils and pharynx are inspected, tonsil size may be graded on a scale of 0–4, with 1 being clearly visible and 4 signifying tonsils that meet or almost meet in the midline.

If the patient has stridor or respiratory distress, do not attempt to force his mouth open; ask for assistance to evaluate him.

The **content and clarity of speech** are assessed. Assessment of content includes estimating the number of single meaningful words in the child's vocabulary, whether or not words are combined into meaningful phrases, and whether or not pronouns or other more complex parts of speech are used. Clarity is assessed by determining how much of the child's speech is comprehensible to strangers (e.g., 50%, almost all) and whether there are mispronunciations. History supplements observations in these areas.

Neck, Thorax, and Upper Limbs

Neck. Beyond infancy, once adequate head control is achieved, assessment for nuchal rigidity as a sign of meningeal irritation becomes a more reliable technique. Nuchal rigidity is stiffness of the neck in the anterior-posterior direction.

Assessment for nuchal rigidity should be performed in any child of toddler age (or older) who is ill or has fever. There are other causes of nuchal rigidity besides meningitis (e.g., cervical spine abnormalities, severe pharyngitis), and not all children with meningitis have nuchal rigidity. When nuchal rigidity is present, it is very important to pursue its cause.

To evaluate for nuchal rigidity, the child, preferably on the examination table, should lie supine. Cradle the back of the child's head in your hands and gently flex the head at the neck until his chin touches his chest. Assess the degree of resistance against this maneuver. When meningeal irritation is present, it will be very difficult to flex the neck. Even healthy children may resist and cry but will allow flexion. It is important to perform this slowly and gently, in a noncrying child if possible. Distraction with your voice or eyes may help (Fig. 15.46).

A child with meningeal irritation will not be able or willing to look down onto his chest, no matter what tricks you attempt. A child who does not really have a stiff neck but simply does not want to be touched can be tricked into looking down at his chest. If a child is old enough to understand it when you say "Hey, you have a spot on your shirt," the child with meningismus will not look down, but the child without it will.

Upper limbs. Older toddlers will cooperate for assessment of grip strength by squeezing your fingers "hard," while younger ones will demonstrate their strength by actively pushing you away! In addition, the older toddler may "help" you count his fingers (simultaneously supplying information about speech and development).

Cardiorespiratory System

Accomplishing either a "quiet" or a recumbent auscultatory examination on the young toddler is not easy. The clinician may need to attempt auscultation at various times during the encounter. An innocent murmur is often first appreciated in this age group. When a heart murmur is suspected, it is especially important to listen to the heart with the patient in both seated and recumbent positions. The cooperative older toddler usually does not mind being examined in both positions. With a less cooperative child, attempt auscultation first in the upright position, deferring the recumbent examination until the abdomen is examined. If the child resists the stethoscope, demonstrate auscultation on either a doll or a parent. Alternately, pretend to auscultate a knee or some other more peripheral body part prior to attempting to get closer to the center of the body.

During auscultation it may be useful to rotate the child's body so that the examiner is facing the child's left side rather than either direct front or back. This is accomplished by asking the parent to turn the child so that the child sits sideways across the lap rather than between the adult's legs. If the child is seated on the exam-

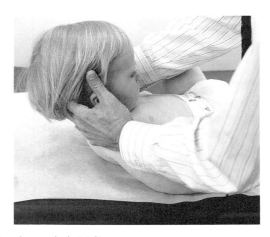

Figure 15.46   Testing for nuchal rigidity.

ination table, the examiner can adopt the same perspective by standing or sitting at the patient's left side rather than standing directly in front of the patient. There are several advantages to performing auscultation in this manner. For the child, this position affords the opportunity to observe all of the clinician's maneuvers. This may be less frightening than having a stethoscope placed on one's back (for lungs) without actually being able to observe the clinician doing so. The patient with a respiratory infection will not be breathing directly at the clinician's face, at least during auscultation. On the other hand, if the child clings to the parent and turns away from the clinician, the opportunity to auscultate the back should be exercised.

At the beginning of the respiratory examination, a cooperative 3- or 4-year-old may try to "help" the examiner by taking a big breath in and then holding it. To avoid this, do not give the child any instruction prior to auscultation. Listen to quiet breathing.

If it is difficult to hear end-expiratory sounds, gently compress the chest between the examining hand (e.g., the one holding the stethoscope on the back) and the other hand placed on the opposite side of the chest (e.g., in the front). This accentuates expiration and makes end-expiratory sounds (e.g., wheezes) easier to hear (Fig. 15.47).

Abdomen

If it is not possible to coax the 2-year-old into a recumbent position (even in a parent's lap), it may be necessary to palpate the abdomen while he is sitting or standing. Fortunately, finding unexpected intra-abdominal pathology in this age group, in the absence of clues from the history, is extremely rare.

Begin palpation superficially and increase pressure gradually. Even though most of the time the abdomen is soft and nontender, the toddler is so wiggly during this examination that he may jump and squirm whenever he is touched. Conversations may help to distract the child (e.g., guessing what he ate for lunch by palpating!). Sometimes, it is helpful to request "help" from an older cooperative,

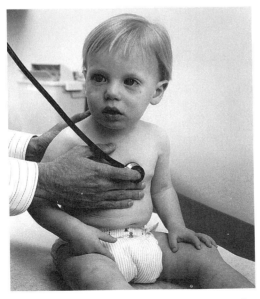

Figure 15.47 During auscultation, chest is compressed between free hand and examining hand to accentuate expiratory sounds, if necessary.

but wiggly patient. If he is supine, have him flex his legs at the hips and the knees so that the soles of his feet grip the surface of the table. Then ask him to place his hand (or hands) on top of yours and request that he "do the pushing" or that he "hold the stethoscope in place for me." The older toddler will enjoy participating in the examination, as is shown in Figure 15.48; in addition, the work of pushing down on your hands often distracts enough to promote relaxing the abdomen.

Percussion of the abdomen in well children is performed only when there is a high index of suspicion for intra-abdominal pathology.

Genitalia

For the genital examination, request that the parent remove the diaper to avoid disturbing the child. For the older child who is lying supine on the examination table and has cooperated up until this point, state matter-of-factly, "Now I am going to check your bottom"; and begin to gently pull down the underpants. If no resistance is encountered, proceed with the examination of the genitals. If resistance is encountered, do not proceed further. Ask the parent to approach the child and assist in calming the child.

Female genitalia. The genitalia are inspected in the **frog leg position.** The labia are gently separated in order to visualize the clitoris, urethra, and vagina. If the child is very frightened, request that the parent position the child and separate the labia. This examination may be performed either on the examining table or in the parent's lap (Fig. 15.49).

The underpants are put back on before proceeding to examination of the lower limbs.

Lower Limbs

If the child refuses to walk, ask the parent to walk to the opposite end of the room or corridor while you gently restrain the patient. When the parent has arrived across the room, let go of the child and watch as he walks or runs over to the

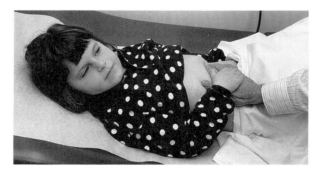

Figure 15.48   Maneuver to relax the abdomen. Ask the patient to "help do the pushing."

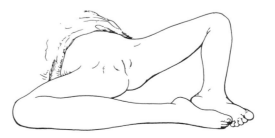

Figure 15.49   Frog-leg position for routine examination of female external genitalia.

waiting parent. Observe whether there is a wide or narrow base to the gait, whether there are bowlegs or knock-knees, and whether the feet are placed flat on the ground or the child is a toe-walker.

Do the child's feet turn in or out when he walks? Estimate the degree of intoeing or outtoeing by **estimating the angle of gait.** The angle of gait is the angle between the line of progression and the long axis of the foot (Fig. 15.50).

The child with an intoeing or outtoeing gait is examined for torsional deformities that may result from excess rotational forces at various points along the lower limbs (e.g., hips, tibiae, feet). Excess forces may impact in isolation at one point along the limb or in combination at several points along the limb. Therefore, each part of the limb must be evaluated separately to determine the reason(s) for the intoeing or outtoeing gait. The feet are examined with the patient in the recumbent position, positioned in the same manner as the infant. The maneuvers to examine for torsional deformities originating in the tibiae and the hips are discussed under Special Maneuvers.

Back

The active toddler provides ample opportunity for inspection of the back, particularly when he turns away and clutches desperately at the parent. If the patient is able to stand quietly, his back is inspected and spine palpated from behind and posture is observed from the side.

Neurologic System and Development

Mentally review these examinations and fill in missing information. Beginning the physical examination with developmental assessment may defuse the child's anxiety (see Fig. 15.8). For the older more cooperative toddler, a large part of the classical neurologic examination begins to resemble that performed in the adult.

Cranial nerves. The younger, uncooperative child is assessed indirectly by using observation (as in the infant). The older child is usually able to actively cooperate in the standard examination.

Motor. Strength and symmetry of muscle groups are assessed by observing the child while he is walking, sitting up, getting on and off the examining table or the floor, heel-walking, etc. Fine motor manipulation is assessed by observing the child playing with blocks, drawing with crayons, or copying a figure.

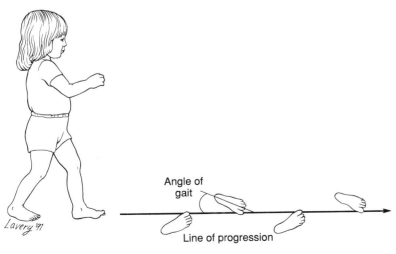

Figure 15.50 Estimating the angle of gait (how much the child toes in or out). The angle of gait is estimated as the average angle that each step makes with the line of progression.

Lower back and pelvic girdle muscle strength are assessed: Ask the patient to squat down on the floor, then get (or jump) up. The clinician may need to squat down at the same time in order to demonstrate the maneuver and to obtain cooperation. Does the child need to brace himself (either against a nearby object or against his own body for support) as he returns to a standing position?

Coordination. Arm swing, fluidity of movement, and balance are observed. The 4-year-old may be asked to imitate rapid thumb-to-forefinger opposition. Coordination is also assessed by observing the child perform gross and fine motor accomplishments (e.g., running, drawing).

Station and gait. The 3–4-year-old may be asked to stand with feet together and maintain balance with eyes open, then with eyes closed (Romberg test). Gait is observed for asymmetries, limp, toe-walking or ataxia.

Sensory system. Formal evaluation of sensation is usually reserved for those in whom there are special neurologic concerns. A few older toddlers can cooperate for evaluation of response to light touch or pin, joint movements, or sensation of tuning fork. Cortical integrity testing may also be difficult, but not impossible, to perform: It may include discriminating objects placed in the hand and/or discriminating simple shapes drawn by the examiner's finger on the body as a "game."

Reflexes. Deep tendon reflexes are assessed in the traditional fashion. It is helpful to have an extra hammer around; offer one to the child. Demonstrate first on a parent, older sibling, or doll.

Completing the Examination

When the physical examination is completed, the patient is complimented on "a job well done." After any other unpleasant procedures have been completed, the patient should be rewarded with a small tangible item (e.g., a sticker or toy). The examination of the young toddler is one of the most challenging experiences in pediatrics. Nevertheless, once the clinician learns some of the special tricks and techniques, it can also be the most satisfying.

Normal and Common Variants and *Clues to Abnormalities*

General Appearance

Toddlers display a full range of typical age-related behaviors in the context of every clinical encounter (e.g., temper tantrums, "me want," lack of impulse control, separation anxiety). Simultaneously, parents respond with a diversity of management strategies (e.g., concern, verbal admonishment, physical punishment, time out, affection). A "good fit" between parents and child is achieved when parents understand their child's temperamental style and developmental abilities (e.g., achieving a balance between flexibility and limit-setting). Extremes of parenting styles and extremes of child behavior are especially important to note and record as accurately as possible.

The toddler who is doing well appears well-nourished, well-developed, and well-cared-for (e.g., clean). He is active and affectionate with his caretaker. Conversely, the appearance of undernourishment, small for stated age, poorly cared for, apathy, and lack of affection to or from caretaker deserve especially careful scrutiny.

Head: Hair, Face, Eyes, Ears, Nose, and Mouth

Eyes. Children before their fifth birthday should read the 20/40 line. *A two-line difference of visual acuity between the eyes, even in the passing range, should be evaluated further. These children are at risk for amblyopia.*

Ears. Failure on audiometric screening equals inability to respond to sounds of 1000 Hz or 2000 Hz at 20 dB or 4000 Hz at 25 dB in either ear if cooperation is judged to be adequate. The child who fails this screening should be referred for formal audiologic evaluation. When parents express concerns about hearing or when language is significantly impaired or delayed in developing, referral for formal audiologic evaluation is indicated.

There are two tympanic membrane conditions that are common findings in asymptomatic or healthy appearing children. **Tympanosclerosis** appears as white plaques in the eardrum. These are usually sequelae of prior infections and are of no consequence unless the entire drum is so scarred that movement with insufflation is inhibited.

Serous otitis media implies the presence of fluid in the middle ear without acute inflammation. The eardrum appears dull, less shiny and translucent than usual and gray, white, or yellow in color. Landmarks may be partly obscured by fluid, and an air-fluid level or bubbles may be visible behind the eardrum. Movement in response to insufflation is reduced or absent. This is more difficult to diagnose than acute otitis media, because the findings are more subtle (Fig. 15.51).

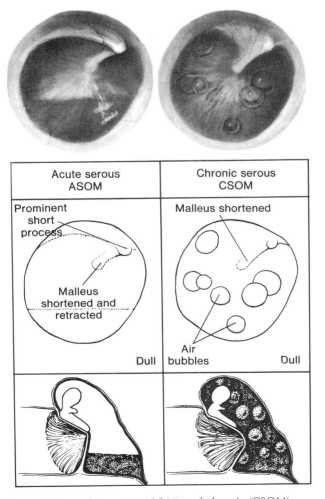

Figure 15.51   Serous otitis media: acute (ASOM) and chronic (CSOM).

Nose. Bilateral nasal drainage secondary to upper respiratory infection is extremely common in this age group. Also common is unilateral nasal drainage, which may be foul smelling and green. The most common explanation for this is a **nasal foreign body**, which is usually a wad of tissue paper, a food remnant, or a bead. Some of the time these are visible and easily retrieved with a forceps; alternately, they may be difficult to visualize without using special instruments and may necessitate otolaryngology referral.

Mouth. In toddlers, tonsils are clearly visible and appear large relative to their size in adults. Maximal development of the lymphoid system occurs prior to puberty. Tonsils and adenoids are involved in this steady normal growth, and therefore, tonsils usually appear progressively larger as children grow older. In addition, because of the high frequency of upper respiratory infections in toddlers, the involved lymph tissues are often further enlarged by hyperplasia. Crypts in the tonsillar tissue are normal. In this age group, large tonsils (e.g., a 2/4 or a 3/4) without signs of inflammation and not interfering with swallowing or breathing functions are not pathologic.

Prior to age 4, an erythematous pharynx, with or without enlarged tonsils and with or without exudate, is usually due to a viral infection.

The epiglottis may be clearly visible when the mouth is wide open. This is a normal finding in a healthy child because the epiglottis does not descend to its final lower position (where it is not usually visible) until puberty. The normal color of the epiglottis is pink. *When the epiglottis is inflamed (e.g., epiglottitis—a serious bacterial infection of childhood), it appears larger, edematous, and bright "cherry red."*

Teeth. By age 2–2½, most children have a full complement of 20 primary teeth (upper and lower, they include central incisors, lateral incisors, cuspids, and first and second molars). *Plaque on teeth and generalized erythema or friability of gingivae usually reflect poor oral hygiene. Any child with colored stains on teeth (even those with orange-pumpkin-colored stains caused by food and plaque) should have a dental checkup.* **Milk bottle caries** *(or BBTD, baby bottle tooth decay) are caused by prolonged contact with a sugar-containing liquid usually secondary to taking a bottle of milk or juice to bed or breast-feeding throughout the night. These appear as brown to black discolorations and holes on the central maxillary incisors (the lower incisors are not involved). Involved maxillary anterior teeth and normal mandibular anterior teeth are pathognomonic of BBTD. If severe, all of the upper teeth may be involved (Fig. 15.52).*

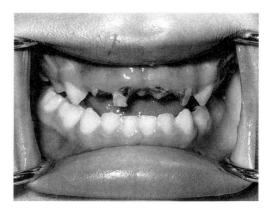

Figure 15.52   Milk bottle caries, severe case.

Speech

Content. By age 2, a child is expected to be able to make his wants known by using his voice, speaking at least several words routinely, and pointing correctly to objects, such as his head or shoe. By age 3, two- or three-word sentences are expected, as is the use of "me" or "you" appropriately and responding to simple commands. By age 4, the child should be able to correctly state his first and last name, discuss aspects of daily life, and use plurals and past tenses.

Clarity. A 2-year-old's speech should be understood approximately 50% of the time. By age 3, a child's speech should be relatively easy to understand. However, certain types of articulation errors (such as substituting "w" for "r" in "rabbit," or "d" for "th" in "that") are normal in the toddler age group. Four-year-olds should be understood most of the time.

Another issue with respect to clarity involves repetition of sounds or words (stuttering) or hesitations. These are called "**disfluencies**" and are a normal process occurring a year or two after the onset of speech development. These are not considered pathologic or "**dysfluencies**" unless they persist for many months or years and interfere with communication (e.g., involve many syllables or words and evoke tension in the child).

Children who fail to communicate within the expected range of normal may require further investigation including complete physical examination, speech and hearing testing, and a developmental evaluation.

Cardiorespiratory System

Heart. The preschool-age group is the most common period for the discovery of an **innocent heart murmur.** Unlike the younger toddler, the older one will usually cooperate for a "quiet" examination. Also, as the chest begins to take on a less rounded, less padded configuration, it becomes somewhat easier to hear heart sounds. There are three innocent murmurs of childhood that are often first heard in this age group: **Still's murmur, venous hum, and carotid bruit.**

Still's murmur is a low-pitched systolic ejection murmur with a musical or vibratory quality (as distinguished from a pathologic harsh or grating sound). It is best heard halfway between the lower left sternal border and the apex, with increased intensity in the supine position. It will sound louder with fever and after exercise.

Venous hum is a continuous (audible in systole and diastole) murmur heard best on the right side of the chest at the level of the clavicles, although it may also be heard at the left infraclavicular area. It may be obliterated or modified by turning the patient's head away from the side of the murmur or compressing the internal jugular vein on the side of the murmur. It disappears in the supine position. The sounds arise from blood flow through the great veins in the neck.

Carotid bruit is a systolic ejection murmur (not louder than a grade 3/6) that is heard over the carotids. It diminishes as the auscultation approaches the aortic or pulmonic areas (which distinguishes it from valvular murmurs) (Table 15.6).

Lungs. One of the pathologic respiratory noises heard particularly often in toddlers is stridor. *Stridor is a harsh sound that occurs when there is obstruction to airflow. The most common cause of stridor in this age group is croup, a viral infection that produces inflammation in the larynx, trachea, and bronchi. Another less common, but extremely dangerous, cause of stridor is epiglottitis, a bacterial infection most commonly caused by Haemophilus influenzae type b. Children with epiglottitis are especially vulnerable to sudden airway obstruction, which can be precipitated by forced pharyngeal examination.* **Therefore, in the ill-appearing toddler with stridor, forced pharynx examination must not be attempted.**

Wheezing is an increasingly common finding in children. Wheezing is due to partial airway obstruction and is most commonly heard during expiration but may also be heard during inspiration. Wheezing is a sign of asthma, although there are many other diseases in which children also wheeze (e.g., foreign-body aspiration, bronchiolitis, congestive heart failure, cystic fibrosis).

Abdomen

As toddlers grow, the trunk gradually slims out, but the protuberant abdomen often remains until abdominal musculature strengthens. Parents frequently inquire about their toddler's "potbelly." The lumbar lordosis of childhood makes the abdomen appear to protrude even farther (Fig. 15.53).

Table 15.6
Innocent Heart Murmurs of Childhood

Definition: An innocent murmur is a murmur that is associated with no underlying heart disease. Except for the venous hum, an innocent murmur is never heard during diastole. An innocent murmur is never associated with adventitious cardiac sounds or with other signs of cardiac disease.

Characteristics: Innocent murmurs are usually **soft, vary in intensity with change in the patient's body position** and are associated with normal S_1 and S_2 sounds.

Murmur	Usual age period when murmur initially audible
Peripheral pulmonic stenosis	**Newborn**
Still's murmur	**Toddler**
Venous hum	**Toddler**
Carotid bruit	**Toddler**
Pulmonary flow	**School-age child**

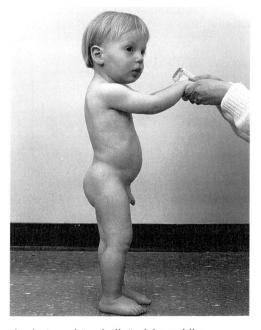

Figure 15.53   Lumbar lordosis and "potbelly" of the toddler.

The liver edge is normally palpable 1–2 cm below the right costal margin. Occasionally, especially in the younger toddler, the spleen tip is slightly palpable at the left costal margin. This finding usually signifies mild splenic enlargement, which is most commonly secondary to a recent or ongoing infection (usually viral in origin). Although it is unlikely to signify a more serious pathologic process, a palpable spleen must be carefully followed until it has resolved or until the underlying etiology has been treated.

The most common palpable abdominal "mass" in this age group is fecal matter in the colon. These are usually felt as firm, freely mobile, circular masses in the left lower quadrant. Alternately, a large sausage-shaped mass that fills the entire descending colon may be palpated.

If abdominal pain is a complaint, ask an older toddler to point to "where it hurts." However, do not expect a lot of information from the answer. The younger the child, the more difficulty he will have in localizing the site of abdominal pain. Not infrequently, a cooperative child will point to the umbilicus. That may mean that it hurts there, but this answer, while an honest one, may also reflect the child's true inability to localize the source of abdominal pain. If the child is truly relaxed and distracted, it is sometimes possible to observe subtle signs of discomfort (e.g., a grimace) in order to locate a more focal site of tenderness.

Genitalia

Female genitalia. Not infrequently, toddler girls develop mild vulvovaginal itching and/or discharge associated with nonspecific irritation. The vulva and perineum may appear red and slightly edematous. There may be an accompanying watery vaginal discharge and a complaint of pain on urination. Poor hygiene secondary to age-appropriate hygiene (e.g., not wiping "front to back") and the use of irritating bubble baths are the most common contributing factors. A vaginal foreign body (e.g., a wad of toilet paper or a toy part) is another common cause of vaginal discharge in this age group. Genital itching and irritation may also accompany pinworm infestation of the gastrointestinal tract. Thin thread-like worms may be seen around the anus, but these are usually not visible, except in the early morning.

Vaginal discharge may also be a sign of a sexually transmitted disease and sexual abuse. If this diagnosis is entertained, an investigation must be conducted under the supervision of an experienced clinician.

Male genitalia. By age 3, 90% of uncircumcised males will have a fully retractable foreskin.

Back

The normal toddler, when viewed from the side, has an exaggerated lumbar lordosis. This forward curvature of the spine is partly responsible for the toddler "potbelly." In school-age children, the curve becomes less prominent.

Lower Limbs

The wide base of the novice walker's gait gradually disappears, and the feet come together. Many toddlers demonstrate an **intoeing gait.** Beyond infancy (in which metatarsus adductus should be identified), the most common explanations for intoeing gaits are secondary to either tibial rotation, known as **internal tibial torsion,** or femoral head rotation, known as **femoral anteversion** (see the Special Maneuvers section under Toddler). Many of these gait "problems" are really non-problems, being developmentally predictable and mostly self-resolving. Persistence of a gait in which the feet point in (–) or out (+) more than 30° from the line of progression is abnormal.

The feet of most toddlers appear to be flat. This is usually related to the presence of fat pads that obscure the longitudinal arch of the foot. Some new walkers walk on their toes initially and within months gradually lose the habit. Some of these children have a family history of toe-walking without any underlying pathology. *Persistence of toe-walking requires a very thorough neuromuscular examination, as children with spastic diplegia or muscular dystrophy may also demonstrate toe-walking.*

Before 2 years of age, it is common for a child to be mildly bowlegged. From age 3–5 years, it is common for a child to be mildly knock-kneed. In most instances, there is a spontaneous correction to a straight-legged stance by age 7 or 8. Severe cases that do not improve require orthopedic attention.

Another common problem, especially in toddlers, is the *child who has a limp or refuses to walk. Even in the absence of a definite history, trauma is a common etiology. The toddler without trauma, who refuses to walk, may have an irritable hip. The child is usually unable to correctly localize the source of the pain. Even an older child with an irritable hip may point to the thigh or knee. This is because hip pain is frequently referred to the thigh and the knee. The child should be examined in the supine position. Observe whether or not the leg in question is held in a different position than the unaffected one. Determine whether there is a difference in range of motion between symmetric joints. Palpate from hip to feet for any tenderness. Palpate the hip joint at the anteromedial thigh immediately distal to the inguinal fold; if there is an inflammatory effusion, there may be signs of swelling and tenderness. The most common cause of an irritable hip in a toddler is* **toxic synovitis,** *an inflammation of the hip joint that is of unknown etiology. As with any hip irritation, there is reduced range of motion at the hip, with the limb held in partial hip flexion, abduction, and external rotation. Full passive internal rotation is difficult to achieve.*

Skin

Birthmarks. "Strawberry" hemangiomas begin to involute in toddlers.

Café-au-lait spots are well-circumscribed, tan macules. Many normal individuals have one or two small spots. *If a prepubertal child has 6 or more café-au-lait spots, especially if these are larger than ½ cm in diameter (in the longest axis), the diagnosis of the neurocutaneous disorder* **neurofibromatosis** *should be considered.*

Depigmented spots are flat spots that have less color than the surrounding skin and are found in many normal individuals.

Sometimes, a depigmented spot may also be the first sign of another neurocutaneous disorder: **tuberous sclerosis.** *In this disease, the classical shape for the depigmented spot is that of an ash leaf. When a concern about a neurocutaneous disease is raised, the entire body should be inspected for spots. Use of a Wood's lamp during inspection may enhance visualization of light or depigmented spots (Figs. 15.54 and 15.55).*

The **nevocellular nevus** is a pigmented lesion with cells in the dermis, epidermis, or both. If a pigmented growth is observed, inquire as to whether or not the child was born with it. Small congenital nevocellular nevi are usually round or oval and may be found in association with hair follicles. *A giant congenital nevocellular nevus that is larger than 10 cm in length carries an increased risk for malignant transformation to malignant melanoma. There is less agreement about the smaller lesions, but many dermatologists believe there is increased risk in individuals with these, too.*

Rashes. Atopic dermatitis (**eczema**) continues to affect children during their toddler years. The dry skin and excoriations may involve any portion of the skin,

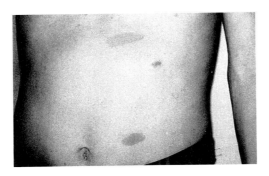

Figure 15.54 Café-au-lait spots.

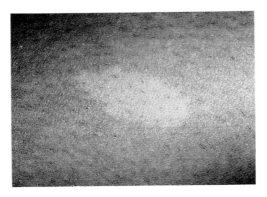

Figure 15.55 Ash leaf-shaped hypopigmented macule.

but from age 2 until adolescence, the rash predominates in the antecubital and popliteal fossae.

Discussion of many other acquired childhood rashes and exanthems is beyond the scope of this book. The reader is referred to textbooks of pediatrics or pediatric dermatology.

Neurologic System and Development

*__Motor.__ A child with muscle weakness in the lower back and pelvic girdle (e.g., a child with **Duchenne muscular dystrophy**) will get up off the floor in a characteristic fashion (called a **Gower's sign**). The child will be unable to jump right up but rather will need to "walk" his hands up the front of his lower limbs, bracing against them until upright.*

Special Maneuvers

MANEUVERS TO DETERMINE THE ETIOLOGY FOR INTOEING OR OUTTOEING

If there is clinically significant intoeing or outtoeing, it is likely that forces at the hip, along the shaft of the tibiae, or at the feet are responsible. Techniques of examination enable the clinician to determine where the source of the problem lies.

The feet are examined in the supine position in the same manner as described for the newborn. The most common cause of intoeing originating at the feet is **metatarsus adductus.** This diagnosis can be made in the newborn and during early infancy.

The feet may also point in because of **internal tibial torsion.** In this condition, the tibiae are rotated inward on their longitudinal axis. An easy way to confirm this is to seat the child on the end of the examining table, with the knees pointing straight at you. Normally, in this position, the malleoli are situated so that the medial malleolus is slightly anterior to the lateral malleolus or a little more of the medial malleolus is visible than the lateral malleolus. If the tibia is internally rotated, the lateral malleolus is positioned so that it is more anterior than usual and the medial malleolus is positioned so that it is more posterior than usual. Internal tibial torsion may be bilateral or unilateral. Mild degrees of this condition may resolve without therapy. More significant degrees, such that the deformity is obvious or interferes with walking, may be corrected with orthoses (Fig. 15.56).

The other common etiology for intoeing is **increased femoral anteversion** (at the hip). In the normal infant and young child, the degree of external rotation of the hip exceeds internal rotation. In patients with increased femoral anteversion, the degree of internal rotation is greater than the 70° normal range. Direct the patient to lie prone on the table. Flex the knees with the hips in extension and determine the arc that each leg circumscribes from the vertical as it falls by gravity into internal rotation and as it crosses the midline in the opposite direction into external rotation. It is helpful to remember that inward and outward rotation refer to the head of the femur. While allowing the leg to fall outward with gravity, you are really rotating the head of the femur inward (internal rotation), and when the leg is moved across the midline, you are really rotating the head of the femur outward (external rotation). If the leg can be moved much farther into internal rotation than into external rotation, then a diagnosis of increased femoral anteversion is established (Fig. 15.57).

Children outtoe for a variety of reasons. By the time a child is walking well, outtoeing is much less common than intoeing. Causes of outtoeing include femoral retroversion (rare) and external tibial torsion (rare in isolation). The maneuvers outlined above may uncover either of these problems.

VISUAL FIELD EVALUATION

Visual field testing is not part of a standard pediatric examination unless a detailed neurologic or ophthalmologic examination is required. If this examina-

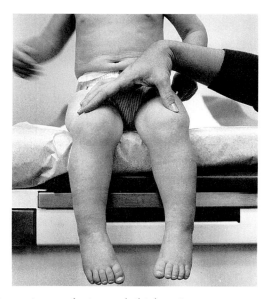

Figure 15.56   Position to inspect for internal tibial torsion.

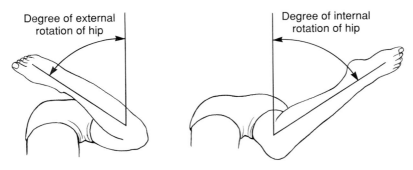

Figure 15.57 Assessment of external and internal rotation at the hip.

tion is necessary, request that the child sit facing a parent who visually distracts him by playing with something directly in between them and right in front of the child. The clinician stands behind the child and brings an attractive object out from behind the child into each of four quadrants in his field of vision. When the child turns his head toward the object, you know he has seen it. This is a very "gross" test of visual fields.

Alternatively, seat the child in the parent's lap. Hold the child's head steady in the midline, and with your free hand, bring an object into the child's field of vision from each of four quadrants. When the eyes deviate toward the object, you know he has seen it.

SCHOOL-AGE CHILD

Techniques of Examination

AREAS OF EMPHASIS

The likelihood of uncovering important covert pathology in the healthy-appearing school-age child is quite small. In addition, most children at this age will cooperate, and the examination is technically easier than on a younger child. Therefore, a routine physical examination on a healthy school-age child should occupy no more than about 5 minutes of a clinical encounter. For the school-age child, a complete examination is performed, with special attention focused on (1) growth pattern, (2) dentition, (3) scoliosis detection, and (4) signs of puberty. The school-age child is frequently examined for minor infectious illnesses. These encounters, as well as those with the hospitalized child, present additional challenges for the student learning to examine children and require knowledge of normal baseline findings. Also, each of these settings provides an opportunity for data gathering about the child's affective development and parent-child relationships.

OVERALL STRATEGIES

By this age, the child generally understands the purpose of the encounter. The patient has memories of prior examinations, is familiar with most instruments and procedures, and can follow the clinician's instructions. Under usual circumstances, the clinician's most difficult tasks in this regard are to engage the child in conversation and diminish anxiety. It will be easy to make friends with an extrovert. More challenge is provided by the encounter with a child who is shy, seriously ill, or fearful of a painful procedure.

As the child grows older an increasing percentage of the entire encounter should include direct clinician-patient (and patient-clinician) discussion without parent intervention. This includes both information gathering and information dispensing. At the older end of the school-age group (the preadolescent or early adolescent), portions of the encounter may be conducted without a parent in the room.

Most of the time, a special or helter-skelter examination sequence should not be necessary. The willing child can be examined in a "head-to-toe" fashion, similar to the adult method. The child who is modest should be offered a gown to wear over underpants. Only one area of the body is exposed at a time, and a drape should be used in addition to the gown. Attention to modesty will also enhance the patient's feeling of being in control. This feeling may be amplified if the clinician (1) provides information as the examination proceeds, (2) alerts the patient as to what is coming next, and (3) continues to offer choices whenever it is realistic to do so.

THE EXAMINATION

When ready to begin, request that the child be seated on the examining table.

General Appearance and Initial Observations

Throughout the encounter do not fail to observe the content of parent-child interaction, both physical and verbal. Are there signs of a supportive relationship, or is there "distance" or excessive criticism?

Measurements

Blood pressure is measured and compared to age and gender norms. If an elevated reading is obtained with a correctly sized cuff, the measurement should be repeated at the conclusion of the examination. If the second reading is abnormal, have the patient lie down in a darkened room for 15 or 20 minutes and repeat the measurement a third time. If the upper limb blood pressure remains elevated, measure it in the lower limbs.

Head: Hair, Face, Eyes, Ears, Nose, and Mouth

Eyes. Vision is first screened subjectively by inquiring about visual difficulties. Objective vision screening is particularly important for children starting school (e.g., at ages 5 and 6). Thereafter, objective vision screening is performed every 2 years unless there are concerns about the eyes or vision. Routine objective screening is omitted at age 10 if prior vision is normal and history about vision and the eye is noncontributory. Color vision is assessed subjectively at least once in this age group. When concerns are raised, objective assessment utilizes special pseudoisochromatic plates.

A routine funduscopic evaluation is usually first successfully accomplished in this age group. The parent may assist by holding aloft an object or a hand for the child to focus on. If it is necessary to turn out the lights during this examination, the clinician should remember to warn the patient ahead of time.

Ears. Hearing is first screened subjectively, by inquiry about hearing difficulties and ear infections. Objective hearing screening is performed at age 5. Thereafter, if prior screens are normal and there is no history to suggest hearing problems, objective screening does not need to be repeated until the beginning of adolescence. Otoscopy is conducted with pinna pulled up and back, using a size "4" otoscope speculum.

Mouth and Pharynx. Oral hygiene, tooth development, spacing, and occlusion are assessed. Occlusion is assessed by directing the patient to bite down. Determine (1) the relationship between the top teeth and the bottom teeth and (2) whether or not the child bites down on the back teeth.

If the child cooperates, visualization of the posterior structures may be accomplished without the use of a tongue depressor. If a depressor is necessary, position it onto the anterior two-thirds of the tongue, in order to avoid stimulating a gag reflex.

Neck, Thorax, and Upper Limbs

Thorax and upper limbs. In particular, the older school-age female will appreciate the clinician's respect for her physical modesty. The sequence for examination maneuvers in this region is the same as for the adult female.

Cardiorespiratory System

The incidence of innocent murmurs in this age group is quite significant. A careful cardiac examination in both upright and recumbent positions is obligatory.

The school-age child can cooperate by "breathing big" for auscultation of the lungs. Demonstrate this with your mouth wide open, and ask the patient to imitate you while you auscultate.

Breasts

A breast examination should always be performed as part of a routine or complete physical examination. The breasts of females *and* males are inspected. The Tanner system of staging pubertal development is a method used to describe and monitor progression of secondary sexual changes during puberty. The Tanner stage of breast development is determined by comparing the appearance of the patient's breasts to the appearance of the models' breasts in Tanner drawings or photos (see Fig. 6.10). Palpation begins whenever breast budding is visible. Only one side at a time is exposed during palpation; the other side is covered by the gown. In addition, the child should be prepared ahead for each subsequent part of the examination (e.g., "now I am going to gently squeeze the nipple"). When the female patient reaches Tanner stage 3, she should be instructed in how to perform breast self-examination. Routine performance of a breast examination during early puberty may subsequently diminish the anxiety that this examination commonly generates.

Abdomen

The abdomen is palpated by the same general approach as is used in adults. The liver edge is often palpable in healthy children. A variation in body habitus or the presence of intrathoracic pathology may increase the amount of palpable liver when, in fact, the actual organ size is normal. When this is suspected, the clinician should add the vertical height of liver palpated inferior to the costal margin to the vertical height of liver superior to the costal margin as estimated by the extent of dullness to percussion in the midclavicular line. As in adults, a bimanual method for palpation of the spleen tip is preferred.

Genitalia

Inform the child that examination of the genitalia is next and that you will be gentle and will not cause any pain. Ask the patient to pull down his or her underpants.

Female genitalia. The lower abdomen and groin are covered by a drape. The genitalia are examined in the frog-leg position. The Tanner stage of pubic hair development is noted (see Fig. 15.60). The genitalia are inspected for inflammation, adhesions, lesions, and vaginal discharge. If the patient is very apprehensive but able to cooperate, she may prefer to "assist" the clinician by separating the labia using her own fingers (with her mother or the clinician guiding her). At the conclusion of the genitalia examination, inform the child that "everything looks normal" (if it does) and direct her to pull her underpants up.

Male genitalia. The penis, scrotum, and testes are inspected. The Tanner stage of genitalia and pubic hair development is noted (see Fig. 15.61). The foreskin is gently retracted. The penis may be buried within the pubic fat pad, making inspection and determination of actual size difficult. The clinician should retract the pubic fat pad with one hand, while gently stretching the penis to its full length with the other hand. It is usually unnecessary to actually measure the penis; estimation is sufficient. When a true objective measurement is required, the penis is measured with a ruler from the pubic ramus to the end of the glans.

The scrotum and testes are palpated. Testicular size is estimated by estimating length. If the testes are not palpable in the scrotum, an attempt is made to "milk" them down into the scrotum. In attempting to locate a testicle, increasing the pressure on lower abdominal contents may be of help: Request that the patient sit with crossed legs, "Indian style."

At the conclusion of the genitalia examination, inform the child that "everything looks normal" (if it does) and direct him to pull his underpants up.

Lower Limbs and Back

For examination of the lower limbs and back, ask the child to stand. Inform the child that you are going to check the back for a curvature of the spine. **Scoliosis** may appear at any age during childhood, but idiopathic scoliosis most commonly presents in the preadolescent and early adolescent age group. Because children entering the growth spurt are at risk for rapid progression of scoliosis, it is especially important that every older school-age child have a thorough back examination (Fig. 15.58).

The shirt or gown should be off so that the entire back may be visualized, as shown in Figure 15.58. Begin by inspecting the spine from behind the patient. Ask

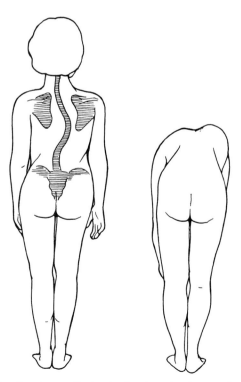

Figure 15.58 Examination for scoliosis: the back and spine are inspected when the patient is upright and bending forward from the waist.

the child to stand with feet together, arms at sides, standing "as straight as possible," with eyes looking straight ahead. Inspect the spine for lateral curvatures and for symmetry in height and prominence of shoulders, scapulae, posterior ribs, and iliac crests. Palpate the spine along its full length for irregularities and tenderness. Scoliosis may be present without an obvious spinal curvature. The only sign may be asymmetric height or prominence of one of the paraspinal structures.

Begin the second half of the examination for scoliosis, which also tests for flexibility of the spine, by asking the patient to bend forward from the waist without bending the knees, letting the arms dangle from the shoulders. Inspect the spine and paraspinal contours from behind the patient; then move to the child's side and repeat the inspection. Observe for straightness of spine and asymmetries of paired bilateral structures. Check carefully for symmetry of paraspinal muscle contour and rib outline.

If the patient's vertebrae are obscured by muscle or fat, a useful adjunct is a ballpoint pen. Feel for each vertebra and put a mark at the site of central prominence. Then ask the child to stand up. The spine will be nicely outlined.

Finally, when the patient is standing straight up, move to the child's side once again and inspect for kyphosis or lordosis. Kyphosis or "hump back" means that the spine curves out posteriorly; lordosis or "sway back" means that the spine curves in anteriorly.

Before the patient returns to the examining table, observe the gait as the child walks across the room.

Neurologic System and Development

The healthy alert school-age child will usually be cooperative for the formal parts of the neurologic examination. At this point in the examination, much of the neurologic examination has been completed. Mentally review the components of the examination and fill in what has been left out.

General appearance and mental status. Observations of the general appearance and mental status include observations of alertness, mood, cognitive skills, and language. Ask the parent, "Do you find him to be generally happy or sad?" or "What kind of mood is he generally in?" or "Do you have any concerns about his mood or attitudes?" etc. In addition, ask the patient questions such as "What kind of things do you enjoy?" "What makes you happy?" "What do you hate?" "What do you feel sad about?" "Are you worried about anything?"

Cognitive functioning is most efficiently assessed by inquiring about school progress. If there are problems with school functioning, inquire about evaluation of the problem, conclusions reached, and plans for remediation. It is especially important to ask for specific data when inquiring about school grades and about school absence.

Development. For the patient approaching adolescence, information about school and athletic performance, as well as pubertal progress, may be used for monitoring development.

Motor. Gross motor movements are observed when the patient walks, sits up, bends down, etc. Fine motor movements are observed when the child ties shoelaces or colors with crayons.

Coordination. These observations are made while assessing large and small motor movements. The school-age child may also be evaluated for ability to perform maneuvers such as finger-to-nose testing.

Station and gait. A Romberg test may be performed. If there are concerns about gait (e.g., limp, clumsiness, asymmetries, posturing), the patient should be observed both walking and running. Running (e.g., down the hall) will accentuate subtle abnormalities in gait.

Sensory examination. Children in middle childhood can cooperate for most types of formal sensory testing if there are special neurologic concerns. Response to light touch, vibration, and position sense may be assessed. Pinprick is deferred unless absolutely necessary because of children's fears. Formal cortical sensation testing may be performed in a manner similar to that used for adults. This may include identifying common objects or shapes or stereognosis.

Normal and Common Variants and *Clues to Abnormalities*

Difficult Interactions

Even though the examination in the school-age child usually proceeds smoothly, there may be some exceptions. Whenever this occurs, the clinician should attempt to uncover the reason for resistance by obtaining further history. **Various children resist examinations: (1) the younger child who is still experiencing difficulties with separation, (2) the extremely shy (or "slow-to-warm-up") child, (3) the child who has had many previous painful or frightening medical experiences, (4) the child who has been physically or sexually abused, (5) the child who is out of control and will not respond to routine limit-setting, and (6) the child who is very ill.** Management should reflect the clinician's hypothesis about the underlying problem. For example, the "slow-to-warm-up" child or the child who is afraid because of previous experiences will respond positively to the clinician who proceeds cautiously, taking care to explain along the way and reassure whenever possible. A child in this age group will understand logical statements and reason.

The child who has been physically or sexually abused may be uncooperative for the general physical examination or uncooperative for only parts of the examination (e.g., the genital examination). It may be very difficult to distinguish between the healthy child who has much natural resistance to having the genitals examined versus the child who has been abused. Often, in the circumstance of abuse, **something in the history** *does not fit, because there are behavioral issues, compliance issues, or other issues. There may be a prior history of neglect or abuse or a history of a sibling having been abused. Some of the time, a successful examination may be accomplished by backing off for a few minutes and explaining what needs to be performed. Keep the child's mother close by. The inexperienced clinician is advised to seek counsel from a supervisor when concern about abuse is raised.*

The uncomfortable, but not critically ill school-age child (e.g., a child with acute abdominal pain or streptococcal pharyngitis) is usually able to cooperate despite being uncomfortable. Attending to the patient's modesty and to the need for explanation should not be overlooked. A child in this age group who resists examination is much more difficult to restrain than a younger child. Therefore, the clinician may choose to omit a nonessential procedure in certain circumstances.

However, when a part of the physical examination is deemed necessary (e.g., examination of the pharynx in a child with a stiff neck), verbally acknowledge its importance, be firm, and ask for assistance if restraining the patient is required.

Measurements

Middle childhood is a period of steady, relatively slow growth with an actual slowing in rate just before adolescence. The beginning of the period of rapid adolescent growth (the "growth spurt") begins as early as age 9½ (range 9½–14½) in girls and age 10½ (range 10½–16) in boys. The growth spurt peaks at approximately age 12 in girls and age 14 in boys. During middle childhood, children tend to grow about 2 inches/year and gain about 7 lbs/year. This is a high-risk period for the development of obesity, especially in inactive children. In an infant, visual assessment for obesity is sometimes inaccurate. By the time the child reaches school age, a child who "looks" obese probably is.

The clinician will encounter some children with excessively short (less than the 5th percentile) or excessively tall (greater than the 95th percentile) stature. There are a variety of etiologies for either, depending on growth pattern, family history, and associated medical problems (e.g., endocrine abnormalities, dysmorphic features, and systemic illness). One of the most important components of the investigation of short or tall stature is a growth curve demonstrating serial longitudinal measurements.

The most common explanation for an elevated blood pressure in a child is inappropriate cuff size selection (too small). The second most common explanation for elevated systolic pressure is anxiety. Lower limb blood pressure is normally higher than upper limb blood pressure. *When lower limb blood pressure is lower than upper limb blood pressure, the possibility of coarctation of the aorta should be investigated.*

Head: Hair, Face, Eyes, Ears, Nose, and Mouth

Head and hair on head. **Alopecia** on the head is not a rare occurrence in this age group. There are a variety of common etiologies for alopecia. During middle childhood, **traction alopecia** is a common cause of localized hair loss. This is secondary to prolonged traction from ponytail holders or tight braiding. Suspect this when isolated localized alopecia is noted, particularly in the female. *Two other common etiologies for localized alopecia on the head are fungal infections (**tinea capitis**) and **alopecia areata**. Alopecia areata presents as a circumscribed patch completely without hair, with a skin surface that is smooth and devoid of stubble (in contrast to tinea capitis). "Exclamation-point hairs," which are short and stubby, may be found at the edge of the bald patch. Alopecia areata is most often idiopathic in etiology, but it may be associated with underlying thyroid or autoimmune disease. Less commonly, a more diffuse thinning of hair is apparent. This type of hair loss is seen in association with a variety of systemic illnesses but may also be idiopathic.*

Face. *The "classic"* ***facies*** *of a child with* **upper respiratory tract allergy** *is so characteristic that pediatricians can make this diagnosis from the doorway. The child has a* **long face with shadows under the eyes** *(from venous engorgement), horizontal skin creases under the lower lids (called* **Dennie's lines***), a horizontal crease just above the tip of the nose (called a* **nasal pleat***) (from wiping the dripping nose in an upward fashion), and an* **open mouth** *(because nasal congestion makes it difficult to breathe through his nose). The shadows under the eyes are called* **allergic shiners,** *and the characteristic upward nose wipe with the palm of the hand is called the a***llergic salute.** *Although the terms are somewhat comical, the condition is not. A similar constellation of facial findings is also seen in children with chronic upper airway obstruction secondary to adenoid enlargement (Fig. 15.59).*

Eyes. *Vision.* Children 5 years of age or older should read a majority of the 20/30 line. *A referral for further evaluation is warranted when the child is unable to read a majority of the figures on the 20/30 line or when there is a two-line difference in vision between the eyes (even if vision is in the normal range).*

Ears. During the summertime, school-age children commonly develop ***otitis externa,*** *or swimmer's ear. In this condition, the external ear canal is red, swollen, and exquisitely tender. The patient complains of pain on manipulation of the auricle. There is purulent material visible in the canal, often obscuring the tympanic membrane.*

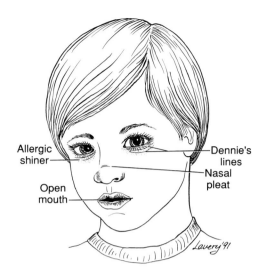

Figure 15.59   Allergic facies.

During an otoscopic examination, it is not unusual for the tympanic membrane to fail to move upon insufflation. If a good seal with the speculum is present (using the largest size speculum that will comfortably fit the canal) and there is no fluid visible behind the eardrum, other causes for a nonmobile tympanic membrane should be considered. One cause is a stiff eardrum that is extremely scarred and thickened. It usually occurs only after a long history of recurrent acute otitis media. This is actually relatively uncommon, perhaps because of the high rate of antibiotic treatment for otitis media. Another cause of a nonmobile tympanic membrane is perforation. *Perforations of the tympanic membrane occur either spontaneously or secondary to trauma. Spontaneous perforations associated with otitis media usually occur in the central portion of the eardrum, although they may occur in other locations also. Traumatic perforations most commonly occur when a child or parent places a foreign body into the ear canal and accidentally perforates the eardrum. This usually occurs when attempting to "clean" the ears using a Q-tip or bobby pin. If the location of a tympanic membrane perforation is somewhere other than the central portion of the eardrum and/or is not associated with an otitis media, suspect an etiology other than infection.*

A **retracted eardrum** is the converse of a bulging eardrum. Like a bulging eardrum, a retracted eardrum may also not move very well upon insufflation (it especially will not move "in" when the bulb on the otoscope attachment is squeezed in). Retraction of the eardrum occurs as a result of negative pressure in the middle ear space. This often accompanies Eustachian tube dysfunction. Eustachian tube dysfunction results from the inflammation that accompanies upper respiratory infections and allergies.

Nose. In this age group, many children suffer from chronic inflammatory processes in the nasal airway (e.g., repeated upper respiratory infection or allergies). As a result, the turbinates may be significantly enlarged (the lower turbinates are visible). These may be confused with nasal polyps, which are much less common than enlarged turbinates in children. *If present, nasal polyps are visible between the lower and middle turbinates. True nasal polyps may be a presenting sign of cystic fibrosis.*

Mouth. The clinician may encounter tonsils at their peak size. "**Kissing tonsils**" are tonsils that meet in the midline and are staged as 4+ in size. If swallowing and breathing are not affected and there is no acute inflammation, "kissing tonsils" may not present a problem for the patient. During adolescence, tonsil size begins to diminish. *A significant enlargement of only one tonsil is distinctly abnormal. This may signify an underlying serious infection (e.g., a peritonsillar abscess) or, rarely, a tumor.*

Pharyngitis is extremely common in this age group. The two most common causes of pharyngitis are viral infections and group A β-hemolytic streptococcal infection. The classic strep throat is heralded by bright red large tonsils and red pharynx, a yellowish tonsillar exudate, petechiae on the posterior palate, and foul-smelling breath. There is fever and enlarged, tender anterior cervical lymph nodes. The difficulty in clinically distinguishing between a strep throat and a case of viral pharyngitis is that viral infections may be accompanied by any or all of the afore-mentioned signs and symptoms classically seen in strep throats. Conversely, infec-tion secondary to strep may be present without many of these signs or symptoms.

Many viral infections of childhood are accompanied by ulcers in the mouth. There may be many ulcers (e.g., Coxsackie, primary herpes simplex, varicella) or only one or a few (e.g., aphthous ulcers ["canker sores"] and recurrent herpes sim-plex). Canker sores occur on fixed mucosa, e.g., palate or gingivae. The ulcers of recurrent herpes simplex are somewhat smaller than canker sores and usually occur on movable mucosa (e.g., on the vermilion border of the lip).

Halitosis may be noted. This may be secondary to poor oral hygiene, pharyngi-tis, or sinusitis.

The child with purulent postnasal drainage, a slight amount of erythema on ton-sils or pharynx, halitosis, and fever (with or without headache or cough) may have sinusitis.

Teeth. When the child bites down, the top teeth should overlap the bottom teeth all the way around. The clinician should also visualize whether the child bites down on the back teeth.

Shedding of primary teeth begins at around age 6, usually with the lower central incisors. Eruption of permanent teeth begins at approximately the same age with replacements for the lower central incisors as well as eruption of the first permanent molars behind the primary molars. During the subsequent 2 years, shedding and eruption of permanent replacements occur for upper central and lower and upper lateral incisors. Following this feverish oral activity, there is a period of quiescence for several years, after which the cuspids and primary molars are shed. The first bicuspids erupt at about age 10.

Neck, Thorax, and Upper Limbs

Neck. The thyroid gland may be slightly palpable (even when not enlarged) in the preadolescent.

Enlarged and tender lymph nodes in the neck are commonly found in the school-age child who is ill with pharyngitis. Enlargement of anterior cervical lymph nodes is commonly seen in strep pharyngitis. Infections caused by viruses will pro-duce enlargement of cervical lymph nodes also, sometimes with predominance of the posterior cervical chains. Epstein-Barr infection (mononucleosis) is classically accompanied by a predominance of enlarged posterior cervical nodes. This is sometimes clinically useful when attempting to distinguish between infection caused by strep and infection caused by mononucleosis. Unfortunately, no one sign is pathognomonic for either problem.

Thorax and upper limbs. During middle childhood, the trunk thins out, the thoracic cage elongates, and with the child in the erect position, the abdomen appears scaphoid. As a result of these changes, sternal deformities become more obvious than in younger children. If the sternum bows in, it is called a **pectus**

excavatum, and if it bows out, it is called a **pectus carinatum.** Occasionally, these abnormalities require surgical correction.

Asymmetry of the chest wall may signify an underlying cardiac or pulmonary problem. In this age group especially, an asymmetry or prominence of one side of the chest may also be secondary to a scoliosis.

Cardiorespiratory System

During middle childhood the PMI gradually changes location. It moves medially and inferiorly so that by approximately age 7 the PMI is felt at the fifth interspace to the right of the midclavicular line.

A third heart sound (in diastole) may be auscultated at the cardiac apex in healthy children. Without an associated pathologic heart murmur, this has no medical significance. A fourth heart sound best appreciated at the apex is pathologic.

Any of the three innocent murmurs that are often appreciated in younger children (i.e., Still's murmur, venous hum, and carotid bruit) may also be heard in a school-age child. A fourth innocent murmur, called a **pulmonary flow murmur,** may first be noted in the school-age child. This is a systolic ejection murmur that is loudest at the upper left sternal border, especially in the recumbent patient. It may disappear completely when the child is sitting up. This is a high-pitched murmur that may be soft or harsh; the intensity may vary from grade I to grade III. S_1 and S_2 are normal; there are no clicks or palpatory abnormalities.

Breasts

In females, normal breast development begins as early as age 8 or as late as age 13. Initial development may be asymmetric. If a patient or her family has not been warned ahead of time, there may be a doctor's visit in middle childhood for a "painful breast lump." This is most often a unilateral, normal breast bud signifying the onset of puberty. A breast bud may also be described as a small tender cyst or cysts underneath the nipple. This is also normal in males. "Tanner 1" (breasts, pubic hair, or genitalia) always signifies a prepubertal appearance. For breast development, this equals flat breasts with elevation of the nipples only. Most females develop Tanner 2 breasts prior to acquiring pubic hair, although the reverse order may also be within normal limits. The papillae and areola become elevated as a small mound, and the areola widens. In the United States, the average age for females to acquire Tanner 2 breasts is 10½, which coincides with the onset of the growth spurt (see Fig. 6.10).

Abdomen

A firm but not hard liver edge may be palpated 1–2 cm below the costal margin in the right midclavicular line. In this age group, the total vertical liver span assessed by using the method of palpation below the costal margin plus percussion over the rib cage should not exceed 9–10 cm.

***Abdominal pain** is a common symptom in middle childhood. Some children with abdominal pain (particularly those with acute pain) have definite, relatively easily identifiable, **intra-abdominal pathology** (e.g., acute appendicitis). Some, especially those with chronic recurring symptoms, have a problem whose source is extremely difficult to discover. Many of these have a multifactorial etiology. A third group of children with abdominal pain has definite, identifiable, **extra-abdominal** pathology. There are many important diseases that fall into the latter category. Two especially common problems in this age group may cause acute abdominal symptoms: group A β-hemolytic streptococcal infections of the pharynx and lower lobe pneumonia. When the chief complaints are fever and abdominal pain and the* *patient says "nothing else hurts," look carefully at the pharynx anyway. It might be beefy red. Also, when the chief complaints are fever and abdominal pain, even if the patient isn't coughing, auscultate the lungs carefully for adventitious sounds.*

Genitalia

Female genitalia. In females, the development of pubic hair (Tanner stage 2) begins between the ages of 8½ and 14 (United States average age is 11), approximately 6 months after the onset of breast budding. Fifteen percent of the time in normal individuals, pubic hair development precedes breast budding.

The onset of puberty in females prior to age 8 is known as precocious puberty (Fig. 15.60).

Premenarcheal females have a normal watery, nonpurulent and non-foul-smelling vaginal discharge. *Bloody, purulent, or foul-smelling vaginal discharge requires investigation for pathologic etiologies, including infection, and consideration of abuse.*

Male genitalia. The first sign of puberty in males (Tanner 2 genitalia) is testicular enlargement and scrotal skin thinning. This begins between ages 9½ and 13½ (average age is 11½). *The onset of puberty in males prior to age 9 is known as precocious puberty.*

Recognizing the beginning of testicular enlargement requires experience. There are special instruments for exact measurement of testicular volume, but these are reserved for cases in which there are special concerns (e.g., suspicion of delayed onset of puberty). The prepubertal testicle measures approximately 1½–2 cm in length.

In males, the onset of pubic hair growth (genital hair Tanner stage 2) occurs between ages 10 and 15. It usually begins with the growth of straight, slightly pigmented hair, 6 months after the onset of testicular enlargement. Since the male growth spurt does not begin until genital Tanner stage 3 (and peaks during stage 4), 2–2½ years after the onset of puberty, the school-age male with early signs of puberty may be reassured that the growth spurt is yet to come. The sequence of male pubertal development is highly predictable. However, for each particular chronologic age in males, the extent of pubertal development is very variable (Fig. 15.61).

Stage 1   No pubic hair.

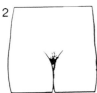

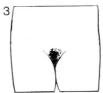

Stage 2   A sparse amount of long, somewhat pigmented hair over labia majora primarily.

Stage 3   Pubic hair darkens, coarsens and curls, and spreads sparsely over the mons pubis.

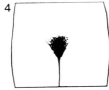

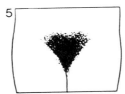

Stage 4   Abundant, coarse, adult-type hair limited to the mons pubis.

Stage 5   Adult type and quantity of hair with spread to the medial aspect of the thighs.

Figure 15.60   Tanner stages of female pubic hair growth.

Stage 1   No pubic hair.
           Genitalia are prepubertal in size.

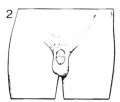

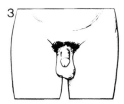

Stage 2   Sparse growth of long, slightly pigmented hair, at and lateral to base of penis. Testes and scrotum begin to enlarge, with pigmentation and thinning of scrotum.

Stage 3   Pubic hair darkens, coarsens and curls, at and lateral to base of penis. Penis lengthens and testes and scrotum further enlarge.

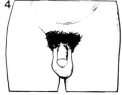

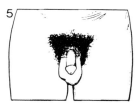

Stage 4   Abundant, coarse adult-type hair limited to the pubic region with no extension to the thighs. Further growth of testes and scrotum, with increased pigmentation of scrotum, and, Increase in width and length of penis.

Stage 5   Adult type and quantity of hair with spread to the medial aspects of the thighs. Adult size and shape of genitalia.

Figure 15.61   Tanner stages of male genital development and pubic hair growth.

Most school-age boys will have a fully retractable foreskin. *If the glans cannot be fully exposed, the patient has phimosis. By this age, most cases of phimosis are no longer developmental; i.e., most will require surgical release to prevent infection.*

Parents may raise the concern that their son has a small penis. In the majority of instances, the concern is not justified. The concern usually stems from either a misunderstanding of the normal sequence of puberty (e.g., testicles enlarge before the penis elongates) or from observing a penis that is hidden within the pubic fat pad. Penile enlargement (genital Tanner stage 3) does not usually begin until age 10½ at the earliest (the normal range is 10½–14½, which is 12–18 months after the onset of testicular enlargement). The average school-age prepubertal male will have a penile length of 6 cm (normal range is 4½–7½ cm).

Back and Lower Limbs

There is normally a mild kyphosis of the upper back and a mild lordosis of the lumbar area. On forward bending the kyphosis appears as a smooth small curve, and the lordosis disappears. Exaggeration of either of these curves requires further investigation.

Skin

Bruising is a very common skin finding, particularly in active toddlers and school-age children. Parents frequently inquire as to whether their child's bruises are normal. Bruising from normal activity is characteristically present on the anterior surfaces of the lower limbs with minimal to no bruising on the rest of the body in the setting of a normal physical examination.

When a **bruise has an unusual appearance** (e.g., linear, looped, or small and round) or an **implausible location** (e.g., on the back, scalp, or in a stocking-glove distribution) or when the **history does not fit either the injury** (e.g., a child with a black eye whose parent tells you "he fell down the stairs") or **the developmental abilities of the child,** the question of **intentional injury** should be raised. If there is a history of **prior injury** or there has been an **unexplained delay in seeking medical care** for a significant injury, such bruises further raise the question of intentional injury. Casually ask the patient or the parent, "How did that bruise happen?" **Observe** him (and his parent) while you listen to the answer.

Neurologic System and Development

Coordination. The school-age child should be able to perform rapid alternating movements such as opposition of thumb to fifth finger (then thumb to each other successive finger) in rapid sequence. By age 8 the child should be able to perform these movements within 5 seconds.

Soft signs. As the patient performs some of the maneuvers requested of him during the neurologic assessment, "soft" neurologic signs may be noted. *These are minor neurologic indicators that, when present, would be considered normal in a younger child but when observed in an older child suggest neuromaturational immaturity. Examples of soft signs in the school-age child include (1) dystonic posturing of the hands and arms while walking across the room on the heels and (2) easily observed movements of the tongue while the child concentrates on writing. Some studies have demonstrated a relationship between the presence of these findings and learning difficulties.*

Unwanted movements. Within this category, unwanted movements, *tics are especially common in the school-age child and adolescent. Tics are rapid, sudden, frequent, irregularly occurring involuntary stereotypical movements or vocalizations. These repetitive movements usually involve a functionally related muscle group or groups. Tics may be simple (e.g., eye blinking, winking, coughing) or more complex (e.g., assumption of a squatting posture). The stereotypical nature of the movements are the main feature distinguishing tics from chorea.*

Reflexes. Several beats of ankle clonus may be within normal limits if the child is not otherwise hyperreflexic and does not have increased muscle tone. The Babinski response is absent; i.e., plantar stimulation leads to flexion of the hallux.

ADOLESCENT

Techniques of Examination

AREAS OF EMPHASIS

The complete physical examination of the adolescent monitors the dramatic physical changes that occur in this age group. Attention is focused on (1) growth and changes in body habitus, (2) skin, (3) breasts and genitalia, and (4) orthopedic concerns. Observation and conversation during the examination also supply data that contribute to the assessment of the patient's affective progress through adolescence.

OVERALL STRATEGIES

The complete examination of the adolescent patient is usually performed in the classic head-to-toe order. The adolescent will be physically cooperative but not necessarily physically comfortable and may be verbally cooperative but not necessarily open. The teenager is acutely aware of his or her body and the changes that may or may not have occurred. The intimate nature of the physical examination has the potential to magnify previously existing anxieties in body image.

Therefore, one of the most important tasks for the clinician is to diffuse anxiety that may be either generated or accentuated by the examination. This may be accomplished by (1) providing thorough explanations as the examination proceeds (e.g., what you are doing and why you are doing it), (2) offering reassurance about findings that are normal, and (3) ensuring privacy and respecting modesty.

THE EXAMINATION

Before the examination, the clinician inquires about the patient's preference for a chaperone. After history is obtained, the patient is provided with a gown and requested to change into it while the clinician waits outside.

General Appearance

The patient's general state of hygiene and grooming is noted.

Measurements

Because of the substantial changes in height, weight, and body proportions, careful attention is focused on plotting measurements on the appropriate growth charts before the patient is examined. Concerns about height, weight, or both are elicited and body habitus is inspected.

Blood pressure is measured in the arm using the adult-sized cuff in a nonobese adolescent. The larger, wide-sized cuff is used in the obese adolescent and for measurement of lower limb pressure.

Skin

Because most teenagers have at least one skin rash or lesion, the skin is inspected carefully. Inquire as to which lesions were "there since birth."

Head: Hair, Face, Eyes, Ears, Nose, and Mouth

Face. Facial appearance and expression are observed closely. Is the patient alert, involved in the encounter, and communicative, or distracted, uninterested, or hostile?

Even at this age there are patients with important but undiagnosed syndromes. An unusual facial appearance may provide the strongest clue to this possibility.

Eyes. During health maintenance visits, vision is screened both subjectively by inquiry and objectively every few years. This is a high-risk period for the development of myopia or nearsightedness.

The lower lid is everted and inspected for pallor of vessels and for evidence of "cobblestoning" or low bumps on the palpebral conjunctivae seen in chronic allergic conjunctivitis.

Ears. During health maintenance visits, hearing is usually screened subjectively unless special concerns exist. When there are none, objective screening is performed once during adolescence.

Mouth. *Teeth.* Because caries and gingival inflammation are more common in this age group than in younger children, special attention is devoted to assessing general oral hygiene. Occlusion and spacing are evaluated as many adolescents require orthodontic treatment.

Neck, Thorax, and Upper Limbs

Special attention is directed toward the examination of the thyroid as problems are more common in teenagers than in younger children. The gland is examined in the same manner as in the adult.

Breasts

Breasts are inspected and palpated in the manner of the adult (see Chapter 6), and the Tanner stage is determined (see Fig. 6.10). Breast self-examination is taught or reviewed. The presence of axillary hair is noted.

Genitalia

Explanations are offered as the examination proceeds. Findings are discussed and, when appropriate, reassurance is offered.

Female genitalia. The principal purposes of the external genital examination in the adolescent female are to monitor pubertal development, search for vaginal and vulvar lesions, and rule out abnormal vaginal discharge. By proceeding slowly and cautiously, the clinician should be successful in securing the patient's cooperation.

The pubic hair is assessed for Tanner stage and inspected for infestations (see Fig. 15.60). The labia are inspected, then separated, in order to visualize the underlying structures. The clitoris is inspected for general size. The color of the vaginal mucosa (pink versus red) is noted. The hymen is assessed to determine that the vaginal orifice is not totally occluded. The vulva is inspected for inflammation, lesions, and vaginal discharges.

A pelvic examination is necessary for the patient who (1) is or wishes to become sexually active, (2) has significant menstrual pain or irregularity, (3) is experiencing abnormal puberty, (4) has lesions of the vulva, (5) has vaginal discharge, (6) has lower abdominal or pelvic pain, (7) has a history of in utero exposure to diethylstilbestrol, or (8) is suspected of being abused.

Male genitalia. The principal purposes of the genital examination in the adolescent male are to monitor pubertal development and search for penile and scrotal lesions, penile discharges, testicular masses, hernias, hydroceles, and varicoceles. Explanations are provided as the clinician proceeds.

Tanner stages of genital and pubic hair development are determined (see Fig. 15.61). Pubic hair is inspected for quantity, texture, distribution, and infestations. The penis is inspected for urethral placement, urethral discharge, and penile lesions. In the uncircumcised patient, the foreskin is retracted to inspect for lesions and to rule out phimosis.

The testicles are palpated for masses by gently rolling the testicle between the thumb and fingers while searching for hard lumps. Testicular self-examination can be taught or reviewed.

The examination for inguinal hernia is performed in the same manner as in the adult.

Rectal examination is reserved for situations in which there is suspicion of rectal, lower abdominal, or pelvic pathology.

Reassurance about the normalcy of findings is offered when appropriate. The adolescent is especially vulnerable to concerns about the genital examination.

Lower Limbs and Back

The back is carefully examined for scoliosis and kyphosis.

A traditional musculoskeletal examination may be performed. Alternately, the quick and easy-to-perform 2-minute orthopedic examination designed by the American Academy of Pediatrics may be used for pre-sports participation. It is designed to be used along with a brief set of questions that screens for major illnesses and conditions that would contraindicate or influence sports participation (Table 15.7).

Table 15.7
The Two-Minute Orthopedic Examination

Instructions	Points of Observation
Stand, facing examiner	Acromioclavicular joints; general habitus
Look at ceiling, floor, over both shoulders; touch ears to shoulders	Cervical spine ROM
Shrug shoulders (examiner resists)	Trapezius strength
Abduct shoulders 90° (examiner resists at 90°)	Deltoid strength
Full external rotation of arms	Shoulder ROM
Flex and extend elbows	Elbow ROM
Arms at sides, elbows 90° flexed; pronate and supinate wrists	Elbow and wrist ROM
Spread fingers; make fist	Hand or finger motion and deformities
Tighten (contract) quadriceps; relax quadriceps	Symmetry and knee effusion; ankle effusion
"Duck walk" four steps (away from examiner with buttocks on heels)	Hip, knee, and ankle ROM
Back to examiner	Shoulder symmetry, scoliosis
Knees straight, touch toes	Scoliosis, hip ROM, hamstring tightness
Raise up on toes, raise heels	Calf symmetry, leg strength

^aROM, range of motion.

Neurologic System and Development

The neurologic examination of the adolescent is similar to the neurologic examination of the adult. For routine encounters with most adolescents, information regarding school performance and athletic involvement, combined with a standard physical examination, provide sufficient information for monitoring development.

At the conclusion of the examination, the patient should be thanked for cooperating. In the outpatient setting, the patient should be requested to change back into street clothes while the clinician steps outside of the examination area. Then, summarize any additional information that needs to be conveyed or discussed. Provide the patient with the opportunity to ask questions or bring forth concerns. If parents have not been present, discuss with the patient whether or not to invite parents into the room and determine beforehand what will be discussed. Close the encounter by reviewing plans for further diagnosis or treatment or future visits. If it is true, tell the patient that you enjoyed the encounter.

Normal and Common Variants and *Clues to Abnormalities*

Measurements and Body Habitus

During puberty, girls grow about 7.5 cm/year for a total of approximately 22.5 cm and gain about 17 kg. Boys grow about 10 cm/year for a total of approximately 33 cm and gain approximately 27 kg. The growth spurt in girls is an early pubertal event that peaks on average at age 12, 1 year after the onset of breast development and about 1¼ years prior to the onset of menarche. In boys, the peak of the growth spurt is a late pubertal event and occurs about 2–2½ years after the onset of puberty. During puberty, body proportions change also: The width of female hips increases, the width of male shoulders increases, and the male leg length exceeds the female leg length.

During a complete examination, it is extremely important for the clinician to have the opportunity to observe the adolescent undressed. Some patients by themselves cannot or will not bring forth concerns about body surfaces or body image. *The adolescent with anorexia nervosa may choose to conceal her body with loose-fitting clothing. Unless she is undressed, the clinician may not appreciate how desperately thin she appears. When her measurements are plotted, the clinician will also appreciate that she has lost 20–50% of her normal body weight.*

In addition to concerns about weight or height, the adolescent may present problems associated with the timing and sequence of pubertal events. Attention to the patient's age, Tanner stage, and sequence in which pubertal events occur and the comparison to established norms should assist in uncovering pathology or providing reassurance. The events of puberty generally proceed in a relatively predictable fashion, with subtle, normal variation. When findings or events exceed established norms, further investigation is indicated. For example, the female who develops pubic hair before beginning breast development may be entirely normal (15% of normals develop in this sequence). There may be a 6- to 12-month separation between these two events. *The circumstance in which a female develops Tanner 5 pubic hair without any breast development is distinctly different and well outside the expected range of normal (e.g., gonadal dysgenesis). The clinician who pays close attention to the growth curve might uncover this problem early, as short stature is an associated finding (Fig. 15.62).*

Skin

Skin problems are extremely common in this age group, e.g., acne; superficial fungal infections, particularly *tinea corporis* or ringworm; *tinea pedis* or athlete's foot; *tinea cruris* or jock itch; and *tinea versicolor*. Atopic dermatitis continues to be a problem. *Psoriasis* may first appear in this age group; it is very uncommon in younger children. These skin problems have the same appearance in adolescents and adults.

Head: Hair, Face, Eyes, Ears, Nose, and Mouth

Face. By adolescence, the sinuses are fully aerated. If sinusitis is suspected, the clinician may attempt to transilluminate the frontal and maxillary sinuses in the same manner as in the adult. This procedure is not feasible in younger children: prior to adolescence, the soft tissues and skull bones are too thick to allow the usual light source to penetrate.

Eyes. Allergic manifestations in the head region are extremely common findings in teenagers. *The child with **allergic conjunctivitis** has red, itchy eyes. There*

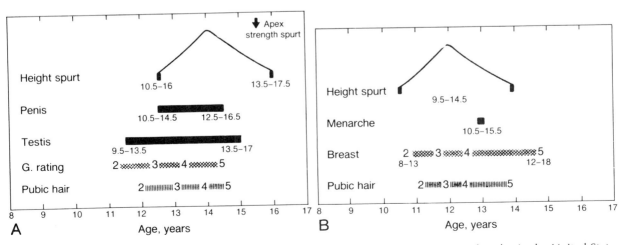

Figure 15.62   Timing of normal pubertal development in males (**A**) and females (**B**). For females in the United States, the entire sequence is displaced to the left by 4–6 months.

may also be a diffuse swelling of the palpebral conjunctivae (called chemosis) and a stringy drainage. Cobblestoning of the conjunctivae is present in chronic cases.

Nose. ***Allergic rhinitis*** *is common in this age group. The nasal mucosa is pale, gray, and boggy (swollen) versus inflamed and friable secondary to an upper respiratory infection. The adolescent with these findings but without infection should be queried about nasal spray overuse and about cocaine.*

Nasal polyps are more common in adolescents than in children. Etiologies include infection of the nose and/or the sinuses, or allergy as part of an association with asthma and aspirin intolerance, or cystic fibrosis.

Mouth. Second molars erupt during early adolescence (ages 12–13). Third molars or, wisdom teeth, erupt during late adolescence (ages 17–21).

Neck, Thorax, and Upper Limbs

Neck. The normal size of the palpable part of the lateral lobe of the thyroid should not exceed the size of the patient's terminal thumb phalanx. If either lobe is larger than this, the patient probably has an enlarged thyroid.

Thorax and upper limbs. Chest pain is a relatively common complaint in this age group. Most healthy adolescents with this complaint do not have underlying heart, lung, or gastrointestinal disease, although these systems do need to be considered in the diagnostic process. *One common etiology for chest pain may be diagnosed during the physical examination:* ***costochondritis.*** *Costochondritis is a problem of musculoskeletal inflammation of one or more of the costochondral junctions. It most commonly involves the upper chest on the left side. The diagnosis is established by palpating, at the site of symptoms, one or more costochondral junctions that are tender and sometimes swollen.*

Breasts

In females, if puberty has not begun by about age 13 or if there is no progression of puberty during a 2-year period after it has begun, puberty is delayed.

Gynecomastia, or breast development in a male, is a common finding during puberty. It is most commonly observed during Tanner genital stage 4 and usually regresses within 1–1½ years. The gynecomastia associated with puberty may be bilateral or unilateral and symmetric or *asymmetric.* This should not be confused with **pseudogynecomastia,** or the appearance of breast development that is commonly seen in obese males.

Axillary hair in both sexes begins to grow approximately 2 years after pubic hair appears.

Cardiorespiratory System

Occasional isolated (less than about 6 or 7/min) premature beats are common and are usually not abnormal, especially if they disappear with exercise.

Still's murmur and venous hum are less common in the adolescent than in the younger child; the pulmonary flow murmur is most common and may be more easily heard in the anxious patient. Heart sounds and murmurs may sound louder than normal in the adolescent who has narrowing in the anterior-posterior dimension of the thoracic cage, without the normal mild kyphosis of the upper back (straight back syndrome).

Recently, there has been increased recognition of mitral valve prolapse. Findings are the same as in the adult (see the Extended Examination section of Chapter 8).

If femoral pulses are delayed or diminished or if upper-limb blood pressure is elevated, ***coarctation of the aorta*** *must be ruled out. Unfortunately, this diagnosis may be delayed until adolescence. The systolic murmur of a coarctation need not* *be louder than a grade 2 or 3 and may be heard along the left sternum or at the apex and, significantly, is also heard in the back between the scapulae. Evidence of collateral circulation must be searched for. The best way to examine for collaterals is to ask the patient to lean over in the same manner as in the scoliosis examination. Palpate for pulsatile collaterals around the scapulae and in the infrascapular areas, as well as between the ribs. Check the systolic pressure in the legs. If it is the same as in the arms, coarctation is ruled out.*

Abdomen

*The incidence of **acute appendicitis** in children peaks in this age group. The classic presentation is one in which the patient initially develops a loss of appetite and diffuse abdominal pain or pain concentrated in the epigastrium or periumbilical area. Subsequently, the pain localizes to the lower right quadrant, and the patient develops fever, nausea, and vomiting. The child may be observed to lie preferentially supine with knees flexed. As the process progresses, examination will reveal diminished bowel sounds, voluntary guarding, and generalized tenderness that is maximal in the right lower quadrant. Eventually, rebound tenderness may be elicited. Late in the course, guarding becomes involuntary, and the abdomen feels rigid. There are many variations in both the history (e.g, the presence of diarrhea, vaginal discharge, or atypical location of pain) and the physical examination (e.g., minimal abdominal tenderness with tenderness in the flank, or tenderness only appreciated during a rectal examination). Just as for the adult, a female adolescent must have gynecologic emergencies considered in the differential diagnosis.*

Genitalia

Female genitalia. The vaginal mucosa in the prepubertal child is thin and red. Under the influence of estrogen, the vaginal mucosa in the pubertal female becomes thicker, dull, and pink. The width of the normal clitoris is 2–4 mm. *If the width of the clitoris approaches 10 mm (or greater), the clitoris is enlarged or masculinized.*

A common normal finding is **physiologic leukorrhea,** a whitish vaginal discharge that results from the influence of estrogen. There are no accompanying signs of inflammation or symptoms of pain or itching.

Male genitalia. The normal prepubertal testicle measures between 1½ and 2 cm. A prepubertal testicle that is smaller or larger than this size may be abnormal. Normal testicular length in normal adult males is 4–5 cm. ***Macro-orchidism*** *(enlarged testes) in adolescents is associated with the fragile X syndrome, a common cause of mental retardation, particularly in males. Other dysmorphic features of this syndrome include large ears, a prominent forehead, and a large jaw.*

Males who have not entered puberty by approximately age 14½ require evaluation for delayed puberty.

Back

Idiopathic scoliosis may be detected at any time during adolescence but most commonly worsens during the period of rapid growth. Occasionally, because the spine is rotated on its vertical axis, it looks as if it is straight when visualized from behind the patient. In this instance, with a true scoliosis, one or more pairs of paraspinal structures will be asymmetric in height or prominence (e.g., shoulders, scapulae, iliac crests).

Lower Limbs

Two problems pertaining to the knee are extremely common: Osgood-Schlatter disease and chondromalacia patellae. ***Osgood-Schlatter disease*** *is a stress injury to the patellar tendon at the site of insertion on the tibial tubercle. This occurs in early-*

to-mid puberty, particularly in the active adolescent. This causes increasing unilateral knee pain. Physical examination will reveal a tender tibial tubercle, which may be swollen. An x-ray will exclude other diagnoses.

Chondromalacia patellae is caused by an instability or maltracking of the patella, which results in softening of the patellar articular cartilage. It is particularly common in the female adolescent who complains of knee pain, particularly during flexion (e.g., sitting, climbing stairs, etc.). On physical examination, the patient will complain of pain when the patella is manipulated laterally or medially with the knee in extension; the examiner may feel crepitation with this maneuver. Further evaluation with special views on x-ray may confirm the diagnosis and rule out others.

The adolescent who develops a limp and has pain referable to the groin, upper thigh, knee, or buttock may have pathology in the hip joint. One problem particularly affecting overweight males in the acceleration phase of the growth spurt, without a preceding history of trauma, is a ***slipped capital femoral epiphysis.*** *This is a slippage of the head of the femur off the metaphysis, usually in a posterior-medial direction. Physical examination may reveal limited range of motion at the hip and/or an outtoeing gait.*

RECOMMENDED READINGS

Algranati PS. The pediatric patient: an approach to history and physical examination. Baltimore: Williams & Wilkins, 1992.

Algranati PS. Pediatric clinical encounter. In: Willms JL, Lewis J, eds. Introduction to clinical medicine. Media, Pennsylvania: Harwal, 1991.

American Academy of Pediatrics Committee on Practice and Ambulatory Medicine. Vision screening and eye exam in children. Pediatrics 1986;77:918–919.

American Academy of Pediatrics Committee on Psychosocial Aspects of Child and Family Health. Guidelines for health supervision. 2nd ed. Elk Grove Village, Illinois: American Academy of Pediatrics, 1988.

Amiel-Tison C. Neurological evaluation of the maturity of newborn infants. Arch Dis Child 1968; 43:89.

Apley J. Listening and talking to patients. Br Med J 1980;281:1116–1117.

Ballard JL, Khoury JC, Wedig K, et al. New Ballard Score, expanded to include extremely premature infants. J Pediatr 1991;119:417–423.

Ballard JL, Novak KK, Driver M. A simplified score for assessment of fetal maturation of newly born infants. J Pediatr 1979;95:769–774.

Comerci GD, Kilbourne KA, Harrison GG. Adolescent nutrition. In: Hofmann AD, Greydanus DE, eds. Adolescent medicine. 2nd ed. Norwalk, Connecticut: Appleton & Lange, 1989:431.

Copeland KC. Variations in normal sexual development. PIR 1986;8:18–25.

Dubowitz L, Dubowitz V, Goldberg C. Clinical assessment of gestational age in the newborn infant. J Pediatr 1970;77:1–10.

Dworkin PH, Wible KL, Sutherland MC, Humphrey N. Manual of pediatric anticipatory guidance. Morgantown, West Virginia: West Virginia University Medical Center, 1986.

Emans SJH, Goldstein DP. Pediatric and adolescent gynecology. 2nd ed. Boston: Little, Brown, 1982.

Engle MA. Heart sounds and murmurs in diagnosis of heart disease. Pediatr Ann 1981;10:21.

Farr V, Mitchell R, Neligan C, et al. The definition of some external characteristics used in the assessment of gestation age of the newborn infant. Dev Med Child Neurol 1966;8:507.

Frankenburg WK, Dodds J, Archer P, Shapiro H, Bresnick B. The Denver II: a major revision and restandardization of the Denver Developmental Screening Test. Pediatrics 1992;89:91–97.

Galazka SS. Clinical magic and the art of examining children. J Fam Pract 1984;18:229–232.

Goldenring JM, Cohen E. Getting into adolescent heads. Contemp Pediatr 1988;July:75–90.

Green M. Twenty interview questions that work. Contemp Pediatr 1992;9:47–71.

Hofmann AD, Greydanus DE. Adolescent medicine. 2nd ed. Norwalk, Connecticut: Appleton & Lange, 1989.

Kaplan SL. Normal growth. In: Rudolph AM, ed. Pediatrics. 17th ed. Norwalk, Connecticut: Appleton-Century-Crofts, 1982:93.

Mahoney CP. Differential diagnosis of goiter. Pediatr Clin North Am 1987;34:891.

McCarthy PL, Lembo RM, Fink HD, Baron MA, Cicchetti DV. Observation, history and physical exam in diagnosis of serious illness in febrile children ≤24 months. J Pediatr 1987;110:29–30.

McCarthy PL, Sharpe MR, Spiesel SZ, et al. Observation scales to identify serious illness in febrile children. Pediatrics 1982;70:802–809.

Moss JR. Helping young children cope with the physical exam. Pediatr Nurs 1981;March/April:17–20.

Moss JR. Teaching adolescents testicular self-exam. Childrens Nurse 1988;6:5.

National Institutes of Health Consensus Development Conference Statement. Neurofibromatosis. Bethesda, Maryland: U S Department of Health and Human Services Publications, 1987;6:1–7.

Nelson LB. Pediatric ophthalmology. Philadelphia: WB Saunders, 1984.

Renshaw TS. Pediatric orthopedics. Philadelphia: WB Saunders, 1986.

Schmitt BD. Preschoolers who refuse to be examined: fearful or spoiled? Am J Dis Child 1984;138:443–446.

Smilkstein G. The pediatric lap exam. J Fam Pract 1977;4;743–745.

Smith J, Felice M. Interviewing adolescent patients: some guidelines for the clinician. Pediatr Ann 1980;9:38–44.

Solomon R. Pediatric experiences in year II clinical sciences. E Lansing, Michigan: Department of Pediatrics and Human Development, College of Human Medicine, Michigan State University, 1986.

Staheli LT. Torsional deformity. Pediatr Clin North Am 1977;24:803–806.

Task Force on Blood Pressure Control in Children. Report of the second task force on blood pressure control in children—1987. Pediatrics 1987;79:1–4.

Telzrow RW. Anticipatory guidance in pediatric practice. J Cont Educ Pediatr 1978;20:14–27.

Walker WA, Mathis RK. Hepatomegaly. Pediatr Clin North Am 1975;22:933.

16

Special Challenges

Clinical problem solving begins with, and is deeply grounded in, the careful and accurate acquisition of the medical history. When the process does not go well, whose fault is it? There is a large body of literature directed at problems in medical history taking: clinician-engendered problems, patient-generated problems, and problems created by the interface. This chapter explores some of the more common and troublesome difficulties encountered (or created) by interviewers. The problems are grouped somewhat arbitrarily, then described with suggestions for solutions.

PROBLEMS RELATED TO FLAWED INTERVIEWER TECHNIQUE

As direct observation by preceptors and/or trained patient instructors has become more commonly practiced in medical education, it has become possible to begin categorizing and analyzing the patient-encounter process and its contribution to history-taking flaws. In 1979, Platt and McMath published the results of their direct observation of medical interviews done by internal medicine residents and began a classification system. Since that time, a number of papers have been published by other investigators. Stillman et al. have created an instrument useful for standardizing specifics of the medical interview that contribute to its strengths and weaknesses.

Absence of Amenities

A fruitful interview demands a setting in which amenities are possible, distractions are minimized, and patient comfort—in so far as possible—is attended to. Privacy and confidentiality have to be established by the clinician-interviewer, and the task to be carried out must be clear to the patient, which requires explanation by the clinician. The common courtesies of human intercourse must be honored.

Inaccurate or Incomplete Database

The clinician has the responsibility for obtaining accurate data. To do so, she needs to press for detailed primary information, i.e., the patient's symptoms—the story of his illness—in his own words. Secondary information, such as that acquired from a third party or from medical records, must be checked whenever possible against the patient's own narrative. Only when the patient cannot, for cognitive (or other valid) reasons, give the medical history, should the interviewer accept other data; and then, the source must be clearly identified. Legitimate barriers to a direct account by the patient include severe dementia, uncontrolled psychiatric difficulty, inability to speak the same language as the interviewer, and willful fabrication. Even in the setting of dementia, the patient's own account has been shown to provide helpful data that cannot be acquired otherwise.

If a patient responds to a question with a medical diagnosis or with a recitation of laboratory results, the clinician then requests a review of the symptoms that led to the particular diagnosis and then *makes her own decision* about that diagnosis based on this primary information. Great patience (and, occasionally, much time) is required to obtain these details, but without them the database is less dependable.

Active listening is essential for garnering accurate data. The clinician must concentrate on each patient response and, while still maintaining the basic structure of the interview, follow the cues that she hears. She explores unexpected leads as far as they contribute to the narrative, reacts appropriately to emotional responses, and checks information periodically for accuracy by summarizing. Maintenance of eye contact and an attentive body position inform the patient that the clinician is interested, involved, and listening to the story. Note-taking is kept to a minimum in order not to interfere with eye contact and active listening but is realistic when types and volume of information exceed unassisted memory capacity. The patient will (rightly) suspect that the clinician is not listening if he finds her repeating requests for information already given (except for further clarification) or notes that she frequently makes errors in summarizing. If the patient feels that the doctor is not listening, his account will become flawed and the relationship jeopardized.

The clinician carefully documents the specifics of the symptoms. Sometimes this requires going back over the parameters in search of clarification. For example, the implications of leg pain that occurs only with exercise and goes away promptly with rest are very different from implications of leg pain made worse by sitting or lying down. The precise location of the pain may also be part of the key to diagnosis. The patient is asked to point to the place(s) in his leg where he experiences the pain. Detailed documentation is pursued until the symptom and all its dimensions are understood.

Poor Organization

Although the patient's narrative is essential to the history process, it is the clinician's responsibility to make an advance plan, to keep it in mind, and to implement it. Even the most alert and cooperative patient will slip into digressions and irrelevancies if the interviewer does not maintain cogent *organization,* signal *transitions* from one aspect of the history to another, maintain a *pace* that allows for exploration of important information without bogging the history down in aimless wandering, and exert proper *control* of content—not so much as to seem tyrannical, nor so little as to allow waste of time.

Failure to Formulate Hypotheses

As the clinician gains experience in diagnosis and patient care, she becomes increasingly adept at formulating hypotheses during the course of the medical history. Certain symptoms and stories of illness evoke a clear impression about the systems or disease processes involved. As a diagnostic hypothesis surfaces, the clinician selects appropriate courses of questioning to test that hypothesis. Questions that would otherwise be relegated to the review of systems (ROS), the past medical history (PMH), the family history (FH), or the personal profile (PP) will require early exploration in hypothesis testing. They are "drawn in" to the present illness. If further questioning leads to refutation of a hypothesis, so be it. Throw it out and formulate another. The active process of formulating, testing, and then retaining or rejecting hypotheses is the mark of a good diagnostician, the problem solver that every clinician must be. Failure to *impose strategy,* order, and hypotheses results in an amorphous mass of uninterpretable history.

Premature Closure

The hazard of hypothesis formulation is premature closure—settling on a final diagnosis before adequate information has been obtained. No matter how appealing the first hypothesis may be, the clinician must avoid jumping to a diagnosis before all pertinent information has been sought. For example, the complaint of chest pain must not be diagnosed as angina pectoris until the major differential possibilities have been considered and tested against the historical facts: Is there a trauma history that could explain the symptom? What are the particular circumstances under which the pain occurs? Is the patient's age, lifestyle, or family history characteristic of coronary artery disease? Are the features pointing to the esophagus, trachea, or sternum rather than to the heart? And so on through the relevant data points in hypothesis testing.

Failure to Summarize

Only by reiterating what she has heard and understood of the patient's narrative—however briefly—can the clinician be assured that all the important information has been obtained and is accurate. When the patient hears his story summarized and responds to the instructions to make additions and corrections, the present illness history becomes complete.

PROBLEMS GENERATED BY THE PATIENT OR HIS SITUATION

It is very easy to blame the patient for a confusing or incomplete history. Every tired intern will sometimes speak of the "poor historian," lack of cooperation, and patient unreliability. Although this plea can also reflect the clinician's own failure, there are certainly situations in which even the most insightful and experienced clinician is unable to obtain satisfactory information. Patients who are cognitively impaired, either intellectually or psychiatrically, or who do not speak or understand the clinician's language or cultural expectations often cannot provide sufficient useful information to allow hypothesis generation and testing.

Cognitively Impaired Patient

The decision to declare a patient unreliable to provide his own history is based on direct observation by the clinician. Obviously, a comatose adult or an infant or small child cannot supply a verbal history, and other means must be employed to obtain the necessary information. Usually, an informant accompanying the patient is chosen, and prior medical records are consulted.

Less obvious are the subtle memory deficits of a mildly demented person or the marginal reliability of a patient with borderline intelligence. The interview is notoriously insensitive at detecting mild-to-moderate intellectual impairment or psychiatrically mediated unreliability. For these purposes formal bedside mental status testing can help distinguish patients who are incapable of accuracy (see Fig. 11.15, Folstein mini-mental status examination). If doubt about reliability persists, the clinician may try reasking an occasional question with altered wording and then to tally the patient's consistency of detail. Ultimately, she may have to cross-validate with third-party verification.

The patient with a *psychosis,* either toxic or functional, presents a different type of challenge. If able to interact with the clinician at all, these patients sometimes provide very detailed, technically convincing, *apparently accurate,* and pseudoinsightful medical histories; however, the history must be viewed with caution until validated by independent observations and accounts from other parties. The clinician thus avoids discounting everything asserted by the patient but maintains a healthy skepticism. In contrast to the situation with the deficits mentioned above, the content and process of the interview itself often provide valuable clues to the nature of the psychosis if it is not already known; effective mental status assessment in this setting begins during the conversation. Unsuspected delusional states, paranoid thoughts, or suicidal ideation, for example, might surface for the first time during the conduct of a medical history. (The psychiatric interview, as a formal entity, is beyond the scope of this text.)

Seductive Patient

An occasional patient communicates, through body language, attire, behavior, or speech, an inappropriate sexualization of the encounter. These behaviors may represent a routine modus operandi for some patients—an innocent flirtatious demeanor used in everyday human interactions. If the clinician is able to remain scrupulously professional, such patients will usually modify the behavior and get to the business at hand.

When the clinician finds seductive behavior disconcerting or interfering with the conduct of the interview, it may become necessary to confront the patient with the discomfort created by the behavior. If the clinician communicates—either explicitly or by careful attention to professional distancing—an interest in and availability to the patient *only* as a clinician, not as an object of sexual interest, most patients will respond appropriately. If the clinician cannot make the patient discontinue seductive behavior, the encounter may have to be terminated.

Language Discrepancies: Jargon and Native Tongue

It is incumbent on the clinician taking a medical history to ascertain the potential for misunderstanding based on language differences between her and her patient. The most common difficulty arises in the realm of medical sophistication: An intelligent, cooperative, English-speaking patient is bewildered by the medical vocabulary that has become familiar to the clinician through daily use. This is a problem only when the clinician either does not recognize or refuses to bridge the gap. She must assess early in the interview how much "jargon" can be used. *When in doubt, use ordinary language.* Many patients, not wishing to appear ignorant, feign understanding, so the burden is on the clinician not to fall into this trap. The potential for inaccurate communication between patient and clinician is very high.

It is demeaning to talk down to the patient. Condescension is not inevitably linked to the avoidance of jargon. In discussing a problem with an adult, a sound alternative, for example, to "you have a lesion of the rectus abdominis" is "I find a problem in the midline of your belly." If your patient understands medical terms and you've ascertained this, you can stay at the level at which he is knowledgeable, but check regularly to make sure that the two of you are continuing to understand one another.

Dialect and/or region-specific word usages present additional potentials for difficulty. In these instances, the clinician must carefully observe answers to questions for language discrepancies and watch the patient's facial and body signs indicating hesitancy or confusion about a word or term. If a patient response doesn't seem to make sense in the context, try another word or draw a simple sketch—even a stick figure—to clarify the word(s). For example, in some regions the word hypertension means high anxiety or hyperactivity, while in other regions it means, as it does for health professionals, high blood pressure. In Boston, many patients call a stroke "a shock"; in Hartford and Missoula they usually do not. Dialect without usage differences generally requires advising the patient to stop you if he doesn't understand your dialect—or you stopping the patient if you don't understand him—and slowing speech somewhat.

Non-English speakers may require a formal translator for the conduct of the medical history. When available, the best translator is one who is medically sophisticated and fluent in both languages. More commonly, medical interviewers rely on family members, often children, to convey information between clinician and patient. This situation is fraught with communication hazards. Some terms are not readily translatable; others have very different overtones across languages. Privacy issues and confidentiality concerns dominate translated questions and answers about "private" bodily functions. The interviewer must choose her words very carefully and ascertain that the translator understands the question and transmits it easily and nonjudgmentally, constantly observing both parties for facial, verbal, or body language indicating discomfort or confusion. It is the clinician, not the patient or the translator, who is responsible for determining the accuracy of the communication. If the responses don't make sense or if the patient appears uncomfortable with a question, it may be necessary to move to sketches, photographs, or hand movements. These interviews are often long and painstaking for all parties, requiring great patience and calm reassurance on the part of the interviewer. Even at that, they often fail, as the translator's beliefs, value system, and hypotheses vitiate both questions and answers.

Third-Party Interviews

When it becomes necessary to rely on a third party to obtain medical history, two precautions apply. First, the relationship and duration of proximity of the informant to the patient must be understood in order to establish the degree and type of information that can reasonably be obtained and relied on. For example, the passerby at the scene of an accident can be expected to give only his version of what he witnessed. At the other end of the spectrum, a spouse or live-in caretaker may be able to provide detailed responses about many dimensions of a disease or disability, both from his or her own observations and from what he or she has learned from the patient's descriptions of the symptoms he is experiencing. The patient's children—commonly called on as translators—will not usually repeat questions about sexual history and practices. Third-party information should not be substituted for direct patient information if the patient is able to provide anything. If there is a discrepancy between two accounts, both must be considered in making diagnostic decisions. For example, if the demented patient moans and points to his belly, but the informant insists that he always complains that it's his chest that hurts, the clinician has to investigate *both* possibilities.

INTERACTIONAL PROBLEMS: THE DIFFICULT DYAD

Although a self-protective tendency exists in all of us—i.e., to blame the patient if things do not go well—increasing attention is being given to the duality of culpability. Some of the instances noted above evoke such negative or frustrated responses in the clinician that communication deteriorates still further. Since the clinician is the professional, she must make the greater effort to bridge the gap when interactional trouble arises.

Gorlin and Zucker attempted to classify clinicians' reactions to various "types" of patients and to demonstrate how clinician behavior accelerated interactional difficulties. Groves selected four models of what he labeled "hateful patients" and made suggestions for improving the relationships between these patients and their medical caregivers. Some of the more commonly experienced difficult dyads and strategies for dealing with them are considered here.

Hostile (Angry) Patient

Hostility represents a prototype of patient attitude and behavior apt to evoke a similar response in the clinician. The immediate human reaction to another's outrage is either flight or fight. The professional who is placed in the caretaking role rarely has "flight" as an immediate option; thus he may respond to hostility with hostility—and the fight is on. An angry exchange inevitably leads to flawed data collection, impaired decision making, and poor patient management.

Why are some patients hostile? Pain, fear, previous bad experiences with the health care system, underlying problems of character and psyche, loss of control over one's body—all of these and many more illness responses may cause a patient to strike out at the clinician.

Why do we, as caregivers, react with anger? Because we are puzzled and hurt, and our need to be liked and respected by our patients is threatened. We resent when the enormous effort poured into our work is met with blame.

What can we do to defuse the hostility of the patient and prevent a nonproductive encounter? First and foremost, refuse to assume responsibility for the problem, unless you have created it. Explicitly acknowledge the hostility of the patient before you respond further. Attempt to learn why it is there. One simple strategy is to stop the interview and deal with the hostility directly: "You look and sound very angry, Mr. Jones. Would you like to talk about what you are feeling?" Once acknowledged openly, hostility is difficult to maintain without exposing its etiology. If the patient erupts, hear out his complaint. If his issue is legitimate, let him know that you can understand why he is angry. If the anger has no apparent basis in reality, hear it anyway and do not quarrel with it. Often, after the patient has been allowed to explode, or to cry, or otherwise to express his anger, he will be ready to proceed with the business at hand. If he continues to be hostile, but you keep your composure and remain gently insistent on carrying through the interaction without fighting, you will usually be successful in obtaining the information needed.

Rarely is the hostility personal and deliberately intended for you. If it is based on a misunderstanding or misinterpretation of something you have said or done, you may attempt to correct the error; if you attempt this, it must be done without anger. When the patient speaks a truth with which you can agree—that you really have done something about which he has every right to be angry—explanation or apology may be in order. Keep it simple. Remember that all clinicians make errors and that this is the nature of human fallibility.

Sometimes, no matter how well you handle the hostile patient, anger continues to be expressed. For example, a patient may have a racist prejudice against your particular ethnic group, or a gender bigotry, or ageism. Do the best you can to cope with the frustration you feel. If you are unable to continue without being engaged in a verbal struggle with the patient, you may have to excuse yourself and either come back at a later time or ask a colleague to carry out the interview.

Mutual Dislike

Some interactions are doomed to failure because of a mutual dislike between clinician and patient. These situations are uncommon, but when they occur, they must be recognized and accepted for what they are. Often, in today's medical practice, a student, house officer, or consultant and a new patient are thrust on each other by the circumstances of the system—and it turns out to be a mismatch. The interview becomes an angry struggle or a cold war. Data collection may be dangerously impaired, the patient's interests may be ill-served, and you may be unable to handle the situation objectively and effectively. If the two of you—

clinician and patient—cannot set aside your mutual dislike in order to accomplish the task at hand, a colleague must be summoned and responsibility transferred.

Gender Barriers

There will be instances in which gender obstructs the relationship between patient and clinician. Even today, when women are commonly found in the clinician role, some patients—*both men and women*—are unable to feel comfortable or secure with a woman as clinician. The inability of a patient to trust or take seriously the clinical competence of a woman constitutes a major barrier to effective history taking.

What can you expect, and how can you respond? A minor variant is the assumption that a white-coated woman physician is a nurse. Most persons who make this presumption in error will learn by being corrected. There is more difficulty with patients who make it clear that they are unwilling to cooperate when the professional woman introduces herself as the clinician designated to take the history and to do the physical examination. They may permit the interview to begin but will display distraction or rudeness or answer questions incompletely. They may laugh inappropriately and try to divert the interview away from the medical information you request and into irrelevant chitchat. For example, they may repeatedly turn the interview around, asking questions about your boyfriend, or children, what your parents think about your choice of profession, etc. If you remain pleasant, but private and firmly insistent on your need to get medical information, some such patients will begin to cooperate. It is your responsibility to determine whether or not you will be able to get a reliable database; if you determine you cannot, you may be forced to seek a colleague to take over the history or care of the patient. There are also patients who prefer or even demand a woman clinician. As with the opposite preference, the man who encounters this barrier must determine if it is powerful enough to prevent an effective history and must respond accordingly.

Mutual sexual attraction—either cross- or same-gender—is an unusual event in the initial professional encounter. The clinician, on recognition of this phenomenon, has the responsibility of making the professional role a priority. The clinician must provide the emotional distancing necessary for effective data collection. If this is not possible, then the clinician must relinquish the role to a colleague.

Age- and Status-Related Barriers

Occasionally, a young clinician will encounter a patient who cannot accept youth as trustworthy or competent. As with the gender-specific preferences of some patients, the age issue may be overt or covert, and its potential for impeding effective data gathering is dealt with similarly. One of the authors (H. S.) grew a beard 20 years ago to minimize this occurrence, but such an external change is fundamentally unnecessary. More sensible is an explicit, simple statement, free of defensiveness, that you possess standard qualifications. Some controlling patients will try a parallel and more pernicious ploy: "You're only the medical student [intern, fellow, new attending]." While formulae are generally to be avoided, a good answer to this is "Yes, I am. Why don't you see how I do?" Such a response conveys being comfortable with and confident in your role and status, and allays the fear that may underlie the question.

Dying Patient

There is an enormous volume of literature on the interactional difficulties created by the patient who knows he is dying and the clinician responsible for obtaining information from and providing care to this patient. Every clinician must be familiar with the psychology and the emotional lability attached to anticipation of death—that of the care-givers as well as that of the patient. While the patient is processing what it means to him to die—a complex, convoluted, and unstable emotional roller-coaster—the clinician is struggling with failure as a lifesaver, her own vulnerability to death, and her pity or sorrow for the patient.

Before entering the room of a dying patient, the clinician must determine how much the patient knows about his diagnosis and prognosis and be prepared to deal openly with mutually shared knowledge. If, for whatever reason, the patient is still ignorant of his prognosis, this is critical constraint on the clinician. Unless charged with giving the bad news, the clinician has the practically and ethically difficult task of feigning ignorance. This is particularly troublesome if the patient suspects he is dying but has not been informed of such.

How do you handle the interview of an informed dying patient? If you enter the room of a patient who knows he is dying, you must be prepared for most anything during the conduct of the medical history. Follow the patient's leads. If he is angry, hostile, and withholding, try empathic silence or, better still, acknowledge that you are aware of his prognosis and realize that he must be very upset. Do not allow yourself to show resentment at his anger—he is not angry at you personally, even though he acts out his anger in your presence. He is much more likely to be angry at God. If he cries, let him do so. Wait, even touch, until he is able to continue—and offer tissues. If he asks you to leave or insists on terminating the interview, do so—but with the promise that you will return soon to resume your task.

These can be very difficult interview situations, especially for the clinician who has no prior relationship with the patient. But with patience and acute awareness of the emotional state of the dying person, the interview can prove gratifying to both parties—informative and satisfying to the clinician and therapeutic for the patient.

Cultural Barriers

It is impossible for any clinician to have a full awareness of all possible cultural nuances attached to illness, but she must be conscious that they can arise in any interview situation. The meaning and value of "dis-ease" varies widely among ethnic cultures, with regional health practices, with religion and with *individual* belief systems, and with the sophistication and protocol within the clinician's own medical culture.

When you encounter a patient who has recently come to your country, particularly if there is an associated language barrier, be especially cognizant of the possibility of both miscommunication and misunderstanding. Observe facial expression and body language closely for signs of discomfort or confusion. Attempt to ascertain the patient's perception of the meaning of his symptoms as they are discussed in order to know that you are both talking about the same phenomena. When you are uncertain about a description given by the patient, retain his own words or gestures, rather than trying to paraphrase, until you can be absolutely sure that you understand what he means. If possible, after obtaining as much information as you can, discuss the case with a colleague who has experience or knowledge of the culture of the patient, or go to library sources that deal with the particular culture and its illness beliefs.

Under no circumstances should you deride, express horror, or laugh at a patient's ideas or methods of describing his symptoms, treatments he has tried, or beliefs he may express about the meaning of the problem. Our particular cultural approach to health and illness, while natural and rational in our own view, is not necessarily correct, trusted, or even comprehended by a significant number of the patients we encounter. To communicate effectively with patients whose views differ from ours, we must first respect and try to understand their need to retain their own cultural autonomy.

Overly Dependent Patient

The situation of the overly dependent patient tends to evolve over time rather than in a single encounter. Personal neediness, often associated with depression, usually underlies the patient's clinging dependency. The clinician is frequently flattered at first, feeling deeply appreciated for her professional skills. However, the dependency eventually becomes a nuisance and dooms the relationship to failure, since the patient's dependency needs require that the clinician's helping attempts fail. Then, guilt, resentment, and impatience replace the gratification initially felt by the provider.

When the clinician senses the first hint of dependency, it is time to set limits. This is most difficult to do when a patient is seriously medically ill, but neither patient nor clinician can benefit from uncontrolled dependency behavior. Tactfully but firmly inform the patient that there are limits to what you can do for him and to the time and energy you can expend on his needs. It is often difficult to admit—to yourself, let alone to others—that you cannot be all things to all people. However, if you don't admit this and follow through with its necessary corollary—*limit-setting*—the therapeutic potential of the relationship is doomed. When limits are not set by the clinician or the patient fails to abide by them, aversion and rejection follow. It is the responsibility of the clinician to control dependency or, failing this, to transfer the care of the patient to someone who can.

Self-destructive Patient

The psychology of the self-abusive patient lies beyond the scope of this chapter. However, relentless self-destruction is familiar to every clinician, as are the responses these behaviors evoke in caregivers. These are the patients who, consciously or unconsciously, do things to themselves that clearly lie opposite to their own best interest. The chronic bronchitic who continues to smoke, the hypertensive who is careless about taking medication, and the diabetic who ignores dangerous weight gain exemplify self-destructive behaviors. The alcoholic and the abuser of intravenous drugs offer still more glaring examples.

The clinician who is responsible for working with these patients is in danger of misassigning blame to herself for failure to change the patient's behavior. Such blame ignores the fundamental nature of adult behavior—that it is not controllable by outside persons no matter how earnest, wise, tireless, and giving the outside persons may be. This error of perception leads to guilt and self-recrimination, to anger at the patient for causing feelings of failure, and thus to further damage to a therapeutic alliance already attenuated by divergent goals.

A few strategies can modify the patient's behavior or at least let the clinician absolve herself of the misguided and fruitless sense of failure. In some instances, *depression* is the basis of self-destructive denial; therefore, evaluation for the presence of treatable depression is worthwhile when the behavior is first recognized. The patient may refuse such evaluation or refuse to cooperate with treatment if depression is diagnosed. Should this occur, the clinician may confront the patient with her recognition of the patient's behavior and the impediments it creates in the professional relationship. Occasionally, a candid exploration of the patient's motives will permit an agreement about sharing responsibility. If the patient is willing to try it, a *contract* may be drawn up in which the actions and obligations

SPECIFIC SEXUAL CONCERNS RAISED BY THE PATIENT

During the course of the routine sexual history or elsewhere during the interview, the patient may have specific questions or concerns about personal sexual function. Below are some of the more common concerns and some amplification questions that the clinician may employ.

Sexual Concerns Specific to Men

Impotence. When a man complains that he is impotent, it is important to define what he means by the word. Is he truly experiencing the inability to attain and maintain an erection long enough for intromission? Or is he describing some other phenomenon, such as loss of sexual desire, anorgasmia, inability to ejaculate, or premature ejaculation? The details of a history of true impotence are critically important to the establishment of its cause and can be obtained from answers to the following questions:

1. How often and under what specific circumstances is the patient unable to attain (or maintain) penile erection?
2. How long has the problem been present?
3. Is is getting better, worse, or not changing?
4. Is he able to masturbate to erection?
5. Does he awaken with erection?
6. Is he taking any medications or recreational drugs? If so, what are the names, doses, and temporal relationship to impotence?
7. How much alcohol does he use?
8. Does he have any known chronic illness?
9. Are there concurrent stresses in the patient's life, particularly in his relationship(s) with his sexual partner(s)?
10. Are there symptoms of aortic vascular insufficiency (e.g., buttock claudication)?
11. Has the man sired a child in the past (establishes prior function)?
12. Is there a history of diabetes mellitus?
13. Is libido preserved or lost?

Premature ejaculation. This refers to the inability to defer ejaculation long enough to satisfy the partner and is the most frequent sexual complaint of younger men. Exactly what happens, and how is it affecting his relationship with his partner(s)? This problem is most often functional and related to mechanics and timing between partners. The interviewer obtains sufficient information to determine the type of counseling indicated.

Ejaculatory incompetence. This is defined as the inability to ejaculate after achieving erection. The follow-up questions are the same as those noted for impotence.

Sexual Concerns Common to Men and Women

Loss of libido (sexual desire). Determine the specifics:

1. What is the chronology of the complaint?
2. Is it partner-specific?
3. Are there stresses in the relationship(s), sexual or otherwise?
4. Are there other life stresses?
5. Does the general medical history raise other health problems as the potential basis for loss of sexual interest?
6. Are there signs and symptoms of depression?

Lack of sexual responsiveness. This is frequently referred to by the patient or partner as "frigidity." Try to determine the following:

1. Precisely what does the patient experience that is being regarded as lack of responsiveness? Is it a lack of interest in sex? If so, the clinician pursues the same line of questioning as outlined for the patient describing loss of desire. Or is it based in some other concern, such as fear of pregnancy or sexually transmitted disease, experience of pain with intercourse, unacceptable sexual practices, emotional reaction to prior unpleasant or brutal sexual encounter, or fear of precipitating or suffering stroke, heart attack, or sudden death?
2. What are the details of past and current sexual practices and dissatisfactions?

Sexual Concerns Specific to Women

Anorgasmia. This refers to the inability to achieve orgasm. Try to determine the specific type:

1. Has the patient ever achieved orgasm, either with masturbation or with a partner? Having never experienced an orgasm is termed **primary anorgasmia**.
2. Does the patient achieve orgasm under certain circumstances (what are they?) and not under others (what are they)? **Situational anorgasmia** is the inability to have an orgasm under very specific circumstances.
3. Is she erratically and unpredictably unable to have an orgasm (**random anorgasmia**)?
4. What is the chronology of the anorgasmia and can it be related by history to physical, pharmacologic, emotional, social, or interpersonal events?

Dyspareunia. This refers to pain or discomfort on intercourse. Ask about the specifics:

1. What are the details of the complaint, e.g., the specific physical location of the pain, the nature and duration of the pain, the timing of the pain relative to the sequence of the sexual act (on intromission, with deep thrusting, postcoital, etc.), relationship to body position during intercourse?
2. What is the chronology of the symptom, e.g., is it new or longstanding? Partner-specific? Cyclic, related to menstrual cycle? To bowel function? To voiding? Getting better, worse, or unchanged? Alleviating or aggravating factors?
3. Does the patient feel she has adequate vaginal lubrication prior to intromission? If not, have lubricants been used, and if so, what is the effect?
4. Is she satisfied with the nonsexual aspects of the relationship(s) with her partner(s)?
5. What are the details of sexual practices, such as use of devices that might be causing perineal or vaginal trauma?
6. Has the patient ever been a victim of rape or other sexual violence?
7. Is the patient able to supply any insights into the cause of the painful intercourse?
8. Is there postcoital vaginal bleeding or spotting (important both for diagnosis and for affective context)?

SEXUAL CONCERNS RAISED BY PHYSICAL EXAMINATION

On routine physical examination, the clinician may note findings that necessitate a return to more detailed sexual history. The patient may have been completely unaware of the problem or may not even have related it to sexual practice. More likely, he consciously chose not to bring it up during the medical history or felt inadequate opportunity or "permission" to do so. Among the physical findings that suggest a need for extended sexual history are (*a*) signs of genital, perianal, perineal, or oral trauma, such as bruises, excoriations, bites, or anal tears; (*b*) evidence of infection, such as urethral or vaginal discharge, condyloma, inguinal or generalized lymphadenopathy, pubic lice (pediculosis pubis), or genital vesicles; (*c*) unexplained pelvic tenderness or mass; (*d*) cervical friability, cervical os discharge, or cervical motion tenderness; or (*e*) vaginal atrophy or estrogen-deficiency vulvovaginitis.

Extended Substance Use History

The clinician decides to seek details of substance use when there is an indication that abuse may be a problem for the patient. This particular portion of the history, when it must be expanded, requires sensitivity to the *possibility of denial* as well as a nonjudgmental approach. Alcohol, since it is the drug most commonly used—and abused—in our society, will be dealt with separately from other chemicals such as marijuana, cocaine, and heroin.

Alcohol, because it is legal, readily available, and an intrinsic part of our social lives, presents particular hazards for the consumer. It is estimated that 10% of the population in the United States has some degree of alcohol-related problem affecting health or social function or both. It is the clinician's responsibility to assess drinking patterns in each patient for whom she is responsible. Every clinician is occasionally humbled by a case where she has missed alcoholism for years.

The screening history for alcohol use is based on the assumption that the patient uses alcohol to some degree; therefore, the introductory question is "How much alcohol do you use?" rather than "Do you use alcohol?" This eliminates the element of judgment and makes it easier for the user to answer candidly; the nonuser should not be offended but can simply correct the interviewer's assumption. Ewing's CAGE screening questions provide a useful device:

• Have you ever felt the need to	**C**ut down on drinking?
• Have you ever felt	**A**nnoyed by criticisms of drinking?
• Have you ever had	**G**uilt feelings about drinking?
• Have you ever taken a morning	**E**ye opener?

Another set of questions has been suggested by Clark:

1. "How do you feel about your drinking?"
2. "Do you ever have negative thoughts or feelings about drinking?"
3. "Has a family member, friend, or physician ever told you he was worried about your drinking?"

If the answers to one or especially to several of these questions are positive, or if the affective nonverbal responses to them are positive, the clinician should have a follow-up strategy in mind. In particular, a history of *morning drinking* has a very high predictive value for alcoholism. The typical patient with an alcohol problem has considerable reluctance to discuss his drinking based on denial, cognitive deficits, and/or painful feelings of anxiety, guilt, and shame. These deterrents to accurate data collection are difficult to overcome. Following are some useful techniques for breaking through these defenses:

1. Focus on the *effects* of alcohol consumption rather than on frequency and quantity. "What happens to you when you drink?" Whether addicted or not, people with alcohol problems drink when they didn't intend to, drink more than they intend to, and suffer some mixture of emotional, physical, social, occupational, financial, and legal difficulty when they drink uncontrollably. Another useful query is, "Have you ever been arrested for driving under the influence of alcohol?"
2. Maintain an accepting attitude of the patient as person while discussing his drinking patterns ("love the sinner; hate the sin"). His self-esteem is low, and

positive reinforcement of his good qualities will greatly facilitate the interview and the therapeutic alliance.

3. As rapport is established, persist in direct questioning. Ask about alcohol- and withdrawal-related physical symptoms, such as blackouts, shakiness, or seizures. Explore conflicts and regrets about drinking. Inquire about family, job problems, and legal problems, especially difficulties with DWI (driving while intoxicated) or DUI (driving under the influence). Be explicit in asking about symptoms of depression and suicidal ideation.

Other than alcohol, the most frequently used substances in the United States are **marijuana, cocaine, amphetamines, and heroin.** The legal ramifications of use of these chemicals adds another dimension to the difficulty in getting accurate information. Again, a nonjudgmental approach to queries will facilitate data collection.

When a patient acknowledges that he uses any of these substances, inquire about the method of use. For example, are amphetamines taken by mouth or intravenously? In what form(s) and by what route(s) is cocaine taken? Additional questions might include the following:

1. Do you use more than one substance at a time?
2. Are you always able to stop using when you want to?
3. Have you had "flashbacks" or "blackouts" as a result of using?
4. Do others express concern about your substance use?
5. Do you ever feel guilty about using?
6. Have you experienced withdrawal symptoms when you've stopped using, or have you been treated to prevent withdrawal symptoms?
7. Have you had medical problems as a result of using, such as convulsions, heart or skin infections, venous clots, memory loss, hepatitis, or a positive HIV test?
8. Have you missed work or lost a job because of using?
9. How do you get the money to purchase the substance(s)?
10. Have you been in trouble with the law as a result of using?
11. Do you skin-pop (a method of injecting drugs that is utilized when there are no longer usable veins)?
12. Do you shoot the pocket? (This is an injection—often by a paid assistant—of the junction of the internal jugular and subclavian veins and is fraught with medical complications.)
13. Do you share needles? Do you clean them?
14. How do you clean your "works?"
15. What water source do you use to dilute (tap, toilet, etc.)?
16. Have you been in any addiction-treatment programs?

If any of the questions is answered in the affirmative, ask the patient to provide details.

Family Violence History

Abuse of children, spouses, or the elderly is estimated to occur in a quarter of the families living in the United States. Therefore, the clinician needs to be prepared to pursue this possibility, particularly in the setting of suspicious injuries. As with other sensitive or potentially threatening content areas, an empathic, nonjudgmental attitude is essential for getting complete and honest information.

When suspicion is raised by trauma as the presenting complaint, the inquiry should be direct: "Tell me exactly what happened when you fell down the stairs." If the response does not make sense or does not correlate with the injuries sustained or the patient is evasive or vague, be more explicit: "Were you pushed by someone?" Persistence in acquiring details of an injury may overcome defenses and finally permit the patient to reveal previously unspoken abuse. If abuse is substantiated by the patient, the history and the pattern of prior abuse, if any, are obtained.

If the patient initially denies abuse, the topic can be raised again as a part of the personal profile: "Who lives in your household?" "How are the relationships among members of the household?" "How do you resolve major disagreements?" "Does anyone ever hit you?"

Family history provides another opportunity to explore the possibility of violence, since violence often appears to be a learned behavior. "Was your mother beaten by your father?" "Were you or your spouse abused as children?" A positive answer indicates the need to return to the presenting injury complaint and restate the possible abuse questions. Follow-up questions include

1. Have bones ever been broken?
2. Does sexual abuse take place along with physical abuse?
3. Have burns, punctures, slashing, whipping, or confining been practiced?
4. What other person has been victimized by the same abuser?
5. Has legal action such as a restraining order ever been implemented?
6. Has help ever been received from social agencies or from a victims' assistance group?
7. Is the abuser likely to remain in the household (or visit the health care site), and what is the potential for further violence?

Mental Health History

Vestiges of our cultural nonacceptance of emotional distress sometimes make the mental health history a difficult content area in the medical interview. There are several clues that a detailed mental health history should be pursued. They include

1. Presenting symptoms that are commonly associated with emotional disturbance, e.g., recent changes in weight, difficulty sleeping, trouble concentrating, memory impairment, fatigue
2. Feelings of worthlessness or hopelessness
3. A history of current substance use
4. A history of recent major change in family or job status
5. A family history of mental illness
6. A history of prior treatment for emotional problems
7. Accelerated or sustained high stress in the patient's environment
8. Chronic illness, disability, or a newly diagnosed serious illness
9. Inappropriate affect—blunted or exaggerated—during the interview
10. Poor personal hygiene or negligence in dress, or extravagant, inappropriately formal, elegant attire
11. Evidence of a thought disorder, difficulty remembering details of the medical history, or an inability to engage in normal conversation

When the clinician determines that an extended mental health history is indicated, the initial questions should be open-ended and phrased so as not to cause defensiveness or incite denial: "How has your mood been?" "How are you sleeping?" "How is your energy?" The patient's responses provide some leads for more detailed, closed questioning, which must always include details of both *prescription and over-the-counter medications.*

Symptoms suggestive of *depression* or situations that the patient perceives as hopeless demand a determination of *suicide risk.* The best way to approach the potential for suicide is by direct questions: "Do you ever think about killing your-self?" "Do you ever wish you were dead?" If the answer is "yes," follow with the question, "Have you thought about how you would kill yourself?" Ask the patient to describe his plan, then determine whether he has the means available to him, and ask "would you go through with it?" Inquire about any past attempts at suicide. The patient at risk for suicide constitutes a medical emergency and should not be allowed to leave the premises. Immediate psychiatric consultation is imperative. Recall that accidentally successful suicide is common even with "mere" suicide gestures. Know also that *elderly men* have the *highest ratio of completed to attempted suicide*. Finally, both adolescents and the aged often present atypically, with a less dysphoric depression. Suicide is such a tragedy and so often preventable that we must never miss the possibility of it—and yet we all do.

SPECIAL CONTENT AREAS

Environmental Health History

Recognition by clinicians of the potential for specific diseases arising from toxic exposures in the environment is a relatively new phenomenon. Following is a systematic approach to the *exposure history* when the present illness or other segments of the history suggest that more detail is necessary.

Because hazardous exposures may cause nondiagnostic symptoms involving any body system and may mimic more ordinary medical diseases, the following points should be incorporated into the screening medical history:

1. Obtain from the development of the HPI any temporal relationship to work or home activities, any history (recent or remote) of toxic exposure, and contributing factors such as smoking or medications. An illness similar in description to that of the patient in a family member or work-colleague may reflect (*a*) a true common exposure (toxic or infective), (*b*) the psychologic tendency to develop or recognize symptoms that an associate has, or (*c*) mere coincidence.
2. Obtain a full employment history, current and remote, with information about duties. Include work done during military service.
3. Even if the HPI has no potential for relationship to toxic exposure, in the ROS explore any history of exposure to fumes, dusts, chemicals, radiation, or loud noise. Remember that *recreation* as well as *occupation* can produce these exposures (e.g., a hobby involving soldering of lead).

If there appears to be a temporal relationship between the patient's symptoms and work or home exposures, detail the timing, e.g., do the symptoms recede or exacerbate in any pattern that would suggest intermittent exposure? Easing of a symptom when the patient is off duty can embody both relief of ongoing exposure and reduction of stress.

When there appears to be a relationship between symptoms and setting, further explore the potential sources.

Work exposure. Obtain the following information:

1. A full list of all jobs held, with the description of duties, duration, and dates
2. A full list of sites of employment and products manufactured
3. A full account of the worker's tasks at each job and, if available, diagnoses
4. A description of any similar symptoms among fellow workers
5. An account of what protective measures were employed, such as noise protection, earguards, ventilation, lead aprons, respirators, and gloves, and how consistently the individual employed them
6. An account of any monitoring that was done of personnel (radiation badges, serial chest radiographs, etc.) or worksite (measurements on air, water)

Other environmental exposure. Obtain the following information:

1. A description of neighborhood pollution, such as nearby industry, exposure to contaminated work clothes of other family members (a recognized mechanism of asbestosis in spouses of insulation workers), and sickness among neighbors
2. A description of possible exposure to household toxins, such as pesticides, chemicals used in hobbies, aerosols, cleaning fluids, or disinfectants, and information about ventilation when using potentially hazardous chemicals and symptoms manifested by any family member

Follow-up information. If any of the other questions yield positive answers, seek more specific information on follow-up:

1. The product or, better yet, the chemical composition of any suspected or possibly harmful substance to which the patient has been or is exposed
2. The physical form in which the chemical is used, e.g., liquid, dust or powder, or gas
3. How the substance is handled, e.g., the protective measures used, operating and cleanup procedures, surveillance procedures, ventilation of the area
4. The potential mode of entry of the substance, e.g., skin exposure, inhalation, eating or smoking with contaminated hands

When a suspicion of hazardous exposure comes from the extended medical history, the sleuthing for cause and effect goes into full swing. Consultation with an occupational health professional or organization may be indicated. For further details on hazards in the work and home environment, see Goldman's paper in the Recommended Readings.

Dietary and Nutritional History

Indications for expanding the screening dietary history may (*a*) arise as part of the HPI, (*b*) be raised by the patient, (*c*) surface during another portion of the routine history, (*d*) result from unexpected physical examination findings, such as inanition, or (*e*) come from results of laboratory tests, such as lymphopenia or hypoalbuminemia.

Symptoms in the HPI. Some symptoms from the dietary and nutritional history that merit attention are

1. A recent loss or gain of greater than 10% of previous weight
2. The presence of a chronic disease such as diabetes mellitus, gastrointestinal disease, hyperlipidemia, vascular disease, or hypertension
3. A condition that increases metabolic demands, such as protracted infection, trauma, malignancy, burns, or bedsores.
4. A condition in which nutrient losses are increased, such as vomiting, diarrhea, chronic blood loss, hemodialysis, or draining sites of infection
5. A change in the ability to cut and handle food, to chew, or to swallow
6. Residence in a nursing home coupled with any of the above

Signals in other portions of the history. Other findings from the history that merit attention are

1. A PMH of food allergies or intolerances
2. A history of difficulty adhering to prior diets prescribed for medical conditions
3. A history of fad or crash dieting, use of appetite depressants or stimulants, anorexia, bulimia, or any substantial and repetitive weight swings
4. A FH of diseases that may genetically predispose the patient to nutritional risk, e.g., diabetes mellitus, breast or colon cancer, hyperlipidemia

5. PP indicators that the patient's lifestyle may place him at risk for nutritional disorders, e.g., alcohol consumption, limited finances, physical disability that may impair food shopping or preparation, or ethnic or cultural food practices that are difficult to follow in the patient's microenvironment

Signs from the physical examination. Physical examination signs that merit closer scrutiny are

1. Body weight varying more than 20% from ideal
2. Unexplained skin or mucous membrane abnormalities such as angular cheilosis, gingival bleeding, glossitis, or diffuse rashes
3. Extensive dental caries, particularly on posterior (lingual) aspects of teeth
4. Subcutaneous or tendinous nodular deposits suggesting xanthomas
5. Poor muscle development and/or tone that is not otherwise explicable

If it is determined that a detailed nutritional history is necessary, several areas may be developed.

A 24-hour dietary recall. The clinician asks the patient to recite in detail what he ate during the past 24 hours. Each meal is described in terms of what foods, what quantities, and how frequently the patient ate. Was this day's food intake typical?

A history of dietary additives. Does the patient take vitamins or food supplements? If so, which ones and what quantities does he take each day? For how long has he supplemented his diet? Does he use laxatives? If so, what type and how often?

A history of dietary aversions or taboos. What types of foods does the patient never eat?

Current use of any prescription or over-the-counter medications. Does the patient take any "medications" that could lead to a nutrient-drug interaction?

Attitude toward eating and toward dietary habits. Does he enjoy food? Does he snack or rely on "fast-food" for nutrition? Can he taste and smell his food? Has there been any change in appetite? Does the patient worry about being too thin or too fat? If so, how does he address the problem?

Nutritional resources. Does the patient have the financial and physical resources—including teeth—to maintain adequate nutrition? Does he possess an understanding of healthy dietary habits?

If the clinician is suspicious of any problem with nutrition, but is unable to gain adequate information from these queries, she may choose to ask the patient to keep a written food diary (quantitative and qualitative) for several days. Alternatively, the patient may be referred to a nutritionist for assessment.

HIV History

The rapidly evolving understanding of HIV disease mandates that this section be considered provisional. The extended history currently related to HIV infection is indicated for risk assessment (*a*) when the patient expresses concerns about exposure or (*b*) when the clinician discovers suspicious abnormalities on physical examination, and (*c*), in modified form, when a patient with known HIV disease is seen.

Risk assessment. To determine the patient's risk for HIV, the clinician needs to elicit

1. An extended sexual history (see Extended Sexual History under the subheading Difficult Interviews: Content Problems, earlier).
2. An intravenous and/or parenteral drug use history including time frame, frequency, and sharing of apparatus (see Extended Substance Abuse History under the subheading Difficult Interviews: Content Problems, earlier).

3. A history of blood product transfusions. What products were received? When and where? Essentially all blood products in the United States since 1985–1986 have been safe. Prior exposures or exposures in other locales represent more risk, e.g., with the French and German scandals.

Occupational exposure is relatively unlikely. However, inquire about whether the patient has been involved in handling bodily secretions of HIV-positive patients? If so, explore the possibility of punctures with contaminated instruments (most commonly needle-stick injuries) or splashes onto open wounds, dermatitic skin, or mucosal surfaces (eyes, mouth). The history of precautions is a variant of that for any other occupational risk.

Patient concerns. If a patient expresses concerns that he may have been exposed to HIV, ask him to share the basis of his concerns, then inquire about any information missing from the risk assessment history. A history of no high-risk behavior coupled with persistent or major concerns may reflect any of four situations: (*a*) ignorance about transmission, often coupled with (*b*) susceptibility to popular hysterical attitudes toward HIV; (*c*) an incomplete database, often resulting from reticence or concealment about risky behavior; (*d*) psychologic disturbance, a gamut from heightened and global anxiety to frank delusions of AIDS.

Unexplained physical examination findings. Almost any organ system may be involved as a result of infection with HIV, although very few findings are absolutely specific for HIV disease. It is unusual to uncover AIDS in an unsuspecting patient, but the clinician should be alert to the possibility if she discovers any of the following not otherwise explicable:

1. Generalized lymphadenopathy
2. Retinal abnormalities, particularly cotton-wool spots in an otherwise healthy young person or the unexplained combination of retinal exudates and hemorrhages coursing along the retinal vessels
3. Mental status abnormalities, most specifically evidence of cognitive impairment *without* psychopathology in a young person
4. Kaposi's sarcoma (KS) of skin (note that KS of the feet or lower legs in elderly men of Jewish or Mediterranean descent does *not* increase suspicion of HIV disease) or of mouth or *strikingly severe* psoriasis, seborrheic dermatitis, or polydermatomal bilateral herpes zoster infection
5. Fever, if it is protracted and unexplained by history
6. Stool samples positive for blood, if otherwise unexplained
7. Severe, extraordinary, necrotic and ulcerative genital and/or oral herpes simplex lesions
8. Unexplained oral lesions of thrush, *any* hairy leukoplakia, or KS

Patient with known HIV disease. In patients known to have HIV disease, the interview serves, among other functions, as assessment for complications. The seven parameters of any new symptom are obtained, and prior symptom status is updated. Ongoing therapy is assessed for complications, side effects, and effectiveness.

Since HIV often causes a chronic and progressive fatal illness, special consideration is given to the following concerns.

Functional status and activities of daily living. How many of the required activities of daily living is the patient able to carry out for himself? Does he have the physical and financial assistance he needs? What additional services would enhance his quality of life? Who is taking care of laundry? Shopping? Food preparation? Cleaning of home? Administration of medications?

Support systems. Are the patient's emotional and social needs being met? Does he have a support network adequate to provide comfort and companionship? Is he in touch with special service organizations, either volunteer or paid?

Nutrition. Inanition is often a major problem. In addition, adverse reactions to medications commonly cause nausea, so the potential for being weakened through malnutrition is commonly amplified in this way.

Bowel function. Refractory diarrhea occurs frequently in patients with AIDS, sometimes from infections or enteric neoplasia, sometimes from medicines, sometimes from HIV itself, and sometimes from treatment. The first step in taking care of this major problem is to find out about its presence and severity.

Preventive therapy and immunizations. Many patients with AIDS will be receiving pills (such as zidovudine), monthly inhalations of pentamidine, and often a host of other treatments. The clinician needs to review these to ascertain supply, cost, consistency of use, and problems. An immunization program is also important and is subject to the same needs. This is also a good time to review, if necessary, the patient's awareness and practice regarding transmission of HIV to others, in particular via needles, blood products, and sex, and nontransmission via social contact and ordinary activities of daily living.

Cough, respiratory status, and supplemental oxygen. Respiratory difficulties may dominate symptoms in AIDS. Routine questioning allows for earliest diagnosis and, at times, best therapy.

Pain control. The presence, locale, and severity of pain depend on particular complications. Your inquiry establishes information and enhances empathy.

Mouth care. Some oral complications such as an especially pernicious gingivitis can be minimized or avoided with good oral hygiene, so the effort of asking and counseling is well justified.

Visual function. Cytomegalovirus (CMV) retinitis can cause blindness, so ask about its earliest symptoms in AIDS—visual floaters and reduced visual acuity.

Nontraditional and unproven therapies. Give the patient a forum to let you know if he's using herbal medicines or other products unapproved in the United States.

Advance directives. Many, but not all, persons with AIDS will have strong preferences about feeding tubes, CPR, and the use of mechanical ventilation. The routine visit is the time to establish these, not when an acute crisis occurs.

Coping with impending death. How much does the patient know about his condition and its anticipated course? What are his fears and concerns about the immediate and the farther future? What plans has he made for dealing with difficulties as they arise? Who are the persons on whom he relies for help in the case of an emergency? When he needs to talk or cry? (See also the subsection Dying Patient under the heading Interactional Problems: The Difficult Dyad, earlier.)

SPECIAL CHALLENGES IN THE PHYSICAL EXAMINATION

There are situations in which the physical examination is made difficult by patient condition or physical setting. The mentally and/or physically impaired patient may need to be examined in a different sequence or by using alternative techniques to those employed for fully mobile and cooperative patients. Under certain circumstances a suboptimal setting is the only one available for physical examination, e.g., the patient's home, an incompletely equipped bedroom in an extended-care facility, or an emergency in a non-health care facility.

EXAMINING THE MENTALLY IMPAIRED PATIENT

Because of limited understanding, or perhaps the memory of a prior bad experience, the **mentally retarded** patient may be fearful of or resistant to standard physical examination maneuvers. Special attention must be paid to the comfort and privacy needs of the patient. Routinely allowing a trusted family member or caregiver to remain in the room during the examination will sometimes alleviate anxiety and enhance cooperation. The examination should be slowly paced and deliberate and may require more than one visit to complete. Careful observation of general appearance and behavior, of responsiveness, and of mobility will guide the clinician in determining which aspects of the physical examination are most crucial. As with children, the more invasive or potentially frightening portions of the examination should be deferred until late in the session so as not to preclude less threatening but essential components.

Mentally Retarded Children

The examination of the **mentally retarded child** must incorporate the following essentials:

1. *Developmental assessment,* e.g., height, weight, growth stage, sexual development in the adolescent, and motor skills
2. Identification of associated abnormalities, e.g., neurologic or cardiac disorders
3. Components of focus when there is no chief complaint include
   a. General body proportions
   b. Head circumference and shape
   c. Hair texture, skin lesions, and rashes
   d. Visual and auditory function
   e. Palatal integrity, tongue size, and dental health
   f. Heart murmurs
   g. Bone and joint deformities
   h. Neurologic dysfunction

Mentally Retarded Adults

The examination of the **mentally retarded adult** in the absence of specific symptom focus should include

1. Determination of *functional capacity*
   a. Motor and cognitive skills to carry out activities of daily living, e.g., eating, personal hygiene, toileting
   b. Language skills including receptive comprehension
   c. Visual and auditory function
   d. Dental health
   e. Nutritional status
2. Routine examination of the physically well, retarded adult includes screening appropriate to the sex and age of the patient, including breast and pelvic examinations, Papanicolaou smear, rectal examination, and stool testing for occult blood
3. Examination components requiring special attention are
   a. General appearance

b. Skin lesions such as those caused by contractures, pressure injury, self-inflicted injury, or fungal infections

c. Hearing assessment—if not possible using routine means, then if indicated, by referral to an audiologist for evoked potential testing

d. Visual acuity, assessed by observing the patient's response to visual stimuli; if funduscopic examination is absolutely required and one attempt fails, gentle restraint or sedation may be necessary

e. Oral examination for caries, periodontal disease, candidal stomatitis

f. Cardiac examination for abnormal heart sounds such as an increased S_2P or murmurs

g. Musculoskeletal examination for muscle tone, joint deformities, and active and passive joint range of motion

h. Neurologic examination including assessment of swallowing, chewing, and sucking; muscle stretch reflexes for symmetry; gait and gross coordination during transfers to and from the examining table (sensory function, individual muscle strength, and fine cerebellar function usually cannot be accurately tested)

EXAMINING THE PSYCHIATRICALLY ILL PATIENT

The examination of the **emotionally disturbed or psychotic** patient may be impaired by hostility or lack of cooperation. Occasionally, a skilled mental health worker or family member may be able to cajole the patient to cooperate with physical examination. If a comprehensive or focused physical examination is imperative to the well-being of a persistently resistant psychotic patient, use of physical or chemical restraint may be appropriate, but the majority of these patients try to cooperate.

EXAMINING THE PHYSICALLY DISABLED PATIENT

The physical examination of the bedridden, wheelchair-bound, or otherwise disabled patient calls for additional time, prioritization of maneuvers, and alterations in technique and sequencing. Assistants may need to be called on to help in lifting, rolling, or repositioning the patient who is unable to help himself.

Special and early attention must be given to examination of the organs most likely implicated in the HPI or raised as particular concerns by the patient or his caregivers, often requiring a change in examination sequence. The positioning of the patient is dictated by the limits of his mobility and may require a change in the usual examination pattern, e.g., the entire examination may have to be done with the patient supine. In such a case the examiner will need to move frequently from side to side of the bed to accomplish her task.

Patients Who Are Unable to Sit or Stand

If the patient is **unable to sit or stand,** there are adaptations that may be made to accomplish indicated portions of the examination.

Funduscopic examination. If the height of the head of the bed permits, the fundi may be visualized by leaning over the patient from above his head, asking him to focus on the ceiling and proceeding as usual (Fig. 16.1). Alternatively, the examiner may have to inspect the right eye from the patient's right side, then move around the bed to examine the left fundus.

Cardiac examination. If special maneuvers are required to assess a murmur, squatting and Valsalva are usually impossible. However, isometric hand grip or passive straight-leg raising, if hip mobility allows, can provide useful manipulation of heart sounds and murmurs. Afterload increase may also be induced by inflating sphygmomanometers on both arms.

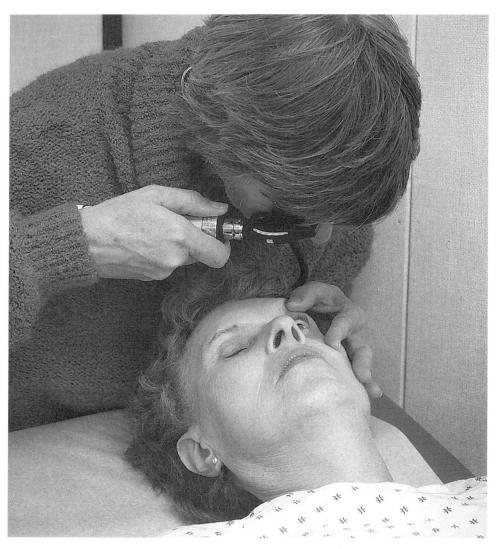

Figure 16.1 The bed-bound patient requires that the examiner optimize funduscopic visualization. One means is examining from the head of the bed, with the patient's neck very slightly passively flexed. Results are inferior to those obtained with seated patients.

Pulmonary examination. Evaluation of the lungs can be accomplished with the help of an assistant to roll the patient onto the left side for assessing the right hemithorax, and then to the right for assessment of the left lung. Percussion is achieved in the same manner as auscultation and fremitus. If the patient cannot be turned, limited auscultation is accomplished by sliding the diaphragm of a stethoscope under the patient's thorax (Fig. 16.2). Turning is, however, preferable (Fig. 16.3).

Rectal examination. The patient is placed, with assistance if required, in the left lateral decubitus position with left hip and knee fully extended, right hip and knee fully flexed, and trunk turned slightly prone. The examiner elevates the right buttock with one hand to expose the anal orifice and inserts the gloved finger of the opposite hand.

Examination of the back. While the patient is in the left lateral decubitus position, the examiner inspects the skin of the lower back and buttocks for any

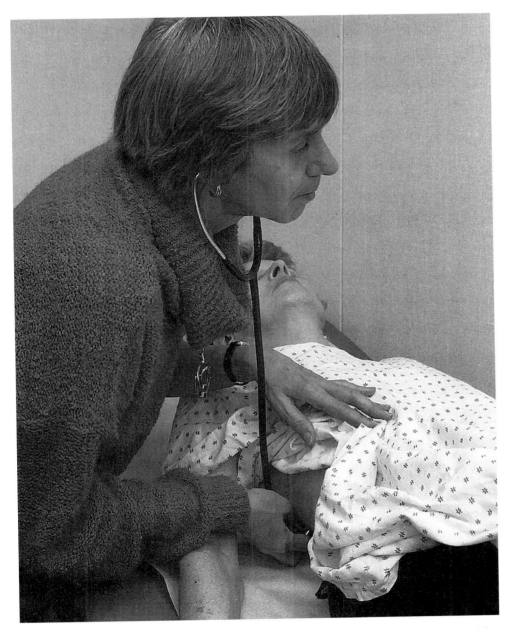

Figure 16.2   Auscultation of the posterior lung fields requires slipping the diaphragm of the stethoscope under the patient's back, i.e., between the back and the bed. Sometimes, the bell must be removed to allow this to proceed more smoothly.

evidence of pressure sores or their precursors. Percussion of the spine can also be carried out at this time.

   Pelvic examination.   When inspection of the perineum and/or bimanual palpation of pelvic organs is indicated, pelvic examination may be accomplished by asking the patient to flex the hips and externally rotate them, if possible, or at least to abduct them. Pillows or folded blankets may be used at the foot of the bed to help the patient maintain the hip flexion, or an assistant may be called to help support the flexed knees. With the examiner standing at the patient's side or at the foot of the bed, perineal inspection and bimanual examination can be done. When

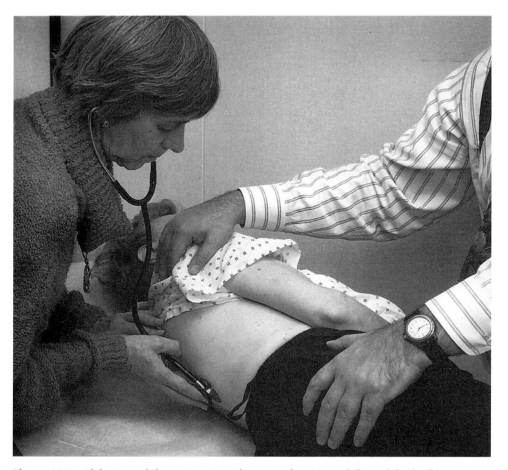

Figure 16.3   If the immobile patient is too heavy and too immobile and the bed is not suitable for one-person repositioning, an assistant can help move the patient into a lateral decubitus position to permit palpation and percussion—otherwise impossible—as well as auscultation and inspection of the entire back and lung fields. Opportunity to assess for pressure sores (bedsores, decubitus ulcers) is another benefit of this maneuver. Examiners are warned against attempting to be both the puller and the listener on the same patient: Bad examinations and muscle strains result.

speculum examination is necessary, an inverted bedpan slipped under the patient's buttocks will elevate them sufficiently to allow insertion of the speculum. However, this will require that the speculum handles point upward rather than down.

Musculoskeletal examination. All joints may be inspected and palpated as usual and put through passive range of motion. In the alert, cooperative patient, some assessment of muscle strength may be made by asking the patient to raise each limb in turn and then the head from the bed. This also allows some assessment of active joint range of motion.

Neurologic examination. Most cranial nerves can be effectively assessed with the patient in a supine position. The gag reflex and swallowing maneuvers are potentially hazardous because of danger of aspiration and should not be attempted unless specifically indicated. Patellar tendon reflexes are elicited as illustrated in Figure 16.4.

Sensory examination of the ventral surface is done as usual; if it is necessary to determine sensory perception dorsally, as in the patient suspected of having a

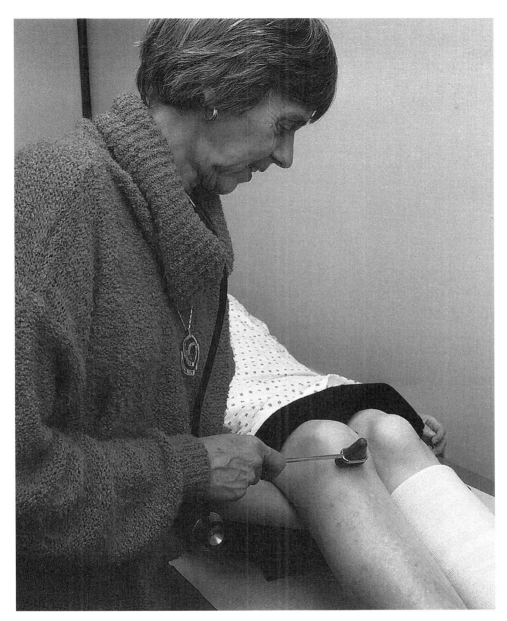

Figure 16.4 For the bedridden patient, the knee jerks are elicited by passively flexing the knees with the nondominant hand. Sometimes, passive elevation and lowering of the knee must be repeated several times in a tense patient or one having marked spasticity.

spinal cord lesion, he may be rolled on his side by an assistant. If the patient can cooperate and can move his extremities, finger-to-nose and heel-to-shin testing will provide an estimate of cerebellar integrity.

Patients in Wheelchairs

The wheelchair-bound patient presents special challenges to the examiner. Assessment of the head and neck, breasts, heart, lungs (posteriorly, accomplished by helping the patient to lean forward in the chair), arms and lower legs, and the bulk of the neurologic and musculoskeletal systems—those portions of the examination usually conducted with the patient seated—are relatively straightforward. Abdomen, rectum, genitalia, lower back, and posterior thighs cannot be satisfactorily examined with the patient in a wheelchair. If assessment of any of these areas is essential, the patient must be transferred to a bed or, preferably, an examination table, and the techniques for examination of the bedridden patient utilized.

Patients with Other Special Needs

Other special needs that may affect the physical examination are discussed below.

Braces or prostheses. Since significant skin, muscle, joint, or neurologic abnormalities may be obscured by the presence of an orthosis, the patient should be asked to remove it and should be positioned comfortably and safely to accommodate its absence.

Hearing loss. Signing, lip reading, or written instructions may be necessary to explain any of the maneuvers requiring active patient participation.

Visual loss. Careful explanation, verbal cuing, and warning before touching or moving the patient will obviate difficulty in examining the visually impaired patient.

Receptive aphasia. Adaptations must be made to such patients' inability to understand instructions. Sometimes, imitation will suffice, with the examiner demonstrating what is wanted of the patient. Gentle manipulation permits completion of other portions of the examination. These patients often have a low threshold for frustration, so patience and a slow, deliberate pace are required. It may not be possible to carry out the more complex assessments, such as those of extraocular movement. Sensory examination is usually unrewarding.

Non-English-speaking patient. Although not impaired, the non-English-speaking patient will have difficulty following instructions given in English. Most maneuvers requiring active patient participation can be demonstrated for imitation; others may require the presence of an interpreter.

Patients in Unusual Situations and Suboptimal Settings

Critical to the success of conducting an examination in the patient's home is a fully equipped "doctor bag" containing the portable items from the equipment and supplies list in Table 1.7. Most homes are not equipped with adjustable beds, so the examination is conducted on a surface that is lower than usual. Request placement of a small table near the bed, on which supplies may be arranged. Bed and lamps may need to be moved to provide access to both right and left sides of the patient and adequate lighting. Bedding and bath towels can be used for draping. The clinician and the patient should agree on the need for third-party presence during the examination.

If the patient is fully mobile and cooperative, either a screening or a symptom-focused extended examination can usually be satisfactorily conducted. If the patient is disabled or bedridden and assistance is required to accomplish the indicated maneuvers, it may be necessary to summon help.

On completion of the examination, remove all used disposable supplies to a closed container and all instruments that must be cleaned before reuse to a second container. Make certain that the room is restored to its normal state and that arrangements are made for disposal of used supplies.

Patients Requiring Unplanned Examinations in Unusual Settings

Most clinicians do not carry medical supplies and equipment to the grocery store, to social events, or on vacation trips. However, it is part of our professional covenant to be responsive to emergency needs when they arise. It is not possible to anticipate or describe here all of the potential predicaments in which a medical professional may be called upon to perform. Some preparatory thinking is suggested.

Basic life support. Every clinician should be trained to provide basic life support in any site at any time. Some carry an oral airway in purse or jacket pocket. Maintain your skills in external cardiac massage and mouth-to-mouth breathing.

Roadside trauma. The priorities for accident victims are

1. Airway management
2. Calling 911 or its equivalent for help
3. Cardiac massage
4. Control of bleeding
5. Minimizing or avoiding movement, unless life is threatened in situ (e.g., pinned underwater) until the nature of the injuries can be ascertained or until ambulance attendants with splints, backboards, cervical collar, and stretchers arrive

Courses in early trauma management are available and are a worthwhile investment for the medical professional.

Taxicab obstetrics, chest pain while traveling in an airplane, and other fearsome events. Ingenuity and common sense guide most clinicians through these crises. A succinct, focused history, with particular attention paid to prior episodes and their alleviating factors, will often allow the clinician to make on-the-spot judgments about necessary immediate physical examination maneuvers. Inspection of the patient's overall color and respiratory rate assists in recognizing the level of emergency in a patient complaining of shortness of breath. An ear pressed against a chest wall serves as a primitive but effective stethoscope. An index finger or a pencil's blunt end can serve as a tongue depressor. One of the authors once sat in the aisle of a Boeing 727, exerting a few pounds of traction on the lower limb of a patient who had just fallen and broken a hip. The diagnosis required only a brief history of the fall and observation of the externally rotated, foreshortened leg. The patient was propped with cushions, her back to the bulkhead, and the comfort provided by the traction enabled continuation of the flight to its planned destination.

RECOMMENDED READINGS

Ardolino A. Examination of the mentally retarded patient. In: Willms JL, Lewis J, eds. Introduction to clinical medicine. Media, Pennsylvania: Harwal, 1991:111–112.

Block MR, Coulehan JL. Teaching the difficult interview in a required course on medical interviewing. J Med Ed 1987;62:35–40.

Clark WD. Alcoholism: blocks to diagnosis and treatment. Am J Med 1981;71:275–285.

Coulehan JL. Who is the poor historian? JAMA 1984;252:221.

Drossman DA. Evaluation and care of medical patients with psychosocial disturbances. Ann Intern Med 1978;88:366–372.

Duffy DL, Hamerman D, Cohen MA. Communication skills of house officers: a study in a medical clinic. Ann Intern Med 1980;93:354–357.

Ewing JA. Detecting alcoholism: The CAGE questionnaire. JAMA 1984;14:1905–1907.

Franks RD. The seductive patient. Am Fam Physician 1980;22:111–114.

Goldman RH, Peters JM. The occupational and environmental health history. JAMA 1981;246:2831–2836.

Gorlin R, Zucker HD. Physicians' reactions to patients: a key to teaching humanistic medicine. N Engl J Med 1983;308:1059–1063.

Gremminger RA. Taking a sexual history. Wis Med J 1983;82:20–24.

Groves JE. Taking care of the hateful patient. N Engl J Med 1978;298:883–887.

Ingelfinger FJ. Arrogance. N Engl J Med 1980;303:1507–1511.

Lazare A. Shame and humiliation in the medical encounter. Arch Intern Med 1987;147:1653–1658.

Mackensie TB. The initial patient interview: identifying when psychosocial factors are at work. Postgrad Med 1983;74:259–265.

Mukaida CS. Dietary and nutritional history. In: Willms JL, Lewis J, eds. Introduction to clinical medicine. Media, Pennsylvania: Harwal, 1991:42–47.

Platt FW, McMath JC. Clinical hypocompetence: the interview. Ann Intern Med 1979;91:898–902.

Quill TE. Partnerships in patient care: a contractual approach. Ann Intern Med 1983;98:228–234.

Schneiderman H. Examination of the bedridden and the disabled patient. In: Willms JL, Lewis J, eds. Introduction to clinical medicine. Media, Pennsylvania: Harwal, 1991:106–111.

Stillman P, Brown D, Redfield D, Sabers D. Construct validation of the Arizona clinical interview rating scale. Educ Psycholog Measurement 1977;77:1031–1038.

Stillman P, et al. Assessment of clinical skills of residents utilizing standardized patients. A follow-up study and recommendations for application. Ann Int Med 1991;5:393–401.

Appendices

Appendix A

ABBREVIATIONS FOUND IN RECORDS OF THE
HISTORY AND PHYSICAL EXAMINATION

Abbreviations are overused in medical records. For any abbreviation with multiple meanings, it is preferable to write out the full term. In general, the clinician should remember that the reader of a record will often lack your specific knowledge base and particular focus. The use of complete terms precludes potentially harmful and even fatal ambiguities and misinterpretations. One example will suffice. A misreading of the abbreviation 5-FC (for 5-fluorocytosine), an antifungal drug, led to the erroneous administration of 5-FU, an anticancer agent whose full name is 5-fluorouracil; the patient, who did not have cancer, died as a result.

Several points need to be made explicitly if the user is to profit maximally from this appendix. Those words marked in *italics* are foreign words, most often Latin; their translations follow immediately, in parentheses. Other parenthetical entries are explanatory. Entries separated by semicolons represent unrelated terms, any of which may be signified by the abbreviation at the left margin; interpretation of the abbreviation thus depends on **context.**

Capitalization of medical abbreviations is variable, and the upper or lower case as shown is usually the most clear (particularly in distinguishing potentially confusing meanings of a set of letters). Periods are not used after medical abbreviations, except in special cases, which are here indicated by the use of periods. Although some terms are marked as applying equally to singular and plural forms, there are others that may be used indiscriminately to abbreviate both singular and plural forms.

The ampersand (&) is treated here as though it were the written-out word "and" for purposes of alphabetizing these abbreviations. By contrast, numbers are treated as nonexistent in alphabetizing this list.

$\bar{a}$	*ante* (before)
A	Asian (with M(an) or W(oman))
A_2	aortic component of the second heart sound (same as S_2A)
AA	Alcoholics Anonymous
AAA	abdominal aortic aneurysm (sometimes abbreviated A^3)
AAAA	atherosclerotic abdominal aortic aneurysm
AAL	anterior axillary line
A&W	alive and well
ab	abortion (spontaneous, i.e., a miscarriage, or otherwise); antibody
ABc	antibiotic
abd	abdomen; abduction
AC	air conduction
ac	*ante cibum* (before meals)
ACEI	angiotensin-converting enzyme inhibitor
ACTH	adrenocorticotropic hormone
AD	primary degenerative dementia: Alzheimer's disease

ADA	American Diabetes Association (usually referring to a diet)
add	adduction
ADL	activities of daily living
ad lib	*ad libitum* (as desired, by the patient not the staff)
AF	atrial fibrillation
AFB	acid-fast bacillus (used as synonym for myco-bacteria)
ag	antigen
AHA	American Heart Association (usually referring to NYHA classes)
AI	aortic insufficiency
AIDS	acquired immunodeficiency syndrome
AJ	ankle jerk (Achilles reflex)
AKA	above-knee amputation; and "also known as"
am	*ante meridiem* (the morning)
AMA	against medical advice; American Medical Association
AMI	acute myocardial infarction; anterior myocardial infarction
ANC	absolute neutrophil count
Ao	aorta
AP	angina pectoris; anteroposterior; apical pulse rate
ARC	AIDS-related complex
ARDS	adult respiratory distress syndrome
AROM	active range of motion
AS	aortic stenosis
ASA	acetylsalicylic acid, i.e. aspirin
ASAP	as soon as possible
ASMI (or ASWMI)	anteroseptal wall myocardial infarction
AV	aortic valve; arteriovenous; atrioventricular
AVF	arteriovenous fistula
AVM	arteriovenous malformation
AWMI	anterior wall myocardial infarction
B	black (with M(an) or W(oman)); bruit
B-II	Billroth II operation, i.e., gastrojejunostomy
BBB	bundle-branch block (with R(ight) or L(eft))
BC	blood culture; bone conduction
BCG	*bacille Calmette-Guèrin* (tuberculosis vaccine)
BCP	birth control pill(s)
BE	barium enema
bid	*bis in dies* (twice daily)
bili	bilirubin
BJ	biceps reflex(es)
BKA (or BK)	below-knee amputation
BM	bone marrow; bowel movement
BP	blood pressure
BPH	benign prostatic hyperplasia
BRBPR	bright red blood per rectum
BRJ	brachioradialis reflex(es)
BRP	bathroom privileges
BS	blood glucose; bowel sounds; breath sounds

BSO	bilateral salpingo-oophorectomy
BSU	Bartholin's and Skene's glands and the female urethra
BUN	blood urea nitrogen
bx	biopsy (singular or plural)
C	(degrees) Celsius; centigrade
c̄	*cum* (with)
Ca	calcium
CA	cancer
CABG	coronary artery bypass graft
CAD	coronary artery disease
C&S	culture and sensitivity testing
CAT	computed (axial) tomography
CBC	complete blood count(s)
CC	chief complaint(s); creatinine clearance
cc	cell count; cubic centimeter(s)
CCB	calcium channel blocker
C/C/E	cyanosis/clubbing/edema
CCU	coronary care unit; critical care unit(s)
CF	cystic fibrosis
CHD	congenital heart disease
chemo	antineoplastic chemotherapy
CHF	congestive heart failure
CHO	carbohydrate
CMV	cytomegalovirus
c/o	complains of; complaints of
COPD	chronic obstructive pulmonary disease
Cor	heart
CPC	clinicopathologic correlation (or a conference about same)
CPR	cardiopulmonary resuscitation
Cr	creatinine
CRF	chronic renal failure
CSF	cerebrospinal fluid
CT	computed tomography
CV	cardiovascular
CVA	costovertebral angle; cerebrovascular accident (the latter is a misnomer for a stroke)
CVAT	costovertebral angle tenderness
CVP	central venous pressure
c/w	consistent with
CXR	chest radiograph
cysto	cystoscopy
D	deceased
d	deciliter(s) (also abbreviated dL)
D&C	dilatation (of the uterine cervix) and curettage (of the endometrium); direct and consensual (pupillary response to light)
DBP	diastolic blood pressure
d/c	discharge; discontinue(d)
ddx, DDx	differential diagnosis
diff	differential cell count

dig	digoxin
DIP	distal interphalangeal (joint)
DJD	degenerative joint disease (osteoarthrosis)
DKA	diabetic ketoacidosis
DM	diastolic murmur; diabetes mellitus
DNR	do not resuscitate if cardiac or respiratory arrest occurs
D/NS, D5W	various dextrose and saline solutions for intravenous administration
DOA	dead on arrival
DOB	date of birth
DOE	dyspnea on exertion
DP	dorsalis pedis artery and its pulse
DPH	phenytoin
DPT	diphtheria, pertussis, and tetanus immunization
DTRs	deep tendon reflex(es) (misnomer for muscle stretch reflex(es))
DTs	delirium tremens
DU	duodenal ulcer
DVT	deep venous thrombosis
D/W	discussed with
dx	diagnosis (singular or plural)
dz	disease(s)
ECG	electrocardiogram (often misabbreviated EKG)
Echo	echocardiogram
ECT	electroconvulsive therapy, shock therapy
EDC	estimated date of confinement (expected date of delivery of a baby)
EEG	electroencephalogram
EGD	esophagogastroduodenoscopy (endoscopic study of the upper digestive tract)
EMG	electromyogram; electromyography
ENT	ear, nose, and throat
EOM	extraocular movement(s)
EOM F&C	extraocular movements are full and conjugate
EOMI	extraocular movements are intact
ER	emergency room; estrogen receptors
EtOH	ethanol
ETT	endotracheal tube; exercise tolerance test
F	(degrees) Fahrenheit; female
FB	foreign body
FBS	fasting blood glucose level
Fe	iron
FET	forced expiratory time
FEV	forced expiratory volume, a pulmonary function test
FH	family history
flex sig	flexible sigmoidoscopy
F → N	finger-to-nose
FROM	full range of motion
FUO	fever of undetermined origin
Fx	fracture; function

g	gallop; gram(s) (also abbreviated gm)
G	gravida
GA	general appearance
G&D	growth and development
GB	gallbladder
GC	gonorrhea or its causative microbe *Neisseria gonorrhoeae*, commonly known as the gonococcus, hence the abbreviation
GDS	geriatric depression scale, a bedside instrument
GI	gastrointestinal
gm	gram(s) (also abbreviated g)
GNID	Gram-negative intracellular diplococci (usually GC)
GNR	Gram-negative rod(s)
GPC	Gram-positive cocci
GSW	gunshot wound
GT (or G-tube)	gastrostomy (feeding) tube
gtt	drop(s)
GTT	glucose tolerance test
GU	gastric ulcer; genitourinary
GXT	graded exercise tolerance test (for coronary disease)
gyn	gynecologic; gynecologist; gynecology
h	hour(s) (also abbreviated hr)
H	hydrogen; Hispanic with M(an) or W(oman)
HA	headache
H&E	hematoxylin and eosin histologic stain; hemorrhage(s) and exudate(s)
H&P	history and physical examination, and record of same
hb	hemoglobin
HBcAb	hepatitis B core antibody
HBP	high blood pressure
HBsAb	hepatitis B surface antibody
HBsAg	hepatitis B surface antigen
HCG	human chorionic gonadotrophin (often erroneously used as a synonym for a pregnancy test)
hct	hematocrit
HCTZ	hydrochlorothiazide
HEENT	head, eyes, ears, nose, (mouth) and throat
heme	blood, hematology
Hg	mercury
hgb	hemoglobin
HH	hiatus hernia
HIV	human immunodeficiency virus
HMD	hyaline membrane disease
HNP	herniated nucleus pulposus (disc disease)
HO	house officer (intern or resident or, in some contexts, postresidency fellow)
HPI	history of the present illness
HR	heart rate
hr	hour(s) (also abbreviated h)
H $\rightarrow$ S	heel-to-shin test of cerebellar function

HS	heart sound(s)
hs	hour of sleep (at bedtime)
HSM	hepatosplenomegaly; holosystolic murmur
HT	hypertension
hx	history
hypo	hypodermic; hypotension
I	iodine
-I	radiographic pulmonary infiltrate (used **only** after an abbreviation for a lung lobe)
IADL	instrumental activities of daily living
IAN	intern's admission note
I&D	incision and drainage
I&O	fluid intake and excretory and other output
ICP	intracranial pressure
ICS	intercostal space
ICU	intensive care unit
ID	infectious disease(s)
IDDM	insulin-requiring diabetes mellitus
Ig	immunoglobulin
IM	intramuscular
IMI	inferior wall myocardial infarction
INH	trade name for one brand of isoniazid
IP	interphalangeal; intraperitoneal
IPN	intern's progress note
IUD	intrauterine contraceptive device
IUP	intrauterine pregnancy
IV	intravenous(ly)
IVDA	intravenous drug abuse(r)
IVF	in vitro fertilization; intravenous fluids
IVP	excretory urogram; intravenous push
IVPB	intravenous piggyback; intravenous push
IWMI	inferior wall myocardial infarction
JAR	junior assistant resident
J-tube	jejunostomy tube
JVD	jugular venous distension
JVP	jugular venous pressure
K	kidney (usually in the form LSK); potassium
kg	kilogram(s)
KJ	knee jerk(s)
KOH	potassium hydroxide
KS	Kaposi's sarcoma
L	left; liter(s); lobe; lymphocyte (in differential counts)
LA	left anterior; left arm; left atrium
L&A	light and accommodation reactions
LE	lower extremity (singular or plural); lupus erythematosus
LICS	left intercostal space
LIH	left inguinal herniorrhaphy
LIQ	lower inner quadrant (usually refers to breast)
LLL	left lower lobe

LLQ	left lower quadrant
LLSB	left lower sternal border
LMD	local medical doctor (sometimes abbreviated PMD for private medical doctor)
LMP	last menstrual period
LN	lymph node(s)
LOC	level of consciousness; loss of consciousness
LOL	little old lady (typically in NAD, a term that can be disparaging but ought not to be)
LOQ	lower outer quadrant (usually refers to breast)
LP	lumbar puncture
LSB	left sternal border (often used imprecisely, without sublocalization such as LLSB)
LSK	liver, spleen, and kidneys
LUL	left upper lobe
LUQ	left upper quadrant
LV	left ventricle
LVH	left ventricular myocardial hypertrophy
M	mother
m	murmur
MAI	*Mycobacterium avium-intracellulare*
MAL	midaxillary line
MCL	midclavicular line
MCP	metacarpophalangeal (usually referring to a joint)
MD	muscular dystrophy; physician
Mg	magnesium
mg	milligram(s)
MG	myasthenia gravis
MI	myocardial infarction
MICU	medical intensive care unit
min	minute(s)
ml (or mL)	milliliter(s)
MMP	multiple medical problems
MMR	measles, mumps, and rubella vaccine/vaccination
MMSE	mini-mental status examination of Folstein
MN	midnight
mo	month(s); mother
Mono	mononuclear cell; mononucleosis
MR	mental retardation or mentally retarded; mitral regurgitation
MRI	magnetic resonance imaging
MRM	modified radical mastectomy
MS	mitral stenosis; morphine sulfate; multiple sclerosis
MSAN	medical student's admission note
MSE	mental status examination
MSL	midsternal line, a part of the anterior midline of the body
MSPN	medical student's progress note
MSR	muscle stretch reflex(es)
MTP	metatarsophalangeal (usually referring to a joint)
MV	mechanical ventilation; mitral valve
MVA	motor vehicle crash (often miscalled an accident)
MVR	mitral valve replacement

N	nausea; nerve; normal
NA	no answer; not applicable
Na	sodium
NAD	no active (or acute) disease; no acute distress
N&V	nausea and vomiting
NAS	no added salt (usually referring to a diet)
NG	nasogastric
NGT	nasogastric tube
NH	nursing home
NIDDM	non-insulin-requiring diabetes mellitus
NKA	no known allergies
NKDA	no known drug allergies
NPO	*nil per os* (nothing by mouth)
NS	normal (0.9%) saline solution
NSAID	nonsteroidal anti-inflammatory drug (refers particularly to prostaglandin inhibitors, usually excepting salicylates)
NT	nontender
NTG	nitroglycerin
NTP	nitrate paste or patches
NYHA	New York Heart Association[a]
O_2	oxygen
OA	osteoarthrosis
Ob	obstetric(s)
OB	occult blood (usually referring to stool testing)
OCA	oral contraceptive agents, i.e., birth control pill(s)
OD	*oculus dexter* (right eye); overdose
OH	occupational history; orthostatic hypotension
OI	opportunistic infection(s)
OM	otitis media
OOB	out of bed
OP	outpatient
OPD	outpatient department
OR	operating room
ORL	otorhinolaryngology
Ortho	orthopedic(s); orthostatic
OS	*oculus sinister* (left eye); opening snap
OT	occupational therapy
OWNL	otherwise within normal limits
P	para; parent; pulse rate; pupil
$\overline{p}$	*post* (after)
P_2	pulmonic component of second heart sound
PA	pernicious anemia; posteroanterior
P&A	percussion and auscultation
PAC	premature atrial contraction
Pap	Papanicolaou-stained cytologic smear (usually of uterine cervical cells but can be of any tissue or fluid)

---

[a]A classification for cardiac disease severity, with class I representing asymptomatic; class II, symptom(s)—usually marked angina pectoris or dyspnea—only with marked exertion; class III, symptom(s) with slight exertion; class IV, symptom(s) at rest.

path	pathologic; pathology
pc	*post cibum* (after meal(s))
PCN	penicillin
PCP	*Pneumocystis carinii* pneumonia
PCV	packed cell volume (hematocrit)
PDx	physical diagnosis
PE	physical examination; pulmonary embolism
PEG	percutaneous endoscopically placed gastrostomy tube
PERRL	pupils equal, round, and reactive to light
PFTs	pulmonary function tests
PGL	persistent generalized lymphadenopathy (associated with HIV infection)
PH	past history
PI	present illness; history of present illness (also HPI)
PIP	proximal interphalangeal (joint(s))
pm	*post meridiem* (afternoon or evening)
PMD	private medical doctor
PMH	past medical history
PMI	point of maximum impulse; posterior wall myocardial infarction
PND	paroxysmal nocturnal dyspnea
PO	*per os* (by mouth)
POMR	problem-oriented medical record
post	postmortem examination, autopsy (a noun, not a verb)
PP	patient profile
PPD	pack per day (of cigarettes smoked); purified protein derivative (of tuberculin) for tuberculosis skin test
prn	*pro re nata* (as needed)
PROM	passive range of motion; premature rupture of fetal membranes
pt	patient
PT	physical therapy; posterior tibial (artery and pulse); prothrombin time
PTA	prior to admission
PTT	partial thromboplastin time
PUD	peptic ulcer disease
PVC	premature ventricular contraction
PWMI	posterior wall myocardial infarction
p-y	pack-years (years of smoking one pack of cigarettes per day)
q	*quisque* (every) (frequently combined with a number and "h," e.g., q2h means "every 2 hours")
$\dot{Q}$	perfusion
qd	every day
qh	every hour
qid	four times a day
qod	every other day
qs	every nursing shift (each of which lasts 8 hours)
qwk	every week

R	respirations; right
RA	rheumatoid arthritis; right anterior; right arm
RAN	resident's admission note
RAS	in the right arm, seated position
RBC	red blood cell(s)
RDS	respiratory distress syndrome (of the newborn)
resp	respiration; respiratory
resp rx	respiratory therapy
RICS	right intercostal space
RLL	right lower lobe
RLQ	right lower quadrant
RML	right middle lobe
ROM	range of motion
ROS	review of systems
RPN	resident's progress note
RR	respiratory rate
RSB	right sternal border
RT	radiotherapy
RUL	right upper lobe
RUQ	right upper quadrant
RUSB	right upper sternal border
RV	right ventricle
rx	therapy; treatment
$\bar{s}$	*sine* (without)
S_1	first heart sound
S_2	second heart sound
S_3	third heart sound
S_4	fourth heart sound
S_2A	aortic component of the second heart sound
SAR	senior assistant resident
s&s	sign(s) and symptom(s)
SBE	infective endocarditis (miscalled subacute bacterial endocarditis)
SBO	small bowel obstruction
SBP	systolic blood pressure; spontaneous bacterial peritonitis
SC	subcutaneous(ly)
SCM	sternomastoid
SDAT	primary degenerative dementia: senile dementia of the Alzheimer type
SEM	systolic ejection murmur
SG	specific gravity
SH	social history
SLE	systemic lupus erythematosus
SMMSE	standardized mini-mental status examination of Molloy
SOB	shortness of breath
S_2P	pulmonic component of the second heart sound
s/p	*status post* (after)
SPT	spinous process tenderness
SQ	subcutaneous(ly)
STA	superficial temporal artery
STD	sexually transmitted disease(s)

SVT	supraventricular tachycardia
sx	symptom(s)
T	temperature
↑T	fever
T_4	T_4 helper lymphocyte count; thyroxine
↑T_4	hyperthyroid(ism)
TA	temporal artery; temporal arteritis
T&A	tonsillectomy and adenoidectomy
TAb	therapeutic abortion
T&C	type and cross-match (blood)
TAH	total abdominal hysterectomy
TB	tuberculosis (also abbreviated tb and tbc)
TFT	thyroid function test(s)
TIA	transient (cerebral) ischemic attack
TJ	triceps reflex(es)
TLC	tender loving care
TM	tympanic membrane(s)
TMJ	temporomandibular joint
TNG	(tri-)nitroglycerin
toxo	*Toxoplasma gondii;* toxoplasmosis
TP	total protein
TUR, TURP	transurethral resection of the prostate
TVF	tactile vocal fremitus
Txn	transplantation; transportation
U	upper
U/A	urinalysis
UA	uric acid
UE	upper extremity (singular or plural)
UGI	upper gastrointestinal (tract; bleeding; or radiographs)
UI	urinary incontinence
UIQ	upper inner quadrant (usually refers to breast)
UL	upper lobe
UOQ	upper outer quadrant (usually refers to breast)
UQ	upper quadrant
URI	upper respiratory tract infection
US	ultrasonic; ultrasound
UTI	urinary tract infection
VD	venereal disease(s)
V̇/Q̇	ventilation/perfusion (ratio or mismatch)
VS	vital sign(s)
W	Caucasian (with M(an) or W(oman))
WA	while awake
WBC	white blood cell(s); or white blood cell count
WD	well developed
wk	week(s)
WN	well nourished
WNL	within normal limits
wt	weight

$\bar{x}$	except
X	times
xrt	radiotherapy
Y	year(s)
YO	year-old

Appendix B

The following is an example of a write-up of a comprehensive history and physical examination. The review of systems in the medical history is deliberately condensed to illustrate a ROS that includes only those systems with positive information that has not been derived from the HPI or PMH. In the recording of the physical examination we employ standardized abbreviations (see Appendix A) that are generally recognized in traditional written case records.

SAMPLE RECORD OF THE COMPREHENSIVE BASIC MEDICAL HISTORY AND PHYSICAL EXAMINATION

H. L. is an 81-YO white widow admitted from her physician's office with
CC:
"I'm bleeding down below."
HPI:
Problem 1: Vaginal bleeding

This woman had an uneventful, natural menopause at age 54, with complete cessation of bleeding until 3 days ago when she first noticed spotting on her underclothes. For the first 24 h she required nothing more than a mini-pad, but then found it necessary to purchase full-sized pads, which she has been changing because they became soaked through about every 4 h. Has tried nothing to alleviate the symptoms and has found nothing that seems to make the bleeding worse. Saw her family doctor today because she had become concerned. Has had no pain. BMs have remained formed, occurring once a day, and painless; bladder function unchanged from usual. Not sexually active since husband died 10 years ago. Does not douche, has had no vaginal discharge or discomfort. Has never taken progestins or estrogen in any form to her knowledge. Last Pap smear about 1 year ago, reported to patient to be normal. Taking no medication other than a diuretic (see Problem 2). Never uses aspirin or other nonprescription drugs. Has been in stable health.

Problem 2: High blood pressure

Has been treated for HBP for 14 years. Takes a diuretic (type unknown) daily, has BP and potassium checked monthly; never advised to take a potassium supplement. No symptoms related to this problem.

Problem 3: Prosthetic heart valve

Six years ago, abrupt onset of DOE, followed within a few days by orthopnea. After investigation by a cardiologist she was referred to Dr. Jones at Providence Hospital, where she underwent AVR with a "pig valve." Takes no anticoagulants or any other medication for her heart, and has remained asymptomatic since surgery. Uses standard antibiotic regimen prescribed by her cardiologist before dental work. Last checkup 3 months ago, was told everything was fine. Activity limited by joint problems, but walks several blocks daily without shortness of breath. No ankle swelling and has never experienced chest pain or palpitations. Sleeps with single pillow, never wakened with breathing difficulty.

Problem 4: "Arthritis"

For 15–20 years, intermittent pain and swelling in both knees, which responds to "drainage" and short-term "Advil." For the past several years, increasing difficulty with right hip, sometimes finding it difficult to go down steps or to walk as far as she would like. Has been told that the hip is "degenerating" but that she will probably never need surgery. No pain in any other joints. No medication for the joint pain for over 6 months.

PMH:

Surgery: (1) appendectomy, about age 14
(2) bilateral vein stripping, age 44
(3) aortic valve replacement, age 75

Other hospitalizations: childbirth only

Major trauma: none

Medications: diuretic, one tablet daily; occasional anti-inflammatory, none in 6 months

Allergies: NKDA. Cephalosporin at time of heart surgery without incident.

Childhood illnesses: "usual"; no known rheumatic fever

Immunizations: Assumes full. "My Dad was a doctor, and he gave us every new shot that came along." Last tetanus 6 years ago; annual "flu" shot; no Pneumovax.

Past medical illnesses: "kidney stones" × 2; last episode 20 years ago; no treatment. Leg vein problems, with subsequent venous ulcers, controlled for the past 4 years with special support stockings.

Pregnancy and delivery: Gr. IV, P II, Ab 2. Uncomplicated pregnancies and deliveries. Both Abs spontaneous in first trimester.

PP:

Master's degree in English, taught high school until retirement at age 65. Lost husband of 48 years 10 years ago, has lived alone in the family home since. Active in several organizations, also volunteer foster grandparent. Many good friends, a strong support system. Two sons live across the continent, sees them and her grandchildren only 2–3 ×/yr. Very health conscious, walks daily as joints permit, eats three small balanced meals each day. No tobacco or recreational drugs ever. One glass of wine with dinner, will take a mixed drink with friends (2–3 ×/mo).

Loves to write letters, "putter" in flower garden, do needlepoint. Still misses husband a great deal. No concerns about sexual inactivity. Days very busy, with social activity, but enjoys solitude for reading and writing. Well-insured, no financial concerns.

FH: No known history of heart disease or diabetes.

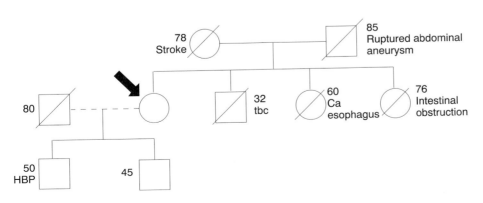

ROS:

HEENT: Glasses for reading. Hearing problem for several years, partially corrected by bilateral hearing aids, still has trouble with telephone communication. Otherwise, negative.

PHYSICAL EXAMINATION

Well-developed, normally nourished woman appearing about stated age of 81. Alert, moves with some caution when getting up from a chair, favoring right hip. Some difficulty understanding instructions unless she can watch lips.

Vital signs:

BP each arm, sitting, 160/88; R arm, standing, 150/92
P, radial, 76 and regular, seated and standing
RR, 14 without effort
T (oral) 36.9°C

Skin: Cool, normal texture and turgor. No cyanosis or icterus. Hair of head gray, with normal thinning for age. No axillary hair; pubic hair sparse, fine. Multiple small nevi over dorsa of both hands and lower forearms. Occasional cherry angiomata on trunk. Single raised grayish keratotic lesion on left breast, ½ × ½ cm in diameter. No petechiae or bruising.

HEENT: Head symmetrical, no evidence of trauma. Facial features symmetrical with equal mobility.

Eyes: Periorbital structures normal. PERRL, D&C. Bilateral arcus cornealis. Visual acuity (with glasses) normal. On funduscope, minimal arterial narrowing without nicking, hemorrhage, or exudate. Disc margins sharp.

Ears: Hearing acuity diminished bilaterally; whisper is only heard to 10 cm. External ears, canals, and tympanic membranes normal. Weber: nonlateralizing. Rinne: BC exceeds AC bilaterally.

Nose: Septum midline; mucosa red-pink and glistening.

Mouth: Oral mucosa without visible lesions. Tongue smooth, normal in color. Good oral hygiene; several restored caries with second and third molars missing. Single crown, left top cuspid. Gingiva pink, healthy. Posterior pharynx unremarkable; tonsils absent. Mouth normal to palpation.

Neck: Head held in normal position. Slight limitation of rotation both left and right, otherwise normal. Thyroid not palpable.

Lymph nodes: No cephalic or cervical nodes palpable. Single small node high in left axilla, under latissimus. Freely mobile, nontender, and less than ½ cm in greatest dimension. No other upper limb nodes felt. A few buckshot-like groin nodes bilaterally, all freely mobile, nontender, and unattached to skin or deep structures.

Breasts: Breasts small, symmetric, and pendulous. No nipple abnormalities or deviation. Move freely and symmetrically with arm elevation and bending forward, without dimpling. Axillae normal except for small left node noted above. Very small amount of breast tissue palpable; no lumps or tenderness. No nipple secretion expressible.

Respiratory (chest and lungs): Midsternal surgical scar with slight keloid formation, well healed. Trachea midline without tug. Respiratory movements easy without use of accessory muscles. Normal TVF. Diaphragmatic excursion 3 cm bilaterally. Percussion note normal over all lobes; breath sounds normal. No crackles, rhonchi, or wheezes.

CV system: No pulsations visible on anterior chest wall. PMI palpable at 5th ICS, in MCL; size, force, and duration normal. No thrills or heaves. On auscultation, $S_2 > S_1$ at base; $S_1 > S_2$ at apex. S_2 single. S_4 at apex. No S_3. Gr II early systolic murmur at 2RICS, RSB, without radiation; intensity decreases with Valsalva maneuver. No diastolic murmur, even with maneuvers for AI. No prosthetic clicks or squeaks. Carotid pulses full and equal bilaterally without bruit or delay. Cervical veins flat at 30°.

Peripheral pulses:

	Radial	Post. Tibial	Dorsalis Pedis
Right	2+	1+	0
Left	2+	1+	0

Abdomen: Flat. RLQ, well-healed 8-cm diagonal surgical scar. Normal bowel sounds. Soft systolic bruit over midepigastrium disappears with light pressure. No tenderness to light or deep palpation. Percussion notes normal throughout. Liver span 7 cm to percussion. Aorta palpable, no enlargement. Liver, spleen, kidneys not felt. No masses, no evidence of fecal impaction, and no suprapubic tenderness.

Limbs: Upper limbs normal to inspection apart from Heberden's nodes on all DIP joints. Lower limbs symmetrical in size and contour. Bilateral surgical scars of superficial vein stripping. Mild medial ankle stasis dermatitis, with well-healed old ulcers bilaterally; no edema or erythema. Hair on both toes. Color and temperature normal and symmetrical. Bilateral bunions and corns on both 5th toes. Toenails and fingernails normal.

Musculoskeletal system:
Upper limbs: ROM normal on rapid joint survey. No tenderness or redness; no swelling other than Heberden's nodes.
Lower limbs: Right hip—flexion limited to 30°; extension normal; external and internal rotation painful at 10°, limited to 30°. Left hip—full ROM except for external rotation limitation to 30°. No tenderness over joint capsules. Both knees—enlarged with marked crepitation, no fluid wave or ballottable fluid, no tenderness, warmth, or redness. Flexion limited to 40°. Extension full. Ankles and feet normal in ROM.
Muscles: Normal tone, nontender on rapid survey. No atrophy.

Back: Cervical spine ROM limited as per Neck, above. Slight excess of dorsal kyphosis. Lumbar curve flattened. No CVAT or SPT.

Neurologic system:
Mental status: 28/30 on SMMSE. Conversation appropriate; affect normal. Limitation in hearing corrects with lipreading.
Cranial nerves: II–XII normal x̄ hearing loss.
Reflexes:

	Biceps	Triceps	BR	Knee	Ankle	Plantar
R	2+	2+	2+	2+	2+	↓
L	2+	2+	2+	2+	2+	↓

Sensation: Pinprick, proprioception normal.

Cerebellar: F→N normal bilaterally. H→S normal on left; unable to test on right because of hip motion limitation. Holds Romberg well; no drift.

Motor: Symmetrical except for mild weakness of quadriceps on right. Gait and stance normal apart from initial cautious positioning. Arises easily from chair, transfers from chair to table easily.

Pelvic and rectal: Vulvar skin atrophic without bleeding or skin lesions. Periurethral area reddened, no discharge. Introitus gaping; on Valsalva, cervix descends to introitus, but no incontinence with this. Speculum insertion difficult, resistance at 5 cm. Vaginal mucosa markedly white, thin, atrophic with some punctate bleeding sites. Cervix slightly open, minimal ectropion. Moderate amount of bright red blood from os cervicis. No vaginal or cervical mass. On bimanual, grade 3 urethrocystocele in conjunction with uterine prolapse. Uterus freely mobile, although enlarged × 2 for age. Anterior and posterior surfaces of fundus easily felt, smooth, nontender; without mass. Neither ovary palpable, adnexal areas unremarkable. No parametrial masses or sense of frozen pelvis.

Rectal: No excoriation or skin lesion. Sphincter tone normal. Scant stool in the vault; negative for occult blood. No masses. Posterior surface of fundus clearly felt through normal rectovaginal septum, smooth, nontender.

PROBLEM LIST

Active problems

Problem 1:   Uterine bleeding, postmenopausal
        A. Uterine enlargement, ?endometrial carcinoma
        B. Atrophic vulvovaginitis
        C. Uterine prolapse with cystourethrocele
Problem 2:   High blood pressure, partly controlled, without evidence of end-organ damage
Problem 3:   Prosthetic heart valve, functional, s/p AVR
        A. Gr. II aortic systolic flow murmur
Problem 4:   "Arthritis", osteoarthrosis pattern
        A. Pain and limited ROM, both hips, R > L
        B. Knee swelling, pain, crepitation, and reduced ROM: 10 yr
        C. Mildly limited motion, neck
        D. Heberden's nodes
Problem 5:   Bilateral hearing loss, conductive, incompletely compensated with hearing aids
Problem 6:   Epigastric bruit, ?origin
Problem 7:   Keratotic skin lesion, breast; minor skin lesions elsewhere
Problem 8:   Smooth tongue, ?vitamin deficiency
Problem 9:   Left axillary lymph node, small and mobile, likely innocuous
Problem 10: Asymptomatic peripheral arterial insufficiency
Problem 11: Venous insufficiency, legs, compensated
        A. Venous ulcers, healed
        B. Dermatitis venosa, mild
Problem 12: Bunions and corns on 5th toes, bilateral
Problem 13: ?Early osteoporosis, back, with kyphosis

Inactive problems
Problem 1:   s/p appendectomy, remote
Problem 2:   s/p bilateral vein stripping, remote
Problem 3:   Kidney stones by history, remote

Appendix C

THE ORAL CASE PRESENTATION

Purpose

The purpose of the oral case presentation is quite different from that of the written patient record. In some ways it is more difficult and demands more careful thought from the presenter. The oral presentation is designed to convey to the listener(s) a concise and carefully edited version of the case. The goal is to permit the listener(s) to arrive at an understanding of the problems the case poses and to begin to formulate plans for their solution. The auditors of the presentation may be peers, supervisors, other members of the team (notably nurses, but sometimes the rehabilitation therapist, pharmacist, social worker, etc.), preceptors, consultants, or a general medical audience.

The specific parameters of an oral case presentation include (a) a time limit that does not exceed the ability of the auditors to maintain concentration and assimilate data (no more than 7 minutes and preferably less), (b) a formulaic framework that is familiar to the audience and that transmits information systematically and efficiently, (c) elimination of any information extraneous to the mission of **immediate problem solving**, and (d) conversely, inclusion of all details necessary to stimulate the problem-formulating and problem-solving processes.

Format

The generally adapted format for oral case presentation follows:

A. Opening remarks

1. The descriptive detail necessary to set the stage for the case that follows includes demographics (age and gender), the reason for the current medical encounter, duration of the presenting problem(s), and any relevant concurrent medical conditions.

2. The patient's chief complaint is paraphrased into medical terms with which the audience is familiar.

B. HPI (events leading to the current encounter)

1. If this is a **new problem**, then the baseline state of health or the patient's status prior to the onset of the presenting problem is iterated.

2. If this encounter represents a **change in the status of a chronic or preexisting condition**, a concise summary of the history of the problem is presented as background to the new event(s). Such a summary is a major achievement if this is the eighth diabetic complication in 30 years, the fifth hospitalization for AIDS, or the hundredth health-care contact with sickle cell disease.

3. If this is a **single-problem HPI**, the events are described chronologically.

4. When the patient's HPI is complicated by **multiple active problems** that must be taken into consideration during the oral development of the case, the presenter chooses between the **chronologic** and the **problem-oriented** approach.

a. The **chronologic approach** offers the sequence of events, beginning with the first departure from good health and interweaving the multiple problems as they appear and change as a narrative in temporal order. The **advantage** of this approach is that it gives the listener a feel for progression of "unwellness" in the patient's story. The **disadvantage** is that the interspersing of details of more than one problem may lead to confusion. This approach is **recommended** for patients with several *closely related problems* in which a single event may simultaneously affect more than one problem.

b. The **problem-oriented approach** precategorizes the problems and develops details of each one separately in chronologic order. The **advantage** of this approach is its organization by problem, which may be a better strategy for oral presentation. The **disadvantage** is that it artificially divides the patient's illness story into diseases rather than giving an overall chronology of his narrative. This may lead to a misinterpretation of the interrelationships of the various problems. This approach is **recommended** for the patient in whom it appears that the multiple active problems are not related or when the interrelationship of problems is not clear. It is also sometimes used as a brief restatement if the problem-oriented approach (strategy *a* above) has met with blank stares.

C. Other parts of the history

The PMI, FH, PP, and ROS are included *only* to the extent that they clarify or refine understanding of the HPI. *Allergies and medicines currently being used are always stated.*

D. Physical examination

The description of the patient's physical examination findings should open with a statement on the patient's general appearance including apparent state of health along with any observable features that help the auditor to gain a general impression of the person being discussed and a full citation of vital signs, including orthostatic pulse and blood pressure changes if appropriate. Subsequently, the physical examination findings are strictly limited to pertinent positives *and* negatives. Positive findings considered unrelated to the problem at hand (e.g., arthritic deformities) should be omitted, as should all normal findings except those that assist in eliminating certain considerations for diagnosis and/or therapy.

Recall that if you, as presenter, eliminate something from the presentation that an auditor considers important, the datum may be requested during the ensuing case discussion. Decisions about just how much historical or physical examination information to include in the oral case presentation are "judgment calls." The power of the group problem-solving resides in pooling of experience and knowledge that may reveal possibilities that the presenter had not considered. There is no disgrace in being asked for a datum you have rationally omitted from an oral case presentation.

E. Laboratory result

This category includes all pertinent normal and abnormal values from **any medical testing** that has been done.

F. Management course to date

This includes all events that have transpired since the patient presented with the problem(s) under consideration: **diagnostic and therapeutic steps, with outcomes,** and **any changes in the patient's condition.**

G. Summary

The summary is a brief wrap-up of the **highlights** of the problem and **questions** that the presenter wishes the listeners to address.

H. Discussion

The discussion of the case usually begins with points of clarification raised by the listeners. The presenter should be prepared to supply any data that she may have chosen to eliminate from the presentation but that an auditor requests. Often, the presenter will restate items that listeners did not catch the first time around. An open discussion of problems and strategies for their solution follows.

SAMPLE ORAL CASE PRESENTATION

The case presented below, in the oral presentation format, is the same case written as a sample for Appendix B. The reader may thus be able to see the difference in organization and detail between the two.

Opening comments: Mrs. L. is an 81-year-old widowed white woman, with known prosthetic aortic valve, mild hypertension, and moderately severe osteoarthrosis, who was in her usual state of health until 3 days ago, when she began to bleed vaginally.

HPI:
Problem 1: Postmenopausal vaginal bleeding

    Patient underwent an uneventful menopause at age 54 and had had no subsequent vaginal bleeding until 3 days ago, when she first noted dark spotting, followed by bright red blood that has required 6–8 pads/day for the past 2 days. She has experienced no pain, malaise, or faintness. There was no apparent antecedent event, and she has not noted anything that alters the flow. She has not been sexually active since the death of her husband 10 years ago and has had no other pelvic problems to her knowledge. She has taken no medications (including OTC preparations) in the past 6 months other than a diuretic for her hypertension. There has been no bleeding from any other site; no increase in bruising. Last Pap smear was 1 year ago and was reported to be normal.

Problem 2: Prosthetic aortic valve

    On the basis of sudden onset of DOE and orthopnea 6 years ago, the patient was diagnosed as having aortic valve (calcific) stenosis with left ventricular decompensation (diagnosis, tests, and treatment confirmed by house staff in telephone conversation with the patient's cardiologist). She underwent an uneventful porcine valve replacement and has remained asymptomatic since, without further DOE, orthopnea, PND, or ankle edema; she takes no cardiac medications and, specifically, no anticoagulants.

Problem 3: Hypertension

    Mrs. L. has taken a diuretic (50 mg of hydrochlorothiazide) daily for many years with moderate control of her hypertension. There are no symptoms of either end-organ damage or complications from the therapy.

Problem 4: Osteoarthrosis

    The patient has experienced progressive limitation of motion with swelling and pain in both knees, controlled by periodic joint aspiration and short-term NSAID treatment. Last course of treatment was 6 months ago. She also has increasing pain and limitation of motion of the right hip, which has been studied by her private physician. No further treatment has been attempted, specifically no recent NSAIDs or aspirin.

PMH, FH, PP, and ROS: Noncontributory.

PHYSICAL EXAMINATION

Mrs. L. is a well-developed, normally nourished lady appearing to be about her stated age of 81. She is hard of hearing but intelligent and interactive. She moves to and from the examining table with some difficulty because of pain and limitation of motion in the right hip.

Vital signs: Temperature 37°C; respirations 16 and easy; blood pressure 160/88 in each arm, sitting; pulse rate 76/minute and regular. No orthostatic hypotension or tachycardia.

Other findings: Bilateral decrease in hearing acuity, assisted very little by hearing aid. No petechiae or bruises seen. A single freely mobile left posterior axillary node, but no breast lesion. Well-healed midsternal surgical scar from valve replacement. PMI is in 5th ICS, at MCL and normal to palpation. No thrills or heaves. Carotid upstroke normal. On auscultation, there is a grade II systolic murmur, loudest at the aortic root. Otherwise, cardiac examination is entirely WNL. Lungs are clear without crackles or wheezes. There is no ankle edema. The abdomen is normal except for a surgical incision in the RLQ and a faint systolic epigastric bruit. Limb examination reveals normal pulses except for bilateral absence of the dorsalis pedis; however, color and temperature of the feet are normal. There is no ankle swelling; there is skin evidence of old venous stasis disease with bilateral saphenous stripping scars. There is notable limitation of motion of the right hip. Both knees are enlarged and crepitant without evidence of fluid accumulation.

Pelvic examination: Reveals severe atrophic vulvovaginitis without bleeding; grade III uterine prolapse with cystourethrocele. Bright red blood issues from a patulous but otherwise normal cervix. On bimanual examination, the uterus is freely mobile and nontender but enlarged to twice its expected size for age. There are no masses. Neither ovary is felt, and the adnexa feel normal. Rectal examination corroborates pelvic. No occult blood in the stool.

Initial workup: Reveals normal urinalysis and CBC, normal platelet count, PT, and PTT. Serum creatinine is 2 mg/100 ml, but all other chemistries including sodium, potassium, uric acid, and glucose are normal. Pelvic ultrasound confirms physical examination findings of symmetric enlargement of the uterus with normal adnexa. Pap smear and endometrial biopsy results pending.

Echocardiogram and Doppler show moderate LVH but normal LV systolic function and a functionally insignificant gradient across the prosthetic aortic valve. Chest film is unremarkable except for surgical clips and wires.

Since admission to hospital 24 hours ago there has been no change in patient's condition. She continues to saturate 4 pads/day and states she feels well.

In summary, this is an 81-year-old woman with an apparently normally functioning porcine aortic valve, mild hypertension with secondary azotemia, and moderately severe osteoarthrosis of both knees and the right hip, who presents with 3 days of new-onset vaginal bleeding and an enlarged uterus by palpation.

This appears to be a case of probable endometrial carcinoma and raises the following questions: While awaiting the results of biopsies, should we seriously consider any other etiologies for the vaginal bleeding? Given the history of aortic valvular disease and venous disease, what preoperative and intraoperative considerations must be foremost? In terms of general medical management, are there other things we need to be working on at this point?

Appendix D

RECORDING THE FOCUSED HISTORY AND PHYSICAL EXAMINATION

The written record of the focused history and physical examination is structured to concentrate on the principal presenting problem(s). Since the setting is usually one of acute care and single-problem orientation, the write-up reflects this orientation. The following sample write-up is that of the case presented in Chapter 1, pages 32–36, in which a previously healthy man comes to the ER with a new, acute problem. The key features in this kind of write-up are (a) rapid but thorough focus on the presenting problem and (b) succinct recording of relevant history, physical examination, and, if appropriate, laboratory data. All information extraneous to the immediate problem and its context is deleted from the record for this visit. If additional considerations are encountered during the course of the visit, they are deferred unless they affect the diagnostic or therapeutic management of the presenting complaint.

SAMPLE FOCUSED CASE RECORD

32-year-old previously healthy man brought to ER by wife because of 2 hours of *severe abdominal pain.* Had been in his usual state of vigorous good health until today.

HPI:
Began this day by competing in a 40-km bicycle race, an activity to which he is accustomed. Rode well, and felt fine until about 1 h after completion of the race when, while repairing a damaged tube in his garage, he noticed sudden gripping discomfort in the periumbilical area and right flank, radiating toward the back. Continued with his task, but within a few minutes the pain became so intense that he couldn't finish. Pain seemed to have moved to right lower abdomen, right testicle, and inner thigh. Tried several body positions and, 15 minutes before being brought into the ER, two aspirin. Neither reduced the pain, nor has anything he done made it worse, although it has progressively increased in intensity. Pain is constant, "tearing," unprecedented in character, and the *worst he has ever experienced.* Normal bowel movement without effect on the pain 1 hour after onset. Has urinated small volume of dark urine twice since onset (claims that the small-volume, dark urine is characteristic of his postcycling urination). Drank a liter of fluid during the ride but has experienced unusual thirst afterward and now.

PMH:
Appendectomy age 6. Only other medical problem is recurrent epigastric "heartburn" with ingestion of ibuprofen, taken episodically for knee pain that impairs cycling. Took both ibuprofen and, for relief of heartburn, Maalox 4 times/day for past 3 days.

FH:
No known family history of renal stones.

PP and ROS:

No pertinent findings. Sexual history nonrevelatory; no history of STDs or of penile drip, prior testicular symptoms, or low-back pain.

PHYSICAL EXAMINATION

In obvious acute distress, restless, asking not to be confined to the examining table, but preferring to pace about. Slightly sweaty and pale. Well-developed, fit young adult who does not appear chronically ill.

Vital signs:

    T (oral) 37.5°C (99.5°F)
    BP 140/88 RAS, 125/75 standing
    P 110/min, regular and full, seated, and 125/min, standing
    RR 18/min, nonlabored

Abdomen: Contour and skin color normal. Well-healed RLQ surgical scar. Bowel sounds normally active; no rubs or bruits. Light and deep palpation reveal no rigidity or guarding. Minimal discomfort on deep palpation in the extreme RLQ, without rebound or point tenderness. No suprapubic tenderness. Liver edge felt on deep palpation, but span and texture normal. No other organs or masses felt. No tenderness to CVA percussion. Femoral pulses normal.

Genitalia: WNL, specifically no scrotal or intrascrotal swelling, discoloration, or tenderness. No urethral tenderness.

Rectal: Normal sphincter tone. No abnormality in vault. Lobes of prostate small, symmetrical, nontender. Scant soft brown stool recovered on glove; test for occult blood negative.

PROBLEM LIST

Problem 1: Acute (2-h duration) abdominal, RLQ, and right scrotal pain—probable ureterolithiasis
Problem 2: Probable acute dehydration secondary to bicycle race today
Problem 3: Dyspepsia with NSAID use, gastropathy

Bibliography

Abrams J. Precordial motion in health and disease. Mod Concepts Cardiovasc Dis 1980;49:55–60.

Ackerman AB, Kornberg R. Pearly penile papules: acral angiofibromas. Arch Dermatol 1973;108: 673–675.

Adams F. The "sheet sign." JAMA 1984;251:891.

Adolph RJ, Fowler NO. Second heart sound: a screening test for heart disease. Mod Concepts Cardiovasc Dis 1970;39:91–96.

Ahola SJ. Unexplained parotid enlargement: a clue to occult bulimia. Conn Med 1982;46:185–186.

Alexander B. Taking the sexual history. Am Fam Physician 1981;23:147–151.

Alibrandi B, Parodi A, Varaldo G. Purpura due to ethanol. N Engl J Med 1990;322:702.

Alpert JS, Krous HF, Dalen JE, O'Rourke RA, Bloor CM. Pathogenesis of Osler's nodes. Ann Intern Med 1976;85:471–473.

Amar D, Attai LA, Gupta SK, Jones A. Bilateral upper extremity blood pressure measurements should be routine prior to coronary artery surgery. Chest 1992;101:882.

Anonymous. Forgotten symptoms and primitive signs. Lancet 1987;1:841–842.

Anthony JC, LeResche L, Niaz U, Von Korff MR, Folstein MF. Limits of the "mini-mental state" as a screening test for dementia and delirium among hospital patients. Psychiatr Med 1982;12: 397–408.

Athreya BH, Silverman BK. Pediatric physical diagnosis. Norwalk, Connecticut: Appleton-Century-Crofts, 1985.

Atkinson K, Austin DE, McElwain TJ, Peckham MJ. Alcohol pain in Hodgkin's disease. Cancer 1976;37:895–899.

Atlee WE Jr. Talc and cornstarch emboli in eyes of drug abusers. JAMA 1972;219:49–51.

Auletta MJ, Headington JT. Purpura fulminans: a cutaneous manifestation of severe protein C deficiency. Arch Dermatol 1988;124:1387–1391.

Balciunas BA, Overholser CD. Diagnosis and treatment of common oral lesions. Am Fam Physician 1987;35:206–220.

Baldwin JG Jr. The healing touch. Am J Med 1986;80:1.

Baraff LJ, Schriger DL. Orthostatic vital signs: variation with age, specificity, and sensitivity in detecting a 450-mL blood loss. Am J Emerg Med 1992;10:99–103.

Barkun AN, Camus M, Meagher T, et al. Splenic enlargement and Traube's space: how useful is percussion? Am J Med 1989;87:562–566.

Barnes TRE. A rating scale for drug-induced akathisia. Br J Psychiatry 1989;154:672–676.

Barness LA. Manual of pediatric physical diagnosis. 6th ed. St Louis: Mosby-Year Book, 1991.

Barnett AJ. The "neck sign" in scleroderma. Arthritis Rheum 1989;32:209–211.

Barrasso R, Brux JD, Croissant O, Orth G. High prevalence of Papillomavirus-associated penile intraepithelial neoplasia in sexual partners of women with cervical intraepithelial neoplasia. N Engl J Med 1987;317:916–923.

Bassett AA. Technique of clinical screening for breast cancer. N Engl J Med 1982;307:826–827.

Bassett AA. Physical examination of the breast and breast self-examination. In: Miller AB, ed. Screening for cancer. New York: Academic Press (Harcourt Brace Jovanovich), 1985:271–291.

Bauman JE. Basal body temperature: unreliable method of ovulation detection. Fertil Steril 1981; 36:729–733.

Beaven DW, Brooks SE. Color atlas of the nail in clinical diagnosis. Chicago: Year Book Medical Publishers, 1984.

Beede SD, Ballard BJ, James EM, Ilstrup DM, Hallet JWJ. Positive predictive value of clinical suspicion of abdominal aortic aneurysm: implications for efficient use of abdominal ultrasonography. Arch Intern Med 1990;150:549–551.

Behrman RE, Vaughan VC III, Nelson WE, eds. Nelson textbook of pediatrics. 13th ed. Philadelphia: WB Saunders, 1987.

Beitman RG, Frost SS, Roth JLA. Oral manifestations of gastrointestinal disease. Dig Dis Sci 1981; 26:741–747.

Benbassat J, Meroz N. The foam sponge as a teaching aid in the examination of the chest. Med Educ 1988;22:554–555.

Bennett HJ. How to survive a case presentation. Chest 1985;88:292–294.

Betts T. Pseudoseizures: seizures that are not epilepsy. Lancet 1990;336:163–164.

Bialecki C, Feder HM, Grant-Kels JM. The six classic childhood exanthems: a review and update. J Am Acad Dermatol 1989;21:891–904.

Bickers DR. The dermatologic manifestations of human porphyria. Ann N Y Acad Sci 1987;514: 261–267.

Blau JN. How to take a history of head or facial pain. Br Med J 1982;285:1249–1251.

Block MR, Coulehan JL. Teaching the difficult interview in a required course on medical interviewing. J Med Educ 1987;62:35–40.

Bloom JN, Palestine AG. The diagnosis of cytomegalovirus retinitis. Ann Intern Med 1988;109:963–969.

Boyle WE Jr, Hoekelman RA. The pediatric history. In: Hoekelman RA, ed. Primary pediatric care. St Louis: CV Mosby, 1987:52–62.

Braun RD, Barnes AE. An evaluation of the roll-over test. J Tenn Med Assoc 1977;70:637–638.

Braverman IM. Skin signs of systemic disease. 2nd ed. Philadelphia: WB Saunders, 1981.

Brewin TB. Alcohol intolerance in neoplastic disease. Br Med J 1966;2:437–441.

Broadmore J, Carr-Gregg M, Hutton JD. Vaginal examinations: women's experiences and preferences. N Z Med J 1986;99:8–10.

Bruce S. Hand dermatitis: annoying and persistent, but treatable. Consultant 1990;30(12):21–27.

Bunker CB, Newton JA, Kilborn J, et al. Most women with acne have polycystic ovaries. Br J Dermatol 1989;121:675–680.

Byrd BF. Close-up: standard breast examination. CA 1974;24:290–293.

Calin A, Porta J, Fries JF, Schurman DJ. Clinical history as a screening test for ankylosing spondylitis. JAMA 1977;237:2613–2614.

Callaham M. Fulminant bacterial meningitis without meningeal signs. Ann Emerg Med 1989;18:90–93.

Callen JP. Skin signs of internal malignancy: fact, fancy and fiction. Semin Dermatol 1984;3:340–357.

Caplan LR. The small corks test: a rapid sensory screening test. JAMA 1981;246:1341–1342.

Carl W. Oral manifestations of systemic chemotherapy and their management. Semin Surg Oncol 1986;2:187–199.

Carlson HE. Gynecomastia. N Engl J Med 1980;303:795–799.

Carroll JL, Clayton JE, Lemen RJ. The physiology and clinical usefulness of common pulmonary physical findings. Ariz Med 1983;40:408–414.

Carter SA. Arterial auscultation in peripheral vascular disease. JAMA 1981;246:1682–1686.

Castell DO, O'Brien KD, Muench H, Chalmers TC. Estimation of liver size by percussion in normal individuals. Ann Intern Med 1969;70:1183–1189.

Cattau ELJ, Benjamin SB, Knuff TE, Castell DO. The accuracy of the physical examination in the diagnosis of suspected ascites. JAMA 1982;247:1164–1166.

Cavanaugh J, Niewoehner CB, Nuttall FQ. Gynecomastia and cirrhosis of the liver. Arch Intern Med 1990;150:563–565.

Chambers BR, Norris JW. Outcome in patients with asymptomatic neck bruits. N Engl J Med 1986;315:860–865.

Christensen JH, Freundlich M, Jacobsen BA, Falstie-Jensen N. Clinical relevance of pedal pulse palpation in patients suspected of peripheral arterial insufficiency. J Intern Med 1989;226:95–99.

Clement PAR. The lymphatic system. Acta Otorhinolaryngol Belg 1983;37:309–323.

Clinch D, Banerjee AK, Ostick G. Absence of abdominal pain in elderly patients with peptic ulcer. Age Ageing 1984;13:120–123.

Cohen A, Reyes R, Kirk M, Fulks RM. Osler's nodes, pseudoaneurysm formation, and sepsis complicating percutaneous radial artery cannulation. Crit Care Med 1984;12:1078–1079.

Cole CW, Barber GG, Bouchard AG, et al. Abdominal aortic aneurysm: consequences of a positive family history. Can J Surg 1989;32:117–120.

Collin J, Gray DW. The eyes closed sign. Br Med J 1987;295:1656.

Connors AF, McCaffree DR, Gray BA. Evaluation of right-heart catheterization in the critically ill patient without acute myocardial infarction. N Engl J Med 1983;308:263–267.

Cordasco EM, Beder S, Coltro A, Bavbek S, Gurses H, Mehta AC. Clinical features of the yellow nail syndrome. Cleve Clin J Med 1990;57:472–476.

Cotter L, Logan RL, Poole A. Innocent systolic murmurs in healthy 40-year-old men. J R Coll Physicians Lond 1980;14:128–129.

Craige E. Should auscultation be rehabilitated? N Engl J Med 1988;318:1611–1613.

Davis GM, Rubin J, Bower JD. Digital clubbing due to secondary hyperparathyroidism. Arch Intern Med 1990;150:452–454.

Davison R, Cannon R. Estimation of central venous pressure by examination of jugular veins. Am Heart J 1974;87(3):279–282.

Dell'Italia LJ, Starling MR, O'Rourke RA. Physical examination for exclusion of hemodynamically important right ventricular infarction. Ann Intern Med 1983;99:608–611.

DeMyer W. Technique of the neurologic examination: a programmed text. 3rd ed. New York: McGraw-Hill, 1980.

Deneke M, Wheeler L, Wagner G, Ling F, Buxton B. An approach to relearning the pelvic examination. J Fam Pract 1982;14:782–783.

Dowdall GG. Five diagnostic methods of John B. Murphy. In: May LA, ed. Classic descriptions of physical signs in medicine. Oceanside, New York: Dabor Science Publications, 1977:269–273.

Dower JC. The pediatric interview. In: Rudolph AM, ed. Pediatrics. 17th ed. Norwalk, Connecticut: Appleton-Century-Crofts, 1982:19–20.

Drife JO. Lateral thinking in gynaecology. Br Med J 1988;296:807–808.

Dukes RJ. Office evaluation of the pulmonary patient (part I). J Indiana State Med Assoc 1982;75: 794–796.

Dworkin PH. Learning and behavior problems of schoolchildren. Philadelphia: WB Saunders, 1985.

Dworkin PH. Pediatrics. 2nd ed. Media, Pennsylvania: Harwal, 1992.

Dworkin PH. The preschool child: developmental themes and clinical issues. Curr Prob Pediatr 1988; 117–119.

Ehrenkranz JRL. A new method for measuring body temperature. N J Med 1986;83:93–96.

Eilen SD, Crawford MH, O'Rourke RA. Accuracy of precordial palpation for detecting increased left ventricular volume. Ann Intern Med 1983;99:628–630.

Ende J, Rockwell S, Glasgow M. The sexual history in general medicine practice. Arch Intern Med 1984;144:558–561.

Fallon TJ, Abell E, Kingsley L, et al. Telangiectasias of the anterior chest in homosexual men. Ann Intern Med 1986;105:679–682.

Fariselli G, Lepera P, Viganotti G, Martelli G, Bandieramonte G, Pietro SD. Localized mastalgia as presenting symptom in breast cancer. Eur J Surg Oncol 1988;14:213–215.

Feussner JR, Linfors EW, Blessing CL, Starmer CF. Computed tomography brain scanning in alcohol withdrawal seizures: value of the neurologic examination. Ann Intern Med 1981;94:519–522.

Fielding JF. Clinical and radiological manifestations of the irritable bowel syndrome. J Ir Coll Physicians Surg 1978;8:11–15.

Filly RA. Ultrasound: the stethoscope of the future, alas. Radiology 1988;167:400.

Fisher MM, Raper RF. Fever in the intensive care unit. Br J Hosp Med 1987;38:109–111.

Fitzgerald F. Physical diagnosis in modern medicine: is the physical examination history? Careers 1989;5(4):5, 14–15.

Fitzgerald FT. The clinical examination—a dying art? Forum Med 1980;May:348–349.

Fitzgerald FT, Tierney LM Jr. The bedside Sherlock Holmes. West J Med 1982;137:169–175.

Fitzpatrick TB, Eisen AZ, Wolff K, Freedberg IM, Austen KF, eds. Dermatology in general medicine: textbook and atlas. 4th ed. New York: McGraw-Hill, 1993.

Fitzpatrick TB, Gilchrest BA. Dimple sign to differentiate benign from malignant pigmented cutaneous lesions. N Engl J Med 1977;296:1518.

Fitzpatrick TB, Polano MK, Suurmond D. Color atlas and synopsis of clinical dermatology. New York: McGraw-Hill, 1983.

Forgacs P. Noisy breathing. Chest 1973;63:38S–41S.

Forman MA, Hetznecker WH, Dunn JM. Assessment and interviewing. In: Vaughan VC, McKay RJ, Behrman RE, eds. Nelson textbook of pediatrics. 11th ed. Philadelphia: WB Saunders, 1979: 80–83.

Fowler NO. Physiology of cardiac tamponade and pulsus paradoxus. I. Mechanisms of pulsus paradoxus in cardiac tamponade. Mod Concepts Cardiovasc Dis 1978;47:109–113.

Friedman RJ, Rigel DS. The clinical features of malignant melanoma. Dermatol Clin 1985;3:271–283.

Friedman RJ, Rigel DS, Kopf AW. Early detection of malignant melanoma: the role of physician examination and self-examination of the skin. CA 1985;35:130–151.

Friedman-Kien AE, Laubenstein LJ, et al. Disseminated Kaposi's sarcoma in homosexual men. Ann Intern Med 1982;96:693–700.

Frohlich ED. Recommendations for blood pressure determination by sphygmomanometry. Ann Intern Med 1988;109:612.

Frohlich ED, Grim C, Labarthe DR, Maxwell MH, Perloff D, Weidman WH. Recommendations for human blood pressure determination by sphygmomanometers. 5th ed. Dallas: American Heart Association, 1987.

Furth PA, Kazakis AM. Nail pigmentation changes associated with azidothymidine (zidovudine). Ann Intern Med 1987;107:350.

Goldstein GD, Dunn MI. Polishing over yellow nails. Chest 1986;90:766–767.

Gooch AS, Cha SD, Maranhao V. The use of the hepatic pressure maneuver to identify the murmur of tricuspid regurgitation. Clin Cardiol 1983;6:277–280.

Grady MJ, Earll JM. Teaching physical diagnosis in the nursing home. Am J Med 1990;88:519–521.

Gray DWR, Dixon JM, Collin J. The closed eyes sign: an aid to diagnosing non-specific abdominal pain. Br Med J 1988;297:837.

Gray DWR, Dixon JM, Seabrook G, Collin J. Is abdominal wall tenderness a useful sign in the diagnosis of non-specific abdominal pain? Ann R Coll Surg Engl 1988;70:233–234.

Gray CS, Walker A. The plantar response: caution in the elderly. Br J Hosp Med 1989;42:105–106.

Gremminger RA. Taking a sexual history. Wis Med J 1983;82:20–24.

Gribbin C, Raghavendra N, Ginsburg HB. Ultrasound diagnosis of jugular venous ectasia. N Y State J Med 1989;89:532–533.

Grob JJ, Bonerandi JJ. Cutaneous manifestations associated with the presence of the lupus anticoagulant. J Am Acad Dermatol 1986;15:211–219.

Guarino JR. Abdominal aortic aneurysm: a new diagnostic sign. J Kansas Med Soc 1975;76(5):108, 15A.

Guarino JR. Auscultatory percussion of the chest. Lancet 1980;1:1332–1334.

Guarino JR. Auscultatory percussion of the urinary bladder. Arch Intern Med 1985;145:1823–1825.

Guinan P, Bush I, Ray V, Vieth R, Rao R, Bhatti R. The accuracy of the rectal examination in the diagnosis of prostate carcinoma. N Engl J Med 1980;303:499–503.

Gump FE, McDermott J. Fibrous disease of the breast in juvenile diabetes. N Y State J Med 1990; 90:356–357.

Gundy JH. The pediatric physical exam. In: Hoekelman RA, ed. Primary pediatric care. St Louis: CV Mosby, 1987:63–109.

Guttenberg SA. Chemical injury of the oral mucosa from verapamil. N Engl J Med 1990;323:615.

Hamilton MS, Dodge EF. Pelvic examination: patient safety and comfort. J Obstet Gynecol Neonatal Nurs 1981;10:344–345.

Hardison JE. "The sky is falling." Am J Med 1980;68:163.

Hardison JE. Whatever happened to the chief complaint? JAMA 1981;245:1942.

Hardison JE. Observations on selected physical findings. Emory Univ J Med 1988;2:205–217.

Hardy WG. How to obtain a history from hard-of-hearing patients. JAMA 1975;232:73.

Hawke M. Clinical pocket guide to ear disease. Philadelphia: Lea & Febiger, 1986.

Hayden GF. Olfactory diagnosis in medicine. Postgrad Med 1980;67:110–118.

Heeren TJ, Lagaay AM, Beek WCAv, Rooymans HGM, Hijmans W. Reference values for the mini-mental state examination (MMSE) in octo- and nonagenarians. J Am Geriatr Soc 1990;38:1093–1096.

Hegde BM. How to detect early splenic enlargement. Practitioner 1985;229:857.

Heinz GJ, Zavala DC. Slipping rib syndrome: diagnosis using the "hooking maneuver." JAMA 1977; 237:794–795.

Henkind SJ, Benis AM, Teichholz LE. The paradox of pulsus paradoxus. Am Heart J 1987;114(1): 198–203.

Henry JA, Altmann P. Assessment of hypoproteinaemic oedema: a simple physical sign. Br Med J 1978; 1:890–892.

Hill NS. The cardiac exam in lung disease. Clin Chest Med 1987;8:273–285.

Hobbs CJ, Wynne JM. Buggery in childhood—a common syndrome of child abuse. Lancet 1986;2: 792–796.

Holzberg M, Walker HK. Terry's nails: revised definition and new correlations. Lancet 1984;1: 896–899.

Hooper PL, Hooper EM, Stehr DE. Guidelines for interviewing. Ann Intern Med 1981;95:238.

Hoppenfeld S. Physical examination of the spine and extremities. Norwalk, Connecticut: Appleton-Century-Crofts, 1976.

Howard R, Turner G. Why don't we take adequate drinking histories from elderly admissions? Br J Addict 1989;84:1374–1375.

Howard RJWM, Valori RM. Hospital patients who wear tinted spectacles—physical sign of psychoneurosis: a controlled study. J R Soc Med 1989;82:606–608.

Humbert P, Dupond JL, Carbillet JP. Pretibial myxedema: an overlapping clinical manifestation of autoimmune thyroid disease. Am J Med 1987;83:1170–1171.

Hurst JW, Hopkins LC, Smith RB. Noises in the neck. N Engl J Med 1980;302:862–863.

Hurwitz S. Clinical pediatric dermatology. Philadelphia: WB Saunders, 1981.

Impallomeni M, Flynn MD, Kenny RA, Kraenzlin M, Pallis CA. The elderly and their ankle jerks. Lancet 1984;1:670–672.

Iwata K. Ophthalmoscopy in the detection of optic disc and retinal nerve fiber layer changes in early glaucoma (summary). Surv Ophthalmol 1989;33:447–448.

Jacobs JW, Bernhard MR, Delgado A, Strain JJ. Screening for organic mental syndromes in the medically ill. Ann Intern Med 1977;86:40–46.

Jacoby R. Loss of memory and concentration. Br J Hosp Med 1985;33:32–34.

Javitt JC. A modified slit lamp for examination of wheelchair-bound patients. Arch Ophthalmol 1989; 107:453–454.

Jenkyn LR, Walsh DB, Culver CM, Reeves AG. Clinical signs in diffuse cerebral dysfunction. J Neurol Neurosurg Psychiatry 1977;40:956–966.

Jones KL. Smith's recognizable patterns of human malformations. 4th ed. Philadelphia: WB Saunders, 1988.

Kampmeier RH. Medicine as an art: the history and physical examination. South Med J 1982; 75:203–210.

Kampmeier RH. The physical examination—an art. South Med J 1988;81:687–690.

Kelly JW, Crutcher WA, Sagebiel RW. Clinical diagnosis of dysplastic melanocytic nevi: a clinicopathologic correlation. J Am Acad Dermatol 1986;14:1044–1052.

Kenik JG, Maricq HR, Bole GG. Blind evaluation of the diagnostic specificity of nailfold capillary microscopy in the connective tissue diseases. Arthritis Rheum 1981;24:885–891.

Kenna C, Murtagh J. Examination of the neck. Aust Fam Physician 1986;15:1015–1020.

Kiernan RJ, Mueller J, Langston JW, Van Dyke C. The neurobehavioral cognitive status examination: a brief but differentiated approach to cognitive assessment. Ann Intern Med 1987;107:481–485.

Kinney EL. Causes of false-negative auscultation of regurgitant lesions: a Doppler echocardiographic study of 294 patients. J Gen Intern Med 1988;3:429–434.

Klein RL. "Miracle cure" of a psychiatric disorder: a case for thorough physical assessment. Arch Intern Med 1984;144:1067.

Koehler JE, LeBoit PE, Egbert BM, Berger TG. Cutaneous vascular lesions and disseminated cat-scratch disease in patients with the acquired immunodeficiency syndrome (AIDS) and AIDS-related complex. Ann Intern Med 1988;109:449–455.

Kraman SS. Lung sounds for the clinician. Arch Intern Med 1986;146:1411–1412.

Kramer DS, French WJ, Criley JM. The postextrasystolic murmur response to gradient in hypertrophic cardiomyopathy. Ann Intern Med 1986;104:772–776.

Kroenke K. The case presentation: stumbling blocks and stepping stones. Am J Med 1985;79:605–608.

Krutchkoff DJ, Eisenberg E, O'Brien JE, Ponzillo JJ. Cocaine-induced dental erosions. N Engl J Med 1990;322:408.

Kurtz KJ. Dynamic vascular auscultation. Am J Med 1984;76:1066–1074.

Kurzrock R, Cohen PR. Erythromelalgia and myeloproliferative disorders. Arch Intern Med 1989;149:105–109.

Lampe RM, Kagan A. Detection of clubbing: Schamroth's sign: closing the window and opening the angle. Clin Pediatr 1983;22:125.

Lamphier TA. Rape. Md State Med J 1982;31:37–43.

Landau WM. Training of the neurologist for the 21st century. Arch Neurol 1989;46:21–22.

Landau WM. Strategy, tactics, and accuracy in neurological evaluation. Ann Neurol 1990;28:86–87.

Langlands AO, Tiver KW. Significance of a negative mammogram in patients with a palpable breast tumour. Med J Aust 1982;1:30–31.

Larkin RF. The callus of crack cocaine. N Engl J Med 1990;323:685.

Leach RM, McBrien DJ. Brachioradial delay: a new clinical indicator of the severity of aortic stenosis. Lancet 1990;335:1199–1201.

Lederle FA, Walker JM, Reinke DB. Selective screening for abdominal aortic aneurysms with physical examination and ultrasound. Arch Intern Med 1988;148:1753–1756.

Lembo NJ, Dell'Italia LJ, Crawford MH, O'Rourke RA. Bedside diagnosis of systolic murmurs. N Engl J Med 1988;318:1572–1578.

Levin J. When doctors question kids. N Engl J Med 1990;323:1569.

Levitt MA. An evaluation of clinical variables in determining the need for pelvic examination in the emergency department. Ann Emer Med 1991;20:351–354.

Lichtenstein MJ, Bess FH, Logan SA. Validation of screening tools for identifying hearing-impaired elderly in primary care. JAMA 1988;259:2875–2878.

Lichtenstein MJ, Schaffner W. Assessing activities of daily living. Hosp Pract 1985;20(May 30):8–9.

Linet OI, Metzler C. Practical ENT: incidence of palpable cervical nodes in adults. Postgrad Med 1977;62:210–211, 213.

Lipkin MJ, Quill TE, Napodano RJ. The medical interview: a core curriculum for residencies in internal medicine. Ann Intern Med 1984;100:277–284.

Lipkin M, Williams ME. Presbycusis and communication. J Gen Intern Med 1986;1:399–401.

Lockhart PB. Gingival pigmentation as the sole presenting sign of chronic lead poisoning in a mentally retarded adult. Oral Surg Oral Med Oral Pathol 1981;52:143–149.

Loo H, Forman WB, Levine MR, Crum ED, Rassiga AL. Periorbital ecchymoses as the initial sign in multiple myeloma. Ann Ophthalmol 1982;14:1066–1068.

Loudon R, Murphy RLHJ. Lung sounds. Am Rev Respir Dis 1984;130:663–673.

Louis S. A bedside test for determining the sub-types of vascular headache. Headache 1981;21:87–88.

Mackenzie TB. The initial patient interview: identifying when psychosocial factors are at work. Postgrad Med 1983;74:259–265.

Mador MJ, Tobin MJ. Apneustic breathing: a characteristic feature of brainstem compression in achondroplasia? Chest 1990;97:877–883.

Magee J. The pelvic examination: a view from the other end of the table. Ann Intern Med 1975;83:563–564.

Mahoney L. Technique of clinical screening for breast cancer. N Engl J Med 1982;307:827.

Mahoney LJ, Bird BL, Cooke GM. Annual clinical examination: the best available screening test for breast cancer. N Engl J Med 1979;301:315–316.

Mann G, Finsterbush A, Frankl U, Yarom J, Matan Y. A method of diagnosing small amounts of fluid in the knee. J Bone Joint Surg (Br) 1991;73B:346–347.

Margolis KL, Money BE, Kopietz LA, Rich EC. Physician recognition of ophthalmoscopic signs of open-angle glaucoma: effect of an educational program. J Gen Intern Med 1989;4:296–299.

Marks R. A diagnostic approach to common dermatology problems. Aust Fam Physician 1982;11:696, 698, 701–702.

Martin CM, Matlow AG, Chew E, Sutton D, Pruzanski W. Hyperviscosity syndrome in a patient with acquired immunodeficiency syndrome. Arch Intern Med 1989;149:1435–1436.

Martin L, Khalil H. How much reduced hemoglobin is necessary to generate central cyanosis? Chest 1990;97:182–185.

Martyn CN, Frier BM, Corrall RJM, McClemont M, French EB. Why palpate the radial artery? Lancet 1981;1:89–90.

Mashberg A, Feldman LJ. Clinical criteria for identifying early oral and oropharyngeal carcinoma: erythroplasia revisited. Am J Surg 1988;156:273–275.

Mashberg A, Samit A. Early detection, diagnosis, and management of oral and oropharyngeal cancer. CA 1989;39:67–88.

Massell TB. Causalgic form of postphlebitic syndrome: a variety of reflex sympathetic dystrophy caused by acute deep thrombophlebitis. West J Med 1988;149:294–295.

McElligott G, Harrington MG. Heart failure and breast enlargement suggesting cancer. Br Med J 1986;292:446.

McFadden JP, Price RC, Eastwood HD, Briggs RS. Raised respiratory rate in elderly patients: a valuable physical sign. Br Med J 1982;284:626–627.

McGinnis LS. The importance of clinical breast examination. Cancer 1989;64(suppl 12):2657–2660.

McMillan JA, Nieburg PI, Oski FA. The whole pediatrician catalogue, vol 1. Philadelphia: WB Saunders, 1977.

McMillan JA, Stockman JA, Oski FA. The whole pediatrician catalogue, vol 2. Philadelphia: WB Saunders, 1979.

McMillan JA, Stockman JA, Oski FA. The whole pediatrician catalogue, vol 3. Philadelphia: WB Saunders, 1982.

McNally D. The technique of physical examination in the ICU. J Crit Illness 1990;5:1305–1312.

Medvei VC, Cattell WR. Mental symptoms presenting in phaeochromocytoma: a case report and review. J R Soc Med 1988;81:550–551.

Mellinkoff SM. "Stethoscope sign." N Engl J Med 1964;271:630.

Messerli FH, Ventura HO, Amodeo C. Osler's maneuver and pseudohypertension. N Engl J Med 1985;312:1548–1551.

Meyer TE, McGregor M. More questions on Kussmaul's sign. Am J Cardiol 1990;66:772.

Meyerowitz BR. Abdominal palpation by stethoscope. Arch Surg 1976;111:831.

Milhorn HT Jr. The genogram: a structured approach to the family history. J Miss State Med Assoc 1981;22:250–252.

Model D. Smoker's face: an underrated clinical sign? Br Med J 1985;291:1760–1762.

Moss AJ. Criteria for diastolic pressure: revolution, counterrevolution, and now a compromise. Pediatrics 1983;71:854–855.

Mulrow CD, Dolmatch BL, Delong ER, et al. Observer variability in the pulmonary examination. J Gen Intern Med 1986;1:364–367.

Munetz MR, Benjamin S. How to examine patients using the abnormal involuntary movement scale. Hosp Community Psychiatry 1988;39:1172–1177.

Murphy RLHJ, Holford SK. Lung sounds. Basics Respir Dis 1980;8(4):1–4.

Murphy RLHJ, Holford SK, Knowler WC. Visual lung-sound characterization by time-expanded wave-form analysis. N Engl J Med 1977;296:968–971.

Murtagh J. Physical signs in low back pain. Aust Fam Physician 1989;18:1561–1562.

Najmaldin A, Burge DM. Acute idiopathic scrotal oedema: incidence, manifestations and aetiology. Br J Surg 1987;74:634–635.

Napodano RJ. The functional heart murmur: a wastebasket diagnosis. J Fam Pract 1977;4:637–639.

Nardone DA. The framework of pathognomonic physical findings. Hosp Pract 1990;25(2):72–76.

Nardone DA, Roth KM, Mazur DJ, McAfee JH. Usefulness of physical examination in detecting the presence or absence of anemia. Arch Intern Med 1990;150:201–204.

Nassar ME. The stethoscopeless cardiologist. J R Soc Med 1988;81:501–502.

Nath AR, Capel LH. Inspiratory crackles: early and late. Thorax 1974;29:223–227.

Naylor CD, McCormack DG, Sullivan SN. The midclavicular line: a wandering landmark. Can Med Assoc J 1987;136:48–50.

Nelson KR, Bicknell JM. Oblique pectoral crease and "scapular hump" in shoulder contour are signs of trapezius muscle weakness. J Neurol Neurosurg Psychiatry 1987;50:1082–1083.

Novack DH. Beyond data gathering: twelve functions of the medical history. Hosp Pract 1985;20(3A):11–12.

Oboler SK, LaForce FM. The periodic physical examination in asymptomatic adults. Ann Intern Med 1989;110:214–226.

Ogren JM. The inaccuracy of axillary temperatures measured with an electronic thermometer. Am J Dis Child 1990;144:109–111.

Oldstone MBA. Stethoscopic treachery. N Engl J Med 1965;272:107.

Parrino TA. Hands on the heart: palpation of the cardiovascular system. Hosp Pract 1989;24(4A): 103–115.

Paton A, Saunders JB. ABC of alcohol: asking the right questions. Br Med J 1981;283:1458–1459.

Pellegrino TR. A faster, focused neurologic exam. Emerg Med 1990;9:71–95.

Perloff JK. The physiologic mechanisms of cardiac and vascular physical signs. J Am Coll Cardiol 1983;1:184–198.

Peterson DS, Barkmeier WW. Oral signs of frequent vomiting in anorexia. Am Fam Physician 1983; 27:199–200.

Phelan JA, Saltzman BR, Friedland GH, Klein RS. Oral findings in patients with acquired immunodeficiency syndrome. Oral Surg Oral Med Oral Pathol 1987;64:50–56.

Phillips CI. Dilate the pupil and see the fundus. Br Med J 1984;288:1779–1780.

Piette WW, Stone MS. A cutaneous sign of IgA-associated small dermal vessel leukocytoclastic vasculitis in adults (Henoch-Schonlein purpura). Arch Dermatol 1989;125:53–56.

Platt FW. Research in medical interviewing. Ann Intern Med 1981;94:405–407.

Platt FW, McMath JC. Clinical hypocompetence: the interview. Ann Intern Med 1979;91:898–902.

Pogson GW, Conn RD. Bedside diagnosis of deep venous thrombosis: a myth exposed. Mo Med 1979;76:203–206.

Ramoska EA, Sacchetti AD, Nepp M. Reliability of patient history in determining the possibility of pregnancy. Ann Emerg Med 1989;18:87–89.

Ratzan RM, Donaldson MC, Foster JH, Walzak MP. The blue scrotum sign of Bryant: a diagnostic clue to ruptured abdominal aortic aneurysm. J Emerg Med 1987;5:323–329.

Reilly DT, Wolfe JHN. The swollen leg. Br Med J 1991;303:1462–1465.

Reinfrank RF, Kaufman RP, Wetstone HJ, Glennon JA. Observations of the Achilles reflex test. JAMA 1967;199:1–4.

Rickford CRK, Negus D. The early detection of postoperative deep vein thrombosis: an assessment of Doppler ultrasound, physical examination and the temperature chart. Br J Surg 1975;62:182–185.

Ridley CM. Principles for the diagnosis of vulvar lesions. Clin Obstet Gynecol 1978;21:963–972.

Riley TL, Ray WF, Massey EW. Gait mechanisms: asymmetry of arm motion in normal subjects. Milit Med 1977;141:467–468.

Roberts REI. Examination of the anus in suspected child sexual abuse. Lancet 1986;2:1100.

Robertson D, Robertson RM. Orthostatic hypotension—diagnosis and therapy. Mod Concepts Cardiovasc Dis 1985;54:7–12.

Robertson TI. Clinical diagnosis in patients with lymphadenopathy. Med J Aust 1979;2:73–76.

Robinson AC, Hawke M. The efficacy of ceruminolytics: everything old is new again. J Otolaryngol 1989;18:263–267.

Rood SR, Johnson JT. Examination for cervical masses. Postgrad Med 1982;71(4):189–194.

Rosemberg SK. Subclinical papilloma viral infection of male genitalia. Urology 1985;26:554–557.

Rosen L. Physical examination of the anorectum: a systematic technique. Dis Colon Rectum 1990; 33:439–440.

Roy CR, Wilson T, Raife M, Horne D. Varicocele as the presenting sign of an abdominal mass. J Urol 1989;141:597–599.

Rudolph AM, Hoffman JIE, eds. Pediatrics. 18th ed. Norwalk, Connecticut: Appleton & Lange, 1987.

Runcie CJ, Dougall JR. Assessment of the critically ill patient. Br J Hosp Med 1990;43:74–76.

Samaranayake LP, Pindborg JJ. Hairy leucoplakia. Br Med J 1989;298:270–271.

Sapira JD. The narcotic addict as a medical patient. Am J Med 1968;45:555–588.

Sapira JD. ...And how big is the spleen? South Med J 1981;74:53–62.

Sapira JD. Why perform a routine history and physical examination? South Med J 1989;82:364–365.

Sapira JD. The art and science of bedside diagnosis. 1st ed. Baltimore: Urban & Schwarzenberg, 1990.

Sapira JD, Kirkpatrick MB. On pulsus paradoxus. South Med J 1983;76:1163–1164.

Sapira JD, Williamson DL. How big is the normal liver? Arch Intern Med 1979;139:971–973.

Scanlon GT, Castellino RA, Rudders R. Lymphographic demonstration of cyclic changes in lymph node size during Pel-Ebstein fever. Cancer 1975;36:2026–2028.

Schamroth L. Personal experience. S Afr Med J 1976;50:297–300.

Schmitt BP, Kushner MS, Wiener SL. The diagnostic usefulness of the history of the patient with dyspnea. J Gen Intern Med 1986;1:386–393.

Schneiderman H. The morgue: a neglected classroom for physical diagnosis. Conn Med 1983;47:8–12.

Schneiderman H. Physical diagnosis versus the oppression of medicine. Consultant 1990;30(6):2,10.

Schneiderman H. Carcinoma of the anus and the value of inspection in the anorectal examination. Consultant 1990;30(9):47–50.

Schneiderman H. Expert selectivity in physical diagnosis. Consultant 1991;31(10):3.

Schneiderman H. Bedside diagnosis: an annotated bibliography of literature on interviewing and physical examination. 2nd ed. Philadelphia: American College of Physicians, 1992.

Schneiderman H. Physical examination of the aged patient. Conn Med 1993;57(5):3–10.

Schneiderman H, Garibaldi RA. Physical examination of HIV-infected patients. Consultant 1990; 30(1):33–38, 41–44, 47–48, 50–51, 55–56, 61–63.

Schulten EAJM, Ten Kate RW, Van Der Waal I. The impact of oral examination on the Centers for Disease Control classification of subjects with human immunodeficiency virus infection. Arch Intern Med 1990;150:1259–1261.

Schwartz RS, Morris JGL, Crimmins D, et al. A comparison of two methods of eliciting the ankle jerk. Aust N Z J Med 1990;20:116–119.

Schwartzman RJ, McLellan TL. Reflex sympathetic dystrophy: a review. Arch Neurol 1987;44:555–561.

Shelley WB, Shelley ED, Burmeister V. Argyria: the intradermal "photograph," a manifestation of passive photosensitivity. J Am Acad Dermatol 1987;16:211–217.

Sherman HI, Hardison JE. The importance of a coexistent hepatic rub and bruit: a clue to the diagnosis of cancer in the liver. JAMA 1979;241:1495.

Shore NA, Schaefer MC. Temporomandibular joint dysfunction. N Y State J Med 1978;78:254–256.

Sickles EA, Greene WH, Wiernik PH. Clinical presentation of infection in granulocytopenic patients. Arch Intern Med 1975;135:715–719.

Silen W. Cope's early diagnosis of the acute abdomen. 18th ed. New York: Oxford University Press, 1991.

Silverman ME, Hurst JW. The hand and the heart. Am J Cardiol 1968;22:718–728.

Simard M, Gumbiner B, Lee A, Lewis H, Norman D. Lithium carbonate intoxication: a case report and review of the literature. Arch Intern Med 1989;149:36–46.

Sofferman RA. Lingual infarction in cranial arteritis. JAMA 1980;243:2422–2423.

Spodick D, Quarry-Pigott VM. Fourth heart sound as a normal finding in older persons. N Engl J Med 1973;288:140–141.

Spodick DH, Kerigan AT, Paz LRdl, Shahamatpour A, Kino M. Clavicular auscultation: preferential clavicular transmission and amplification of aortic valve murmurs. Chest 1976;70:337–340.

Sprackling PD. Alternative to "aaah." Lancet 1988;1:769.

Stearns MW. Digital rectal examination. CA 1974;24(March–April):100–103.

Steel K. History taking from elderly patients. Hosp Pract 1985;20(5A):70–71.

Stevenson RWD, Szasz G, Maurice WL, Miles JE. How to become comfortable talking about sex to your patients. Can Med Assoc J 1983;128:797–800.

Strauss RE. Ocular manifestations of Crohn's disease: literature review. Mt Sinai J Med 1988;55:353–356.

Sturman MR. Pelvic examination versus fiberoptic laparoscopy: a fictional study of patient preference in 1534 women. J Clin Gastroenterol 1988;10:612–613.

Sullivan S, Williams R. Reliability of clinical techniques for detecting splenic enlargement. Br Med J 1976;2:1043–1044.

Sulzbach LM. Measurement of pulsus paradoxus. Focus Crit Care 1989;16(2):142–145.

Sunderland T, Hill JL, Mellow AM, et al. Clock drawing in Alzheimer's disease: a novel measure of dementia severity. J Am Geriatr Soc 1989;37:725–729.

Sykes D, Dewar R, Mohanaruban K, et al. Measuring blood pressure in the elderly: does atrial fibrillation increase observer variability? Br Med J 1990;300:162–163.

Tager RM. Simulated disability. J Occup Med 1985;27:915–916.

Talbot T, Jewell L, Schloss E, Yakimets W, Thomson ABR. Cheilitis antedating Crohn's disease: case report and literature update of oral lesions. J Clin Gastroenterol 1984;6:349–354.

Tanner JM. Growth at adolescence. 2nd ed. Oxford, England: Blackwell Scientific Publications, 1962.

Thomson H, Francis DMA. Abdominal-wall tenderness: a useful sign in the acute abdomen. Lancet 1977;2:1053–1054.

Tinetti ME, Ginter SF. Identifying mobility dysfunctions in elderly patients: standard neuromuscular examination or direct assessment? JAMA 1988;259:1190–1193.

Tunnessen WW. Cutaneous infections. Pediatr Clin North Am 1983;30:515–518.

Tyberg TI, Goodyer AVN, Langou RA. Genesis of pericardial knock in constrictive pericarditis. Am J Cardiol 1980;46:570–575.

Uhlmann RF, Rees TS, Psaty BM, Duckert LG. Validity and reliability of auditory screening in demented and non-demented older adults. J Gen Intern Med 1989;4:90–95.

Verghese A, Dison C, Berk SL. Courvoisier's "law"—an eponym in evolution. Am J Gastroenterol 1987;82:248–250.

Verghese A, Gallemore G. Kernig's and Brudzinski's signs revisited. Rev Infect Dis 1987;9:1187–1192.

Verghese A, Krish G, Howe D, Stonecipher M. The harlequin nail: a marker for smoking cessation. Chest 1990;97:236–238.

von Noorden GK. Binocular vision and ocular motility. St Louis: CV Mosby, 1980.

Wald ER. Diagnosis and management of acute sinusitis. Pediatr Ann 1988;17:629–638.

Walshe TM. Neurologic examination of the elderly patient: signs of normal aging. Postgrad Med 1987;81:375–378.

Walzer A, Koenigsberg M. Examining the anterior right kidney: frequent lack of appreciation in examination of the right upper quadrant. JAMA 1979;242:2320–2321.

Wartenberg R. The Babinski reflex after fifty years. JAMA 1947;135:763–767.

Watanakunakorn C, Hayek F. High fever (greater than 39°C) as a clinical manifestation of pulmonary embolism. Postgrad Med J 1987;63:951–953.

Weinstein C, Littlejohn GO, Miller MH, Dorevitch AP, Axtens R, Buchanan R. Lupus and non-lupus cutaneous manifestations in systemic lupus erythematosus. Aust N Z J Med 1987;17:501–506.

Werner SC. Modification of the classification of the eye changes of Graves' disease: recommendations of the Ad Hoc Committee of the American Thyroid Association. J Clin Endocrinol Metab 1977;44: 203–204.

Wertheimer AJ. Examination of the rape victim. Postgrad Med 1982;71:173–176, 179–180.

Williams DRR. Family history and the risk of complications in diabetes mellitus. Ann Intern Med 1986;105:795.

Witkowski JA, Parish LC. The touching question. Int J Dermatol 1981;20:426.

Wolner-Hanssen P, Holmes KK. Clinical manifestations of vaginal trichomoniasis. JAMA 1989; 261:571–576.

Wong M, Tei C, Shah PM. Degenerative calcific valvular disease and systolic murmurs in the elderly. J Am Geriatr Soc 1983;31:156–163.

Wood NK, Goaz PW. Differential diagnosis of oral lesions. 3rd ed. St Louis: CV Mosby, 1985.

Yaffe ME. Rectal examination in adolescent males. Ann Intern Med 1983;99:574.

Van Ruiswyk J, Noble H, Sigmann P. The natural history of carotid bruits in elderly persons. Ann Intern Med 1990;112:340–343.

Wylie EJ, Mitchell DB. Case report: iodide mumps following intravenous urography with iopamidol. Clin Radiol 1991;43:135–136.

Zaun H. Leukonychias. Semin Dermatol 1991;10(1):17–20.

Figure and Table Credits

Figure	Source
11.15	Reproduced with permission from Marshall Folstein, M.D.
15.1	Reproduced with permission from Algranati PS. The pediatric patient: an approach to history and physical examination. Baltimore: Williams & Wilkins, 1992:17.
15.2	Adapted from Hamill PVV, Drizd TA, Johnson CL, Reed RB, Roche AF, Moore WM. Physical growth: National Center for Health Statistics percentiles. Am J Clin Nutr 1979;32:607–629. Data from the Fels Longitudinal Study, Wright State University School Of Medicine, Yellow Springs, Ohio. ©1982 Ross Laboratories.
15.3	Adapted from Hamill PVV, Drizd TA, Johnson CL, Reed RB, Roche AF, Moore WM. Physical growth: National Center for Health Statistics percentiles. Am J Clin Nutr 1979;32:607–629. Data from the Fels Longitudinal Study, Wright State University School Of Medicine, Yellow Springs, Ohio. ©1982 Ross Laboratories.
15.4	Reproduced with permission from Algranati PS. The pediatric patient: an approach to history and physical examination. Baltimore: Williams & Wilkins, 1992:18.
15.5	Reproduced with permission from Nellhaus G. Head circumference from birth to eighteen years. Pediatrics 1968;41:106–114.
15.6	Reproduced with permission from Algranati PS. The pediatric patient: an approach to history and physical examination. Baltimore: Williams & Wilkins, 1992:20.
15.7	Reproduced with permission from Task Force on Blood Pressure Control in Children. Report of the Second Task Force on Blood Pressure Control in Children—1987. Pediatrics 1987;79:1–30.
15.8	Reproduced with permission from Frankenburg WK, Dodds J, Archer P, Shapiro H, Bresnick B. The Denver II: a major revision and restandardization of the Denver Developmental Screening Test. Pediatrics 1992;89:91–97.
15.9	Reproduced with permission from Algranati PS. The pediatric patient: an approach to history and physical examination. Baltimore: Williams & Wilkins, 1992:35.
15.10	Reproduced with permission from Algranati PS. The pediatric patient: an approach to history and physical examination. Baltimore: Williams & Wilkins, 1992:36.
15.11	Reproduced with permission from Algranati PS. Pediatric clinical encounter. In: Willms JL, Lewis J, eds. Introduction to clinical medicine. Media, Pennsylvania: Harwal, 1991:138.
15.12	Reproduced with permission from DeMyer W. Technique of the neurologic examination: a programmed text. 3rd ed. New York: McGraw-Hill, 1980:3.
15.13	Reproduced with permission from Algranati PS. The pediatric patient: an approach to history and physical examination. Baltimore: Williams & Wilkins, 1992:30.
15.14	Reproduced with permission from Algranati PS. The pediatric patient: an approach to history and physical examination. Baltimore: Williams & Wilkins, 1992:29.

15.15   Reproduced with permission from Algranati PS. The pediatric patient: an approach to history and physical examination. Baltimore: Williams & Wilkins, 1992:39.

15.16   Reproduced with permission from Algranati PS. The pediatric patient: an approach to history and physical examination. Baltimore: Williams & Wilkins, 1992:44.

15.17   Reproduced with permission from Algranati PS. Pediatric clinical encounter. In: Willms JL, Lewis J. Introduction to clinical medicine. Media, Pennsylvania: Harwal, 1991:137.

15.18A   Reprinted with permission from Ballard JL, Khoury JC, Wedig K, et al. New Ballard Score, expanded to include extremely premature infants. J Pediatr 1991;119:417–423, and Ross Laboratories, Columbus, Ohio, 43216. ©1991 Ross Laboratories.

15.18B   Used with permission from Dubowitz L, Dubowitz V, Goldberg C. Clinical assessment of gestational age in the newborn infant. J Pediatr 1970;77:1–10.

15.19   Reprinted with permission from Battaglia FC, Lubchenco LO. A practical classification of newborn infants by weight and gestational age. J Pediatr 1967;71:159–163, and Lubchenco LO, Hansman C, Boyd E. Intrauterine growth in length and head circumference as estimated from live births at gestational ages from 26 to 42 weeks. Pediatrics 1966;37:403–408, and Ross Laboratories, Columbus, Ohio, 43216. ©1991 Ross Laboratories.

15.20   Reproduced with permission from Algranati PS. The pediatric patient: an approach to history and physical examination. Baltimore: Williams & Wilkins, 1992:51.

15.21   Reproduced with permission from Algranati PS. The pediatric patient: an approach to history and physical examination. Baltimore: Williams & Wilkins, 1992:27.

15.22   Reproduced with permission from Algranati PS. The pediatric patient: an approach to history and physical examination. Baltimore: Williams & Wilkins, 1992:26.

15.23   Reproduced with permission from Algranati PS. Pediatric clinical encounter. In: Willms JL, Lewis J. Introduction to clinical medicine. Media, Pennsylvania: Harwal, 1991:140.

15.24   Reproduced with permission from Algranati PS. The pediatric patient: an approach to history and physical examination. Baltimore: Williams & Wilkins, 1992:38.

15.25   Reproduced with permission from Algranati PS. The pediatric patient: an approach to history and physical examination. Baltimore: Williams & Wilkins, 1992:39.

15.26   Reproduced with permission from Hurwitz S. Clinical pediatric dermatology. Philadelphia: WB Saunders, 1981:191.

15.27   Reproduced with permission from Hurwitz S. Clinical pediatric dermatology. Philadelphia: WB Saunders, 1981:195.

15.28   Reproduced with permission from Hurwitz S. Clinical pediatric dermatology. Philadelphia: WB Saunders, 1981:11.

15.29   Courtesy of Stanley F. Glazer, M.D.

15.30   Reproduced with permission from Algranati PS. The pediatric patient: an approach to history and physical examination. Baltimore: Williams & Wilkins, 1992:43.

15.31 Reproduced with permission from Algranati PS. Pediatric clinical encounter. In: Willms JL, Lewis J. Introduction to clinical medicine. Media, Pennsylvania: Harwal, 1991:137.

15.32 Reproduced with permission from Algranati PS. The pediatric patient: an approach to history and physical examination. Baltimore: Williams & Wilkins, 1992:78.

15.33 Reproduced with permission from Algranati PS. The pediatric patient: an approach to history and physical examination. Baltimore: Williams & Wilkins, 1992:79.

15.34 Reproduced with permission from Algranati PS. The pediatric patient: an approach to history and physical examination. Baltimore: Williams & Wilkins, 1992:79.

15.35 Reproduced with permission from Algranati PS. The pediatric patient: an approach to history and physical examination. Baltimore: Williams & Wilkins, 1992:81.

15.36 Reproduced with permission from Algranati PS. The pediatric patient: an approach to history and physical examination. Baltimore: Williams & Wilkins, 1992:81.

15.37 Reproduced with permission from Algranati PS. The pediatric patient: an approach to history and physical examination. Baltimore: Williams & Wilkins, 1992:75.

15.38 Adapted with permission from Algranati PS. Pediatric clinical encounter. In: Willms JL, Lewis J. Introduction to clinical medicine. Media, Pennsylvania: Harwal, 1991:146.

15.39 Reproduced with permission from Algranati PS. The pediatric patient: an approach to history and physical examination. Baltimore: Williams & Wilkins, 1992:78.

15.40 Reproduced with permission from Fleisher GR. Infectious disease emergencies. In: Fleisher GR, Ludwig S, eds. Textbook of pediatric emergency medicine. 2nd ed. Baltimore: Williams & Wilkins, 1988:428.

15.41 Reproduced with permission from Fleisher GR. Infectious disease emergencies. In: Fleisher GR, Ludwig S, eds. Textbook of pediatric emergency medicine. 2nd ed. Baltimore: Williams & Wilkins, 1988:428.

15.42 Reproduced with permission from Algranati PS. The pediatric patient: an approach to history and physical examination. Baltimore: Williams & Wilkins, 1992:69.

15.43 Reproduced with permission from Hurwitz S. Clinical pediatric dermatology. Philadelphia: WB Saunders, 1981:27.

15.44 Reproduced with permission from Hurwitz S. Clinical pediatric dermatology. Philadelphia: WB Saunders, 1981:29.

15.45 Reproduced with permission from Algranati PS. The pediatric patient: an approach to history and physical examination. Baltimore: Williams & Wilkins, 1992:68.

15.46 Reproduced with permission from Algranati PS. The pediatric patient: an approach to history and physical examination. Baltimore: Williams & Wilkins, 1992:101.

15.47 Reproduced with permission from Algranati PS. The pediatric patient: an approach to history and physical examination. Baltimore: Williams & Wilkins, 1992:103.

15.48   Reproduced with permission from Algranati PS. The pediatric patient: an approach to history and physical examination. Baltimore: Williams & Wilkins, 1992:104.

15.49   Reproduced with permission from Paradise JE. Pediatric and adolescent gynecology. In: Fleisher GR, Ludwig S, eds. Textbook of pediatric emergency medicine. 2nd ed. Baltimore: Williams & Wilkins, 1988:711.

15.50   Redrawn with permission from Staheli LT. Torsional deformity. Pediatr Clin North Am 1977;24:802.

15.51   Reproduced with permission from Fleisher GR. Infectious disease emergencies. In: Fleisher GR, Ludwig S, eds. Textbook of pediatric emergency medicine. 2nd ed. Baltimore: Williams & Wilkins, 1988:428.

15.53   Reproduced with permission from Algranati PS. The pediatric patient: an approach to history and physical examination. Baltimore: Williams & Wilkins, 1992:106.

15.54   Courtesy of Stanley F. Glazer, M.D.

15.55   Reproduced with permission from Hurwitz S. Clinical pediatric dermatology. Philadelphia: WB Saunders, 1981:416.

15.56   Reproduced with permission from Algranati PS. The pediatric patient: an approach to history and physical examination. Baltimore: Williams & Wilkins, 1992:75.

15.57   Redrawn with permission from Staheli LT. Torsional deformity. Pediatr Clin North Am 1977;24:803.

15.58   Reproduced with permission from Avery ME, First LR., eds. Pediatric medicine. Baltimore: Williams & Wilkins, 1989:1283.

15.59   Reproduced with permission from Algranati PS. The pediatric patient: an approach to history and physical examination. Baltimore: Williams & Wilkins, 1992:128.

15.60   Adapted with permission from Marshall WA, Tanner JM. Variations in patterns of pubertal changes in girls. Arch Dis Child 1969;44:291–303, and Root AW. Endocrinology of puberty. 1. Normal sexual maturation. J Pediatr 1973;83:1–19. Illustrations from Collins M. Adolescent emergencies. In: Fleisher GR, Ludwig S. Textbook of pediatric emergency medicine. 2nd ed. Baltimore: Williams & Wilkins, 1988:1207.

15.61   Adapted with permission from Marshall WA, Tanner JM. Variations in patterns of pubertal changes in boys. Arch Dis Child 1970;45:13–23, and Root AW. Endocrinology of puberty. 1. Normal sexual maturation. J Pediatr 1973;83:1–19. Illustrations from Collins M. Adolescent emergencies. In: Fleisher GR, Ludwig S. Textbook of pediatric emergency medicine. 2nd ed. Baltimore: Williams & Wilkins, 1988:1205.

15.62   Adapted with permission from Tanner JM. Growth and endocrinology of the adolescent. In: Gardner LI, ed. Endocrinology and genetic diseases of childhood and adolescents. 2nd ed. Philadelphia: WB Saunders, 1975:20, 31.

Table	Source
2.5	Adapted with permission from American Heart Association. Recommendations for human blood pressure determination by sphygmomanometers. Dallas, Texas: American Heart Association, 1988. Copyright American Heart Association.

2.6   Adapted with permission from American Heart Association. Recommendations for human blood pressure determination by sphygmomanometers. Dallas, Texas: American Heart Association, 1988. Copyright American Heart Association.

10.1   Adapted from Saphira JP. The art and science of bedside diagnosis. Baltimore: Urban & Schwarzenberg, 1990.

10.2   Adapted from Saphira JP. The art and science of bedside diagnosis. Baltimore: Urban & Schwarzenberg, 1990.

15.1   Reproduced with permission from Lowrey GH. Growth and development of children. 8th ed. Chicago: Mosby-Year Book, 1986:246.

15.2   Reproduced with permission from Cloutier MM. Pulmonary disease. In: Dworkin PH, ed. Pediatrics. 2nd ed. Baltimore: Williams & Wilkins, 1992:314.

15.3   Reproduced with permission from Apgar V, Holoday DA, James LS, Weisbrot IM, Berrien C. Evaluation of the newborn infant—second report. JAMA 1958;168:1985–1988. ©1958, American Medical Association.

15.5   Reproduced with permission from McCarthy PL, Shapre MR, Spiesel SZ, et al. Observation scales to identify serious illness in febrile children. Pediatrics 1982;70:802–809.

15.7   Adapted with permission from American Academy of Pediatrics, Committee on Sports Medicine and Fitness. Sports medicine: health care for young athletes. 2nd ed. Elk Grove Village, Illinois: American Academy of Pediatrics, 1991:54.

Index

Page numbers in *italics* denote figures; those followed by "t" denote tables.